T0191502

Lecture Notes in Computer Science 12963

More information about this series at https://link.springer.com/bookseries/558

Alessandro Crimi · Spyridon Bakas (Eds.)

Brainlesion: Glioma, Multiple Sclerosis, Stroke and Traumatic Brain Injuries

7th International Workshop, BrainLes 2021
Held in Conjunction with MICCAI 2021
Virtual Event, September 27, 2021
Revised Selected Papers, Part II

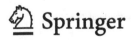 Springer

Editors
Alessandro Crimi 🆔
Sano Centre for Computational Personalized
Kraków, Poland

Spyridon Bakas 🆔
University of Pennsylvania
Philadelphia, PA, USA

ISSN 0302-9743 ISSN 1611-3349 (electronic)
Lecture Notes in Computer Science
ISBN 978-3-031-09001-1 ISBN 978-3-031-09002-8 (eBook)
https://doi.org/10.1007/978-3-031-09002-8

This Springer imprint is published by the registered company Springer Nature Switzerland AG
The registered company address is: Gewerbestrasse 11, 6330 Cham, Switzerland

In loving memory of Prof. Christian Barillot

Preface

This volume contains articles from the 7th International Brain Lesion Workshop (BrainLes 2021), as well as the RSNA-ASNR-MICCAI Brain Tumor Segmentation (BraTS 2021) Challenge, the Federated Tumor Segmentation (FeTS 2021) Challenge, the Cross-Modality Domain Adaptation (CrossMoDA 2021) Challenge, and the challenge on Quantification of Uncertainties in Biomedical Image Quantification (QUBIQ 2021). All these events were held in conjunction with the Medical Image Computing and Computer Assisted Intervention (MICCAI) conference on September 27, 2021, in Strasbourg, France, taking place online due to COVID-19 restrictions.

The presented manuscripts describe the research of computational scientists and clinical researchers working on glioma, multiple sclerosis, cerebral stroke, traumatic brain injuries, vestibular schwannoma, and white matter hyper-intensities of presumed vascular origin. This compilation does not claim to provide a comprehensive understanding from all points of view; however, the authors present their latest advances in segmentation, disease prognosis, and other applications in the clinical context.

The volume is divided into five chapters: the first chapter comprises invited papers summarizing the presentations of the keynotes during the full-day BrainLes workshop and the FeTS challenge, the second includes the accepted paper submissions to the BrainLes workshop, and the third through the sixth chapters contain a selection of papers regarding methods presented at the RSNA-ASNR-MICCAI BraTS, FeTS, CrossMoDA, and QUBIQ challenges, respectively.

The content of the first chapter with the invited papers covers the current state-of-the-art literature on federated learning applications for cancer research and clinical oncology analysis, as well as an overview of the deep learning approaches improving the current standard of care for brain lesions and current neuroimaging challenges.

The aim of the second chapter, focusing on the accepted BrainLes workshop submissions, is to provide an overview of new advances of medical image analysis in all the aforementioned brain pathologies. It brings together researchers from the medical image analysis domain, neurologists, and radiologists working on at least one of these diseases. The aim is to consider neuroimaging biomarkers used for one disease applied to the other diseases. This session did not have a specific dataset to be used.

The third chapter focuses on a selection of papers from the RSNA-ASNR-MICCAI BraTS 2021 challenge participants. BraTS 2021 made publicly available the largest ever manually annotated dataset of baseline pre-operative brain glioma scans from 20 international institutions in order to gauge the current state of the art in automated brain tumor segmentation using skull-stripped multi-parametric MRI sequences (provided in NIfTI file format) and to compare different methods. To pinpoint and evaluate the clinical relevance of tumor segmentation, BraTS 2021 also included the prediction of the MGMT methylation status using the same skull-stripped multi-parametric MRI sequences but provided in the DICOM file format to conform to the clinical standards (https://www.rsna.org/education/ai-resources-and-training/ai-image-challenge/brain-tumor-ai-challenge-2021).

The fourth chapter contains a selection of papers from the Federated Tumor Segmentation (FeTS 2021) challenge participants. This was the first computational challenge focussing on federated learning, and ample multi-institutional routine clinically-acquired pre-operative baseline multi-parametric MRI scans of radiographically appearing glioblastoma were provided to the participants, along with splits on the basis of the site of acquisition. The goal of the challenge was two-fold: i) identify the best way to aggregate the knowledge coming from segmentation models trained on the individual institutions, and ii) find the best algorithm that produces robust and accurate brain tumor segmentations across different medical institutions, MRI scanners, image acquisition parameters, and populations. Interestingly, the second task was performed by actually circulating the containerized algorithms across different institutions, leveraging the collaborators of the largest real-world federation to date (www.fets.ai).

The fifth chapter contains a selection of papers from the CrossMoDA 2021 challenge participants. CrossMoDA 2021 was the first large and multi-class benchmark for unsupervised cross-modality domain adaptation for medical image segmentation. The goal of the challenge was to segment two key brain structures involved in the follow-up and treatment planning of vestibular schwannoma (VS): the VS tumour and the cochlea. The training dataset provides annotated T1 scans ($N = 105$) and unpaired non-annotated T2 scans ($N = 105$). More information can be found on the challenge website (https://crossmoda-challenge.ml/).

The sixth chapter contains a selection of papers from the QUBIQ 2021 challenge participants. QUBIQ 2021 continued the success of the first challenge on uncertainty quantification in medical image segmentation (QUBIQ 2020). The goal of the challenge was to model the uncertainty in diverse segmentation tasks in which the involved images include different modalities, e.g., CT and MRI scans and varied organs and pathologies. QUBIQ 2021 included two new 3D segmentation tasks, pancreas segmentation and pancreatic lesion segmentation.

We heartily hope that this volume will promote further exciting computational research on brain related pathologies.

December 2021

Alessandro Crimi
Spyridon Bakas

Organization

BrainLes Organizing Committee

Spyridon Bakas	University of Pennsylvania, USA
Alessandro Crimi	Sano Science, Poland

BrainLes Program Committee

Bhakti V. Baheti	University of Pennsylvania, USA
Ujjwal Baid	University of Pennsylvania, USA
Florian Kofler	Technical University of Munich, Germany
Hugo Kuijf	University Medical School of Utrecht, The Netherlands
Jana Lipkova	Technical University of Munich, Germany
Andreas Mang	University of Houston, USA
Raghav Mehta	McGill University, Canada
Sarthak Pati	University of Pennsylvania, USA
Szymon Plotka	Warsaw University of Technology, Poland
Zahra Riahi Samani	University of Pennsylvania, USA
Aristeidis Sotiras	Washington University at St. Louis, USA
Siddhesh Thakur	University of Pennsylvania, USA
Benedikt Wiestler	Technical University of Munich, Germany

Challenges Organizing Committees

Brain Tumor Segmentation (BraTS) Challenge

Ujjwal Baid	University of Pennsylvania, USA
Spyridon Bakas (Lead Organizer)	University of Pennsylvania, USA
Evan Calabrese	University of California San Francisco, USA
Christopher Carr	Radiological Society of North America, USA
Errol Colak	Unity Health Toronto, Canada
Keyvan Farahani	National Cancer Institute, National Institutes of Health, USA
Adam E. Flanders	Thomas Jefferson University Hospital, USA
Felipe C. Kitamura	Diagnósticos da América SA and Universidade Federal de São Paulo, Brazil
Bjoern Menze	University of Zurich, Switzerland
Luciano Prevedello	The Ohio State University, USA

| Jeffrey Rudie | University of California, San Francisco, USA |
| Russell Taki Shinohara | University of Pennsylvania, USA |

Federated Tumor Segmentation (FeTS) Challenge

Ujjwal Baid	University of Pennsylvania, USA
Spyridon Bakas (Task 1 Lead Organizer)	University of Pennsylvania, USA
Yong Chen	University of Pennsylvania, USA
Brandon Edwards	Intel, USA
Patrick Foley	Intel, USA
Alexey Gruzdev	Intel, USA
Jens Kleesiek	University Hospital Essen, Germany
Klaus Maier-Hein	DKFZ, Germany
Lena Maier-Hein	DKFZ, Germany
Jason Martin	Intel, USA
Bjoern Menze	University of Zurich, Switzerland
Sarthak Pati	University of Pennsylvania, USA
Annika Reinke	DKFZ, Germany
Micah J. Sheller	Intel, USA
Russell Taki Shinohara	University of Pennsylvania, USA
Maximilian Zenk (Task 2 Lead Organizer)	DKFZ, Germany
David Zimmerer	DKFZ, Germany

Cross-Modality Domain Adaptation (CrossMoDA) Challenge

Spyridon Bakas	University of Pennsylvania, USA
Jorge Cardoso	King's College London, UK
Reuben Dorent (Lead Organizer)	King's College London, UK
Ben Glocker	Imperial College London, UK
Samuel Joutard	King's College London, UK
Aaron Kujawa	King's College London, UK
Marc Modat	King's College London, UK
Nicola Rieke	NVIDIA, Germany
Jonathan Shapey	King's College London, UK
Tom Vercauteren	King's College London, UK

Quantification of Uncertainty in Biomedical Image Quantification (QUBIQ) Challenge

Spyridon Bakas	University of Pennsylvania, USA
Anton Becker	Memorial Sloan Kettering Cancer Center, USA
Andras Jakab	University Children's Hospital Zürich, University of Zürich, Switzerland

Leo Joskowicz   The Hebrew University of Jerusalem, Israel
Ender Konukoglu   ETH Zürich, Switzerland
Hongwei (Bran) Li   Technical University of Munich, Germany
Bjoern Menze   University of Zurich, Switzerland

Contents – Part II

FeTS

CrossMoDA

QUBIQ

Contents – Part I

BraTS

BiTr-Unet: A CNN-Transformer Combined Network for MRI Brain Tumor Segmentation

Qiran Jia and Hai Shu$^{(\boxtimes)}$

Department of Biostatistics, School of Global Public Health,
New York University, New York, NY 10003, USA
hs120@nyu.edu

Abstract. Convolutional neural networks (CNNs) have achieved remarkable success in automatically segmenting organs or lesions on 3D medical images. Recently, vision transformer networks have exhibited exceptional performance in 2D image classification tasks. Compared with CNNs, transformer networks have an appealing advantage of extracting long-range features due to their self-attention algorithm. Therefore, we propose a CNN-Transformer combined model, called BiTr-Unet, with specific modifications for brain tumor segmentation on multimodal MRI scans. Our BiTr-Unet achieves good performance on the BraTS2021 validation dataset with median Dice score 0.9335, 0.9304 and 0.8899, and median Hausdorff distance 2.8284, 2.2361 and 1.4142 for the whole tumor, tumor core, and enhancing tumor, respectively. On the BraTS2021 testing dataset, the corresponding results are 0.9257, 0.9350 and 0.8874 for Dice score, and 3, 2.2361 and 1.4142 for Hausdorff distance. The code is publicly available at https://github.com/JustaTinyDot/BiTr-Unet.

Keywords: Brain tumor · Deep learning · Multi-modal image segmentation · Vision transformer

1 Introduction

As one of the most complicated tasks in computer vision, automated biomedical image segmentation plays an important role in disease diagnosis and further treatment planning. It aims to act like experienced physicians to identify types of tumors and delineate different sub-regions of organs on medical images such as MRI and CT scans [15,27]. Earlier segmentation systems were based on traditional approaches such as edge detection filters, mathematical methods, and machine learning algorithms, but the heavy computational complexity hindered their progress [9]. In recent years, remarkable breakthroughs have been made to computer hardware and deep learning. Deep learning is a derivation of machine learning, which implements multiple processing layers to build a deep neural network to extract representations from data by mimicking the working

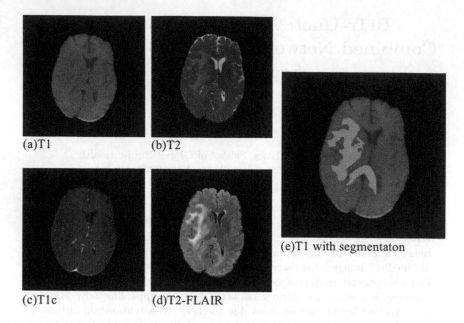

(a)T1   (b)T2

(c)T1c   (d)T2-FLAIR

(e)T1 with segmentaton

Fig. 1. Visualization of one case from the BraTS2021 training data.

mechanism of human brains [12]. Deep learning has succeeded in various difficult tasks including image classification and speech recognition, and also has become the most prevailing method for automated biomedical image segmentation [9,11,17,19]. While many challenges and limitations such as the shortage of annotated data persist, deep learning exhibits its superiority over traditional segmentation methods in processing speed and segmentation accuracy [9].

To promote the development of biomedical image segmentation techniques, many relevant challenges and conferences are held each year for researchers to propose innovative algorithms and communicate new discoveries. Year 2021 is the tenth anniversary of the Brain Tumor Segmentation Challenge (BraTS), which has been dedicated to being the venue of facilitating the state-of-the-art brain glioma segmentation algorithms [1–4,16]. Due to privacy protection issues, biomedical image data are notoriously difficult to obtain and usually in a comparatively small scale. However, this year the number of the well-curated multi-institutional multi-parametric MRI scans of glioma provided by the organizer have been updated from 660 to 2000, which largely benefits setting the new benchmark and exploring the potential of algorithms [1]. The training dataset provides four 3D MRI modalities, including native T1-weighted (T1), post-contrast T1-weighted (T1c), T2-weighted (T2), and T2 Fluid Attenuated Inversion Recovery (T2-FLAIR), together with the "ground-truth" tumor segmentation labeled by physicians; see Fig. 1. For the validation and testing datasets, the "ground-truth" tumor segmentation is not open to participants. The ranking criterion in BraTS2021 consists of the Dice score, Hausdorff distance (95%),

Sensitivity, and Specificity for the respective segmentation of the whole tumor, tumor core, and enhancing tumor.

The invention of U-Net, which supplements the contracting network by successive layers to build an encoder-decoder with skip connections architecture, successfully makes the feature extraction in biomedical images more precise and efficient [18]. U-Net has become the baseline network that is frequently modified for better performance in BraTS ever since, and one of U-Net's modified versions, nnU-Net, took the first place in BraTS2020 [10], which again proves the excellent performance of the fully convolutional network and the structure of successive upsampling layers. Some other top-ranked networks in BraTS2020 also add innovative modules such as the variational autoencoder (VAE), attention gate (AG), as well as Convolutional Block Attention Module (CBAM) into U-net like structures to regularize the feature extraction process and boost generalization performance [8,10,15]. Overall, it is generally acknowledged that modifying and enhancing U-Net architecture is an efficient and elegant way to obtain good results for biomedical image segmentation.

Another important network structure, Transformer [22], which displays successful improvement on performances of networks in the Natural Language Processing (NLP) realm, is also proved to be useful in the domain of computer vision. Vision Transformer (ViT) [6] proposes the idea that divides an image into several equivalent patches and then applies the self-attention mechanism of Transformer to each patch to capture the long-range dependencies. Compared with networks that are built solely on convolutional layers, ViT overcomes their limitation of locality and therefore makes predictions with more considerations. To boost the performance of ViT and continually set the state-of-the-art benchmark of image classification tasks, various modifications of ViT have been proposed [5,21,25]. Furthermore, to alleviate the high computational cost of the original Transformer on high-resolution images, the architecture design of CNN is introduced to the networks that adopt Transformer [7,23].

Even though many works have been done to apply Transformer to the computer vision realm, only a small number of researches on utilizing Transformer to 3D biomedical image segmentation are available. NVIDIA proposed UNETR [7], which uses a modified ViT as the encoder, and adopts the successive upsampling layers from U-Net as the decoder. Since there are 12 Transformer layers in the encoder of UNETR, the sequence representations of different layers are upsampled by CNN and then concatenated with the decoder layers to create the skip connections. Another Transformer-based network designed for 3D biomedical image segmentation is TransBTS [23], which explores another possibility of incorporating Transformer into CNN-based network. Like a conventional U-Net, there are downsampling and upsampling layers with skip connections in TranBTS, but the unique part is that at the bottom of the network, the encoder and decoder are connected by the following 4 types of layers: a linear projection layer, a patch embedding layer to transfer the image tensor to sequence data, ViT layers to extract long-range dependencies, and a feature mapping layer to fit the sequence data back to the 3D CNN decoder. The benefit of arranging

ViT in this way into the U-Net architecture is that at the end of the 3D CNN encoder the ViT can compute long-range dependencies with a global receptive field.

Given that several studies have incorporated Transformer into the task of 3D medical image segmentation and yielded satisfactory results, we believe that such a type of algorithms has the potential to succeed in BraTS2021. TransBTS and UNETR both displayed great potentials to be applied to this challenge with specific modifications and improvement, but TransBTS's arrangement of the ViT layers is more suitable for the BraTS data (we will discuss it in detail in the Method section). Therefore, we decide to borrow the backbone and the core idea from TransBTS to propose a refined version for BraTS2021, called Bi Transformer U-Net (BiTr-Unet). The prefix "Bi" means that we have two sets of ViT layers in our modified model while TransBTS only has one.

2   Method

2.1   Basic Structure of BiTr-Unet

Figure 2 provides an overview of the proposed BiTr-Unet, which contains the main characteristics and core backbone of TransBTS. Overall, the proposed deep neural network f takes the multi-modal MRI scans X as the input, and outputs the predicted segmentation image Y, which can be simply written as

$$Y = f(X). \tag{1}$$

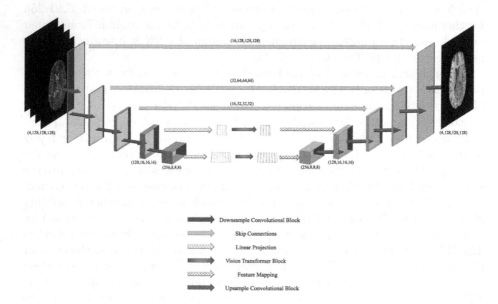

Fig. 2. The basic architecture of BiTr-Unet.

Preprocessing. The BraTS MRI scans with four modalities including T1, T1c, T2, and T2-FLAIR, and the extra "ground-truth" segmentation label for the training data are stored as separate NIfTI files (.nii.gz). For each patient, the four NIfTI files of MRI images are imported as NumPy arrays and stacked along a new axis to recreate the volumetric information in one NumPy array X. For the training data, the NIfTI file of segmentation label is imported as one NumPy array Y. Then, X, or X and Y for the training data only, will be stored as one Pickle file (.pkl). Details of the implementation of other conventional preprocessing steps are provided in the Implementation Details Section.

3D CNN Encoder with Attention Module. BiTr-Unet has an encoder with 3D CNN downsample layers. The preprocessed input of MRIs $X \in \mathbb{R}^{C \times H \times W \times D}$ is fed into the network. After the initial convolutional block with a stride of 1 to increase the dimension of feature map F to $4C \times H \times W \times D$, there are four consecutive $3 \times 3 \times 3$ convolutional blocks with a stride of 2 in the encoder to extract the feature representation of the input image. The resulting output dimension of the feature representation is $(64C, \frac{H}{16}, \frac{W}{16}, \frac{D}{16})$. The Convolutional Block Attention Module (CBAM) is proposed in [24] to improve the performance of CNN models on various tasks. This efficient and lightweight CBAM can be seamlessly integrated into a CNN architecture for adaptive feature refinement by computing attention maps. The original CBAM in [24] is designed for 2D CNN, and in [8] the CBAM is expanded for 3D CNN. Given the intermediate feature map F, 3D CBAM produces the channel attention map $M_c \in \mathbb{R}^{C \times 1 \times 1 \times 1 \times 1}$ and the 3D spatial attention map $M_s \in \mathbb{R}^{1 \times H \times W \times D}$. The process of computing the 3D spatial attention maps is written as

$$F' = M_c(F) \otimes F, \tag{2}$$
$$F'' = M_S(F') \otimes F', \tag{3}$$

where $\otimes$ is the element-wise multiplication between maps, and F'' represents the refined feature map after the CBAM block. We integrate the 3D CBAM into the encoder by replacing the regular 3D CNN block with 3D CBAM block.

Feature Embedding of Feature Representation. Since Transformer takes sequence data as the input, the most common way of changing image input into sequence data is to divide an image into several equivalent patches. However, since the input of Transformer in BiTr-Unet is the intermediate feature map $F_{int} \in \mathbb{R}^{K \times M \times M \times M}$, a more convenient way introduced by TransBTS is used. F_{int} firstly go through a $3 \times 3 \times 3$ convolutional block to increase its channel dimension K to d. In this way the spatial and depth dimensions of the feature representations are flattened to one dimension of size N. This process is named linear projection, and the resulting feature map f has a dimension of $d \times N$, so it can be regarded as N d-dimensional tokens to be input of the Transformer block. For the positional embedding of these N d-dimensional tokens, TransBTS utilizes learnable position embeddings and adds them to the tokens directly by

$$z_0 = f + PE = W \times F + PE, \tag{4}$$

where W is the linear projection, $PE \in \mathbb{R}^{d \times N}$ is the position embeddings, and $z_0 \in \mathbb{R}^{d \times N}$ is the whole operation of feature embeddings of the feature representations.

Transformer Layers. Figure 3 illustrates the workflow of the Transformer block in our model. After feature embedding, the tokenized and position embedded sequence of feature representations goes through the typical Transformer layers with a Multi-Head Attention (MHA) block and a Feed Forward Network (FFN). For the best result, Layer Normalization (LN) is performed before MHA and FFN, and the number of Transformer layers L can be modified. The output of the lth ($l = 1, \ldots, L$) Transformer layer is denoted by z_l and calculated as

$$z_l' = MHA(LN(z_{l-1})) + z_{l-1}, \tag{5}$$
$$z_l = FFN(LN(z_l')) + z_l'. \tag{6}$$

Feature Mapping. Since the outputs of the Transformer layers are the sequence data, it should be transferred back to the intermediate feature representation $F_{int} \in \mathbb{R}^{K \times M \times M \times M}$ for the 3D CNN upsample layer. To achieve this, the output $z_L \in \mathbb{R}^{d \times N}$ of the Transformer layers are reshaped to $z_L \in \mathbb{R}^{d \times M \times M \times M}$ and then go through a 3×3×3 convolutional block to reduce the

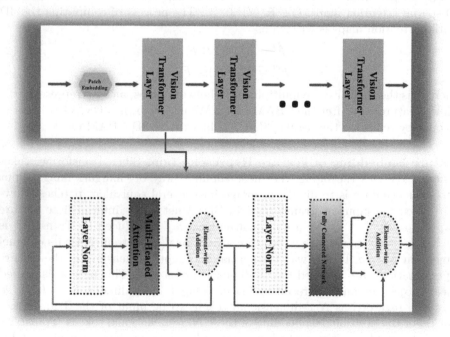

Fig. 3. The basic structure of the vision transformer block.

channel dimension from d to K. After this process, the feature representation $F_{int} \in \mathbb{R}^{K \times M \times M \times M}$ is ready for the 3D CNN upsample layer.

3D CNN Decoder. BiTr-Unet has a decoder with 3D CNN upsample layers. There are four consecutive 3×3×3 convolutional blocks with a stride of 2, and one final convolutional block with a stride of 1 to decrease the dimension of the feature map F_{final} to $C \times H \times W \times D$ in the decoder to construct the final segmentation image. The resulting output segmentation label is $Y \in \mathbb{R}^{C \times H \times W \times D}$.

Skip Connections. The output of the first three layers of the 3D CNN layers are directly sent to the last three layers of the 3D CNN layers to create the skip connections. Unlike the output of the first three 3D downsample CNN layers which are concatenated directly with the input of the last three 3D upsample CNN layers, the output of the fourth and the fifth 3D downsample CNN layers go through a feature embedding of feature representation layer, transformer layers, and a feature mapping layer, and then go through the corresponding 3D upsample CNN layer.

Postprocessing and Model Ensemble. The champion model of BraTS2020, nnU-Net, applies a BraTS-specific postprocessing strategy to achieve a higher Dice score, which eliminates a volume of predicted segmentation if this volume is smaller than a threshold [10]. We borrow this postprocessing technique to maximize the Dice score of the resulting segmentation. Majority voting is an effective and fast method of model ensemble, which may result in a significant improvement in prediction accuracy [15]. We adopt majority voting to ensemble differently trained models of BiTr-Unet. Specifically, for each voxel, every model votes for the voxel's category, and the category with the highest number of votes is used as the final prediction of the voxel. Given n differently trained BiTr-Unet models $f_i(X)$ $(i = 1, \ldots, n)$, the output of the majority voting for each j-th voxel is

$$C(X)[j] = \mathrm{mode}(f_1(X)[j], \ldots, f_n(X)[j]). \tag{7}$$

If the j-th voxel has more than one category with the highest number of votes, its final predicted label is the category with the largest averaged prediction probability over all trained models, i.e.,

$$y_j = \underset{k \in C(X)[j]}{\arg\max} (p_{jk}), \tag{8}$$

where p_{jk} is the averaged prediction probability of the k-th category for the j-th voxel over the n trained models.

2.2 Comparison with Related Work

Modifications from TransBTS. BiTr-Unet is a variant of TransBTS, but our modifications are significant and make the network well-prepared for BraTS2021.

We keep all the innovative and successful attributes of TransBTS, including the combination of CNN and Transformer, feature embedding, and feature mapping. Meanwhile, we also notice that the CNN encoder and decoder in TransBTS can be refined by adding the attention module. We also increase the depth of the whole network for a denser feature representation. TransBTS only utilizes Transformer at the end of the encoder, so it is an operation of the whole feature representation after the fourth layer of the encoder. Since the depth of the encoder layers is increased to five, we use Transformer for both the fourth and the fifth layers. For the fourth layer, Transformer works as an operation to build a skip connection so that its output is concatenated with the input of the fourth decoder layer.

Differences from UNETR. A recently proposed network for 3D medical image segmentation, UNETR, also uses Transformer to extract long-range spatial dependencies [7]. Unlike TransBTS and our BiTr-Unet, which involve 3D convolutional blocks in both encoder and decoder of the network, UNETR does not assign any convolutional block to the encoder. ViT [6] is designed to operate on 2D images, and UNETR expands it for 3D images but keeps the original ViT's design that divides an image into equivalent patches and treats each patch as one token for the operation of attention mechanism. It is an elegant way that using a pure Transformer for the encoding of 3D medical image segmentation, but removing convolutional blocks in the encoder may lead to the insufficiency in extracting local context information for the volumetric BraTS MRI data. Moreover, UNETR stacks Transformer layers and keeps the sequence data dimension unchanged during the whole process, which results in expensive computation for high-resolution 3D images.

3   Result

3.1   Implementation Details

Our BiTr-Unet model is implemented in Pytorch and trained on four NVIDIA RTX8000 GPUs for 7050 epochs with a batch size of 16. For the optimization, we use the Adam optimizer with an initial learning rate of 0.0002. The learning rate decays by each iteration with a power of 0.9 for better convergence. We adopt this training strategy to avoid overfitting, but it also needs a high number of training epochs. The four modalities of the raw BraTS training data for each case are randomly cropped from $240 \times 240 \times 155$ voxels to $128 \times 128 \times 128$ voxels. We also randomly shift the intensity in the range of $[-0.1, 0.1]$ and scale in the range of $[0.9, 1.1]$. Test Time Augmentation (TTA), which is proved to increase the prediction accuracy in [20], is applied when using the trained model to generate the segmentation images of the validation data. During TTA, we create 7 extra copies of the input X by flipping all the possible combinations of directions H, W and D.

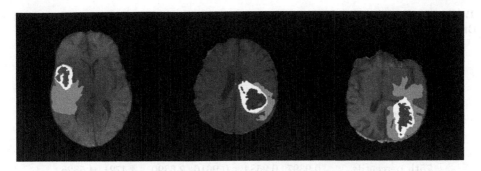

Fig. 4. Visualization of the segmentation results from the ensembled BiTr-Unet for three cases in BraTS2021 Validation data.

3.2 Segmentation Result

During the validation phase, the segmentation images of BraTS2021 validation data from our BiTr-Unet are evaluated by the BraTS2021 organizer through the Synapse platform (https://www.synapse.org/#!Synapse:syn25829067/wiki). We validate three checkpoints with different numbers of trained epochs and also validate the ensemble model of these three checkpoints. Table 1 shows the mean score on the validation data. Figure 4 presents the segmentation results from the ensembled model for three validation cases.

In the testing phase, we are required to encapsulate the execution environment dependencies and the trained model in an Docker image, and push the built Docker image into Synapse for the testing evaluation. Automated model ensemble through Docker may lead to increased Docker image size, longer processing time, and even unstable result. To avoid risks, we skip the model ensemble and only select the 7050-epoch BiTr-Unet model for the testing Docker submission. Table 2 shows the detailed segmentation result of the 7050-epoch BiTr-Unet on BraTS2021 validation data, and Table 3 shows the result on the testing data.

Table 1. Mean segmentation result of differently trained BiTr-Unet models on BraTS2021 validation data.

Model	Mean dice			Mean Hausdorff95 (mm)		
	ET	WT	TC	ET	WT	TC
4800-epoch	0.8139	0.9070	0.8466	16.7017	4.5880	13.3968
6050-epoch	0.8237	0.9079	0.8383	15.3014	4.5883	13.9110
7050-epoch	0.8187	0.9097	0.8434	17.8466	4.5084	16.6893
Ensemble by majority voting	0.8231	0.9076	0.8392	14.9963	4.5322	13.4592

Table 2. Detailed segmentation result of the 7050-epoch BiTr-Unet model on BraTS2021 validation data.

Statistics	Dice			Hausdorff95 (mm)		
	ET	WT	TC	ET	WT	TC
Mean	0.8187	0.9097	0.8434	17.8466	4.5084	16.6893
Standard deviation	0.2327	0.08837	0.2305	73.6517	7.6621	65.5411
Median	0.8899	0.9366	0.9338	1.4142	2.8284	2.2361
25th percentile	0.8289	0.8903	0.8610	1	1.4142	1
75th percentile	0.9397	0.9584	0.9616	2.6390	4.4721	4.5826

Table 3. Detailed segmentation result of the 7050-epoch BiTr-Unet model on BraTS2021 testing data.

Statistics	Dice			Hausdorff95 (mm)		
	ET	WT	TC	ET	WT	TC
Mean	0.7256	0.7639	0.7422	65.2966	62.1576	69.006318
Standard deviation	0.3522	0.3426	0.3738	139.003958	133.4915	140.8401
Median	0.8874	0.9257	0.9350	1.4142	3	2.2361
25th percentile	0.7313	0.8117	0.7642	1	1.4142	1
75th percentile	0.9512	0.9600	0.9708	3.7417	9.1647	8.2002

4 Discussion

We propose a new deep neural network model called BiTr-Unet, a refined version of TransBTS, for the BraTS2021 tumor segmentation challenge. The result on the validation data indicates that BiTr-Unet is a stable and powerful network to extract both local and long-range dependencies of 3D MRI scans. Compared to models with U-Net alike architectures but without attention modules that are successful in BraTS2020, BiTr-Unet takes the advantage of the novel Transformer module for potentially better performance. The way we incorporate Transformer into a CNN encoder-decoder model is inspired by TransBTS, but we propose more innovative and suitable modifications such as making feature representations of the skip connection to go through a ViT block. However, there is plenty more room for further explorations to incorporate Transformer into networks for 3D medical image segmentation. The result on the testing data shares similar median and 75th percentile with that on the validation data, but has an inferior mean, standard deviation, and 25th percentile. With the fact that testing data is more dissimilar to the training data than the validation data, this discrepancy result indicates that BiTr-Unet may still struggle when processing unseen patterns. Due to the time limit, we did not finish the experiment to test the performance of the model with more encoder and decoder layers that are connected by a skip connection going through a ViT Block, or to test ViT with different embedding dimensions. Also, inspired by the recent work of innovative Transformer models for image classification or segmentation that reduces computation complexity by special algorithms [13,14,26], we would also try to introduce them into our model in the future to improve the performance and decrease the computation complexity.

Acknowledgements. This research was partially supported by the grant R21AG0 70303 from the National Institutes of Health and a startup fund from New York University. The content is solely the responsibility of the authors and does not necessarily represent the official views of the National Institutes of Health or New York University.

References

1. Baid, U., et al.: The RSNA-ASNR-MICCAI BraTs 2021 benchmark on brain tumor segmentation and radiogenomic classification. arXiv preprint arXiv:2107.02314 (2021)
2. Bakas, S., et al.: Segmentation labels and radiomic features for the pre-operative scans of the TCGA-GBM collection, July 2017. https://doi.org/10.7937/K9/TCIA.2017.KLXWJJ1Q
3. Bakas, S., et al.: Segmentation labels and radiomic features for the pre-operative scans of the TCGA-LGG collection. Cancer Imaging Arch. **286** (2017)
4. Bakas, S., et al.: Advancing the cancer genome atlas glioma MRI collections with expert segmentation labels and radiomic features. Sci. Data 4(1), 1–13 (2017)
5. Chen, C.F., Fan, Q., Panda, R.: Crossvit: cross-attention multi-scale vision transformer for image classification. arXiv preprint arXiv:2103.14899 (2021)
6. Dosovitskiy, A., et al.: An image is worth 16x16 words: transformers for image recognition at scale. arXiv preprint arXiv:2010.11929 (2020)
7. Hatamizadeh, A., Yang, D., Roth, H., Xu, D.: UnetR: transformers for 3D medical image segmentation. arXiv preprint arXiv:2103.10504 (2021)
8. Henry, T., et al.: Brain tumor segmentation with self-ensembled, deeply-supervised 3D u-net neural networks: a BraTs 2020 challenge solution. arXiv preprint arXiv:2011.01045 (2020)
9. Hesamian, M.H., Jia, W., He, X., Kennedy, P.: Deep learning techniques for medical image segmentation: achievements and challenges. J. Digit. Imaging **32**(4), 582–596 (2019). https://doi.org/10.1007/s10278-019-00227-x
10. Isensee, F., et al.: nnu-Net: self-adapting framework for u-net-based medical image segmentation. arXiv preprint arXiv:1809.10486 (2018)
11. Krizhevsky, A., Sutskever, I., Hinton, G.E.: ImageNet classification with deep convolutional neural networks. In: Pereira, F., Burges, C.J.C., Bottou, L., Weinberger, K.Q. (eds.) Advances in Neural Information Processing Systems, vol. 25. Curran Associates, Inc. (2012). https://proceedings.neurips.cc/paper/2012/file/c399862d3b9d6b76c8436e924a68c45b-Paper.pdf
12. LeCun, Y., Bengio, Y., Hinton, G.: Deep learning. Nature **521**, 436–44 (2015). https://doi.org/10.1038/nature14539
13. Lin, H., et al.: Cat: cross attention in vision transformer. arXiv preprint arXiv:2106.05786 (2021)
14. Liu, Z., et al.: Swin transformer: hierarchical vision transformer using shifted windows. arXiv preprint arXiv:2103.14030 (2021)

15. Lyu, C., Shu, H.: A two-stage cascade model with variational autoencoders and attention gates for MRI brain tumor segmentation. In: Crimi, A., Bakas, S. (eds.) BrainLes 2020. LNCS, vol. 12658, pp. 435–447. Springer, Cham (2021). https://doi.org/10.1007/978-3-030-72084-1_39
16. Menze, B.H., et al.: The multimodal brain tumor image segmentation benchmark (brats). IEEE Trans. Med. Imaging **34**(10), 1993–2024 (2014)
17. Noda, K., Yamaguchi, Y., Nakadai, K., Okuno, H.G., Ogata, T.: Audio-visual speech recognition using deep learning. Appl. Intell. **42**(4), 722–737 (2014). https://doi.org/10.1007/s10489-014-0629-7
18. Ronneberger, O., Fischer, P., Brox, T.: U-net: convolutional networks for biomedical image segmentation. In: Navab, N., Hornegger, J., Wells, W.M., Frangi, A.F. (eds.) MICCAI 2015. LNCS, vol. 9351, pp. 234–241. Springer, Cham (2015). https://doi.org/10.1007/978-3-319-24574-4_28
19. Shu, H., et al.: A deep learning approach to re-create raw full-field digital mammograms for breast density and texture analysis. Radiol. Artif. Intell. **3**(4), e200097 (2021). https://doi.org/10.1148/ryai.2021200097
20. Simonyan, K., Zisserman, A.: Very deep convolutional networks for large-scale image recognition (2015)
21. Touvron, H., Cord, M., Douze, M., Massa, F., Sablayrolles, A., Jégou, H.: Training data-efficient image transformers & distillation through attention. In: International Conference on Machine Learning, pp. 10347–10357. PMLR (2021)
22. Vaswani, A., et al.: Attention is all you need. In: Advances in Neural Information Processing Systems, pp. 5998–6008 (2017)
23. Wang, W., Chen, C., Ding, M., Li, J., Yu, H., Zha, S.: TransBTS: multimodal brain tumor segmentation using transformer. arXiv preprint arXiv:2103.04430 (2021)
24. Woo, S., Park, J., Lee, J.Y., Kweon, I.S.: CBAM: convolutional block attention module. In: Proceedings of the European conference on computer vision (ECCV), pp. 3–19 (2018)
25. Wu, H., et al.: CVT: introducing convolutions to vision transformers. arXiv preprint arXiv:2103.15808 (2021)
26. Xie, Y., Zhang, J., Shen, C., Xia, Y.: COTR: efficiently bridging CNN and transformer for 3D medical image segmentation. arXiv preprint arXiv:2103.03024 (2021)
27. Zhong, L., et al.: 2WM: tumor segmentation and tract statistics for assessing white matter integrity with applications to glioblastoma patients. Neuroimage **223**, 117368 (2020)

Optimized U-Net for Brain Tumor Segmentation

Michał Futrega[✉], Alexandre Milesi, Michał Marcinkiewicz, and Pablo Ribalta

NVIDIA, Santa Clara, CA 95051, USA
{mfutrega,alexandrem,michalm,pribalta}@nvidia.com

Abstract. We propose an optimized U-Net architecture for a brain tumor segmentation task in the BraTS21 challenge. To find the optimal model architecture and the learning schedule, we have run an extensive ablation study to test: deep supervision loss, Focal loss, decoder attention, drop block, and residual connections. Additionally, we have searched for the optimal depth of the U-Net encoder, number of convolutional channels and post-processing strategy. Our method won the validation phase and took third place in the test phase. We have open-sourced the code to reproduce our BraTS21 submission at the NVIDIA Deep Learning Examples GitHub Repository (https://github.com/NVIDIA/DeepLearningExamples/blob/master/PyTorch/Segmentation/nnUNet/notebooks/BraTS21.ipynb).

Keywords: U-Net · Brain tumor segmentation · Deep learning · MRI

1 Introduction

One of the most challenging problems in medical image processing is automatic brain tumor segmentation. Obtaining a computational model capable of surpassing a trained human-level performance would provide valuable assistance to clinicians and would enable a more precise, reliable, and standardized approach to disease detection, treatment planning and monitoring. Gliomas are the most common type of brain tumors in humans [1]. Their accurate segmentation is a challenging medical image analysis task due to their variable shape and appearance in multi-modal magnetic resonance imaging (MRI). Manual segmentation of such brain tumors requires a great deal of medical expertise, is time-consuming, and prone to human error. Moreover, the manual process lacks consistency and reproducibility, which negatively affects the results and can ultimately lead to incorrect prognosis and treatment.

The rapid progress in development of deep learning (DL) algorithms shows great potential for application of deep neural networks (DNNs) in computer-aided automatic or semi-automatic methods for medical data analysis. The drastic improvements of convolutional neural networks (CNNs) resulted in models being able to approach or surpass the human level performance in plethora

© The Author(s), under exclusive license to Springer Nature Switzerland AG 2022
A. Crimi and S. Bakas (Eds.): BrainLes 2021, LNCS 12963, pp. 15–29, 2022.
https://doi.org/10.1007/978-3-031-09002-8_2

of applications, such as image classification [2] or microscope image segmentation [3], among many others. DL-based models are great candidates for brain tumor segmentation, as long as sufficient amount of training data is supplied. The Brain Tumor Segmentation Challenge (BraTS) provides a large, high-quality dataset consisting of multi-modal MRI brain scans with corresponding segmentation masks [4–8].

The state-of-the-art models in brain tumor segmentation are based on the encoder-decoder architectures, with U-Net [9] being the most popular for medical image segmentation, based on the citations number. In recent years, U-Net-like architectures were among top submissions to the BraTS challenge. For instance, in 2018, Myronenko *et al.*, modified a U-Net model by adding a variational autoencoder branch for regularization [10]. In 2019, Jiang *et al.*, employed a two-stage U-Net pipeline to segment the substructures of brain tumors from coarse to fine [11]. In 2020, Isensee *et al.*, applied the nnU-Net framework [12] with specific BraTS designed modifications regarding data post-processing, region-based training, data augmentation, and minor modifications to the nnU-Net pipeline [13].

Those achievements prove that well-designed U-Net based architectures have the ability to perform very well on tasks such as brain tumor segmentation. In order to design a competitive solution for challenges like BraTS21, both optimal neural network architecture and training schedule has to be selected. However, there exists a plethora of U-Net variants, for example: Attention U-Net [14], Residual U-Net [15], Dense U-Net [16], Inception U-Net [17], U-Net++ [18], SegResNetVAE [10] or UNETR [19], just to name a few. A wide range of U-Net architectures makes the selection of the optimal one a difficult task. Furthermore, once the neural network architecture is selected, designing a proper training schedule is critical for getting optimal performance. Designing a training schedule is associated with selecting optimal components, such as a loss function, data augmentation strategy, learning rate and its schedule, number of epochs to train, and many more. Also, it is not trivial to decide which model extensions to add, for example, deep-supervision [20] or drop-block [21].

The fact that datasets for medical image segmentation are small (usually around 100 examples), and there is no common benchmark for measuring improvements of different architecture tweaks, often makes such comparisons unreliable. However, the dataset released for BraTS21 provides 2,040 examples (respectively 1251, 219, 570 examples in the training, validation, and test set), which makes it the largest dataset for medical image segmentation at the moment, and a perfect candidate to measure performance improvements for different U-Net variants.

In this paper, we have run extensive ablation studies to select both an optimal U-Net variant and training schedule for the BraTS21 challenge. We have tested U-Net[9], Attention U-Net [14], Residual U-Net [15], SegResNetVAE [10] and UNETR [19] for U-Net variants, and experimented with Deep Supervision [20], Drop-Block [21], and different loss functions (combinations of Cross Entropy, Focal, and Dice). Furthermore, we have optimized our model further by increas-

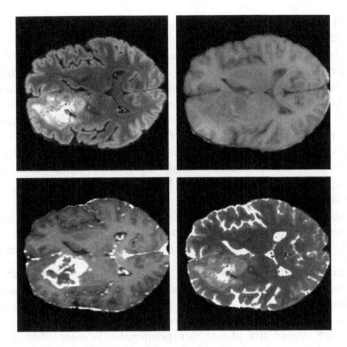

Fig. 1. Example with ID 00000 from the BraTS21 training dataset. Each subplot presents a different modality. From top left to bottom right: FLAIR, T1, T1Gd T2.

ing the encoder depth, adding one-hot-encoding channel for the foreground voxels to the input data, and increasing the number of convolutional filters.

2   Method

2.1   Data

The training dataset provided for the BraTS21 challenge [4–8] consists of $1,251$ brain MRI scans along with segmentation annotations of tumorous regions. The 3D volumes were skull-stripped and resampled to $1\,mm^3$ isotropic resolution, with dimensions of $(240, 240, 155)$ voxels. For each example, four modalities were given: native (T1), post-contrast T1-weighted (T1Gd), T2-weighted (T2), and T2 Fluid Attenuated Inversion Recovery (T2-FLAIR). Example images of each modality are presented on Fig. 1. Segmentation labels were annotated manually by one to four experts. Annotations consist of four classes: enhancing tumor (ET), peritumoral edematous tissue (ED), necrotic tumor core (NCR), and background (voxels that are not part of the tumor).

2.2   Data Preprocessing and Augmentations

Each example of the BraTS21 dataset consists of four NIfTI [22] files with different MRI modalities. As a first step of data pre-processing, all four modalities were stacked such that each example has a shape of $(4, 240, 240, 155)$ (input tensor is in the (C, H, W, D) layout, where C-channels, H-height, W-width and D-depth). Then redundant background voxels (with voxel value zero) on the borders of each volume were cropped, as they do not provide any useful information and can be ignored by the neural network. Subsequently, for each example, the mean and the standard deviation were computed within the non-zero region for each channel separately. All volumes were normalized by first subtracting the mean and then divided by the standard deviation. The background voxels were not normalized so that their value remained at zero. To distinguish between background voxels and normalized voxels which have values close to zero, an additional input channel was created with one-hot encoding for foreground voxels and stacked with the input data.

Data augmentation is a technique that alleviates the overfitting problem by artificially extending a dataset during the training phase. To make our method more robust, the following data augmentations were used during training phase:

1. **Biased crop:** From the input volume, a patch of dimensions $(5, 128, 128, 128)$ was randomly cropped. Additionally, with probability of 0.4 the patch selected via random biased crop is guaranteed that some foreground voxels (with positive class in the ground truth) are present in the cropped region.
2. **Zoom:** With probability of 0.15, a random value is sampled uniformly from $(1.0, 1.4)$ and image size is resized to its original size times the sampled value with the cubic interpolation, while the ground truth with the nearest neighbour interpolation.
3. **Flips:** With probability of 0.5, for each x, y, z axis independently, volume was flipped along that axis.
4. **Gaussian Noise:** With probability of 0.15, random Gaussian noise with mean zero and standard deviation sampled uniformly from $(0, 0.33)$ is sampled for each voxel and added to the input volume.
5. **Gaussian Blur:** With probability of 0.15, Gaussian blurring with standard deviation of the Gaussian Kernel sampled uniformly from $(0.5, 1.5)$ is applied to the input volume.
6. **Brightness:** With probability of 0.15, a random value is sampled uniformly from $(0.7, 1.3)$ and then input volume voxels are multiplied by it.
7. **Contrast:** With probability of 0.15, a random value is sampled uniformly from $(0.65, 1.5)$ and then input volume voxels are multiplied by it and clipped to their original value range.

2.3 Model Architecture

In order to select the most optimal neural network architecture, we have run ablation studies for the following models: U-Net [9], Attention U-Net [14], Residual U-Net [15], SegResNetVAE [10] and UNETR [19]. Below, we present a short description of each model.

U-Net [9] architecture (shown in the Fig. 2) is characterised by a symmetric U-shape, and can be divided into two parts, i.e., encoder and decoder. The first part is the contracting path (encoder) which is transforming the input volume into lower dimensional space. The encoder has a modular structure consisting of repeating convolution blocks. Each block has two smaller blocks of transformations (dark and light blue blocks on the Fig. 2). The first smaller block is reducing the spatial dimensions of the input feature map by a factor of two via convolutional layer with kernels $3 \times 3 \times 3$ and stride $2 \times 2 \times 2$, then instance normalization and Leaky ReLU activation with negative slope if 0.01 are applied (dark blue block). Next feature map is transformed with almost the same set of operations except that the convolutional layer has stride $1 \times 1 \times 1$ (light blue).

After the spatial dimensions of the feature map are transformed to the size of $2 \times 2 \times 2$, then the decoder part starts. The decoder also has a modular structure, but its goal is to increase the spatial dimensions by reducing the encoder feature map. The block in the decoder is built from three smaller blocks. The first one is transposed convolution with kernels $2 \times 2 \times 2$ and stride $2 \times 2 \times 2$, which is increasing the spatial dimensions of the feature map by a factor of two. Then upsampled feature map is concatenated with encoder feature map from the equivalent spatial level and then transformed by two identical blocks with convolutional layer with kernels $3 \times 3 \times 3$ and stride $1 \times 1 \times 1$, instance normalization and Leaky ReLU activation with negative slope if 0.01 are applied (light blue). Additionally, deep-supervision (Subsect. 2.4) can be used, which is computing loss functions for outputs from lower decoder levels.

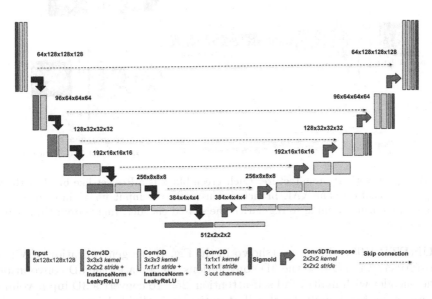

Fig. 2. U-Net architecture. The encoder is transforming the input by reducing its spatial dimensions, and then the decoder is upsampling it back to the original input shape. Additional two output heads are used for deep supervision loss (green bars). (Color figure online)

SegResNetVAE [10] is a residual U-Net with autoencoder (shown in the Fig. 3) regularization that has won the BraTS 2018 challenge and modifies U-Net by designing new architecture for encoder blocks and by adding a variational autoencoder (VAE) [23] branch in the decoder, which reconstructs the input and has a regularization effect.

The encoder part uses ResNet like blocks, where each block consists of two convolutions with group normalization and ReLU activation, followed by additive identity skip connection. The decoder structure is similar to the encoder, but only with a single block per each spatial level. Each decoder block begins with reducing the number of channels by a factor of 2 (with $1 \times 1 \times 1$ convolution) and doubling the spatial dimension (using 3D bilinear), followed by an addition with encoder feature map from the equivalent spatial level.

In the VAE branch in the decoder, first the feature map from the bottleneck is reduced into a low dimensional space of 256 (128 to represent mean, and 128 to represent std). Then, a sample is drawn from the Gaussian distribution with the given mean and std, and reconstructed into the input image dimensions following the same architecture as the decoder.

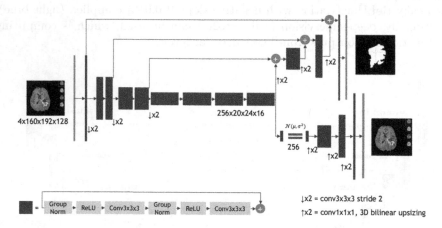

Fig. 3. SegResNetVAE architecture. Each green block is a ResNet-like block with the group normalization. The VAE branch reconstructs the input image into itself, and is used only during training to regularize the shared encoder. Image from [10]. (Color figure online)

UNETR [19] architecture (shown in the Fig. 4) is a generalization of Vision Transformer (ViT) [24] to the 3D convolutions—it replaces the 3D convolutions in the encoder with multi-head self-attention [25]. To convert a 3D input volume into an input for a multi-head self-attention it is divided into a sequence of uniform non-overlapping patches (with $16 \times 16 \times 16$ shape) and projected into an embedding space (with 768 dimensions) using a linear layer, and added with a positional embedding. Such input is then transformed by a multi-head self-attention encoder.

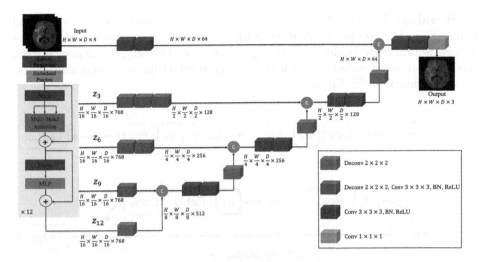

Fig. 4. UNETR architecture. Instead of using 3D convolution in the encoder, UNETR is transforming the input volume via multi-head self-attention blocks known from the Transformer model. Image from [19].

Attention U-Net [14] is extending base U-Net by adding an attention gate (shown in the Fig. 5) in the decoder part. Attention gate is transforming the feature map from the encoder before the concatenation in the decoder block. It learns which regions of the encoder feature map are the most important, considering the context of the feature map from the previous decoder block. This is achieved by multiplication of the encoder feature map with the weights computed by the attention gate. The weight values are in the $(0, 1)$ range and represent the attention level that the neural network is paying to a given pixel.

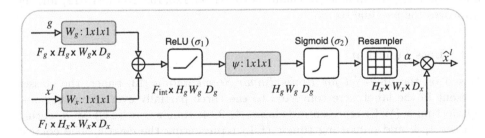

Fig. 5. The architecture of the attention gate. Input features (x^l) are multiplied by attention weights (α). To compute α, input features (x^l), and feature map from corresponding encoder level are first transformed by $1 \times 1 \times 1$ convolution, and the summed. Next, ReLU activation and another $1 \times 1 \times 1$ convolution are applied. Finally, attention weights are upsampled with trilinear interpolation. Image from [14].

Residual U-Net [15] is inspired by a ResNet model [15] where residual connections were proposed. Adding residual connections is helping with training a deep neural network due to better gradient flow. The only difference between basic U-Net and Residual U-Net is the computation within a convolutional block, which is shown in the Fig. 6.

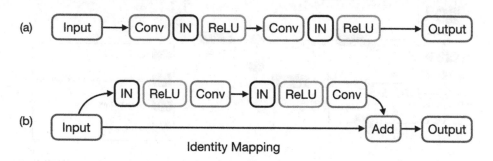

Fig. 6. Difference between blocks in basic U-Net (a) and Residual U-Net (b). Conv block (orange) corresponds to a convolutional layer with $3 \times 3 \times 3$ kernels, IN (green) is instance normalization and ReLU (blue) is a Rectified Linear Unit activation. (Color figure online)

Based on our experiments (the detailed results are shown in Subsect. 3.3), a basic U-Net achieves the best results, and was selected for further exploration. The next optimization was adjusting the encoder depth and optimal selection of the convolution channels. As a baseline, a default U-Net architecture from the nnU-Net framework was used, i.e., the depth of the network was 6, and the convolution channels at each encoder level were: $32, 64, 128, 256, 320, 320$. Our experiments have demonstrated that increasing the depth of the encoder to 7, and modifying the number of channels to: $64, 96, 128, 192, 256, 384, 512$, further improves the baseline score.

2.4 Loss Function

Based on the *nnU-Net for Brain Tumor Segmentation* [13] paper, the classes present in the label were converted to the three partially overlapping regions: whole tumor (WT) representing classes 1, 2, 4; tumor core (TC) representing classes 1, 4; and enhancing tumor (ET) representing the class 4. The contest leaderboard is computed based on those overlapping regions instead of classes present in the labels. It is beneficial to construct the loss function based on classes used for ranking calculation, thus we designed the output feature map to have three channels (one per class) which at the very end are transformed via the sigmoid activation.

Each region was optimized separately with a sum of binary cross-entropy or Focal loss [26] (with gamma parameter set to 2) with the Dice loss [27]. For Dice loss, its batched variant was used, i.e., Dice loss was computed over all samples in the batch instead of averaging the Dice loss over each sample separately.

Deep Supervision [20] is a technique that helps with a better gradient flow by computing loss function on different decoder levels. In this work, we added two additional output heads, marked by green bars on Fig. 2. To compute the deep supervision loss, labels were first downsampled using nearest neighbor interpolation to the $(64, 64, 64)$ and $(32, 32, 32)$ spatial shapes such that they match the shapes of additional outputs. For labels y_i and predictions p_i for $i = 1, 2, 3$, where $i = 1$ corresponds to the last output head, $i = 2$ is the output head on the penultimate decoder level and $i = 3$ is before the penultimate, final loss function is computed as follows:

$$\mathcal{L}(y_1, y_2, y_3, p_1, p_2, p_3) = \mathcal{L}(y_1, p_1) + \frac{1}{2}\mathcal{L}(y_2, p_2) + \frac{1}{4}\mathcal{L}(y_3, p_3). \quad (1)$$

2.5 Inference

During inference, the input volume can have arbitrary size, instead of the fixed patch size $(128, 128, 128)$ as during the training phase. Thus, we used a sliding window inference[1], where the window has the same size as the training patch, i.e., $(128, 128, 128)$ and adjacent windows overlap by half the size of a patch. The predictions on the overlapping regions are then averaged with Gaussian importance weighting, such that the weights of the center voxels have higher importance, as in the original nnU-Net paper [12].

One of the known ways to improve robustness of predictions is to apply test time augmentations. During inference, we have created eight versions of the input volume, such that each version corresponds to one of eight possible flips along the x, y, z axis combination. Then we run inference for each version of the input volume and transform the predictions back to the original input volume orientation by applying the same flips to predictions as were used for the input volume. Finally, the probabilities from all predictions were averaged.

By optimizing the three overlapping regions (ET, TC, WT) we had to convert them back to the original classes (NCR, ED, ET). The strategy for transforming classes back to the original one is the following: if the WT probability for a given voxel is less than 0.45 then its class is set to 0 (background), otherwise if the probability for TC is less than 0.4 the voxel class is 2 (ED), and finally if probability for ET is less than 0.45 voxel has class 1 (NCR), or otherwise 4 (ET).

Furthermore, we applied the following post-processing strategy: find ET connected components, for components smaller than 16 voxels with mean probability smaller than 0.9, replace their class to NCR (such that voxels are still considered part of the tumor core), next if there is overall less than 73 voxels with ET and their mean probability is smaller than 0.9 replace all ET voxels to NCR. With such post-processing we avoided the edge case where the model predicted a few voxels with enhancing tumor, but there were not any in the ground truth. Such post-processing was beneficial to the final score as if there were no enhancing

---

[1] MONAI sliding window implementation was used.

tumor voxels in the label, then the Dice score for zero false positive prediction was 1, and 0 otherwise.

That methodology was tested on the validations sets from the 5-fold cross-validation. Hyperparameters were selected to yield the highest score combined on all the folds. The threshold value was selected via a grid search method with a step of 0.05 in the range (0.3, 0.7). Similarly, the number of voxels was searched in the range (0, 100) and selected by maximizing score on the 5-fold cross-validation.

3 Results

3.1 Implementation

Our solution is written in PyTorch [28] and extends NVIDIA's implementation of the nnU-Net. The code is publicly available on the NVIDIA Deep Learning Examples GitHub repository[2]. Proposed solution is using the NVIDIA NGC PyTorch 21.07 Docker container[3] which allows for the full encapsulation of dependencies, reproducible runs, as well as easy deployment on any system. All training and inference runs were performed with use of Mixed Precision [29], which speeds-up the model and reduces the GPU memory consumption. Experiments were run on NVIDIA DGX A100 (8×A100 80 GB) system.[4]

3.2 Training Schedule

Each experiment was trained for $1,000$ epochs using the Adam optimizer [30] with three different learning rates: 0.0005, 0.0007, 0.0009 and a weight decay equal to 0.0001. Additionally, during the first 1000 steps, we used a linear warm-up of the learning rate, starting from 0 and increasing it to the target value, and then it was decreased with a cosine annealing scheduler [31]. The weights for 3D convolutions were initialized with Kaiming initialization [32].

For model evaluation, we used 5-fold cross validation and compared the average of the highest Dice score reached on each of the 5-folds. The evaluation on the validation set was run after every epoch. For each fold, we have stored the two checkpoints with the highest mean Dice score on the validation set reached during the training phase. Then during the inference phase, we ensembled the predictions from stored checkpoints by averaging the probabilities.

3.3 Experiments

To select the model architecture, we experimented with three U-Net variants: baseline U-Net [9] which architecture follows the nnU-Net [12] architecture heuristic, UNETR [19] which replaces the U-Net encoder with a Vision

---

[2] https://github.com/NVIDIA/DeepLearningExamples/tree/master/PyTorch/ Segmentation/nnUNet.

[3] https://ngc.nvidia.com/catalog/containers/nvidia:pytorch.

[4] https://www.nvidia.com/en-us/data-center/a100.

Transformer (ViT) [24] generalization for the 3D convolutions, and U-Net with autoencoder regularization (SegResNetVAE) which extends U-Net architecture with variational autoencoder (VAE) [23] branch for input reconstruction in the decoder.

Table 1. Averaged Dice scores of ET, TC, WT classes for each 5-folds comparing the baseline U-Net, UNETR, SegResNetVAE models.

Model	U-Net	UNETR	SegResNetVAE
Fold 0	**0.9087**	0.9044	0.9086
Fold 1	**0.9100**	0.8976	0.9090
Fold 2	**0.9162**	0.9051	0.9140
Fold 3	**0.9238**	0.9111	0.9219
Fold 4	**0.9061**	0.8971	0.9053
Mean Dice	**0.9130**	0.9031	0.9118

Presented results in the Table 1 have shown that baseline U-Net achieves the highest score. Although the score of SegResNetVAE is similar to the plain U-Net, the training time is three times longer compared to U-Net, because of the additional VAE branch. Thus, we decided to select U-Net architecture for further exploration.

In the next phase of experiments we tested various U-Net architecture tweaks: decoder attention [14], deep supervision [20], residual connections [15] and drop block [21]. Additionally, we have experimented with the modified loss function with Focal loss [26] instead of cross-entropy, so that the loss function was Focal+Dice.

The experimental results presented in the Table 2 have shown that the only extension which significantly improves the 5-fold average Dice score over the baseline U-Net (0.9130) was the deep supervision (0.9149).

Table 2. Averaged Dice scores of ET, TC, WT classes for each 5-folds comparing the decoder attention (attention), deep supervision (DS), residual connections (residual), drop block (DB) and focal loss (focal).

Model	Baseline	Attention	DS	Residual	DB	Focal
Fold 0	0.9087	0.9091	**0.9111**	0.9087	0.9096	0.9094
Fold 1	0.9100	0.9110	**0.9115**	0.9103	0.9114	0.9026
Fold 2	0.9162	0.9157	**0.9175**	**0.9175**	0.9159	0.9146
Fold 3	0.9238	0.9232	**0.9268**	0.9233	0.9241	0.9229
Fold 4	0.9061	0.9061	**0.9074**	0.9070	0.9071	0.9072
Mean Dice	0.9130	0.9130	**0.9149**	0.9134	0.9136	0.9133

Finally, for the U-Net with deep supervision, we tested the modification of the U-Net encoder. The baseline U-Net architecture follows the architecture heuristic from the nnU-Net [12] framework for which the depth of the network was 6, and the convolution channels at each encoder level were: $32, 64, 128, 256, 320, 320$. We experimented with an encoder of depth 7, modified the number of channels to: $64, 96, 128, 192, 256, 384, 512$, and checked the input volume with an additional channel with one-hot encoding for foreground voxels.

Table 3. Averaged Dice scores of ET, TC, WT classes for each 5-folds comparing the deep supervision (DS), deeper U-Net encoder, modified number of convolution channels, additional input channel with one-hot encoding for foreground voxels, and all modification applied together (D+C+O) i.e., deeper U-Net with changed number of convolution channels and one-hot encoding channel for foreground voxels.

Model	DS	Deeper	Channels	One-hot	D+C+O
Fold 0	0.9111	**0.9118**	0.9107	0.9109	**0.9118**
Fold 1	0.9115	0.9140	0.9135	0.9132	**0.9141**
Fold 2	0.9175	0.9170	0.9173	0.9174	**0.9176**
Fold 3	**0.9268**	0.9256	0.9265	0.9263	**0.9268**
Fold 4	0.9074	**0.9079**	0.9072	0.9075	0.9076
Mean Dice	0.9149	0.9152	0.9150	0.9050	**0.9156**

The results in the Table 3 have shown that applying each of the modifications separately is slightly improving the score over baseline U-Net with deep supervision (0.9149), however if using all modifications together then the score is further improved (0.9156).

Finally, we experimented with a post-processing strategy. It is known from previous BraTS editions that removing small regions with enhanced tumor can be beneficial to the final score. It is so because if there is no enhancing tumor in the label, then the Dice score for zero false positive prediction is 1, and 0 otherwise. The best strategy we found for our 5-fold cross-validation is the following: find ET connected components, for components smaller than 16 voxels

Table 4. Averaged Dice scores of ET, TC, WT classes for each 5-folds without and with post-processing.

Post-processing	Without	With
Fold 0	0.9118	**0.9132**
Fold 1	0.9141	**0.9142**
Fold 2	0.9176	**0.9189**
Fold 3	**0.9268**	0.9268
Fold 4	0.9076	**0.9086**
Mean Dice	0.9156	**0.9163**

with mean probability smaller than 0.9, replace their class to NCR, next if there is overall less than 73 voxels with ET and their mean probability is smaller than 0.9 replace all ET voxels to NCR.

The best model, i.e., deeper U-Net with deep supervision, modified number of channels and additional input one-hot encoding channel for foreground voxels was the winner of the challenge validation phase. The detailed scores are shown in the Table 5.

Table 5. Top 9 normalized statistical ranking scores for BraTS21 validation phase.

1	2	3	4	5	6	7	8	9
0.267	0.272	0.287	0.289	0.298	0.305	0.306	0.312	0.316

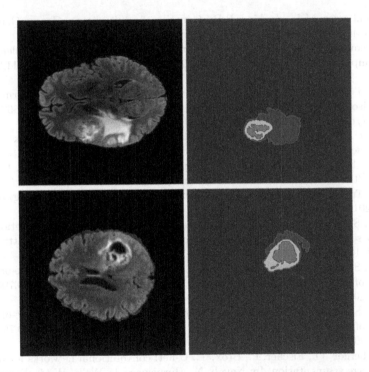

Fig. 7. Predictions on the challenge validation dataset. On the left column FLAIR modality is visualized while on the right model predictions where the meaning of colors is the following: purple - background, blue - NCR, turquoise - ED, yellow - ET. (Color figure online)

# 4	Conclusions

We have experimented with various U-Net variants (basic U-Net [9], UNETR [19], SegResNetVAE [10], Residual U-Net [15], and Attention U-Net [14]), architecture modifications and training schedule tweaks like: deep supervision [20], drop block [21], and Focal loss [26]. Based on our experiments, U-Net with deep supervision yields the best results which can be further improved by adding an additional input channel with one-hot encoding for foreground, increasing encoder depth together with a number of convolutional channels and designing a post-processing strategy.

References

1. Goodenberger, M.L., Jenkins, R.B.: Genetics of adult glioma. Cancer Genet. **205** (2012). https://doi.org/10.1016/j.cancergen.2012.10.009
2. Russakovsky, O., et al.: ImageNet large scale visual recognition challenge. Int. J. Comput. Vision **115**(3), 211–252 (2015). https://doi.org/10.1007/s11263-015-0816-y
3. Zeng, T., Wu, B., Ji, S.: DeepEM3D: approaching human-level performance on 3D anisotropic EM image segmentation. Bioinformatics **33**(16), 2555–2562 (2017). https://doi.org/10.1093/bioinformatics/btx188
4. Baid, U., et al.: The RSNA-ASNR-MICCAI BraTS 2021 benchmark on brain tumor segmentation and radiogenomic classification (2021)
5. Menze, B.H., Jakab, A., Bauer, S., Kalpathy-Cramer, J., Farahani, K., Kirby, J., et al.: The multimodal brain tumor image segmentation benchmark (BRATS). IEEE Trans. Med. Imaging **34**(10), 1993–2024 (2015). https://doi.org/10.1109/TMI.2014.2377694
6. Bakas, S., et al.: Advancing the cancer genome atlas glioma MRI collections with expert segmentation labels and radiomic features. Sci. Data **4** (2017). https://doi.org/10.1038/sdata.2017.117
7. Bakas, S., et al.: Segmentation labels and radiomic features for the pre-operative scans of the TCGA-GBM collection, July 2017. https://doi.org/10.7937/K9/TCIA.2017.KLXWJJ1Q
8. Bakas, S., et al.: Segmentation labels and radiomic features for the pre-operative scans of the TCGA-GBM collection, July 2017. https://doi.org/10.7937/K9/TCIA.2017.GJQ7R0EF
9. Ronneberger, O., Fischer, P., Brox, T.: U-net: convolutional networks for biomedical image segmentation. In: Navab, N., Hornegger, J., Wells, W.M., Frangi, A.F. (eds.) MICCAI 2015. LNCS, vol. 9351, pp. 234–241. Springer, Cham (2015). https://doi.org/10.1007/978-3-319-24574-4_28
10. Myronenko, A.: 3D MRI brain tumor segmentation using autoencoder regularization. In: Crimi, A., Bakas, S., Kuijf, H., Keyvan, F., Reyes, M., van Walsum, T. (eds.) BrainLes 2018. LNCS, vol. 11384, pp. 311–320. Springer, Cham (2019). https://doi.org/10.1007/978-3-030-11726-9_28
11. Jiang, Z., Ding, C., Liu, M., Tao, D.: Two-stage cascaded U-net: 1st place solution to BraTS challenge 2019 segmentation task. In: Crimi, A., Bakas, S. (eds.) BrainLes 2019. LNCS, vol. 11992, pp. 231–241. Springer, Cham (2020). https://doi.org/10.1007/978-3-030-46640-4_22

12. Isensee, F., Jäger, P.F., Kohl, S.A., Petersen, J., Maier-Hein, K.H.: nnU-Net: a self-configuring method for deep learning-based biomedical image segmentation. Nat. Methods 1–9 (2020)
13. Isensee, F., Jäger, P.F., Full, P.M., Vollmuth, P., Maier-Hein, K.H.: nnU-Net for brain tumor segmentation. In: Crimi, A., Bakas, S. (eds.) BrainLes 2020. LNCS, vol. 12659, pp. 118–132. Springer, Cham (2021). https://doi.org/10.1007/978-3-030-72087-2_11
14. Oktay, O., et al.: Attention U-net: learning where to look for the pancreas (2018)
15. He, K., Zhang, X., Ren, S., Sun, J.: Deep residual learning for image recognition (2015)
16. Huang, G., Liu, Z., van der Maaten, L., Weinberger, K.Q.: Densely connected convolutional networks (2016)
17. Szegedy, C., et al.: Deep residual learning for image recognition (2014)
18. Zhou, Z., Rahman Siddiquee, M.M., Tajbakhsh, N., Liang, J.: UNet++: a nested U-net architecture for medical image segmentation. In: Stoyanov, D., et al. (eds.) DLMIA/ML-CDS -2018. LNCS, vol. 11045, pp. 3–11. Springer, Cham (2018). https://doi.org/10.1007/978-3-030-00889-5_1
19. Hatamizadeh, A., Yang, D., Roth, H., Xu, D.: UNETR: transformers for 3D medical image segmentation (2021)
20. Zhu, Q., Du, B., Turkbey, B., Choyke, P.L., Yan, P.: Deeply-supervised CNN for prostate segmentation (2017)
21. Ghiasi, G., Lin, T.Y., Le, Q.V.: DropBlock: a regularization method for convolutional networks (2018)
22. Cox, R., Ashburner, J., et al.: A (sort of) new image data format standard: NiFTI-1, vol. 22, January 2004
23. Kingma, D.P., Welling, M.: Auto-encoding variational Bayes (2014)
24. Dosovitskiy, A., et al.: An image is worth 16x16 words: transformers for image recognition at scale (2021)
25. Vaswani, A., et al.: Attention is all you need (2017)
26. Lin, T.-Y., Goyal, P., Girshick, R., He, K., Dollár, P.: Focal loss for dense object detection. In: International Conference on Computer Vision (ICCV) (2017)
27. Milletari, F., Navab, N., Ahmadi, S.A.: V-Net: fully convolutional neural networks for volumetric medical image segmentation. In: International Conference on 3D Vision (3DV) (2016)
28. Paszke, A., Gross, et al.: Pytorch: an imperative style, high-performance deep learning library. In: Wallach, H., Larochelle, H., Beygelzimer, A., d'Alché-Buc, F., Fox, E., Garnett, R. (eds.) Advances in Neural Information Processing Systems, vol. 32, pp. 8024–8035. Curran Associates, Inc. (2019). http://papers.neurips.cc/paper/9015-pytorch-an-imperative-style-high-performance-deep-learning-library.pdf
29. Micikevicius, P., et al.: Mixed precision training (2018)
30. Kingma, D.P., Ba, J.: Adam: a method for stochastic optimization (2017)
31. Loshchilov, I., Hutter, F.: SGDR: Stochastic gradient descent with warm restarts (2017)
32. He, K., Zhang, X., Ren, S., Sun, J.: Delving deep into rectifiers: surpassing human-level performance on imagenet classification (2015)

MS UNet: Multi-scale 3D UNet for Brain Tumor Segmentation

Parvez Ahmad[1]([✉]) [ID], Saqib Qamar[2], Linlin Shen[3,4], Syed Qasim Afser Rizvi[5], Aamir Ali[6], and Girija Chetty[7] [ID]

[1] School of Computer Science and Technology,
Huazhong University of Science and Technology, Wuhan, China
parvezamu@hust.edu.cn
[2] Department of Computer Applications,
Madanapalle Institute of Technology and Science, Madanapalle, India
[3] AI Research Center for Medical Image Analysis and Diagnosis,
Shenzhen University, Shenzhen, China
[4] Computer Vision Institute, School of Computer Science and Software Engineering,
Shenzhen University, Shenzhen, China
llshen@szu.edu.cn
[5] Guangzhou University, Guangzhou, China
[6] Central University of Punjab, Bathinda, India
[7] School of IT and Systems Faculty of Science and Technology,
University of Canberra, Bruce, Australia
Girija.Chetty@canberra.edu.au

Abstract. A deep convolutional neural network (CNN) achieves remarkable performance for medical image analysis. UNet is the primary source in the performance of 3D CNN architectures for medical imaging tasks, including brain tumor segmentation. The skip connection in the UNet architecture concatenates multi-scale features from image data. The multi-scaled features play an essential role in brain tumor segmentation. Researchers presented numerous multi-scale strategies that have been excellent for the segmentation task. This paper proposes a multi-scale strategy that can further improve the final segmentation accuracy. We propose three multi-scale strategies in MS UNet. Firstly, we utilize densely connected blocks in the encoder and decoder for multi-scale features. Next, the proposed residual-inception blocks extract local and global information by merging features of different kernel sizes. Lastly, we utilize the idea of deep supervision for multiple depths at the decoder. We validate the MS UNet on the BraTS 2021 validation dataset. The dice (DSC) scores of the whole tumor (WT), tumor core (TC), and enhancing tumor (ET) are 91.938%, 86.268%, and 82.409%, respectively.

Keywords: CNN · UNet · Contextual information · Dense connections · Residual inception blocks · Brain tumor segmentation

1   Introduction

A brain tumor is the growth of irregular cells in the central nervous system that can be life-threatening. Primary and secondary are two types of brain tumors. Primary brain tumors originate from brain cells, whereas secondary tumors metastasize into the brain from other organs. Gliomas are primary brain tumors. Gliomas can be subdivided into high-grade glioblastoma (HGG) and low-grade glioblastoma (LGG). In the diagnosis and treatment planning of glioblastomas, brain tumor segmentation results are required to derive quantitative measurements. However, the manual 3D image segmentation is a time-consuming task due to the variations of each patient's shapes, sizes, and locations. Conversely, Convolutional Neural Networks (CNNs) can be applied to MRI images for developing automatic segmentation methods. Deep CNNs have achieved remarkable performances for brain tumor segmentation [9,10,16,20,30]. A $3D$ UNet is a popular CNN architecture for automatic brain tumor segmentation [12,17,27]. The multi-scale contextual information of the encoder-decoder is effective for the accurate brain tumor segmentation task. Researchers have presented variant forms of the $3D$ UNet to extract the enhanced contextual information from MRI [19,21].

Inspired by the multi-scale concepts, we propose MS UNet with three blocks. First, we suggest dense blocks in the encoder-decoder to reduce the number of learnable parameters. We replace the residual learning function [13] with a dense connection [14] in each dense block to provide multi-scale features to its adjacent block. As a result, feature maps with different receptive scales are sent into the blocks. A residual-inception block comprising two parallel dilated convolution layers is proposed in the decoder. As a result, the multi-scale features are available to the dense blocks of the decoder. In addition, a deep supervision concept is presented in the decoder to acquire new semantic features and improve the segmentation maps of multiple tumor sub-types. The key contributions of this study are given below:

- A novel densely connected $3D$ encoder-decoder architecture is proposed to extract context features at each level of the network.
- Residual-inception block (RIB) is used to extract local and global information by merging features of different kernel sizes.
- Deep supervision for faster convergence and better segmentation accuracy is proposed. In the decoder, dense blocks create multiscale segmentation maps. Aggregating these multiscale segmentation maps speeds up processing and improves accuracy.
- Our network achieves state-of-the-art performance as compared to other recent methods.

2   Proposed Method

Figure 1 shows our proposed architecture for brain tumor segmentation. We used dense connections in MS UNet while enhancing the maximum features' size to

32 in the final output layer. Therefore, the number of features is twice compared
to the previous architecture [1]. The output features at the levels of the encoder
are 32, 64, 128, and 256. Inspired by the KiUNet [32], we redesigned strided convolutions in the encoder for high input resolution. MS UNet can be divided into
(i) dense blocks, which are building blocks of the encoder-decoder, (ii) residual-
inception blocks, which are used with the upsampling layers at the decoder, and
(iii) deep supervision approach, which is proposed for faster convergence and
better segmentation accuracy.

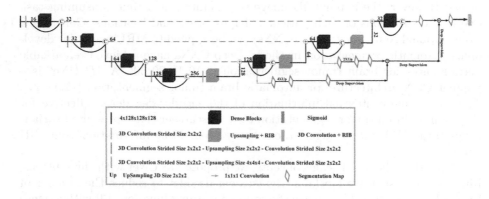

Fig. 1. Proposed MS UNet.

2.1   Dense Blocks

As depicted in Fig. 2, a dense block has three convolution layers, in which feature
maps of all previous layers are concatenated and passed as input to the current
layer. In addition, after the first convolution layer in each dense block, the spatial
dropout layer is employed at a rate of 0.2 to avoid overfitting problems. The
concept of dense connections in a dense block can be summarized as

$$x_{l+1} = g\left(x_l\right) \copyright x_l \tag{1}$$

where x_l denotes the output of a current layer l, $g(.)$ represents a sequence of
Conv-IN-LeakyReLU and $\copyright$ denotes a concatenation operation. Furthermore,
the input feature maps of a lth convolution layer can be summarized as

$$x_{l+1} = X_{-1} + \sum_{j=1}^{l} X_j \tag{2}$$

where X_{-1} is the input feature maps for each layer of a dense block.

A growth-rate 2 (X_j) is used in a dense block to reduce the number of
parameters in each convolution layer. The input layer uses the feature re-usability
property to have more significant features. In this way, dense networks decrease

the number of training parameters and the redundant features of a standard 3D convolution. A $1 \times 1 \times 1$ convolution is also utilized to keep an equal number of input and output channels of a dense block.

The advantages of dense connections in the encoder-decoder are 1) Flow of gradients information easily propagates to all preceding lower layers through short-skip connections. In contrast, the layers without residual and dense connections have an issue of gradients vanishing/exploding. 2) Each dense block offers multi-scale features to its neighbour block. Therefore, feature maps of different receptive scales are input to the blocks. In the proposed architecture, the first dense block has multi-scale inputs resulting from a residual-inception block. 3) Fewer learnable parameters are sufficient for improving the final segmentation scores.

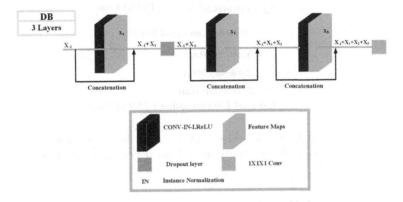

Fig. 2. Overview of the proposed dense block. X_1, X_2, and X_3 denote the feature maps of the convolution layer in terms of growth-rate. Additionally, each convolution layer's input and output channels are subjected to a concatenation operation.

2.2 Residual-Inception Blocks

Figure 3 illustrates a residual-inception block. In this block, we utilize dilation rates 2 and 3 in the top and last parallel layers, respectively. Different dilation rates increase the receptive field sizes of parallel convolution layers by adding zeros between kernel elements without incrementing parameters. As a result, the proposed residual-inception blocks use large receptive field sizes to learn more local and global contexts. In addition, having multiple dilation rates helps to avoid the gridding implications that erupt with equal dilation rates [33]. We concatenate input and output feature maps of each receptive scale. Meanwhile, we aggregate feature maps convolved by two receptive scales, such as $5 \times 5 \times 5$ and $7 \times 7 \times 7$.

In the decoder, we also propose a deep supervision technique [11] on the output feature maps of several dense blocks for faster convergence and superior segmentation accuracy. As a result of deep supervision technique, in addition to the final layer's segmentation map, the MS UNet has two more same-resolution segmentation maps to improve the final segmentation results.

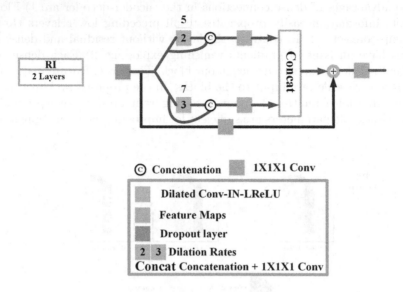

Fig. 3. Proposed residual-inception block. IN refers to instance normalization. The numbers at the top of each dilated convolution layer denote receptive field sizes.

3   Experimental Results

3.1   Dataset

The BraTS aims to bring the research communities together, along with their brilliant ideas for different tasks. Especially for the segmentation task, public benchmark datasets are provided by the organizers. In BraTS challenges, organizers provide various independent datasets for training, validation, and testing. In this paper, we use BraTS 2018, BraTS 2019, BraTS 2020 [4–7,25], and BraTS 2021 datasets [3–6,25] to train and evaluate our proposed work. In addition, we validate our proposed work for FeTS 2021 challenge [4–6,28,29,31]. Details of different BraTS datasets are shown in Table 1. Here, we can further classify some training datasets into high-grade glioblastoma (HGG) and low-grade glioblastoma (LGG). Furthermore, we have access only to the training and validation datasets of BraTS 2018, BraTS 2019, BraTS 2020, and FeTS 2021. Four different types of modalities, i.e., native (T1), post-contrast T1-weighted (T1Gd), T2-weighted (T2), and T2 Fluid Attenuated Inversion Recovery (T2-FLAIR), are related to each patient in the training, validation, and testing datasets. For each training patient, the annotated labels have the values of 1 for the necrosis and non-enhancing tumor (NCR/NET), 2 for peritumoral edema (ED), 4 for enhancing tumor (ET), and 0 for the background. The segmentation accuracy is measured by several metrics, where the predicted labels are evaluated by merging three regions, namely whole tumor (Whole Tumor or Whole: label 1, 2 and 4), tumor core (Tumor Core or Core): label 1 and 4), and enhancing tumor (Enhancing Tumor or Enhancing: label 4). The organizers performed necessary pre-processing steps for simplicity. However, the truth label is not provided for the patients of the validation and testing datasets.

Table 1. Details of BraTS datasets.

Dataset	Type	Patients	HGG	LGG
BraTS 2018	Training	285	210	75
	Validation	66		
BraTS 2019	Training	335	259	76
	Validation	125		
BraTS 2020	Training	369	293	76
	Validation	125		
BraTS 2021	Training	1251	-	-
	Validation	219		
	Testing	530		
FeTS 2021	Training	340	-	-
	Validation	111		

3.2 Implementation Details

Since 19 institutes are involved in data collection, these institutes used multiple scanners and imaging protocols in the acquisition of the brain scans. Thus, normalization would be a necessary step to establish a similar range of intensity for all the patients and their various modalities to avoid the network's initial biases. Here, normalization of entire data may degrade the segmentation accuracy. Therefore, we normalize each MRI of each patient independently. We extract patches of size $128 \times 128 \times 128$ from 4 MRI modalities to feed them into the network. We used five-fold cross-validation, in which each time our network is trained 200 epochs. The batch size is 1. Adam is the optimizer with the initial learning rate 7×10^{-5}, which is dropped by 50% if validation loss not improved within 30 epochs. Moreover, we used augmentation techniques during the training by randomly rotating the images within a range of $[-1°, 1°]$ and random mirror flips (on the x-axis) with a probability of 0.5.

During the designing of our network, we have tuned several hyperparameters, such as the number of layers for the dense and residual-inception blocks, the initial number of channels for training, the growth rate's value, and the number of epochs, etc. Hence, to avoid any further hyperparameter tunning and inspired by a non-weighted loss function's potential, we employed the previously proposed multi-class dice loss function [26]. Thus, the earlier mentioned dice loss function can be easily adapted with our proposed model and summarized as

$$Loss = -\frac{2}{D} \sum_{d \in D} \frac{\sum_j P_{(j,d)} T_{(j,d)}}{\sum_j P_{(j,d)} + \sum_j T_{(j,d)}} \qquad (3)$$

where $P_{(j,d)}$ and $T_{(j,d)}$ are the prediction obtained by softmax activation and ground truth at voxel j for class d, respectively. D is the total number of classes.

3.3   Qualitative Analysis

Figure 4 is shown the segmentation results of our proposed architecture. Figure 4 depicts the $T1ce$ sagittal and coronal slices of four different patients. Figure 4a and c shows the truth labels overlaid on $T1ce$ sagittal and coronal slices, while the overlaying of the segmented labels on $T1ce$ sagittal and coronal slices is shown in Fig. 4b and d, respectively. Our proposed model can accurately segment the truth labels of axial, sagittal, and coronal slices based on the visualized slices.

3.4   Quantitative Analysis

We now evaluate our proposed work. In this paper, our main contribution is to suggest a variant form of 3D UNet, improving context information. Hence, a simple training procedure is performed to check the potential of the proposed model. For deep learning models, cross-validation is a powerful strategy, which helps reduce the variance. Therefore, we perform a five-fold cross-validation procedure on the BraTS training datasets. After training, a single model has been used to evaluate the validation datasets. The scores of unseen validation and testing datasets are shown in Table 2.

Table 3 shows the comparisons between the proposed model and the state-of-the-art methods in the previous MICCAI BraTS validation datasets. Our proposed model has obtained excellent mean dice scores for the whole tumor. In the meantime, our proposed work has secured the competitive enhancing tumor scores than several ensembles works [2, 15, 17–19, 23, 24, 34, 35]. However, our model has obtained lower scores for tumor core than the ensembles works. Overall, our proposed model has secured the best mean dice scores in all tumors than our previous work (Ahmad [1]). This improvement is due to the full utilization of multi-scale context features.

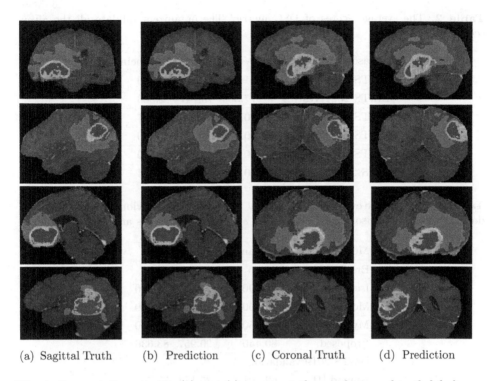

(a) Sagittal Truth   (b) Prediction   (c) Coronal Truth   (d) Prediction

Fig. 4. Segmentation results. (*a*) and (*c*) represent the overlaying of truth labels on $T1ce$ sagittal and coronal slices. Simultaneously, (*b*) and (*d*) shows the segmented labels overlaid on $T1ce$ sagittal and coronal slices. Different colors represent different parts of the tumor: red for TC, green for WT, and yellow for ET. (Color figure online)

We chose several cutting-edge methods, including Isensee [17], Liu [22], and Ben naceur [8]. We begin with a 5-fold cross-validation on the BraTS 2021 training set. Each fold contains 996 cases chosen at random for training and 249 cases selected at random for validation. Following training, we evaluate the BraTS 2021 validation dataset. As shown in Table 4, the results (of MS UNet) are competitive for the DSC metric. Our proposed model's enhancing tumor score is 12.6% higher than Isensee [17]. On the other hand, our proposed model has an 8% lower whole tumor score and an 11.5% lower tumor core score than Isensee [17]. The higher tumor core score in Isensee [17] could be due to an ensembling approach. Furthermore, our proposed method outperforms Liu [22], and Ben naceur [8] for the DSC metric. Furthermore, unlike Isensee [17], and Ben naceur [8], our proposed model results have not been subjected to any post-processing steps.

Table 2. The average scores of DSC metric. The organizers validate all the given scores.

Dataset	Whole	Core	Enhancing
BraTS 2021 Validation	91.938	86.268	82.409
BraTS 2021 Testing	77.309	73.747	72.503
BraTS 2020 Validation	90.242	83.095	77.877
BraTS 2019 Validation	90.469	84.588	78.000
BraTS 2018 Validation	90.957	83.636	80.440
FeTS 2021 Validation	90.516	85.266	76.124

Table 3. Performance evaluation of different methods on the previous BraTS validation datasets. For comparison, only DSC scores are shown. All scores are evaluated online.

Methods	Enhancing	Whole	Core
BraTS 2018 validation			
Isensee [17]	79.590	90.800	84.320
McKinley [23]	79.600	90.300	84.700
Myronenko [27]	81.450	90.420	85.960
Proposed	80.440	90.957	83.636
BraTS 2019 validation			
Ahmad [1]	62.301	85.184	75.762
Zhao [19]	73.700	90.800	82.300
McKinley [24]	75.000	91.000	81.000
Proposed	78.000	90.469	84.588
BraTS 2020 validation			
Ahmad [2]]	75.635	90.678	84.248
Isensee [15]	79.450	91.190	85.240
Jia [18]	78.492	91.261	84.428
Wang [34]	78.700	90.800	85.600
Yuan [35]	79.270	91.080	85.290
Proposed	77.877	90.242	83.095

Table 4. Performance evaluation of state-of-the-art methods on the BraTS 2021 validation dataset. For comparison, only DSC scores are shown. All scores are evaluated online.

Methods	Enhancing	Whole	Core
Isensee [17]	81.149	92.751	87.415
Liu [22]	81.628	91.047	84.300
Ben naceur [8]	81.637	91.511	85.921
Proposed	82.409	91.938	86.268

4   Discussion and Conclusion

This paper proposes MS UNet for brain tumor segmentation. To reduce the training parameters and efficient gradient flow, we implemented densely connected blocks in the proposed MS UNet. Meanwhile, dense connections used the feature-reusability property for multi-scaled features. The MS UNet also used residual-inception blocks to learn multi-scale contexts. For multi-scale contexts, in the decoder, we proposed the residual-inception blocks. Additionally, we employed a deep supervision approach for faster convergence and superior segmentation accuracy. Simultaneously, the deep supervision approach enhances segmentation accuracy by combining various depths' segmentation maps. The proposed MS UNet achieved considerable segmentation scores on various brain MRI datasets. In the future, we would like to combine MS UNet with deep reinforcement learning approaches as the current MS UNet has consumed a significant amount of time in hyper-parameters tunning that is usually done using grid search.

Acknowledgment. This work is supported by the National Natural Science Foundation of China under Grant No. 91959108.

References

1. Ahmad, P., Qamar, S., Hashemi, S.R., Shen, L.: Hybrid labels for brain tumor segmentation. In: Crimi, A., Bakas, S. (eds.) BrainLes 2019. LNCS, vol. 11993, pp. 158–166. Springer, Cham (2020). https://doi.org/10.1007/978-3-030-46643-5_15
2. Ahmad, P., Qamar, S., Shen, L., Saeed, A.: Context aware 3d unet for brain tumor segmentation. CoRR abs/2010.13082 (2020), https://arxiv.org/abs/2010.13082
3. Baid, U., et al.: The RSNA-ASNR-MICCAI brats 2021 benchmark on brain tumor segmentation and radiogenomic classification. CoRR abs/2107.02314 (2021). https://arxiv.org/abs/2107.02314
4. Bakas, S., et al.: Segmentation labels and radiomic features for the pre-operative scans of the TCGA-GBM collection. Cancer Imaging Arch. **2017** (2017)
5. Bakas, S., et al.: Segmentation labels and radiomic features for the pre-operative scans of the TCGA-LGG collection. Cancer Imaging Arch. **286** (2017)
6. Bakas, S., et al.: Advancing the cancer genome atlas glioma MRI collections with expert segmentation labels and radiomic features. Sci. Data **4**, 170117 (2017). https://doi.org/10.1038/sdata.2017.117
7. Bakas, S., et al.: Identifying the best machine learning algorithms for brain tumor segmentation, progression assessment, and overall survival prediction in the BRATS challenge. CoRR abs/1811.0 (2018). http://arxiv.org/abs/1811.02629
8. Ben Naceur, M., Akil, M., Saouli, R., Kachouri, R.: Fully automatic brain tumor segmentation with deep learning-based selective attention using overlapping patches and multi-class weighted cross-entropy. Med. Image Anal. **63**, 101692 (2020). https://doi.org/10.1016/j.media.2020.101692, https://www.sciencedirect.com/science/article/pii/S1361841520300578
9. Chen, L., Bentley, P., Mori, K., Misawa, K., Fujiwara, M., Rueckert, D.: DRINet for medical image segmentation. IEEE Trans. Med. Imaging **37**(11), 2453–2462 (2018). https://doi.org/10.1109/TMI.2018.2835303

10. Dolz, J., Gopinath, K., Yuan, J., Lombaert, H., Desrosiers, C., Ayed, I.B.: HyperDense-Net: a hyper-densely connected CNN for multi-modal image segmentation. CoRR abs/1804.0 (2018). http://arxiv.org/abs/1804.02967

11. Dou, Q., Chen, H., Jin, Y., Yu, L., Qin, J., Heng, P.: 3D deeply supervised network for automatic liver segmentation from CT volumes. CoRR abs/1607.00582 (2016). http://arxiv.org/abs/1607.00582

12. Feng, X., Tustison, N., Meyer, C.: Brain tumor segmentation using an ensemble of 3D U-nets and overall survival prediction using radiomic features. In: Crimi, A., Bakas, S., Kuijf, H., Keyvan, F., Reyes, M., van Walsum, T. (eds.) BrainLes 2018. LNCS, vol. 11384, pp. 279–288. Springer, Cham (2019). https://doi.org/10.1007/978-3-030-11726-9_25

13. He, K., Zhang, X., Ren, S., Sun, J.: Deep residual learning for image recognition. CoRR abs/1512.0 (2015). http://arxiv.org/abs/1512.03385

14. Huang, G., Liu, Z., Weinberger, K.Q.: Densely connected convolutional networks. CoRR abs/1608.0 (2016). http://arxiv.org/abs/1608.06993

15. Isensee, F., Jaeger, P.F., Full, P.M., Vollmuth, P., Maier-Hein, K.H.: nnu-Net for brain tumor segmentation. CoRR abs/2011.00848 (2020). https://arxiv.org/abs/2011.00848

16. Isensee, F., Kickingereder, P., Wick, W., Bendszus, M., Maier-Hein, K.H.: Brain tumor segmentation and radiomics survival prediction: contribution to the BRATS 2017 challenge. CoRR abs/1802.1 (2018). http://arxiv.org/abs/1802.10508

17. Isensee, F., Kickingereder, P., Wick, W., Bendszus, M., Maier-Hein, K.H.: No new-net. In: Crimi, A., Bakas, S., Kuijf, H., Keyvan, F., Reyes, M., van Walsum, T. (eds.) BrainLes 2018. LNCS, vol. 11384, pp. 234–244. Springer, Cham (2019). https://doi.org/10.1007/978-3-030-11726-9_21

18. Jia, H., Cai, W., Huang, H., Xia, Y.: H2NF-net for brain tumor segmentation using multimodal MR imaging: 2nd place solution to brats challenge 2020 segmentation task. CoRR abs/2012.15318 (2020). https://arxiv.org/abs/2012.15318

19. Jiang, Z., Ding, C., Liu, M., Tao, D.: Two-stage cascaded U-net: 1st place solution to BraTS challenge 2019 segmentation task. In: Crimi, A., Bakas, S. (eds.) BrainLes 2019. LNCS, vol. 11992, pp. 231–241. Springer, Cham (2020). https://doi.org/10.1007/978-3-030-46640-4_22

20. Kamnitsas, K., et al.: Ensembles of multiple models and architectures for robust brain tumour segmentation. CoRR abs/1711.0 (2017). http://arxiv.org/abs/1711.01468

21. Kamnitsas, K., et al.: Efficient multi-scale 3D CNN with fully connected CRF for accurate brain lesion segmentation. Med. Image Anal. 36, 61–78 (2017)

22. Liu, Z., et al.: CANet: context aware network for brain glioma segmentation. IEEE Trans. Med. Imaging 40(7), 1763–1777 (2021). https://doi.org/10.1109/TMI.2021.3065918

23. McKinley, R., Meier, R., Wiest, R.: Ensembles of densely-connected CNNs with label-uncertainty for brain tumor segmentation. In: Crimi, A., Bakas, S., Kuijf, H., Keyvan, F., Reyes, M., van Walsum, T. (eds.) BrainLes 2018. LNCS, vol. 11384, pp. 456–465. Springer, Cham (2019). https://doi.org/10.1007/978-3-030-11726-9_40

24. McKinley, R., Rebsamen, M., Meier, R., Wiest, R.: Triplanar ensemble of 3D-to-2D CNNs with label-uncertainty for brain tumor segmentation. In: Crimi, A., Bakas, S. (eds.) BrainLes 2019. LNCS, vol. 11992, pp. 379–387. Springer, Cham (2020). https://doi.org/10.1007/978-3-030-46640-4_36

25. Menze, B.H., et al.: The multimodal brain tumor image segmentation benchmark (BRATS). IEEE Trans. Med. Imaging 34(10), 1993–2024 (2015). https://doi.org/10.1109/TMI.2014.2377694

26. Milletari, F., Navab, N., Ahmadi, S.A.: V-net: fully convolutional neural networks for volumetric medical image segmentation. CoRR abs/1606.0 (2016). http://arxiv.org/abs/1606.04797

27. Myronenko, A.: 3D MRI brain tumor segmentation using autoencoder regularization. CoRR abs/1810.1 (2018). http://arxiv.org/abs/1810.11654

28. Pati, S., et al.: The federated tumor segmentation (FETS) challenge. CoRR abs/2105.05874 (2021). https://arxiv.org/abs/2105.05874

29. Reina, G.A., et al.: OpenFL: an open-source framework for federated learning. CoRR abs/2105.06413 (2021). https://arxiv.org/abs/2105.06413

30. Ronneberger, O., Fischer, P., Brox, T.: U-net: convolutional networks for biomedical image segmentation. CoRR abs/1505.0 (2015). http://arxiv.org/abs/1505.04597

31. Sheller, M.J., et al.: Federated learning in medicine: facilitating multi-institutional collaborations without sharing patient data. Sci. Rep. **10**(1), 12598 (2020). https://doi.org/10.1038/s41598-020-69250-1

32. Valanarasu, J.M.J., Sindagi, V.A., Hacihaliloglu, I., Patel, V.M.: KiU-net: overcomplete convolutional architectures for biomedical image and volumetric segmentation. IEEE Trans. Med. Imaging 1 (2021). https://doi.org/10.1109/TMI.2021.3130469

33. Wang, P., et al.: Understanding convolution for semantic segmentation. CoRR abs/1702.08502 (2017). http://arxiv.org/abs/1702.08502

34. Wang, Y., et al.: Modality-pairing learning for brain tumor segmentation. CoRR abs/2010.09277 (2020). https://arxiv.org/abs/2010.09277

35. Yuan, Y.: Automatic brain tumor segmentation with scale attention network. CoRR abs/2011.03188 (2020). https://arxiv.org/abs/2011.03188

Evaluating Scale Attention Network for Automatic Brain Tumor Segmentation with Large Multi-parametric MRI Database

Yading Yuan[✉]

Department of Radiation Oncology,
Icahn School of Medicine at Mount Sinai, New York, NY, USA
yading.yuan@mssm.edu

Abstract. Automatic segmentation of brain tumors is an essential but challenging step for extracting quantitative imaging biomarkers for accurate tumor detection, diagnosis, prognosis, treatment planning and assessment. This is the 10th year of Brain Tumor Segmentation (BraTS) Challenge that utilizes multi-institutional multi-parametric magnetic resonance imaging (mpMRI) scans for tasks: 1) evaluation the state-of-the-art methods for the segmentation of intrinsically heterogeneous brain glioblastoma sub-regions in mpMRI scans; and 2) the evaluation of classification methods to predict the MGMT promoter methylation status at pre-operative baseline scans. We participated the image segmentation task by applying a fully automated segmentation framework that we previously developed in BraTS 2020. This framework, named as scale-attention network, incorporates a dynamic scale attention mechanism to integrate low-level details with high-level feature maps at different scales. Our framework was trained using the 1251 challenge training cases provided by BraTS 2021, and achieved an average Dice Similarity Coefficient (DSC) of 0.9277, 0.8851 and 0.8754, as well as 95% Hausdorff distance (in millimeter) of 4.2242, 15.3981 and 11.6925 on 570 testing cases for whole tumor, tumor core and enhanced tumor, respectively, which ranked itself as the second place in the brain tumor segmentation task of RSNA-ASNR-MICCAI BraTS 2021 Challenge (id: deepX).

1 Introduction

Glioblastoma, and diffuse astrocytic glioma with molecular features of glioblastoma (WHO grade 4 astrocytoma), are the most common and aggressive primary tumor of the central nervous system in adults, with extreme intrinsic heterogeneity in appearance, shape and histology. Glioblastoma patients have very poor prognosis, and the current standard of care treatment includes neurosurgery followed by radiotherapy and chemotherapy. Quantitative assessment of multi-parametric Magnetic Resonance Imaging (mpMRI) plays an essential step of tumor detection, diagnosis, prognosis, treatment planning and outcome

A. Crimi and S. Bakas (Eds.): BrainLes 2021, LNCS 12963, pp. 42–53, 2022.
https://doi.org/10.1007/978-3-031-09002-8_4

evaluation [1]. However, proper interpretation of mpMRI images is a challenging task not only because of the large amount of three-dimensional (3D) or four-dimensional (4D) image data generated from mpMRI sequences that characterize different tissue properties and tumor spreads, but also because of the intrinsic heterogeneity of brain tumor. While manual delineation of brain tumor is still irreplaceable in brain MRI image analysis, it is time-consuming and suffers from inter- and intra-operator variations, therefore, automatic segmentation of brain tumor and its sub-regions has been of great demand to assist clinicians in quantitative image analysis for better interpretation of mpMRI images of brain tumor.

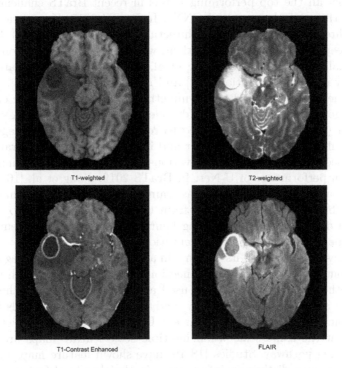

Fig. 1. An example of MRI modalities used in BraTS 2021 challenge

The brain tumor segmentation challenge (BraTS) [2–6] aims to accelerate the research and development of reliable methods for automatic brain tumor segmentation by providing a large 3D mpMRI dataset with ground truth annotated by multiple physicians. This year, BraTS 2021 provides 1251 cases for model training, 219 cases for model validation and 570 cases for the final testing. The MRI scans were collected from different institutions and acquired with different protocols, magnetic field strengths and manufacturers. For each patient, a native T1-weighted, a post-contrast T1-weighted, a T2-weighted and a T2 Fluid-Attenuated Inversion Recovery (FLAIR) were provided, as an example shown in Fig. 1. These images were rigidly registered, skull-stripped and resampled to

$1 \times 1 \times 1$ mm isotropic resolution with image size of $240 \times 240 \times 155$. Three tumor subregions, including the enhancing tumor, the peritumoral edema and the necrotic and other non-enhancing tumor core, were manually annotated by one to four raters following the same annotation protocol and finally approved by experienced neuro-radiologists.

2   Related Work

With the success of convolutional neural networks (CNNs) in biomedical image segmentation, all the top performing teams in recent BraTS challenges exclusively built their solutions around CNNs. In BraTS 2017, Kamnitsas et al. [7] combined three different network architectures, namely 3D FCN [8], 3D U-Net [10], and DeepMedic [9] and trained them with different loss functions and different normalization strategies. Wang et al. [11] employed a FCN architecture enhanced by dilated convolutions [12] and residual connections [13]. In BraTS 2018, Myronenko [14] utilized an asymmetrical U-Net with a large encoder to extract image features, and a smaller decoder to recover the label. A variational autoencoder (VAE) branch was added to reconstruct the input image itself in order to regularize the shared encoder and impose additional constraints on its layers. Isensee et al. [15] introduced various training strategies to improve the segmentation performance of U-Net. In BraTS 2019, Jiang et al. [16] proposed a two-stage cascaded U-Net, which was trained in an end-to-end fashion, to segment the subregions of brain tumor from coarse to fine, and Zhao et al. [17] investigated different kinds of training heuristics and combined them to boost the overall performance of their segmentation model.

The success of U-Net and its variants in automatic brain tumor segmentation is largely contributed to the skip connection design that allows high resolution features in the encoding pathway be used as additional inputs to the convolutional layers in the decoding pathway, and thus recovers fine details for image segmentation. While intuitive, the current U-Net architecture restricts the feature fusion at the same scale when multiple scale feature maps are available in the encoding pathway. Studies [18,19] have shown feature maps in different scales usually carry distinctive information in that low-level features represent detailed spatial information while high-level features capture semantic information such as target position, therefore, the full-scale information may not be fully employed with the scale-wise feature fusion in the current U-Net architecture.

To make full use of the multi-scale information, we propose a novel encoder-decoder network architecture named scale attention network (SA-Net) [27], where we re-design the inter-connections between the encoding and decoding pathways by replacing the scale-wise skip connections in U-Net with full-scale skip connections. This allows SA-Net to incorporate low-level fine details with the high-level semantic information into a unified framework. In order to highlight the important scales, we introduce the attention mechanism [20,21] into SA-Net such that when the model learns, the weight on each scale for each feature channel will be adaptively tuned to emphasize the important scales while suppressing the less important ones. Figure 2 shows the overall architecture of SA-Net.

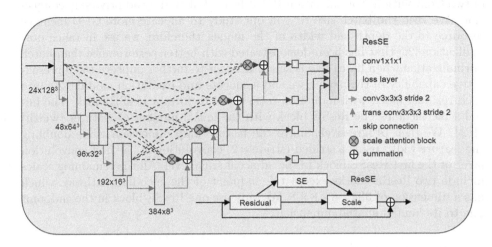

Fig. 2. Architecture of SA-Net. Input is a 4 × 128 × 128 × 128 tensor followed by one ResSE block with 24 features. Here ResSE stands for a squeeze-and-excitation block embedded in a residual module [20]. By progressively halving the feature map dimension while doubling the feature width at each scale, the endpoint of the encoding pathway has a dimension of 384 × 8 × 8 × 8. The output of the decoding pathway has three channels with the same spatial size as the input, i.e., 3 × 128 × 128 × 128.

3   Methods

3.1   Overall Network Structure

SA-Net follows a typical encoding-decoding architecture with an asymmetrically larger encoding pathway to learn representative features and a smaller decoding pathway to recover the segmentation mask in the original resolution. The outputs of encoding blocks at different scales are merged to the scale attention blocks (SA-block) to learn and select features with full-scale information. Due to the limit of GPU memory, we randomly crop the input image from 240 × 240 × 155 to 128 × 128 × 128, and concatenate the four MRI modalities of each patient into a four channel tensor to yield an input to SA-Net with the dimension of 4 × 128 × 128 × 128. The network output includes three channels, each of which presents the probability that the corresponding voxel belongs to WT, TC, and ET, respectively.

3.2   Encoding Pathway

The encoding pathway is built upon ResNet [13] blocks, where each block consists of two Convolution-Normalization-ReLU layers followed by additive skip connection. We keep the batch size to 1 in our study to allocate more GPU memory resource to the depth and width of the model, therefore, we use instance normalization [26] that has been demonstrated with better performance than batch normalization when batch size is small. In order to further improve the representative capability of the model, we add a squeeze-and-excitation module [20] into each residual block with reduction ratio $r = 4$ to form a ResSE block. The initial scale includes one ResSE block with the initial number of features (width) of 24. We then progressively halve the feature map dimension while doubling the feature width using a strided (stride $= 2$) convolution at the first convolution layer of the first ResSE block in the adjacent scale level. All the remaining scales include two ResSE blocks except the endpoint of the encoding pathway, which has a dimension of $384 \times 8 \times 8 \times 8$. We only use one ResSE block in the endpoint due to its limited spatial dimension.

3.3   Decoding Pathway

The decoding pathway follows the reverse pattern as the encoding one, but with a single ResSE block in each spatial scale. At the beginning of each scale, we use a transpose convolution with stride of 2 to double the feature map dimension and reduce the feature width by 2. The upsampled feature maps are then added to the output of SA-block. Here we use summation instead of concatenation for information fusion between the encoding and decoding pathways to reduce GPU memory consumption and facilitate the information flowing. The endpoint of the decoding pathway has the same spatial dimension as the original input tensor and its feature width is reduced to 3 after a $1 \times 1 \times 1$ convolution and a sigmoid function.

In order to regularize the model training and enforce the low- and middle-level blocks to learn discriminative features, we introduce deep supervision at each intermediate scale level of the decoding pathway. Each deep supervision subnet employs a $1 \times 1 \times 1$ convolution for feature width reduction, followed by a trilinear upsampling layer such that they have the same spatial dimension as the output, then applies a sigmoid function to obtain extra dense predictions. These deep supervision subnets are directly connected to the loss function in order to further improve gradient flow propagation.

3.4   Scale Attention Block

The proposed scale attention block consists of full-scale skip connections from the encoding pathway to the decoding pathway, where each decoding layer incorporates the output feature maps from all the encoding layers to capture fine-grained details and coarse-grained semantics simultaneously in full scales. As an example illustrated in Fig. 3, the first stage of the SA-block is to transform the input feature maps at different scales in the encoding pathway, represented as $\{S_e, e = 1, ..., N\}$ where N is the number of total scales in the encoding pathway except the last block ($N = 4$ in this work), to a same dimension, i.e., $\bar{S}_{ed} = f_{ed}(S_e)$. Here e and d are the scale level at the encoding and decoding pathways, respectively. The transform function $f_{ed}(S_e)$ is determined as follows. If $e < d$, $f_{ed}(S_e)$ downsamples S_e by $2^{(d-e)}$ times by maxpooling followed by a Conv-Norm-ReLU block; if $e = d$, $f_{ed}(S_e) = S_e$; and if $e > d$, $f_{ed}(S_e)$ upsamples S_e through tri-linear upsampling after a Conv-Norm-ReLU block for channel number adjustment. After summing these transformed feature maps as $P_d = \sum_e \bar{S}_{ed}$, a spatial pooling is used to average each feature to form a information embedding tensor $G_d \in R^{C_d}$, where C_d is the number of feature channels in scale d. Then a $1 - to - N$ Squeeze-Excitation is performed in which the global feature embedding G_d is squeezed to a compact feature $g_d \in R^{C_d/r}$ by passing through a fully connected layer with a reduction ratio of r, then another N fully connected layers with sigmoid function are applied for each scale excitation to recalibrate the feature channels on that scale. Finally, the contribution of each scale in each feature channel is normalized with a softmax function, yielding a scale-specific weight vector for each channel as $w_e \in R^{C_d}$, and the final output of the scale attention block is $\widetilde{S}_d = \sum_e w_e \cdot \bar{S}_{ed}$.

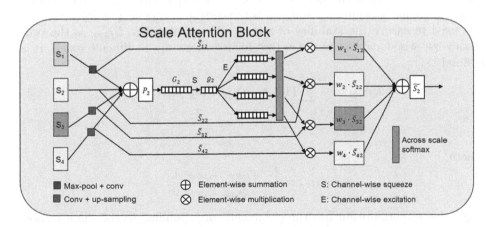

Fig. 3. Scale attention block. Here $S1, S2, S3$ and $S4$ represent the input feature maps at different scales from the encoding pathway. $d = 2$ in this example.

3.5   Implementation

Our framework was implemented with Python using Pytorch package. As for pre-processing, since MRI images are non-standarized, we simply normalized each modality from each patient independently by subtracting the mean and dividing by the standard deviation of the entire image. The model was trained with randomly sampled patches of size $128 \times 128 \times 128$ voxels and batch size of 1. Training the entire network took 300 epochs from scratch using Adam stochastic optimization method. The initial learning rate was set as 0.003, and learning rate decay and early stopping strategies were utilized when validation loss stopped decreasing. In particular, we kept monitoring both the validation loss ($L^{(valid)}$) and the exponential moving average of the validation loss ($\widetilde{L}^{(valid)}$) in each epoch. We kept the learning rate unchanged at the first 150 epochs, but dropped the learning rate by a factor of 0.3 when neither $L^{(valid)}$ nor $\widetilde{L}^{(valid)}$ improved within the last 30 epochs. The models that yielded the best $L^{(valid)}$ and $\widetilde{L}^{(valid)}$ were recorded for model inference.

Our loss function used for model training includes two terms:

$$L = L_{jaccard} + L_{focal} \tag{1}$$

$L_{jaccard}$ is a generalized Jaccard distance loss [22–25], which we developed in our previous work for single object segmentation, to multiple objects. It is defined as:

$$L_{jaccard} = 1 - \frac{\sum\limits_{i,j,k} (t_{ijk} \cdot p_{ijk}) + \epsilon}{\sum\limits_{i,j,k} (t_{ijk}^2 + p_{ijk}^2 - t_{ijk} \cdot p_{ijk}) + \epsilon}, \tag{2}$$

where $t_{ijk} \in \{0, 1\}$ is the actual class of a voxel x_{ijk} with $t_{ijk} = 1$ for tumor and $t_{ijk} = 0$ for background, and p_{ijk} is the corresponding output from SA-Net. ϵ is used to ensure the stability of numerical computations. L_{focal} is the two-class voxel-wise focal loss function that focuses more on the difficult voxels. It is defined as:

$$L_{focal} = - \sum\limits_{i,j,k} (1 - p_{ijk}(t_{ijk}))^2 log(p_{ijk}(t_{ijk})), \tag{3}$$

where

$$p_{ijk}(t_{ijk}) = \begin{cases} p_{ijk}, & t_{ijk} = 1 \\ 1 - p_{ijk}, & t_{ijk} = 0 \end{cases}. \tag{4}$$

Since the network output has three channels corresponding to the whole tumor, tumor core and enhanced tumor, respectively, we used the weighed sum of the three loss functions corresponding to each channel as the final loss function for model training.

In order to reduce overfitting, we randomly flipped the input volume in left/right, superior/inferior, and anterior/posterior directions on the fly with a probability of 0.5 for data augmentation. We also adjusted the contrast in each image input channel by a factor randomly selected from [0.9, 1.1]. We used 5-fold cross validation to evaluate the performance of our model on the training dataset, in which a few hyper-parameters were also experimentally determined. All the experiments were conducted on Nvidia GTX 1080 TI GPU with 11 GB memory.

During inference, we applied the sliding window around the brain region and extracted 8 patches with a size $128 \times 128 \times 128$ (2 windows in each dimension), and averaged the model outputs in the overlapping regions before applying a threshold of 0.5 to obtain a binary mask of each tumor region.

4   Results

We trained SA-Net with the training set (1251 cases) provided by the BraTS 2021 challenge, and evaluated its performance on the same set via 5-fold cross validation, as well as on the validation set, which includes 219 cases with unknown segmentation. Figure 4 shows an example of segmentation results. Table 1 shows the segmentation results in terms of Dice similarity coefficient (DSC) for each region. For comparison, we also listed the results we obtained from BraTS 2020 challenge. It is clear to see that the segmentation performance can be significantly improved with larger dataset.

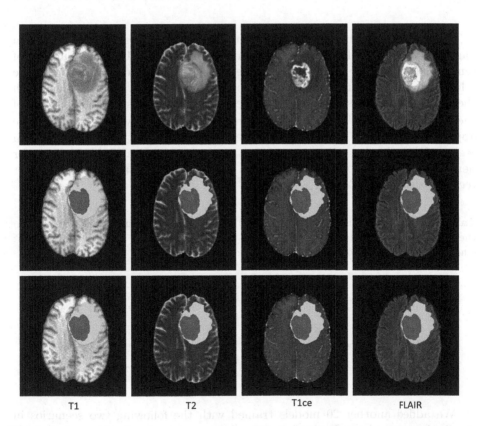

| T1 | T2 | T1ce | FLAIR |

Fig. 4. An example of auto segmentation on different MRI sequences. The second and third row show the ground truth and the segmentation results, respectively. The labels include edema (yellow), necrotic and non-enhancing tumor (blue), and enhanced tumor (green). (Best view with color figure online)

Table 1. Comparison between BraTS 2020 and BraTS 2021 segmentation results (DSC) in 5-fold cross validation using training image sets in each challenge. WT: whole tumor; TC: tumor core; ET: enhanced tumor.

		fold-0	fold-1	fold-2	fold-3	fold-4	ALL
BraTS 2020 (369 cases)	WT	0.9218	0.9003	0.9104	0.9021	0.9113	0.9092
	TC	0.8842	0.8735	0.8772	0.8307	0.8700	0.8671
	ET	0.7982	0.7672	0.7922	0.7955	0.8007	0.7908
	AVG	0.8680	0.8470	0.8599	0.8428	0.8607	0.8557
BraTS 2021 (1251 cases)	WT	0.9413	0.9336	0.9346	0.9376	0.9389	**0.9372**
	TC	0.9265	0.9116	0.9164	0.9164	0.9296	**0.9211**
	ET	0.8910	0.8895	0.8831	0.8831	0.8830	**0.8843**
	AVG	0.9116	0.9116	0.9114	0.9114	0.9172	**0.9142**

When applying the trained models on the challenge validation dataset, a bagging-type ensemble strategy was implemented to combine the outputs of ten models to further improve the segmentation performance. In particular, we selected two models from each fold during the 5-fold cross validation - one with the best validation loss ($L^{(valid)}$) and the other with the best moving average of the validation loss ($\widetilde{L}^{(valid)}$). The outputs of these models were averaged before applying a threshold of 0.5 to generate binary segmentation masks for each region. We uploaded our segmentation results to the BraTS 2021 server for performance evaluation in terms of DSC and Hausdorff distance for each tumor region, as shown in Table 2.

Table 2. Comparison between BraTS 2020 and BraTS 2021 segmentation results on the validation sets in terms of Mean DSC and 95% Hausdorff distance (mm). WT: whole tumor; TC: tumor core; ET: enhanced tumor.

		DSC			HD95		
		WT	TC	ET	WT	TC	ET
BraTS 2020 (125 cases)	The best single model	0.9044	0.8422	0.7853	5.4912	8.3442	20.3507
	Ensemble of 10 models	0.9108	0.8529	0.7927	4.0975	5.8879	18.1957
BraTS 2021 (219 cases)	The best single model	0.9234	0.8838	0.8342	4.1176	4.4067	16.3184
	Ensemble of 10 models	**0.9265**	**0.8655**	**0.8479**	**3.6747**	**11.1890**	**12.7501**

We added another 20 models trained with the following two scenarios in the final testing phase. In the first scenario, we assigned different random seeds to different folds to allow a more dynamic model initialization. In the second scenario, we reshuffled the training set and evenly distributed those cases without enhanced tumor to the new five folds. It took two minutes to segment one case with the SA-Net ensemble in our experimental environment using a single NVidia GTX 1080 TI GPU. Table 3 summarizes the results of SA-Net on the testing dataset, which ranked our method as the second place in the BraTS 2021 challenge.

Table 3. Segmentation results of SA-Net on the BraTS 2021 testing set in terms of Mean DSC and 95% Hausdorff distance (mm). WT: whole tumor; TC: tumor core; ET: enhanced tumor.

	DSC			HD95		
	WT	TC	ET	WT	TC	ET
Mean	0.9277	0.8851	0.8754	4.2242	15.3981	11.6925
StdDev	0.0945	0.2320	0.1910	7.6970	65.1213	57.7321
Median	0.9575	0.9655	0.9414	1.7321	1.4142	1.0000
25quantile	0.9148	0.9184	0.8582	1.0000	1.0000	1.0000
75quantile	0.9764	0.9834	0.9698	4.1231	2.9571	2.0000

5   Summary

In this work, we further evaluated SA-Net, a fully automated segmentation model, on a larger dataset for the task of brain tumor segmentation from multi-modality 3D MRI images. Our SA-Net replaces the long-range skip connections between the same scale in the vanilla U-Net with full-scale skip connections in order to make maximum use of feature maps in full scales for accurate segmentation. Attention mechanism is introduced to adaptively adjust the weights of each scale feature to emphasize the important scales while suppressing the less important ones. As compared to the vanilla U-Net structure with scale-wise skip connection and feature concatenation, the proposed scale attention block not only improved the segmentation performance by 1.47%, but also reduced the number of trainable parameters from 17.8M (U-Net) to 16.5M (SA-Net) [27]. Our results demonstrate the importance of collecting more training data in improving segmentation for automated image segmentation models. On the BraTS 2021 online evaluation with 570 testing cases, our model achieved an average DSC of 0.9277, 0.8851 and 0.8754 for whole tumor, tumor core and enhanced tumor, respectively, which ranked itself as the second place in the brain tumor segmentation task of RSNA-ASNR-MICCAI BraTS 2021 Challenge.

Acknowledgment. This work is supported by a research grant from Varian Medical Systems (Palo Alto, CA, USA), UL1TR001433 from the National Center for Advancing Translational Sciences, and R21EB030209 from the National Institute of Biomedical Imaging and Bioengineering, National Institutes of Health, USA. The content is solely the responsibility of the authors and does not necessarily represent the official views of the National Institutes of Health.

References

1. Kotrotsou, A., et al.: Radiomics in brain tumors: an emerging technique for characterization of tumor environment. Magn. Reson. Imaging Clin. N. Am. **24**, 719–729 (2016)
2. Menze, B.H., et al.: The multimodal brain tumor image segmentation benchmark (BRATS). IEEE Trans. Med. Imaging **34**(10), 1993–2024 (2015)
3. Bakas, S., et al.: Advancing the cancer genome atlas glioma MRI collections with expert segmentation labels and radiomic features. Nat. Sci. Data **4**, 170117 (2017)
4. Baid, U., et al.: The RSNA-ASNR-MICCAI BraTS 2021 benchmark on brain tumor segmentation and radiogenomic classification. arXiv preprint arXiv:2107.02314 (2021)
5. Bakas, S., et al.: Segmentation labels and radiomic features for the pre-operative scans of the TCGA-GBM collection. Cancer Imaging Arch. (2017)
6. Bakas, S., et al.: Segmentation labels and radiomic features for the pre-operative scans of the TCGA-LGG collection. Cancer Imaging Arch. (2017)
7. Kamnitsas, K., et al.: Ensembles of multiple models and architectures for robust brain tumour segmentation. In: Crimi, A., Bakas, S., Kuijf, H., Menze, B., Reyes, M. (eds.) BrainLes 2017. LNCS, vol. 10670, pp. 450–462. Springer, Cham (2018). https://doi.org/10.1007/978-3-319-75238-9_38
8. Long, J., et al.: Fully convolutional networks for semantic segmentation. In: CVPR, pp. 3431–3440 (2015)
9. Kamnitsas, K., et al.: Efficient multi-scale 3D CNN with fully connected CRF for accurate brain lesion segmentation. Med. Image Anal. **36**, 61–78 (2017)
10. Ronneberger, O., Fischer, P., Brox, T.: U-net: convolutional networks for biomedical image segmentation. In: Navab, N., Hornegger, J., Wells, W.M., Frangi, A.F. (eds.) MICCAI 2015. LNCS, vol. 9351, pp. 234–241. Springer, Cham (2015). https://doi.org/10.1007/978-3-319-24574-4_28
11. Wang, G., Li, W., Ourselin, S., Vercauteren, T.: Automatic brain tumor segmentation using cascaded anisotropic convolutional neural networks. In: Crimi, A., Bakas, S., Kuijf, H., Menze, B., Reyes, M. (eds.) BrainLes 2017. LNCS, vol. 10670, pp. 178–190. Springer, Cham (2018). https://doi.org/10.1007/978-3-319-75238-9_16
12. Chen, L.-C., et al.: DeepLab: semantic image segmentation with deep convolutional nets, atrous convolution, and fully connected CRFs. IEEE Trans. Pattern Anal. Mach. Intell. **40**(4), 834–848 (2018)
13. He, K., et al.: Deep residual learning for image recognition. In: Proceedings of CVPR 2016, pp. 770–778 (2016)
14. Myronenko, A.: 3D MRI brain tumor segmentation using autoencoder regularization. In: Crimi, A., Bakas, S., Kuijf, H., Keyvan, F., Reyes, M., van Walsum, T. (eds.) BrainLes 2018. LNCS, vol. 11384, pp. 311–320. Springer, Cham (2019). https://doi.org/10.1007/978-3-030-11726-9_28
15. Isensee, F., Kickingereder, P., Wick, W., Bendszus, M., Maier-Hein, K.H.: No new-net. In: Crimi, A., Bakas, S., Kuijf, H., Keyvan, F., Reyes, M., van Walsum, T. (eds.) BrainLes 2018. LNCS, vol. 11384, pp. 234–244. Springer, Cham (2019). https://doi.org/10.1007/978-3-030-11726-9_21
16. Jiang, Z., Ding, C., Liu, M., Tao, D.: Two-stage cascaded U-net: 1st place solution to BraTS challenge 2019 segmentation task. In: Crimi, A., Bakas, S. (eds.) BrainLes 2019. LNCS, vol. 11992, pp. 231–241. Springer, Cham (2020). https://doi.org/10.1007/978-3-030-46640-4_22

17. Zhao, Y.-X., Zhang, Y.-M., Liu, C.-L.: Bag of tricks for 3D MRI brain tumor segmentation. In: Crimi, A., Bakas, S. (eds.) BrainLes 2019. LNCS, vol. 11992, pp. 210–220. Springer, Cham (2020). https://doi.org/10.1007/978-3-030-46640-4_20

18. Zhou, Z., et al.: Unet++: redesigning skip connections to exploit multiscale features in image segmentation. IEEE Trans. Med. Imaging **39**(6), 1856–1867 (2019)

19. Roth, H., et al.: Spatial aggregation of holistically-nested convolutional neural networks for automated pancreas localization and segmentation. Med. Imaging Anal. **45**, 94–107 (2018)

20. Hu, J., et al.: Squeeze-and-excitation networks. In: Proceedings of CVPR 2018, pp. 7132–7141 (2018)

21. Li, X., et al.: Selective kernel networks. In: Proceedings of CVPR 2019, pp. 510–519 (2019)

22. Yuan, Y., et al.: Automatic skin lesion segmentation using deep fully convolutional networks with Jaccard distance. IEEE Trans. Med. Imaging **36**(9), 1876–1886 (2017)

23. Yuan, Y.: Hierachical convolutional-deconvolutional neural networks for automatic liver and tumor segmentation. arXiv preprint arXiv:1710.04540 (2017)

24. Yuan, Y.: Automatic skin lesion segmentation with fully convolutional-deconvolutional networks. arXiv preprint arXiv:1703.05154 (2017)

25. Yuan, Y., et al.: Improving dermoscopic image segmentation with enhanced convolutional-deconvolutional networks. IEEE J. Biomed. Health Inf. **23**(2), 519–526 (2019)

26. Wu, Y., He, K.: Group normalization. In: Ferrari, V., Hebert, M., Sminchisescu, C., Weiss, Y. (eds.) ECCV 2018. LNCS, vol. 11217, pp. 3–19. Springer, Cham (2018). https://doi.org/10.1007/978-3-030-01261-8_1

27. Yuan, Y.: Automatic brain tumor segmentation with scale attention network. In: Crimi, A., Bakas, S. (eds.) BrainLes 2020. LNCS, vol. 12658, pp. 285–294. Springer, Cham (2021). https://doi.org/10.1007/978-3-030-72084-1_26

Orthogonal-Nets: A Large Ensemble of 2D Neural Networks for 3D Brain Tumor Segmentation

Kamlesh Pawar[1,2](✉) (iD), Shenjun Zhong[1,6] (iD), Dilshan Sasanka Goonatillake[5], Gary Egan[1,2,3] (iD), and Zhaolin Chen[1,4] (iD)

[1] Monash Biomedical Imaging, Monash University, Melbourne, VIC, Australia
kamlesh.pawar@monash.edu
[2] School of Psychological Sciences, Monash University, Melbourne, VIC, Australia
[3] ARC Center of Excellence for Integrative Brain Functions, Monash University, Melbourne, VIC, Australia
[4] Department of Data Science and AI, Faculty of Information Technology, Monash University, Melbourne, VIC, Australia
[5] Department of Electrical and Computer System Engineering, Monash University, Melbourne, VIC, Australia
[6] National Imaging Facility, Melbourne, Australia

Abstract. We propose Orthogonal-Nets consisting of a large number of ensembles of 2D encoder-decoder convolutional neural networks. The Orthogonal-Nets takes 2D slices of the image from axial, sagittal, and coronal views of the 3D brain volume and predicts the probability for the tumor segmentation region. The predicted probability distributions from all three views are averaged to generate a 3D probability distribution map that is subsequently used to predict the tumor regions for the 3D images. In this work, we propose a two-stage Orthogonal-Nets. Stage-I predicts the brain tumor labels for the whole 3D image using the axial, sagittal, and coronal views. The labels from the first stage are then used to crop only the tumor region. Multiple Orthogonal-Nets were then trained in stage-II, which takes only the cropped region as input. The two-stage strategy substantially reduces the computational burden on the stage-II networks and thus many Orthogonal-Nets can be used in stage-II. We used one Orthogonal-Net for stage-I and 28 Orthogonal-Nets for stage-II. The mean dice score on the testing datasets was 0.8660, 0.8776, 0.9118 for enhancing tumor, core tumor, and whole tumor respectively.

Keywords: Brain tumor segmentation · Convolutional neural network · Medical imaging

1 Introduction

Segmentation of glioma sub-regions is the process of pixel-wise labeling of the multimodal 3D magnetic resonance imaging (mpMRI) scans from glioblastoma patients,

A. Crimi and S. Bakas (Eds.): BrainLes 2021, LNCS 12963, pp. 54–67, 2022.
https://doi.org/10.1007/978-3-031-09002-8_5

which is critical for treatment planning. Automating the process is a challenging problem in medical image analysis, due to the heterogeneous biological properties and structural variations of the glioma tumors. The Brain Tumor Segmentation (BraTS) challenge [1] aims to validate automated segmentation methods on a collection of the manually annotated dataset [1–6]. The dataset is limited in size, compared to those in natural images, such as ImageNet [7], which may lead to poor generalization power in these methods.

Since the start of the BraTS challenges, many computer vision (CV) algorithms, particularly deep learning models, have been developed to improve prediction accuracy. Most of the recent state-of-the-art (SOTA) methods apply 3D models, e.g. 3D U-Net [8], SA-Net [9], paired training with two 3D U-Nets [10], N2NF-Net [11], 3D nnU-Net (the 1st place in BraTS 2020) [12] and Squeeze-and-Expansion transformer with I3D backbone (the current SOTA of the BrasTS dataset) [13]. 3D models are a natural candidate for the brain tumor segmentation task as they can relate pixels in all three spatial dimensions thus providing a better estimation of segmented tumor regions. However, there are certain limitations of using 3D models including (i) they require a large amount of GPU memory which limits the complexity (depth, width, and the number of parameters) of the DL network; (ii) number of training samples are reduced as compared to 2D models since the number of samples is equal to the number of subjects for the 3D model while the number of samples is equal to the number of subjects times the number of slice per subject for 2D model; (iii) the computational complexity of 3D convolutions is higher than the 2D convolution which makes the 3D models computationally expensive. The limitation of relatively small number of samples can be partially addressed using techniques such as regularization, data augmentation and model ensemble that were proven to improve the model performance on the BraTS dataset [14, 15].

On the other hand, some of the previous work has shown that deeper 2D models [16, 17] perform well for the brain tumor segmentation task. However, 2D networks suffer from a lack of knowledge of the third spatial dimension. In this work, we propose a method for brain tumor segmentation called Orthogonal-Nets that builds upon the strengths of both 2D and 3D models. The Orthogonal-Net consists of an ensemble of 2D networks acting on the orthogonal planes (axial, sagittal, and coronal planes). Since three 2D models are applied in the orthogonal planes, the ensemble is aware of all three directions for better estimation of the 3D tumor region. The 2D models required relatively less memory hence more complex models (deeper and wider) can be used. Additionally, we propose a two-stage strategy for training and validation which involves applying an Orthogonal-Net on the full image, to get coarse labels and using those labels to crop the region of the image containing only the tumor. The cropped regions are further processed through an ensemble of Orthogonal-Nets in stage-II. The two-stage strategy results in better delineation of the tumor boundaries.

2   Methods

2.1   Datasets

There were a total of 2000 cases (i.e. mpMRI scans) in the 2021 BraTS challenge, which was further divided into 1251 cases for training, 219 for online validation, and the remaining for challenge ranking. These mpMRI scans were acquired from different clinical procedures and scanners across multiple imaging sites consisting of T1, post-contrast T1-weighted (T1Gd), T2, and T2 Fluid Attenuated Inversion Recovery (T2-FLAIR) scans. All the scans were firstly annotated by an ensemble of previously top-performed methods [15, 18, 19], and then manually reviewed and refined by neuroradiology experts. The annotated glioma sub-regions were: (i) the enhancing tumor (ET), (ii) the tumor core (TC), and (iii) the whole tumor (WT).

Compared with the BraTS 2020 dataset (660 cases), the 2021 dataset had more data for developing and validating methods. In our work, we further divided the 1251 annotated datasets into local training (1051 cases) and local validation (200 cases). This reduced the amount of data for model training but provided a mechanism to examine the generalization performance from the model.

2.2   Model Architecture

We proposed a two-stage approach using Orthogonal-Nets, which consisted of a large ensemble of 2D neural networks trained on orthogonal slices for the segmentation of 3D tumor volumes. The segmentation processing pipeline is depicted in Fig. 1, in which an averaged ensemble of 2D models on axial, sagittal, and coronal slices constitute an Orthogonal-Net. In stage-I, a single ResUNet-50 was trained on orthogonal slices to predict segmentation labels, this label is then used to crop a region of interest (ROI) consisting of only the tumor region. The actual crop was 125% of the tumor bounding box. In stage-I, many Orthogonal-Nets (28 in total) are trained on the cropped ROI as depicted in Fig. 1. Table 1 shows the architectures and encoder backbone used along with the number of parameters and FLOPs. The architectures included were U-Net [20], U-Net plus-plus [21], Manet [22], PSP-Net [23], PAN [24], FPN [25] and Linknet [26]. Also, different encoders were used in pairs with different network architectures, e.g. Resnet-50 [27], InceptionResNetV2 [28] and EfficientNet-B5 [29].

2.3   Training

Each slice from the orthogonal views was normalized to standardize the dynamic range of the image intensity before feeding to the training pipeline. The normalization consisted of subtracting the mean and dividing by the standard deviation of each input sample (image slice). On-the-fly data augmentation was applied to individual slices of all contrasts with (i) 50% probability to have one of the random spatial transformations, e.g. rotation, mirroring, and cropping; (ii) 50% probability to apply one of random affine (including scaling, translation, shearing), perspective and grid distortion transformations; (iii) 50% probability to add one of the Gaussian blurring, motion blurring or random contrast scaling.

Table 1. The stage-I and stage-II models in the proposed approach.

Type	Encoder	Params (M)	FLOPs (G)
	Stage-I Model		
Unet	Resnet50	33.8	3.90
	Stage-II Models		
Unet	Resnet50	33.8	3.90
MAnet	Resnet50	147.4	7.88
PSPNet	Resnet50	2.0	2.15
PAN	Resnet50	2.0	2.15
FPN	Resnet50	26.1	4.23
FPN	Se-Resnet50	28.6	4.01
FPN	Dpn92	37.9	0.79
FPN	InceptionResNetV2	56.7	4.12
FPN	Densenet169	14.1	0.96
FPN	EfficientNet-B5	29.1	2.43
FPN	Dpn68	13.1	0.27
FPN	Timm-regnetx64	26.9	0.39
UnetPP	Resnet50	33.8	3.90
UnetPP	Se-Resnet50	36.5	3.68
UnetPP	Dpn92	49.4	0.33
UnetPP	InceptionResNetV2	62.9	3.88
UnetPP	Densenet169	21.4	0.62
UnetPP	EfficientNet-B5	30.3	2.40
UnetPP	Dpn68	17.3	0.08
UnetPP	Timm-regnetx64	32.7	0.17
Linknet	Resnet50	31.8	3.87
Linknet	Se-Resnet50	33.7	3.65
Linknet	Dpn92	49.2	0.31
Linknet	InceptionResNetV2	59.4	3.85
Linknet	Densenet169	18.2	0.59
Linknet	EfficientNet-B5	27.7	2.37
Linknet	Dpn68	13.3	0.05
Linknet	Timm-regnetx64	29.3	0.13

The two stages were trained separately. The input to all the networks was $224 \times 224 \times$ 4 with the last dimension being different image contrasts (T1, T2, T2-Flair, T1Gd). The preprocessing and data augmentation was applied by the Pytorch data generator on the fly. To train the networks of stage-II, ground truth labels were used for cropping the ROI (125% of the tumor bounding box) and 28 separate networks (Table 1) were trained. Slices from the ROI were first resized to 224×224 before feeding them to the model for training. The training was performed on the Nvidia DGX computing cluster with 8 V100 GPUs, the batch sizes were empirically optimized for each model and the models were trained separately for 40 epochs. We used Adam optimizer and logarithmic soft dice loss for training while the learning rate for each model was tuned with the learning rate finder [28]. The best model for each architecture was selected based on the lowest validation loss.

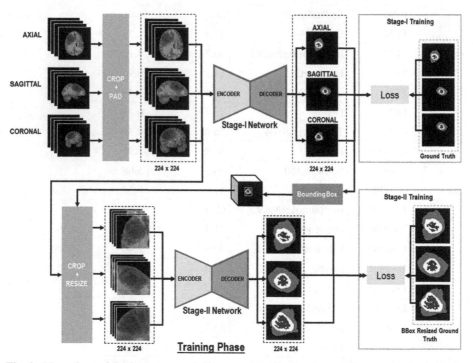

Fig. 1. Flow chart of the two-stage training process; stage-I and stage-II are trained separately. In stage-I, a Unet with Reset50 encoder was trained on 2D slices in all three orientations (axial, sagittal, and coronal). In stage-II, multiple Unets (28 in total) were trained using the cropped images resized to 224×224 in all the orientations.

2.4 Inference

In the inference stage, 2D trained models were used to predict segmentation labels for 3D volume. As shown in Fig. 2, the inference workflow was similar to the training phase, but had several differences:

1. Given a 3D volume, the 2D slices were pre-processed and fed into the stage-I network to obtain a series of 2D probability maps, which were then concatenated to form a 3D probability map (step 6 in Algorithm 1).
2. The same process repeated for the axial, sagittal, and coronal slices, and outputs were averaged to obtain the coarse segmentation labels (step 9 in Algorithm 1).
3. Both the bounding box and the ROI, i.e. the patch containing tumors were constructed in 3D space, unlike the training phase. The 3D patch size was 125% of the tumor bounding box.
4. The 3D patches were resized to match the stage-II network input dimension, 224 × 224 (step 14 in Algorithm 1).
5. In stage 2, the 3D probability map was also aggregated by averaging the probability maps for each orthogonal direction (step 21 in algorithm 1).
6. The aggregated 3D probability map was weighted averaged over the predictions from all the models in the ensemble (step 18 in Algorithm 1). The weights were calculated using the 200 validation dataset.
7. The final segmentation labels were determined from the 3D probability map obtained in step 6 using the argmax operation.

Algorithm 1. Inference workflow

// Stage One

INPUT: mpMRI image => [240x240x155x4]

1: **FOR** volume in [axial, sagittal, coronal] **DO**
2:   **FOR** slice in volume.depth **DO**
3:   Crop and Pad the slice to be [224x224x4]
4:   Feed to Stage-I network to Compute logits
5:   **ENDFOR**
6:   Concatenate the logits for each slice to form 3D logits
7: **ENDFOR**
8:
9: Compute 3D probability map by averaging in orthogonal directions
10: Compute bounding box with 125% coverage
11: Crop the volume by the bounding box to generate an ROI

// Stage Two

INPUT: ROI from the first stage

12: **FOR** ROI in [axial, sagittal, coronal] **DO**
13:   **FOR** slice in ROI.depth **DO**
14:   Resample the slice to be [224x224x4]
15:   **FOR** model in Ensemble **DO**
16:   Compute logits by feeding into the model
17:   **ENDFOR**
18:   Average the logits computed by all models
18:   **ENDFOR**
19:   Concatenate the logits to form a 3D probability map
20: **ENDFOR**
21: Average the 3D probability map over all orthogonal directions
22: Resize and realign the 3D probability map in the original space

---

// Final Output

INPUT: 3D probability map from stage I
        3D probability map from stage II

23: Weighted average of the 3D probability map from both stages where weights were estimated using local validation dataset.
24: Compute final segmentation labels with argmax operation

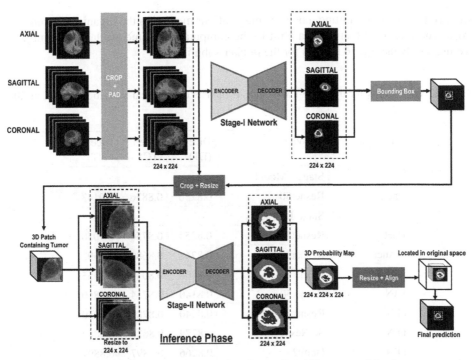

Fig. 2. During the inference phase the networks of stage-I and II were combined to compute the final predictions. Using the stage-I network, coarse labels were obtained which were used to crop the input images; the cropped images were processed using the stage-II networks (28 in total). The predicted probabilities from all the predictions were weighted averaged to get a 3D probability map, and the final labels were obtained from the aggregated probability map.

3   Results and Discussion

The models with the best performance on the local validation dataset (200 samples) were selected to submit to the online validation portal and obtain the results. The metrics used were dice score, Hausdorff distance (95%), sensitivity, and specificity measurements. Table 2 shows the results of the proposed method on the 200 samples local dataset for individual models and the ensemble of the two-stage network. The dice scores for the ensemble were substantially better than the individual models, particularly for the enhancing tumor. Table 3 shows the scores on the 219 samples for the online validation dataset of the challenge. The dice scores were 0.913 for the whole tumor label, 0.849 for the tumor core, and 0.8320 for the enhancing tumor sub-regions. Compared to the local validation dataset there was a slight decrease in all the dice scores on the validation dataset, we attribute this to a slight mismatch in both the data distribution. The method achieved high specificity scores for all the sub-regions, and also achieved sensitivity scores of 90.9% for the whole tumor, 82.5% for the tumor core, and 83.4% for the enhancing tumor. Table 4 shows the scores on the test dataset consisting of more than 500 images, all the scores were improved compared to the small number of images (~200) in both local validation and validation datasets. The results for the test dataset were obtained by submitting a docker image of our method to the organizers' compute infrastructure, since there was a limit to the computational time available per subject, we used only the top 16 models for the docker submission.

Table 2. Dice scores for the stage-I and stage-II models on the local validation dataset of 200 images

Type	Encoder	Dice (ET)	Dice (TC)	Dice (WT)
	Stage-I Model			
Unet	Resnet50	0.8256	0.8876	0.9143
	Stage-II Models			
Unet	Resnet50	0.8254	0.8750	0.9050
MAnet	Resnet50	0.8248	0.8689	0.8992
PSPNet	Resnet50	0.8700	0.8079	0.8955
PAN	Resnet50	0.8140	0.8714	0.8860
FPN	Resnet50	0.8240	0.8780	0.9030
FPN	Se-Resnet50	0.8279	0.8826	0.9067
FPN	Dpn92	0.8266	0.8897	0.8897
FPN	InceptionResNetV2	0.8303	0.8841	0.9127
FPN	Densenet169	0.8300	0.8785	0.9039
FPN	EfficientNet-B5	0.8370	0.8868	0.8997
FPN	Dpn68	0.8320	0.8745	0.9009
FPN	Timm-regnetx64	0.8298	0.8831	0.9042
UnetPP	Resnet50	0.8353	0.8799	0.8932
UnetPP	Se-Resnet50	0.8326	0.8834	0.9152
UnetPP	Dpn92	0.8391	0.8827	0.9074
UnetPP	InceptionResNetV2	0.8414	0.8917	0.9069
UnetPP	Densenet169	0.8317	0.8865	0.9101
UnetPP	EfficientNet-B5	0.8403	0.8978	0.9104
UnetPP	Dpn68	0.8343	0.8878	0.9081
UnetPP	Timm-regnetx64	0.8351	0.8911	0.9143
Linknet	Resnet50	0.8276	0.8714	0.8980
Linknet	Se-Resnet50	0.8406	0.8885	0.9120
Linknet	Dpn92	0.8400	0.8934	0.8935
Linknet	InceptionResNetV2	0.8340	0.8811	0.9060

(continued)

Table 2. (*continued*)

Type	Encoder	Dice (ET)	Dice (TC)	Dice (WT)
Linknet	Densenet169	0.8392	0.8861	0.9025
Linknet	EfficientNet-B5	0.8439	0.8907	0.9098
Linknet	Dpn68	0.8309	0.8737	0.8981
Linknet	Timm-regnetx64	0.8348	0.8851	0.9107
ENSEMBLE		**0.8531**	**0.9076**	**0.9243**

After visual inspection of the segmentation results, we observed that fragmented tumor regions were not accurately detected by the proposed method, as shown in Fig. 3, with the dice scores of 0.7260 (ET), 0.7890 (TC), and 0.8869 (WT), which were significantly lower than the average performance obtained over all the validation dataset in Table 2. On the other hand, the method performed well on the non-fragmented tumor regions as shown in Fig. 4 where all the sub-regions were accurately segmented with high dice scores of 0.9440 (ET), 0.9521 (TC), and 0.9626 (WT).

Table 3. Performance of the model on the 219 samples in the BraTS 2021 validation dataset.

Metric	ET	TC	WT
Dice	0.8320	0.8499	0.9138
Hausdorff (95%)	20.97	9.81	5.43
Sensitivity	0.8342	0.8252	0.9089
Specificity	0.9998	0.9998	0.9993

Other related work that uses a model ensemble, such as the bag-of-tricks method having an ensemble of five models and won second place in BraTS'19 challenge [14], self-ensemble models (a solution for BraTS'20) where the same architecture was trained differently and merged [30]. Our method was inspired by these methods which aimed at maximizing the number of models in an ensemble. The use of 2D models in orthogonal directions, instead of 3D models enabled us to implement a large number of models in an ensemble that improve the model's accuracy without missing the 3D spatial information.

Another advantage of using 2D based approaches in medical image analysis is to take advantage of more public datasets for pre-training and perform transfer learning from other imaging modalities. On the other hand, there are very limited 3D medical imaging datasets publicly available with high-quality annotations. Recent work showed that using pre-trained models had an around 2.5% accuracy improvement (i.e. dice score) for transformer-based architecture and 1% for U-Net variants on BraTS20 dataset [13]. The proposed framework was able to capture 3D contexts using Orthogonal-Nets and benefits from large-scale 2D pre-training.

Table 4. Performance of the model on the BraTS 2021 test dataset.

Metric	ET	TC	WT
Dice	0.8660	0.8776	0.9118
Hausdorff (95%)	13.09	14.98	8.36
Sensitivity	0.8795	0.8833	0.9210
Specificity	0.9998	0.9997	0.9993

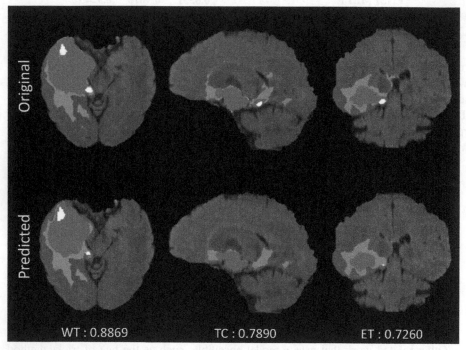

Fig. 3. Image overlay showing FLAIR image with original segmentation mask (top row) and predicted segmentation mask (bottom row). An example case where the algorithm underperformed with low Dice similarity scores.

The two-stage design improves detection of small anatomical structures, but at the same time, a biased coarse prediction in the first stage may become the bottleneck of delivering accurate final segmentations. The first stage of the approach estimates a rough ROI containing the brain tumor, and the second stage models only view the ROI. One limitation of the proposed approach is that if the predictions from the first stage did not capture the right location or partially cover the tumor area, the stage-II networks will not be able to process the region left out by the first stage which will result in the less accurate final segmentations. Another factor affecting the performance of the method is the artifact in the images such as motion or accelerated imaging artifact that can result in

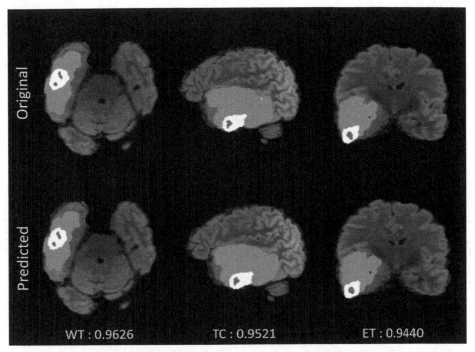

Fig. 4. Image overlay showing FLAIR image with original segmentation mask (top row) and predicted segmentation mask (bottom row). An example case where the algorithm performed well with high Dice similarity scores.

reduced accuracy. The problem of image quality can partly be solved by pre-processing the images through the image enhancement [31–33] deep learning methods.

4   Conclusion

In this work, we have developed a two-stage approach for segmenting 3D brain glioma sub-regions using a large number of 2D model ensembles. The proposed network has been trained and validated using the BraTS21 dataset. The high dice scores of 0.8660, 0.8776, and 0.9118 for enhancing tumor, tumor core, and whole tumor respectively, on the unseen testing dataset demonstrate that a carefully trained ensemble to 2D networks can perform at par the 3D networks.

References

1. Menze, B.H., et al.: The multimodal brain tumor image segmentation benchmark (BRATS). IEEE Trans. Med. Imaging (2015)
2. Bakas, S., et al.: Advancing the cancer genome atlas glioma MRI collections with expert segmentation labels and radiomic features. Sci. Data **4**, 170117 (2017)

3. Bakas, S., et al.: Identifying the best machine learning algorithms for brain tumor segmentation, progression assessment, and overall survival prediction in the BRATS challenge. arXiv preprint arXiv:1811.02629 (2018)
4. Bakas, S., et al.: Segmentation labels and radiomic features for the pre-operative scans of the TCGA-LGG collection. The Cancer Imaging Archive **286** (2017)
5. Baid, U., et al.: The RSNA-ASNR-MICCAI BraTS 2021 benchmark on brain tumor segmentation and radiogenomic classification. arXiv preprint arXiv:2107.02314 (2021)
6. Bakas, S., et al.: Segmentation labels and radiomic features for the pre-operative scans of the TCGA-GBM collection. The Cancer Imaging Archive (2017)
7. Deng, J., Dong, W., Socher, R., Li, L.-J., Li, K., Fei-Fei, L.: Imagenet: a large-scale hierarchical image database. In: 2009 IEEE Conference on Computer Vision and Pattern Recognition, pp. 248–255. IEEE (2009)
8. Ballestar, L.M., Vilaplana, V.: MRI brain tumor segmentation and uncertainty estimation using 3D-UNet architectures. arXiv preprint arXiv:2012.15294 (2020)
9. Hu, J., Wang, H., Wang, J., Wang, Y., He, F., Zhang, J.: SA-Net: a scale-attention network for medical image segmentation. PLoS ONE **16**, e0247388 (2021)
10. Wang, Y., et al.: Modality-pairing learning for brain tumor segmentation. arXiv preprint arXiv:2010.09277 (2020)
11. Jia, H., Cai, W., Huang, H., Xia, Y.: H2NF-Net for Brain Tumor Segmentation using Multimodal MR Imaging: 2nd Place Solution to BraTS Challenge 2020 Segmentation Task (2020)
12. Isensee, F., Jäger, P.F., Full, P.M., Vollmuth, P., Maier-Hein, K.H.: Nnu-net for brain tumor segmentation. In: Crimi, A., Bakas, Spyridon (eds.) Brainlesion: Glioma, Multiple Sclerosis, Stroke and Traumatic Brain Injuries: 6th International Workshop, BrainLes 2020, Held in Conjunction with MICCAI 2020, Lima, Peru, October 4, 2020, Revised Selected Papers, Part II, pp. 118–132. Springer International Publishing, Cham (2021). https://doi.org/10.1007/978-3-030-72087-2_11
13. Li, S., Sui, X., Luo, X., Xu, X., Liu, Y., Goh, R.S.M.: Medical image segmentation using squeeze-and-expansion transformers. arXiv preprint arXiv:2105.09511 (2021)
14. Zhao, Y.-X., Zhang, Y.-M., Liu, C.-L.: Bag of tricks for 3D MRI brain tumor segmentation. In: Crimi, A., Bakas, S. (eds.) Brainlesion: Glioma, Multiple Sclerosis, Stroke and Traumatic Brain Injuries: 5th International Workshop, BrainLes 2019, Held in Conjunction with MICCAI 2019, Shenzhen, China, October 17, 2019, Revised Selected Papers, Part I, pp. 210–220. Springer International Publishing, Cham (2020). https://doi.org/10.1007/978-3-030-46640-4_20
15. Kamnitsas, K., et al.: Efficient multi-scale 3D CNN with fully connected CRF for accurate brain lesion segmentation. Med. Image Anal. **36**, 61–78 (2017)
16. Pawar, K., Chen, N.Z., Shah, J., Egan, G.F.: An ensemble of 2D convolutional neural network for 3D brain tumor segmentation. In: Crimi, A., Bakas, S. (eds.) Brainlesion: Glioma, Multiple Sclerosis, Stroke and Traumatic Brain Injuries: 5th International Workshop, BrainLes 2019, Held in Conjunction with MICCAI 2019, Shenzhen, China, October 17, 2019, Revised Selected Papers, Part I, pp. 359–367. Springer International Publishing, Cham (2020). https://doi.org/10.1007/978-3-030-46640-4_34
17. Pawar, K., Chen, Z., Shah, N.J., Egan, G.: Residual encoder and convolutional decoder neural network for glioma segmentation. In: Crimi, A., Bakas, S., Kuijf, H., Menze, B., Reyes, M. (eds.) Brainlesion: Glioma, Multiple Sclerosis, Stroke and Traumatic Brain Injuries BrainLes 2017 Third International Workshop, BrainLes 2017, Held in Conjunction with MICCAI 2017, Quebec City, QC, Canada, September 14, 2017, Revised Selected Papers. LNCS, vol. 10670, pp. 263–273. Springer, Cham (2018). https://doi.org/10.1007/978-3-319-75238-9_23

18. McKinley, R., Meier, R., Wiest, R.: Ensembles of densely-connected CNNs with label-uncertainty for brain tumor segmentation. In: Crimi, A., Bakas, S., Kuijf, H., Keyvan, F., Reyes, M., van Walsum, T. (eds.) Brainlesion: Glioma, Multiple Sclerosis, Stroke and Traumatic Brain Injuries: 4th International Workshop, BrainLes 2018, Held in Conjunction with MICCAI 2018, Granada, Spain, September 16, 2018, Revised Selected Papers, Part II, pp. 456–465. Springer International Publishing, Cham (2019). https://doi.org/10.1007/978-3-030-11726-9_40

19. Isensee, F., Jaeger, P.F., Kohl, S.A., Petersen, J., Maier-Hein, K.H.: nnU-Net: a self-configuring method for deep learning-based biomedical image segmentation. Nat. Methods **18**, 203–211 (2021)

20. Ronneberger, O., Fischer, P., Brox, T.: U-Net: convolutional networks for biomedical image segmentation. In: Navab, N., Hornegger, J., Wells, W.M., Frangi, A.F. (eds.) MICCAI 2015. LNCS, vol. 9351, pp. 234–241. Springer, Cham (2015). https://doi.org/10.1007/978-3-319-24574-4_28

21. Zhou, Z., Siddiquee, M.M.R., Tajbakhsh, N., Liang, J.: Unet++: a nested u-net architecture for medical image segmentation. Deep Learning in Medical Image Analysis and Multimodal Learning for Clinical Decision Support, pp. 3–11. Springer (2018)

22. Li, R., et al.: Multiattention network for semantic segmentation of fine-resolution remote sensing images. IEEE Transactions on Geoscience and Remote Sensing (2021)

23. Zhao, H., Shi, J., Qi, X., Wang, X., Jia, J.: Pyramid scene parsing network. In: Proceedings of the IEEE conference on computer vision and pattern recognition, pp. 2881–2890 (2017)

24. Khosravan, N., Mortazi, A., Wallace, M., Bagci, U.: Pan: projective adversarial network for medical image segmentation. In: Shen, D., Liu, T., Peters, T.M., Staib, L.H., Essert, C., Zhou, S., Yap, P.-T., Khan, A. (eds.) Medical Image Computing and Computer Assisted Intervention – MICCAI 2019: 22nd International Conference, Shenzhen, China, October 13–17, 2019, Proceedings, Part VI, pp. 68–76. Springer International Publishing, Cham (2019). https://doi.org/10.1007/978-3-030-32226-7_8

25. Lin, T.-Y., Dollár, P., Girshick, R., He, K., Hariharan, B., Belongie, S.: Feature pyramid networks for object detection. In: Proceedings of the IEEE conference on computer vision and pattern recognition, pp. 2117–2125 (2017)

26. Chaurasia, A., Culurciello, E.: Linknet: Exploiting encoder representations for efficient semantic segmentation. In: 2017 IEEE Visual Communications and Image Processing (VCIP), pp. 1–4. IEEE (2017)

27. He, K.M., Zhang, X.Y., Ren, S.Q., Sun, J.: Deep residual learning for image recognition. Proc. CVPR IEEE, 770–778 (2016)

28. Szegedy, C., Ioffe, S., Vanhoucke, V., Alemi, A.A.: Inception-v4, inception-resnet and the impact of residual connections on learning. In: Thirty-First AAAI Conference on Artificial Intelligence (2017)

29. Tan, M., Le, Q.: Efficientnet: rethinking model scaling for convolutional neural networks. In: International Conference on Machine Learning, pp. 6105–6114. PMLR (2019)

30. Henry, T., et al.: Brain tumor segmentation with self-ensembled, deeply-supervised 3D U-net neural networks: a BraTS 2020 challenge solution. arXiv preprint arXiv:2011.01045 (2020)

31. Pawar, K., Chen, Z., Shah, N.J., Egan, G.F.: Suppressing motion artefacts in MRI using an Inception-ResNet network with motion simulation augmentation. NMR Biomed. e4225 (2019)

32. Pawar, K., Egan, G.F., Chen, Z.: Domain knowledge augmentation of parallel MR image reconstruction using deep learning. Comput. Med. Imaging Graph. 101968 (2021)

33. Pawar, K., Chen, Z., Shah, N.J., Egan, G.F.: A Deep learning framework for transforming image reconstruction into pixel classification. IEEE Access **7**, 177690–177702 (2019)

Feature Learning by Attention and Ensemble with 3D U-Net to Glioma Tumor Segmentation

Xiaohong Cai[1], Shubin Lou[2], Mingrui Shuai[2], and Zhulin An[3(✉)]

[1] Xiamen Institute of Data Intelligence, Xiamen, China
[2] School of Compute Science and Technology, Anhui University, Hefei, China
[3] Institute of Computing Technology, Chinese Academy of Sciences, Beijing 100190, China
anzhulin@ict.ac.cn

Abstract. BraTS2021 Task1 is research on segmentation of intrinsically heterogeneous brain glioblastoma sub-regions in mpMRI scans. Base on BraTS 2020 top ten team's solution (open brats2020, ranked among the top ten teams work), we proposed a similar as 3D U-Net neural network, called as TE U-Net, to differentiate glioma sub-regions class. According that automatically learns to focus on sub-regions class structures of varying shapes and sizes, we proposed TE U-Net which is similar with U-Net++ network architecture. Firstly, we reserved encoder second and third stage's skip connect design, then also cut off first stage skip connect design. Secondly, multiple stage features through attention gate block before features skip connect, so as to ensemble channels and space region information to suppress irrelevant regions. Finally, in order to improve model performance, on network post-processing stage, we ensemble multiple similar 3D U-Net with attention module. On the online validation database, the TE U-Net architecture get best result is that the GD-enhancing tumor (ET) dice is 83.79%, the peritumoral edematous/invaded tissue (TC) dice is 86.47%, and the necrotic tumor core (WT) dice is 91.98%, Hausdorff(95%) values is 6.39,7.81,3.86and Sensitivity values is 82.20%, 83.99%, 91.92% respectively. And our solution achieved a dice of 85.62%,86.70%,90.64% for ET,TC and WT, as well as Hausdorff(95%) is 18.70,21.06,10.88 on final private test dataset.

Keywords: Glioma · Brain tumor · Machine learning · Deep learning · Transfer learning · Medical image segmentation

1 Introduction

1.1 Glioma Research

Glioblastoma, and diffuse astrocytic glioma with molecular features of glioblastoma (WHO Grade 4 astrocytoma), are the most common and aggressive malignant primary tumor of the central nervous system in adults, with extreme intrinsic heterogeneity in appearance, shape, and histology. Glioblastoma patients have very poor prognosis and the current standard of care treatment comprises surgery, followed by radiotherapy and chemotherapy [1]. Ordinary have an approximate 5-year survival rate of 10% in their highest grade. Regard of the poor clinical outcomes associated with malignant tumor and the high cost of treatment, researching brain tumor screening through magnetic resonance imaging (MRI) has been a hot research highlights topic.

MRI screening in healthy asymptomatic adults can detect both early gliomas and other benign central nervous system abnormalities [2]. General structure image usually have native (T1), post-contrast T1-weighted (T1ce), T2-weighted (T2) and T2 Fluid Attenuated Inversion Recovery (Flair) multi-modality of patient brain scans and see in Fig. 1.

Associating with Glioblastoma, there have Four distinct tumor subregions in MRI volumes which plays import role for identify benign or malignant tumor. In detail, the enhancing tumor (ET) which corresponds to area of relative hyperintensity in the T1Gd with respect to the T1 sequence; the non-enhancing tumor (NET) and the necrotic tumor (NCR) which are both hypointense in T1-Gd when compared to T1; and the last peritumoral edema (ED) which is hyper-intense in FLAIR sequence. These almost homogeneous subregions can be clustered together to compose three "semantically" meaningful tumor subparts: ET is the first cluster, addition of ET, NET and NCR represents the "tumor core" (TC) region, and addition of ED to TC represents the "whole tumor" (WT) [3]. Example of each sequence and tumor sub-volumes is provided in Fig. 1. In BraTS2021 segmentation task, label 1 mean NET, label 2 mean ED, label 4 mean ET.

1.2 RSNA-ASNR-MICCAI BraTS Challenge 2021

The RSNA-ASNR-MICCAI BraTS 2021 challenge utilizes multi-institutional multi-parametric magnetic resonance imaging (mpMRI) scans, and Task 1 is focuses on the evaluation of state-of-the-art methods for the segmentation of intrinsically heterogeneous brain glioblastoma sub-regions in mpMRI scans. In addition, this year's challenge also organized Task 2 that evaluated the classification methods for predicting the MGMT promoter methylation status at pre-operative baseline scans. In this work, we only participate in the segmentation Task 1.

In contrasting with BraTS Challenge 2020, the datasets used in this year's challenge have been updated, since BraTS2020, with many more routine clinically-acquired mpMRI scans from institutions that have not previously contributed to BraTS, increasing the demographic diversity of the represented patient population. Ground truth annotations of the tumor sub-regions are created and approved by expert neuroradiologists for every subject included in the training, validation, and testing datasets to quantitatively evaluate the predicted tumor segmentations of Task 1.

Therefore, one of biggest change to The BraTS2021 Task 1 is dataset [4–8] comprises 1251 training cases and 219 validation cases. As usually, participants can't available to the ground truth annotations for the validation set. And participants can use the online evaluation platform [1] to evaluate their models. Through online Submission Dashboard participants can compare their scores with other teams. Besides, BraTS2021 add docker file submissions operation.

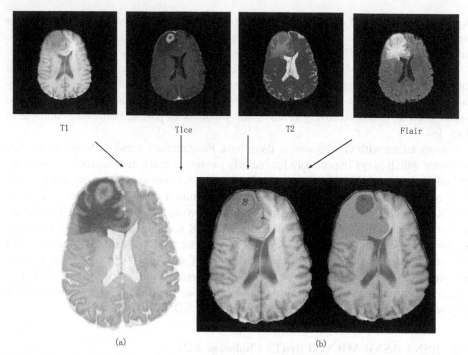

T1   T1ce   T2   Flair

(a)   (b)

Fig. 1. Example of a brain tumor from the BraTS2021 training dataset (BraTS2021_00062). Top line is General structure MRI, such as T1 weighted sequence, T1-weighted contrast enhanced sequence, T2 weighted sequence, Flair weighted sequence. Botton line (a): fusion of T1, T1ce, T2 and Flair by opencv tool. Botton line (b): T1 weighted sequence with label mark's contours, Blue contours surrounding region is enhancing tumor (ET), Red surrounding region is non enhancing tumor/ necrotic tumor (NET/NCR) and Green surrounding region is peritumoral edema (ED).

2   Method

2.1   Metric for BraTS Challenge 2021 Rank

In recent years, more and more deep learning technologies have shown very promising performance in solving various medical image segmentation tasks, such as pathology, X-ray, Computed Tomography (CT), Magnetic Resonance Imaging (MRI) and ultrasound. With a good performance medical image segmentation model can help doctor then reduce their workloads.

Consequently, selecting best model is an essential part of medical segmentation task. Most challenges in evaluating medical segmentation uses metric to choose suitable model. There had an overview of 20 evaluation metrics selected based on a comprehensive literature review [9].

BraTS2021 segmentation task is use MRI database to research brain glioma subregion segment. The MRI data size is extremely large as in the case of whole head MRI volume. Therefore, BraTS2021 task 1 use a "rank then aggregate" approach, most likely because it is well suited to combine different types of segmentation metrics (as Dice, HD95, Sensitivity and Specificity) [10]. Each online submission obtains twelve math metric values for three subregion class in per patient's case. The final rank is normalized by the number of participating algorithms to form the ranking score, which ranges from 0 (best) to 1 (worst).

The Dice similarity coefficient (DSC, also named Dice) was proposed by Dice [11]. Dice is a spatial overlap index and a reproducibility validation metric. The ranges of Dice value is from zero to one, and dice equal zero indicating no spatial overlap between two sets of binary segmentation results, to one indicating complete overlap. The detail description is displayed in Fig. 2.

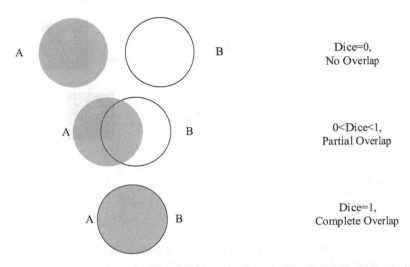

(a) Spatial Overlap of Target A and Predict Segmentations   (b) Dice(DSC) = 2(A∪B)/(A∪B)

Fig. 2. The detail description for dice metric. (a) Dice representing spatial overlap that between target with predict segmentations and reproducibility, (b) Dice responding by set calculate.

2.2 TE U-Net Neutral Network Architecture

The BraTS Challenge have hold 10th anniversary. For brain tumor segmentation task, many methods with machine learning and deep learning had proposed and attempt to focus on data preprocess stage, design the architecture of model, study the strategy of model training and model inference procedure.

After research about relative work [2, 12–17], we proposed 3D U-Net like neural network architecture, named as TE U-Net, to identify glioma lesion area and differentiate sub-regions class. It is heavily inspired by the 2D U-Net++ architecture [12, 13], 3D U-Net architecture [14] and the block of attention 2D U-Net [15]. Eventually, the TE U-Net architecture used is show in Fig. 3.

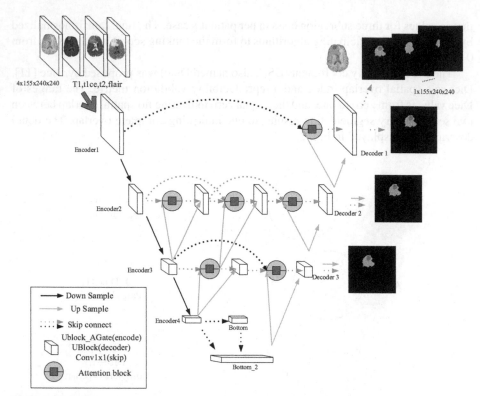

Fig. 3. The architecture scheme of TE Net Network. 3D U-Net [2] combined with the nest block of UNet++ and attention U-Net that had made minor modifications.

Inspired by the conciseness of the 2019 and 2020 winning solution. It's a good choose to transfer general structure MRI (multi-modality, T1, T1ce, T2, Flair volumes) into 4D channels data, as $4 \times 155 \times 2540 \times 240$. In the next up description, a stage structure is same with Neugut et al. [2] works, each stage block defined as an arbitrary number of convolutions that does not change the spatial dimensions of the feature maps. All convolutions blocks were combined a normalization layer with a nonlinear activation (ReLU layer [18]), then to reduce gradient diffusion when gradient back propagation in training phase. Given that input data had 4D channels, then a small batch size always used during training, had proved that can get a good theoretical performance on non-medical datasets. Consequently, group normalization [19] were used as a replacement for Batch Normalization in convolution block, such as UBlock and UBlock_AGate.

As Fig. 3 show, encoder and decoder stages both of convolution block. Remarkably, each encoder section placed an UBlock_AGate convolution block which is consisted of two $3 \times 3 \times 3$ UBlock in the above described and AGate (Attention Gate) block either. AGate block is Oktay O et al. [15] proposed a novel self-attention gating module in attention U-Net [15] used to focus on attention coefficients learning, then model will to be more specific to local regions that was beneficial to get enhancing tumor (ET) sub-regions features information. Additionally, AGate attention block can be used for deep supervision in U-Net architecture owe to it had not perform adaptive pooling as Fig. 4 described.

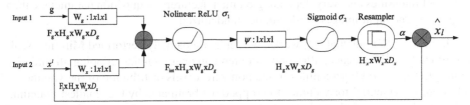

Fig. 4. Attention Block: A block diagram of the paper [15] proposed Attention U-Net segmentation model. Schematic of the proposed additive attention gate (AG). Input features (x^l) are scaled with attention coefficients (α) computed in AG. Spatial regions are selected by analysing both the activations and contextual information provided by the gating signal (g) which is collected from a coarser scale. Grid resampling of attention coefficients is done using trilinear interpolation.

Encoder Part. The number of filters for first convolution in four stages were increased by the predefined value for the stage (48 or 24 for stage 1), while the second one in the block was kept the number of output channels unchanged. In order enlarge the space of texture features, spatial down sampling was performed by a MaxPool layer with a kernel size of $2 \times 2 \times 2$ with stride 2 between in each stage. After each spatial downsampling, with the number of filters was doubled. After the last stage, place two $3 \times 3 \times 3$ dilated convolutions (Bottom, Bottom_2, as Fig. 3) with a dilation rate of 2 were performed, and then concatenated with the last stage output.

Decoder Part. The decoder part of the TE U-Net network was almost symmetrical to the encoder. Between each stage, Conversely, spatial upsampling operation was performed using a trilinear interpolation. Shortcut and skip connections between encoder and decoder stages that shared the same spatial sizes were performed by concatenation. Furthermore, as Zhou Z et al. [13] ideas that the encoder and decoder sub-networks are connected through a series of nested, dense skip pathways, reducing the semantic gap between the feature maps of encoder output and responding upsampling output. Similar that, we add the Agate block and convolution 1×1 sequence with skip connection in two and three decoder stages, detail in Fig. 3. Finally, decoder stage one was performing last convolutional layer used a $1 \times 1 \times 1$ kernel with 3 output channels and a sigmoid activation in decoder stage one, two and three. Then it can get deeply supervison for segmentation mask information.

2.3 Data Augmentation Techniques

There have many strategies for increasing generalization performance focus on the model's architecture itself. In contrast to the model design techniques mentioned above, data pre-processing and data augmentation approaches prevent overfitting from the root of the problem in the train or validation dataset.

Data Pre-Processing: Although the MRI database were created by some pre-processing operation, i.e., multiple modalities were co-registered to the same anatomical template, interpolated to the same resolution (1 × 1 × 1 mm) and also skull-stripped [1], MRI intensities also vary depending on manufacturers, acquisition parameters, then sequences and input images needed to be standardized.

Following Neugut et al. [2] works, we remain separately performed Min-max scaling of each MRI sequence, after only adopted clip operation that clipping all intensity values to the 1 and 99 percentiles of the non-zero voxels distribution of the volume. In addition, it's essential for volumes to cropped out brain area by the smallest bounding box containing the whole brain, then also randomly re-cropped to a fixed patch size of 128 × 128 × 128 before model training. And this allowed to remove most of the useless background that was present black in the original volume.

Data Augmentation: Some traditional data augmentation methods [16, 17], example that improves the image quality as noise suppression, or changes the image intensity such as brightness, saturation, and contrast, or changes the image layout such as rotation, distortion, and scaling. Above augment operations could be effectively enlarge the training set, then improves the robust of model.

In our work, we adopted to random combinatorial augment operations which had predefined probability during model training, thus increased the robustness of our models. The augmentations and their respective probability of application were:

- 75% probability for input channel to rescale: multiplying each voxel by a factor uniformly sampled between 0.9 and 1.1.
- input channel intensity shift: Adding each voxel a constant uniformly sampled between 0.1 and 0.1.
- additive gaussian noise, using a centered normal distribution with a standard deviation of 0.1.
- 16% probability for input channel to drop: all voxel values of one of the input channels were randomly set to zero.
- 80% probability for volumes to random flip along each spatial axis.

2.4 Training Details

The experiment environment was under Ubuntu18.04 OS. TE U-Net network was built and trained with Pytorch v1.7 (which has native FP16 training capability) on Python 3.6, The model could fit on one or more graphic card (GPU).

It's late for us to participate competition due to some reasons in twenty days ago. In the beginning, we plan to train models by a five-fold cross-validation method and one of fold dataset used to monitor network's performance during training. In actually, model was trained with full database then produced final model parameters. During model training, it was monitored by lowest dice loss values and optimizer was select ranger [20–22] and also SGD [23].

In conclusion, we totally trained four kind of segmentation network, as 3D U-Net model [2], Attention 3D U-Net model [2], TE Net Network model and 3D U-Net that encoder backbone using efficientnet-b2 [24, 25] convolutional block.

2.5 Ensemble Inference

Ultimately, we adopted ensemble learning [2, 26] method to improve the predictive performance of a single model by training multiple models, then regard as last predictions.

First, we retrain the TE Net Network best parameters gained in full database using five-fold cross-validation, and retrain method adopted "self-ensembled" [2] with SGD optimizer. After that, we ensemble four model in model inference stage since time had limited.

3 Result

3.1 Online Validation Dataset

As the following Table 1 show, our TE Net Network get a better result than others that we had trained using the same environment in online validation data. Our TE Net models produced a best Dice and Hausdorff metric greater than others. Remarkably, TE Net Network's parameters only half of 3D U-Net (or Attention 3D U-Net and 3D-Unet efficient-net-b2), using define the number of convolutional filters since we left just rarely time. The encoder stage of TE Net was predefined 24 and 3D U-Net was 48.

Table 1. Performance on the RSNA BraTs'21 online validation data.

Model	Dice (%)			Hausdorff (95%)		
	ET	TC	WT	ET	TC	WT
3D-Unet	82.63	86.56	91.77	16.10	7.89	4.21
Attention 3D-Unet	83.39	86.58	91.22	17.51	7.80	4.74
3D-Unet efficient-net-b2	80.77	85.28	89.87	20.00	8.40	6.31
TE net	81.47	86.11	91.07	18.35	10.00	4.33
TE Net ensemble	83.79	86.47	91.99	6.39	7.81	3.86

3.2 Private Test Dataset

The Private Test dataset has 570 cases. Our submission, however, the docker file was successful on 561 out of 570 cases in test dataset owing that the CUDA memory issue still remained in challenge platform. Given the timeline, organizer move forwarded with our submission (eval cases = 561) and assigned the penalty scores (Dice = 0 and Hausdorff = 374) to the cases that could not be evaluated.

Finally, our model in Private Test dataset achieved dice and hausdorff results is displayed in Table 2, sensitivity and specificity as Table 3 show.

Table 2. Performance on the RSNA BraTs'21 private test data.

model	Dice (%, mean)			Hausdorff (95%, mean)		
	ET	TC	WT	ET	TC	WT
TE Net ensemble	85.62	86.70	90.64	18.70	21.06	10.88

Table 3. Performance on the RSNA BraTs'21 private test data.

Model	Sensitivity (%, mean)			Specificity (%, mean)		
	ET	TC	WT	ET	TC	WT
TE Net ensemble	84.86	86.41	90.42	98.40	98.40	98.37

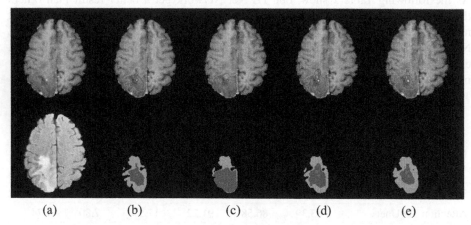

(a)   (b)   (c)   (d)   (e)

Fig. 5. The performance of our models inferenced in BraTS2021 Validation database. we select three cases (BraTS2021:01735_106), and also filtered some scans. In detail that had (a)–(e) five columns (a)cross-section of patient's t1ce (top row) and flair (bottom row) scan; (b) 3D U-Net model's result; (c) the result of Attention 3D U-Net; (d) the result of TE Net Network; (e) the result of 3D-Unet efficient-net-b2.

4   Discussion

As the Table 1 display, our solution for RSNA BraTS2021 segmentation task had a potential to obtain a better result if we setting filters number as same much with 3D U-Net [2]. Notably, it's interested found that the nest structure of TE Net maybe detected critical lesion about glioma but it perhaps not a ground label actually, just like Fig. 5 descripted, TE Net in d-column had acquired more features that lower the values of Hausdorff metric. Furthermore, we also discovered that different architecture of networks to ensemble then enable acquires complementary feature for glioma lesions. In the Fig. 6 show, the performance of 3D-Unet efficient-net-b2 with 3D-Unet (in Fig. 6 e-columns), had better than TE-Net Network ensemble with 3D-Unet (in Fig. 6 f-columns).

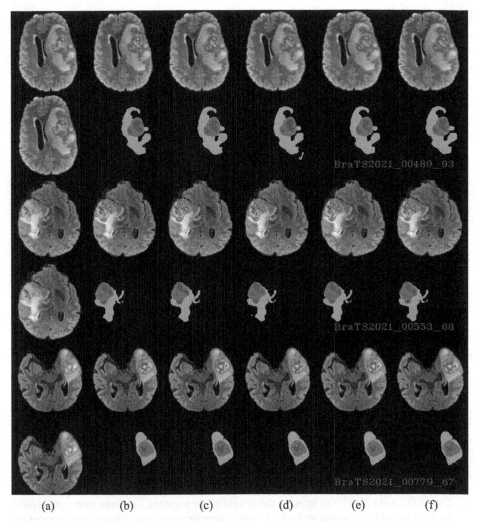

Fig. 6. The performance of our models inferenced in BraTS2021 Validation database. we select three cases (BraTS2021:00489,00553,00779), and also filtered some scans. In detail that had (a)–(f) six columns (a)cross-section of patient's flair scan; (b) 3D U-Net model's result; (c) result of 3D-Unet efficient-net-b2; (d) result of TE-Net Network; (e) result of ensemble of model (b) with model (c); (f) result of ensemble of model (b) with d model.

5   Conclusion

Given all that a nest of structure had ability automatically learns to focus on sub-regions class structures of varying shapes and sizes. Due to the time problem, we had a good idea could not achieved that replaced TE Net encoder with a series of pretrained efficient-net backbone, just that using RSNA-MICCAI Brain Tumor Radiogenomic Classification Task 2 [27] database. Unfortunately, classification task's data had a lot of problem, it's necessary takes some time to data clean.

References

1. https://www.synapse.org/#!Synapse:syn25829067/wiki/610865
2. Neugut, A.I., et al.: Magnetic resonance imaging-based screening for asymptomatic brain tumors: a review. Oncologist **24**(3), 375 (2019)
3. Henry, T., et al.: Brain tumor segmentation with self-ensembled, deeply-supervised 3D U-net neural networks: a BraTS 2020 challenge solution. arXiv preprint arXiv:2011.01045 (2020)
4. Baid, U., et al., The RSNA-ASNR-MICCAI BraTS 2021 benchmark on brain tumor segmentation and radiogenomic classification. arXiv:2107.02314 (2021)
5. Menze, B.H., et al.: The multimodal brain tumor image segmentation benchmark (BRATS). IEEE Trans. Med. Imaging **34**(10), 1993–2024 (2015). https://doi.org/10.1109/TMI.2014.2377694
6. Bakas, S., et al.: Advancing the cancer genome atlas glioma MRI collections with expert segmentation labels and radiomic features. Nat. Sci. Data **4**, 170117 (2017). https://doi.org/10.1038/sdata.2017.117
7. Bakas, S., et al.: segmentation labels and radiomic features for the pre-operative scans of the TCGA-GBM collection. Cancer Imaging Arch. (2017). https://doi.org/10.7937/K9/TCIA.2017.KLXWJJ1Q
8. Bakas, S., et al.: Segmentation labels and radiomic features for the pre-operative scans of the TCGA-LGG collection. Cancer Imaging Arch. (2017). https://doi.org/10.7937/K9/TCIA.2017.GJQ7R0EF
9. Taha, A.A., Hanbury, A.: Metrics for evaluating 3D medical image segmentation: analysis, selection, and tool. BMC Med. Imaging **15**(1), 1–28 (2015)
10. Isensee, F., et al.: nnU-Net for brain tumor segmentation. International MICCAI Brainlesion Workshop, pp. 118–132. Springer, Cham (2020)
11. Dice, L.R.: Measures of the amount of ecologic association between species. Ecology **26**(3), 297–302 (1945)
12. Ronneberger, O., Fischer, P., Brox, T.: U-net: convolutional networks for biomedical image segmentation. In: International Conference on Medical image computing and computer-assisted intervention, pp. 234–241. Springer, Cham (2015)
13. Zhou, Z., et al.: UNet++: a nested U-Net architecture for medical image segmentation. Deep Learning in Medical Image Analysis and Multimodal Learning for Clinical Decision Support, pp. 3–11. Springer, Cham (2018)
14. Çiçek, Ö., et al.: 3D U-Net: learning dense volumetric segmentation from sparse annotation. In: International conference on medical image computing and computer-assisted intervention, pp. 424–432. Springer, Cham (2016)
15. Oktay, O., et al.: Attention U-Net: Learning where to look for the pancreas. arXiv preprint arXiv:1804.03999 (2018)
16. Liu, Z., et al.: Deep learning based brain tumor segmentation: a survey. arXiv preprint arXiv:2007.09479 (2020)
17. Lei, T., et al.: Medical image segmentation using deep learning: a survey. arXiv preprint arXiv:2009.13120 (2020)
18. Nair, V., Hinton, G.E.: Rectified Linear Units Improve Restricted Boltzmann Machines. ICML (2010)
19. Wu, Y., He, K.: Group normalization. In: Ferrari, V., Hebert, M., Sminchisescu, C., Weiss, Y. (eds.) ECCV 2018. LNCS, vol. 11217, pp. 3–19. Springer, Cham (2018). https://doi.org/10.1007/978-3-030-01261-8_1
20. Liu, L., et al.: On the variance of the adaptive learning rate and beyond. arXiv preprint arXiv:1908.03265 (2019)

21. Zhang, M.R., et al.: Lookahead optimizer: k steps forward, 1 step back. arXiv preprint arXiv: 1907.08610 (2019)
22. Yong, H., et al.: Gradient centralization: A new optimization technique for deep neural networks. In: European Conference on Computer Vision, pp 635–652. Springer, Cham (2020)
23. Ruder, S.: An overview of gradient descent optimization algorithms. arXiv preprint arXiv: 1609.04747 (2016)
24. Tan, M., Le, Q.: Efficientnet: Rethinking model scaling for convolutional neural networks. In: International Conference on Machine Learning, pp. 6105–6114. PMLR (2019)
25. https://github.com/shijianjian/EfficientNet-PyTorch-3D
26. Sagi, O., Rokach, L.: Ensemble learning: a survey. Wiley Interdiscip. Rev.: Data Min. Knowl. Discov. **8**(4), e1249 (2018)
27. https://www.kaggle.com/c/rsna-miccai-brain-tumor-radiogenomic-classification/overview

MRI Brain Tumor Segmentation Using Deep Encoder-Decoder Convolutional Neural Networks

Benjamin B. Yan, Yujia Wei, Jaidip Manikrao M. Jagtap, Mana Moassefi,
Diana V. Vera Garcia, Yashbir Singh, Sanaz Vahdati, Shahriar Faghani,
Bradley J. Erickson, and Gian Marco Conte$^{(\boxtimes)}$ ⓘ

Mayo Clinic, Rochester, MN 55901, USA
Conte.gianmarco@mayo.edu

Abstract. In this study, we focus on Task 1 of the 2021 Multimodal Brain Tumor
Segmentation (BraTS) challenge. We present a modified U-net model aimed at
improving the segmentation of glioblastomas, reducing the computation time without compromising detection sensitivity. Our automated approach takes multimodal
MR images as input, generates a bounding box of the brain volume, and combines
the model predictions at the 2D slice level into a full 3D segmentation that is
written into a NIfTI file. On the official 2021 BraTS test set of 570 cases, the
model obtained median Dice scores of 0.80, 0.87, and 0.87, as well as median
95% Hausdorff distances of 2.45, 4.64, and 6.40 for the enhancing tumor, tumor
core, and whole tumor regions, respectively.

Keywords: MRI · Glioblastoma · Segmentation

1 Introduction

Brain tumors are one of the most aggressive forms of malignancies [1]. Gliomas are
the most frequent type of primary brain cancer, and they are caused by the carcinogen-
esis of glial cells in the spinal cord and brain [2]. Gliomas show variable aggressiveness, reflected in variable prognosis, with glioblastomas (GBMs) being one of the most
aggressive subtypes [2, 3].

Magnetic resonance imaging (MRI) is a non-invasive technique commonly used
in radiology to diagnose GBMs, characterize their inherent heterogeneity, and monitor
their progression; MRI is also widely applied for radiotherapy planning and patients'
follow-up [4].

GBMs typically show heterogeneous histological subregions, such as a necrotic
core, a tumor core, and peritumoral edema. The histological heterogeneity of GBMs
is reflected in their imaging phenotype, with sub-regions characterized by different
MRI intensity profiles [2, 5]. Differentiating between cancerous and normal tissue
and between sub-regions is challenging since tumor boundaries, shape, location, and

extent vary significantly between patients and are frequently hazy. Therefore, identifying and measuring the various tumor sub-regions is essential for radiotherapy planning, monitoring progression, and follow-up investigations [6].

Manual GBMs segmentation has traditionally been time-consuming and limited to qualified radiologists, whereas automatic segmentation offers the advantages of speed, consistency, and fatigue resistance. As a result, a robust semi-automated or automated glioma segmentation approach is in high demand to aid GBMs diagnosis and treatment strategies.

Automatic and semi-automatic segmentation of brain tumors has amassed much attention in the last 20 years because of its clinical importance and difficulty, resulting in the publication of several methods [7, 8]. Before the institution of the BraTS challenge, researchers evaluated their algorithms on local datasets, and there was no worldwide gold standard for the fair evaluation of techniques [9]. The BraTS challenge has offered a global forum for researchers to test their proposed algorithms on publicly available datasets, complete with a leaderboard. Over the years, many computational methods for tumor segmentation have been presented, including texture analysis, probabilistic models, and active contours, advancing the field of neuro-oncology [9–11].

The 2021 BraTS challenge focuses on the evaluation of state-of-the-art methods for the accurate segmentation of GBMs sub-regions (Task 1) and the classification of these tumors as MGMT methylated (MGMT+) and unmethylated (MGMT−) (Task 2) [8].

In the present study, we focus on Task 1 of the challenge, presenting a modified U-net model aiming at improving the segmentation of GBMs, reducing the computation time without compromising detection sensitivity.

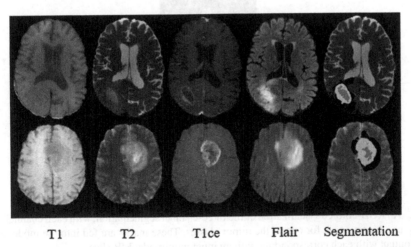

     T1   T2   T1ce   Flair   Segmentation

Fig. 1. Sample 2D MR slices from the BraTS training dataset and the corresponding manual segmentation of the necrotic tumor core (red), the peritumoral edematous/invaded tissue (green), and the enhancing tumor region (yellow). (Color figure online)

2 Methods

2.1 A Subsection Sample

We used the data available for the 2021 BraTS challenge (Fig. 1) [8], which is comprised of routine clinically acquired multi-parametric (mpMRI) scans of gliomas. The scans consist of four MRI sequences—pre-contrast T1-weighted, post-contrast T1-weighted with gadolinium contrast, T2-weighted, and T2-weighted fluid-attenuated inversion recovery (T2-FLAIR). All mpMRI images had a dimension of $240 \times 240 \times 155$, were skull-stripped, and had been resampled to an isotropic resolution of $1 \times 1 \times 1$ mm^3.

For each case, we stacked the four available MRI sequences and the target segmentation mask into a singular five-channel volume with dimensions $240 \times 240 \times 155 \times 5$. Then, we extracted a minimal bounding box surrounding the entire brain region, identified using a global threshold, and used it for training. Next, we normalized all MR voxels to [0,1] and extracted two-dimensional axial slices from the brain volume. Finally, we randomly cropped each MR slice to patches with a fixed size of $128 \times 128 \times 4$. We used these patches and the corresponding $128 \times 128 \times 1$ segmentation patches as input data to train our model. We performed one-hot encoding on each segmentation patch to obtain a three-channel $128 \times 128 \times 3$ slice, with each channel designed as a binary mask for the necrotic and non-enhancing tumor core (TC), peritumoral edema (ED), and enhancing tumor (ET), in this order (Fig. 2).

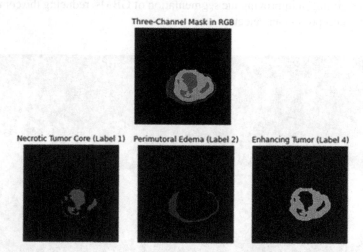

Fig. 2. An RGB-colored visualization of the three-channel segmentation, with each channel functioning as a binary mask for one of the tumor classes. These masks are fed into the model as the target output with each corresponding with an input multimodal MR slice.

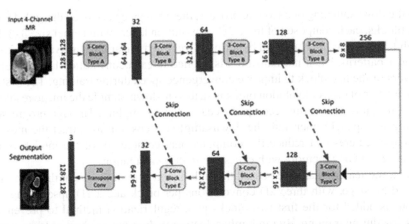

Fig. 3. Convolutional neural network (CNN) architecture, composed of 3-convolution blocks and a final 2D transpose convolution layer to create the one-hot encoded segmentation mask. Skip connections were used to transport information in shortcuts across the network.

2.2 Model Architecture

Our segmentation model (Figs. 3 and 4) is an adapted version of the prominent U-net model developed by Ronneberger et al. in 2015 [12].

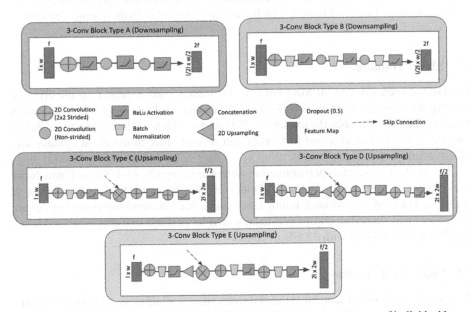

Fig. 4. Decomposition of each 3-convolution block in Fig. 1 into its sequence of individual layers (convolution, activation, normalization, etc.) and alteration of the feature map dimensions and feature width.

In the downsampling or encoding process, the input patch is passed through 4 convolution blocks, each composed of three 2D convolution layers with kernel size 3x3. Each convolution layer is accompanied by a ReLU (rectified linear unit) activation to extract nonlinear patterns; batch normalization is applied to each convolution layer except for the layers of the first block to improve convergence speed during training. The first convolution layer of each convolution block is strided to down-sample the image resolution. A doubling in feature width accompanies each down-sampling. Through progressively reducing the spatial dimension, the downsampling steps aim to extract the most crucial image features and reduce the computational complexity of the model to avoid inundating the GPU memory with excessive matrix calculations.

Next, the feature maps are passed through 3 convolution blocks in the upsampling or decoding stage, with three 2D convolutions per block and a 2D upsampling layer. Dropout is added for the first two blocks as a regularization method to prevent data overfitting during training. By randomly selecting to drop out a subset of layer outputs, the aim is to empower the network to learn multiple data representations in parallel, configuring it to be more generalizable and hence less likely to overfit the training data.

Each feature map in the upsampling stage is concatenated with a corresponding feature map in the downsampling stage using skip connections, as visualized in the model architecture scheme (Fig. 3). The purpose is to prevent excessive spatial information loss across the large network and bulwark against the vanishing gradient problem. The final layer is a transpose 2D convolution layer with a hyperbolic tangent activation function that produces the final $128 \times 128 \times 3$ segmentation mask. There was a total of 6,590,067 parameters in the full CNN model, which was implemented in Python using Tensorflow (v. 2.5) and Keras.

2.3 Model Training

In total, we used 150 and 50 MRI volumes for training and testing, respectively. The training data represents around 10% of the total data available from the 2021 BraTS training dataset. We trained the model for 200 epochs, with a batch size of 32, and Adam optimizer, which uses adaptive first-order and second-order moments to dynamically adjust its gradient descent process.

The gradient descent hyperparameters were a learning rate of 0.001 and beta decay rates of 0.9 and 0.999 for the 1st and 2nd moments. We calculated the loss function as an aggregate Dice loss across each tumor label in the three-channel segmentation output. The model was trained in end-to-end fashion and its performance was evaluated using an NVIDIA Tesla GPU with 32 GB of RAM.

2.4 End to End Pipeline

We used the validation data to build the end-to-end pipeline and evaluate the performance of our model. The pipeline was developed in Python and featured the NiBabel, Numpy, Tensorflow, and Keras libraries. First, we obtained a bounding box for the brain after reading the MR volume data from the NIfTI files. The intent was to reduce the relevant search space for the model for more efficient and computationally affordable region segmentation.

Then, we resized each axial slice to 128 × 128 using bicubic interpolation and passed it through the trained segmentation model as input. To create the final segmentation output for the whole volume, each voxel of the output slice was translated from the one-hot encoded vector to labels 0 (background), 1 (necrotic tumor core), 2 (peritumoral edematous tissue), or 4 (enhancing tumor) by applying sigmoid activation element-wise to the vector returning the label with the highest value. The purpose was to select the class with the highest predicted probability for each voxel, as reflected by the sigmoid function output.

We used label 0 (background) in case none of the three vector entries for the tumor labels were above 0.5 after the sigmoid activation. We then resized each slice to the original MR dimension and concatenated them along the z-axis; we set the regions outside the brain bounding to the background label. Finally, we saved the 240 × 240 × 155 volume as a NIfTI file, using the original affine matrix of the input scans to align the MR coordinates properly. The end-to-end segmentation process takes approximately 11–12 s for each patient. For the BraTS challenge, this pipeline was harnessed by a Docker image with an NVIDIA cuDNN CUDA (Deep Neural Network library) base to allow the segmentation to be expedited on graphics cards.

3 Results

Table 1. Results from the 2021 BraTS Validation Dataset (219 cases) for the enhancing tumor (ET), tumor core (TC), and whole tumor (WT) regions.

	Dice Score			95% Hausdorff			Sensitivity			Specificity		
	ET	TC	WT	ET	TC	WT	ET	TC	WT	ET	TC	WT
Median	0.79	0.87	0.89	3.00	4.90	4.58	0.73	0.82	0.93	1.00	1.00	1.00
25th Quantile	0.62	0.65	0.83	1.73	2.29	3.00	0.52	0.58	0.85	1.00	1.00	1.00
75th Quantile	0.86	0.92	0.92	6.88	10.37	8.63	0.84	0.90	0.97	1.00	1.00	1.00
Mean	0.68	0.72	0.85	28.27	17.75	8.47	0.63	0.68	0.87	1.00	1.00	1.00
SD	0.28	0.29	0.13	85.03	56.25	11.09	0.29	0.31	0.17	0.00	0.00	0.00

The model was evaluated on the BraTS validation dataset for 2021 using the BraTS challenge dashboard, with the results presented in Table 1 and Figs. 5 and 6. Here, the model achieved mean dice scores of 0.68, 0.72, and 0.85 for the enhancing tumor (ET), tumor core (TC), and whole tumor (WT) regions, respectively, and the median dice scores were 0.79, 0.87, and 0.89, respectively. The model also attained 95% Hausdorff distances of 28.27, 17.75, and 8.47 for the three regions in the aforementioned order.

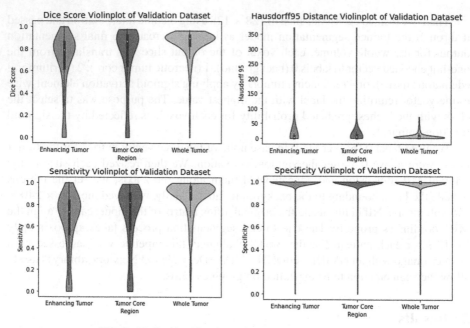

Fig. 5. Violin plots for the validation dataset (219 cases).

The provided classes in the training data are the enhancing tumor, necrotic tumor core, and peritumoral edematous tissue. However, the categories in the BraTS challenge evaluation are the hierarchically organized enhancing tumor, tumor core (enhancing tumor and necrotic core), and whole tumor (all three classes), as visualized below. One future approach could entail training the model to segment the ET, TC, and WT classes directly from the MR image, and allowing overlap in classes for each image voxel when rendering the final segmentation from the three-channel binary mask predictions (Fig. 7).

The model generally performed the best in segmenting the whole tumor, with an average Dice score of 0.85, sensitivity of 0.93, and specificity of 1.00, as well as a Dice median and interquartile range of 0.89 [0.83,0.92]. Meanwhile, the model was the least robust on the enhancing tumor class, with an average Dice score of 0.68, sensitivity of 0.63, and specificity of 1.00, and a median and interquartile Dice score range of 0.79 [0.62,0.86]. For all three classes, the mean specificity was 1.00, which suggests that the model performed well in classifying non-tumor voxels accurately. A visual sample of segmentation outcomes on the 2021 BraTS validation dataset is illustrated in Fig. 6.

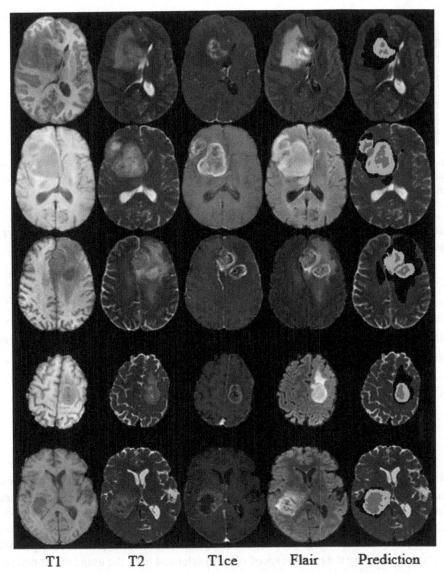

T1   T2   T1ce   Flair   Prediction

Fig. 6. Visual results from the 2021 BraTS validation dataset. Each row features the four MR sequences and corresponding segmentation prediction from the model. The red area represents the necrotic tumor core, the green is the peritumoral edema and the yellow is the enhancing tumor region. (Color figure online)

The model's final results are also provided for the 2021 BraTS test dataset, which is comprised of a larger set of 570 cases. Our approach obtained mean Dice scores of 0.67, 0.79, and 0.72, as well as median Dice scores of 0.80, 0.87, and 0.87 for the ET, TC, and WT regions, respectively (Table 2). We observe that similar to the validation set, the ET region was generally the most difficult region for the model to segment.

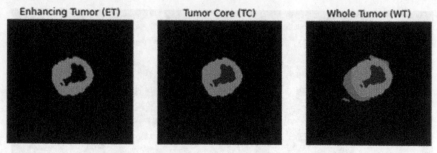

Fig. 7. Glioma regions for performance evaluation, with the enhancing tumor (yellow), necrotic tumor core (red), and peritumoral edema (green) sub-regions from the training data annotation. (Color figure online)

Table 2. Results from the 2021 BraTS test dataset (570 cases) for the enhancing tumor (ET), tumor core (TC), and whole tumor (WT) regions.

	Dice Score			95% Hausdorff			Sensitivity			Specificity		
	ET	TC	WT	ET	TC	WT	ET	TC	WT	ET	TC	WT
Median	0.80	0.87	0.87	2.45	4.64	6.40	0.74	0.85	0.93	1.00	1.00	1.00
25th Quantile	0.63	0.67	0.77	1.41	2.24	3.46	0.50	0.59	0.81	1.00	1.00	1.00
75th Quantile	0.87	0.93	0.91	6.69	12.08	20.22	0.84	0.93	0.97	1.00	1.00	1.00
Mean	0.67	0.72	0.79	32.32	31.34	23.13	0.63	0.70	0.83	1.00	1.00	1.00
SD	0.29	0.31	0.22	93.57	87.34	53.61	0.29	0.32	0.25	0.00	0.00	0.00

4 Discussion

Obtaining a fast and accurate segmentation of gliomas subregions has several implications in clinical practice: it is a crucial step when defining the diagnosis, prognosis, and treatment selection for these patients [13]. In this paper, we adapted the U-net model [12] to perform the segmentation of the whole tumor, the tumor core, and the enhancing tumor areas in a cohort of glioblastomas, using multiple MRI sequences as input. We were able to increase the training speed of our model and limit the usage of our computational resources by automatically drawing a bounding box around the brain and use it as the starting point to generate the inputs for our model. We obtained promising results when evaluating our model on the official validation and test sets from the 2021 Brats competition (Tables 1 and 2).

Based on our preliminary results, our model seems to struggle with the segmentation of the enhancing tumor areas; this is a particularly challenging task, although considering that we trained our model using only 10% of the available training data, we anticipate a significant improvement in our model performance using the training dataset in full.

References

1. Ferlay, J., Shin, H.-R., Bray, F., Forman, D., Mathers, C., Parkin, D.M.: Estimates of worldwide burden of cancer in 2008: GLOBOCAN 2008. Int. J. Cancer **127**(12), 2893–2917 (2010). https://doi.org/10.1002/ijc.25516
2. Van Meir, E.G., Hadjipanayis, C.G., Norden, A.D., Shu, H.-K., Wen, P.Y., Olson, J.J.: Exciting new advances in neuro-oncology: the avenue to a cure for malignant glioma. CA Cancer J. Clin. **60**(3), 166–193 (2010)
3. Bakas, S., et al.: Advancing The Cancer Genome Atlas glioma MRI collections with expert segmentation labels and radiomic features. Sci. Data **4**, 170117 (2017)
4. Wen, P.Y., et al.: Updated response assessment criteria for high-grade gliomas: response assessment in neuro-oncology working group. J. Clin. Oncol. **28**(11), 1963–1972 (2010)
5. Seow, P., Wong, J.H.D., Ahmad-Annuar, A., Mahajan, A., Abdullah, N.A., Ramli, N.: Quantitative magnetic resonance imaging and radiogenomic biomarkers for glioma characterisation: a systematic review. Br. J. Radiol. **91**(1092), 20170930 (2018)
6. Liu, L., et al.: Overall survival time prediction for high-grade glioma patients based on large-scale brain functional networks. Brain Imag. Behav. **13**(5), 1333–1351 (2018). https://doi.org/10.1007/s11682-018-9949-2
7. Angelini, E.D., Clatz, O., Mandonnet, E., Konukoglu, E., Capelle, L., Duffau, H.: Glioma dynamics and computational models: a review of segmentation, registration, and in silico growth algorithms and their clinical applications. Curr. Med. Imag. Rev. **3**(4), 262–276 (2007)
8. Baid, U., et al.: The RSNA-ASNR-MICCAI BraTS 2021 benchmark on brain tumor segmentation and radiogenomic classification. arXiv [cs.CV]. http://arxiv.org/abs/2107.02314 (2021)
9. Bakas, S., et al.: Identifying the best machine learning algorithms for brain tumor segmentation, progression assessment, and overall survival prediction in the BRATS challenge. arXiv [cs.CV]. http://arxiv.org/abs/1811.02629 (2018)
10. Menze, B.H., et al.: The multimodal brain tumor image segmentation benchmark (BRATS). IEEE Trans. Med. Imag. **34**(10), 1993–2024 (2015)
11. Bakas, S., et al.: Segmentation labels and radiomic features for the pre-operative scans of the TCGA-GBM collection. Cancer Imag. Arch. (2017). https://doi.org/10.7937/K9/TCIA.2017.KLXWJJ1Q
12. Ronneberger, O., Fischer, P., Brox, T.: U-Net: convolutional networks for biomedical image segmentation. arXiv [cs.CV]. http://arxiv.org/abs/1505.04597 (2015)
13. Fink, J.R., Muzi, M., Peck, M., Krohn, K.A.: Multimodality brain tumor imaging: MR imaging, PET, and PET/MR imaging. J. Nucl. Med. **56**(10), 1554–1561 (2015)
14. Bakas, S., et al.: Segmentation labels and radiomic features for the pre-operative scans of the TCGA-LGG collection. Cancer Imag. Arch. (2017). https://doi.org/10.7937/K9/TCIA.2017.GJQ7R0EF

Brain Tumor Segmentation with Patch-Based 3D Attention UNet from Multi-parametric MRI

Xue Feng[1]([✉]) [ORCID], Harrison Bai[2], Daniel Kim[3], Georgios Maragkos[4], Jan Machaj[5], and Ryan Kellogg[4]

[1] Biomedical Engineering, University of Virginia, Charlottesville, VA, USA
xf4j@virginia.edu
[2] Radiology and Radiological Science, Johns Hopkins University, Baltimore, MD, USA
[3] Diagnostic Imaging, Rhode Island Hospital and Alpert Medical School of Brown University, Providence, RI, USA
[4] Neurosurgery, University of Virginia, Charlottesville, VA, USA
[5] Neurosurgery, Prisma Health, Greenville, SC, USA

Abstract. Accurate segmentation of different sub-regions of gliomas including peritumoral edema, necrotic core, enhancing and non-enhancing tumor core from multiparametric MRI scans has important clinical relevance in diagnosis, prognosis and treatment of brain tumors. However, due to the highly heterogeneous appearance and shape, segmentation of the sub-regions is very challenging. Recent development using deep learning models has proved its effectiveness in the past several brain segmentation challenges as well as other semantic and medical image segmentation problems. In this paper we developed a deep-learning-based segmentation method using a patch-based 3D UNet with the attention block. Hyperparameters tuning and training and testing augmentations were applied to increase the model performance. Preliminary results showed effectiveness of the segmentation model and achieved mean Dice scores of 0.806 (ET), 0.863 (TC) and 0.918 (WT) in the validation dataset.

Keywords: Brain tumor segmentation · 3D U-Net · Attention block · Deep learning

1 Introduction

Gliomas are the most common primary brain malignancies, with different degrees of aggressiveness, variable prognosis and various heterogeneous histological sub-regions, i.e. peritumoral edema, necrotic core, enhancing and non-enhancing tumor core. This intrinsic heterogeneity of gliomas is also portrayed in their radiographic phenotypes, as their sub-regions are depicted by different intensity profiles disseminated across multi-parametric MRI (mpMRI) scans, reflecting differences in tumor biology. Quantitative analysis of imaging features such as volumetric measures after manual/semi-automatic segmentation of the tumor region has shown advantages in image-based tumor phenotyping over traditionally used clinical measures such as largest anterior-posterior, transverse, and inferior-superior tumor dimensions on a subjectively-chosen slice [1, 2]. Such phenotyping may enable assessment of reflected biological processes and assist in surgical and treatment planning. To compare and evaluate different automatic segmentation algorithms, the Multimodal Brain Tumor Segmentation Challenge (BraTS) 2021 was organized using multi-institutional pre-operative MRI scans for the segmentation of intrinsically heterogeneous brain tumor sub-regions [3–7]. More specifically, the dataset used in this challenge includes multiple-institutional clinically-acquired pre-operative multimodal MRI scans of glioblastoma (GBM/HGG) and low-grade glioma (LGG) containing a) native (T1) and b) post-contrast T1-weighted (T1Gd), c) T2-weighted (T2), and d) Fluid Attenuated Inversion Recovery (FLAIR) volumes. 1251 training volumes with annotated GD-enhancing tumor, peritumoral edema and necrotic and non-enhancing tumor were provided. The main goal of this study is to develop a deep learning-based method trained from the provided cases for automatic segmentation of these subregions. **Our Team ID is xf4j.**

2   Methods

For the brain tumor segmentation task, the steps in our proposed method include pre-processing of the images, patch extraction, building and training 3D U-Net structure with attention blocks, patch-based deployment with sliding window. Details are described as follows.

2.1   Image Pre-processing

As MR images do not have standard pixel intensity values, to reduce the effects from different contrasts and different subjects, each 3D image was normalized to 0-mean, unit variance by subtracting the mean value and dividing by the standard deviation, which are calculated on all voxels of the 3D image. After normalization, for each subject, images of all contrast were fused to form the last dimension so that the whole input image size becomes 155x240x240x4 following the order of T1, T1Gd, T2 and FLAIR.

2.2   Non-uniform Patch Extraction

For simplicity, we will use foreground to denote all tumor pixels and background to denote the rest. There are several challenges in directly using the whole images as the input to a 3D U-Net: 1) the memory of a moderate GPU is often 12 Gb so that in order to fit the model into the GPU, the network needs to greatly reduce the number of features and/or the layers, which often leads to a significant drop in performance as the expressiveness of the network is much reduced; 2) the training time will be greatly prolonged since more voxels contribute to calculation of the gradients at each step and the number of steps cannot be proportionally reduced during optimization; 3) as the background voxels dominate the whole image, the class imbalance will cause the model to focus on background if trained with uniform loss, or prone to false positives if trained with weighted loss that favors the foreground voxels. Therefore, to more effectively utilize the training data, smaller patches were extracted from each subject. As the foreground labels contain much more variability and are the main targets to segment, more patches from the foreground voxels should be extracted.

In implementation, during each epoch, a random patch was extracted from each subject using non-uniform probabilities. The valid patch centers were first calculated by removing edges to make sure each extracted patch was completely within the whole image. Instead of fixing the patch selection, we randomly select one patch from each training sample during each epoch. Specifically, we used a probability of 0.9 to select the patch whose center is a foreground voxel and choose the voxel randomly from all foreground voxels; for the remaining probability of 0.1 we randomly select the patch center from all voxels.

2.3   Network Structure and Training

A 3D U-Net based network was used as the general structure, as shown in Fig. 1. Zero padding was used to make sure the spatial dimension of the output is the same with the input. For each encoding block, a VGG like network with two consecutive 3D convolutional layers with kernel size 3 followed by the activation function and batch norm layers were used. The number of features was doubled while the spatial dimension was halved with every encoding block, as in conventional U-Net structure. To improve the expressiveness of the network, a large number of features were used in the first encoding block. Symmetric decoding blocks were used with skip-connections from corresponding encoding blocks. Features were concatenated to the de-convolution outputs. The extracted segmentation map of the input patch was expanded to the multi-class the ground truth labels (3 foreground classes and the background). The loss function was chosen as the summation of weighted cross entropy and Dice loss.

In the decoding blocks, the attention layers were added to help the network to better focus on the regions-of-interest spatially.

The number of encoding/decoding blocks, the weights in the loss function and the patch size were chosen as the tunable hyper-parameters when constructing multiple models. detailed parameters shown in Table 1. N denotes the input size, M denotes the number of encoding/decoding blocks and f denotes the input features at the first layer. For weighted loss, 1.0 was used for background and 2.0 was used for each class of foreground voxels.

Training was performed on a Nvidia Titan Xp GPU with 12 Gb memory. 4000 epochs were used. As mentioned earlier, during each epoch, only one patch was extracted every subject. To better control the training time, each epoch is defined to sample 100 cases randomly from all training samples, resulting in a total of 400000 iterations. The Tensorflow framework was used with stochastic gradient descent (SGD) optimizer with learning rate decay. Batch size was set to 1 during training. Augmentations applied include random shift, rotation, and left-right mirroring. The total training time was about 96 h. Figure 2 shows the training loss and Dice scores at each iteration (blue) and the average value (orange). Due to random patch sampling, the fluctuations during training is high.

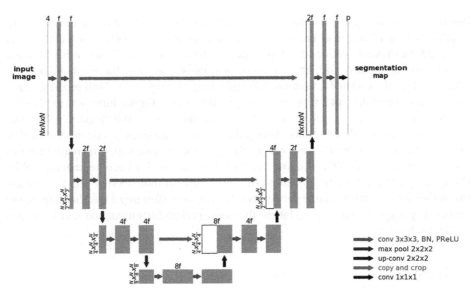

Fig. 1. 3D U-Net structure with 3 encoding and 3 decoding blocks.

Table 1. Detailed parameters for the 3D U-Net models

Batch size	M	N	f	Weights
1	5	128 * 128 * 128	32	1.0 (background), 4.0, 4.0, 4.0

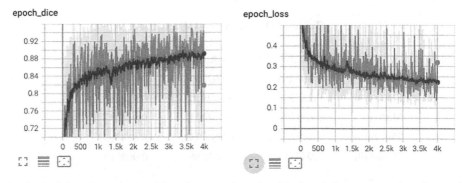

Fig. 2. Training dice scores and loss for every iteration (blue) and the average values (orange). (Color figure online)

2.4 Deployment

Due to the fact that the entire image cannot fit into the memory during deployment, a sliding window approach needs to be used to get the output for each subject. However, as significant padding was made to generate the output label map at the same size as the input, boundary voxels of a patch were expected to yield unstable predictions when sliding the window across the whole image without overlaps. To alleviate this problem, a stride size at a fraction of the window size was used and the output probability was averaged. In implementation, the deployment window size was chosen to be the same as the training window size, and the stride was chosen as ½ of the window size. For each window, the original image and left-right flipped image were both predicted, and the average probability after flipping back the output of the flipped input was used as the output. Therefore, each voxel, except for a few on the edge, will be predicted 16 times when sliding across all directions. Although smaller stride sizes can be used to further improve the accuracy with more averages, the deployment time will be increased 8 times for every ½ reduction of the window size and thus will quickly become unmanageable. Using the parameters as mentioned on the same GPU, it took about 1 min to generate the output for the entire volume per subject. Instead of performing a thresholding on the probability output to get the final labels, the direct probability output was saved for each model to the disk.

3   Results

3.1   Brain Tumor Segmentation

All 1251 training subjects were used in training the final model. 219 subjects were provided as validation. The dice indexes, sensitivities and specificities, 95 Hausdorff distances of the enhanced tumor (ET), whole tumor (WT) and tumor core (TC) were automatically calculated after submitting to the challenge website (https://www.synapse.org/#!Synapse:syn25829067/wiki/611501). Tables 2 and 3 show the statistics of the Dice scores and Hausdorff distances for validation.

Table 2. Dice scores for validation

	Dice_ET	Dice_TC	Dice_WT
Mean	0.80628597	0.86306681	0.91779557
SD	0.25757809	0.19942057	0.07751627
Median	0.891156	0.934305	0.941277
25quantile	0.81325675	0.86070525	0.89430325
75quantile	0.9437155	0.965066	0.962915

Figure 3 shows the segmentation results for one case overlayed on T1ce images in the validation dataset containing 8 slices around the region of segmented tumor. Red shows the whole tumor, blue corresponds to label 2 and yellow corresponds to label 4. The contours align well with the hyperintensity regions of on this contrast.

Table 3. Hausdorff distances for validation

	Hausdorff95_ET	Hausdorff95_TC	Hausdorff95_WT
Mean	20.8288482	6.38856155	5.31638349
SD	77.8010076	26.1483438	9.92331121
Median	1.414214	2	2.236068
25quantile	1	1	1.414214
75quantile	2.828427	4.472136	4.472136

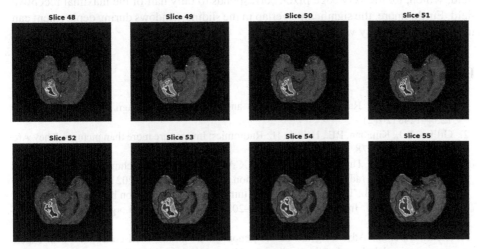

Fig. 3. Segmentation results on T1ce images for one validation case.

Testing was performed by uploading a docker image and running on unseen dataset. The results are shown in Table 4.

Table 4. Dice scores for testing

	Dice_ET	Dice_TC	Dice_WT
Mean	0.85851705	0.8701169	0.9228672
SD	0.2008376	0.24114078	0.08065181
Median	0.923919	0.9572755	0.946424
25quantile	0.851321	0.902946	0.910828
75quantile	0.95989275	0.97857825	0.96915025

4 Discussion and Conclusions

In this paper we developed a brain tumor segmentation method using a patch-based 3D U-Net with attention block. Intensity normalization was applied in pre-processing. In selecting patches for training, the tumor voxels are heavily biased to increase the sensitivity of the model.

Compared with the patch-based model that only predicts the center pixel, when predicting the segmentation label maps for the full patch, different pixels are very likely to have different effective receptive field sizes due to the zero padding in the edge. We argue that a pixel should still be able to be predicted even based on partial receptive field, which, for the very edge pixel, corresponds to only half of the maximal receptive field. Furthermore, the significant overlap in the sliding windows during deployment can improve the accuracy with more averages.

References

1. Kumar, V., et al.: Radiomics: the process and the challenges. Magn. Reson. Imaging **30**, 1234–1248 (2012)
2. Gillies, R.J., Kinahan, P.E., Hricak, H.: Radiomics: images are more than pictures. They Are Data Radiology **278**, 563–577 (2015)
3. Baid, U., et al., The RSNA-ASNR-MICCAI BraTS 2021 benchmark on brain tumor segmentation and radiogenomic classification. arXiv:2107.02314 (2021)
4. Menze, B.H., et al.: The multimodal brain tumor image segmentation benchmark (BRATS). IEEE Trans. Med. Imaging **34**(10), 1993–2024 (2015). https://doi.org/10.1109/TMI.2014. 2377694
5. Bakas, S., et al.: Advancing the cancer genome atlas glioma MRI collections with expert segmentation labels and radiomic features. Nat. Sci. Data **4**, 170117 (2017). https://doi.org/ 10.1038/sdata.2017.117
6. Bakas, S., et al.: Segmentation labels and radiomic features for the pre-operative scans of the TCGA-GBM collection. The Cancer Imaging Archive (2017). https://doi.org/10.7937/K9/ TCIA.2017.KLXWJJ1Q
7. Bakas, S., et al.: Segmentation labels and radiomic features for the pre-operative scans of the TCGA-LGG collection. The Cancer Imaging Archive (2017). https://doi.org/10.7937/ K9/TCIA.2017.GJQ7R0EF
8. Bakas, S., et al.: Identifying the best machine learning algorithms for brain tumor segmentation, progression assessment, and overall survival prediction in the BRATS challenge. arXiv preprint arXiv:1811.02629 (2018)
9. Gal, Y., Ghahramani, Z.: Dropout as a bayesian approximation: representing model uncertainty in deep learning. arXiv preprint. arXiv:1506.02142 (2015)
10. Pan, H., Feng, Y., Chen, Q., Meyer, C., Feng, X.: Prostate segmentation from 3D MRI using a two-stage model and variable-input based uncertainty measure. arXiv preprint. arXiv:1903. 02500 (2019)

Dice Focal Loss with ResNet-like Encoder-Decoder Architecture in 3D Brain Tumor Segmentation

Hai Nguyen-Truong[1,2,3] and Quan-Dung Pham[1(✉)]

[1] VinBrain, Ho Chi Minh City, Vietnam
{v.haing,v.dungpham}@vinbrain.net
[2] University of Science, Ho Chi Minh City, Vietnam
[3] Vietnam National University, Ho Chi Minh City, Vietnam

Abstract. Accurate identification of brain tumor sub-regions boundaries in MRI plays a profoundly important role in clinical applications, such as surgical treatment planning, image-guided interventions, monitoring tumor growth, and the generation of radiotherapy maps. However, manual delineation practices has suffered from many problems such as requiring anatomical knowledge, taking considerable time for annotation, showing inaccuracy due to human error. To tackle these issues, automated segmentation of brain tumors from 3D magnetic resonance images (MRIs) has been used in recent years. In this work, a ResNet-like Encoder-Decoder architecture is trained on the Multimodal Brain Tumor Segmentation Challenge (BraTS) 2021 training dataset. Experimental results demonstrate that this work shows a faily good performance in brain tumor segmentation.

Keywords: Seg resnet · Brain tumor segmentation · Glioma · Glioblastoma · Segmentation · Machine learning · Radiomics · Medical image segmentation

1 Introduction

Recently, deep neural networks have become a standard tool for solving a wide range of computer vision problems in general, in particular segmentation tasks. In the last decade, based on the success of U-Net [1], the application of deep neural networks for medical image segmentation has attracted huge attention; with the goal of saving physicians time and providing an accurate reproducible solution for further analysis and monitoring.

In medical domain, brain tumor segmentation is considered one of the most challenging task. The most common and aggressive malignant primary tumor of the central nervous system in adults are Glioblasttoma (GBM) [2] and diffuse astrocytic glioma with molecular features of GBM. Nowadays, Magnetic Resonance Imaging (MRI) plays a pivotal role in brain tumor analysis, monitoring tumor growth and surgical treatment planning. To fully assess tumor

A. Crimi and S. Bakas (Eds.): BrainLes 2021, LNCS 12963, pp. 97–105, 2022.
https://doi.org/10.1007/978-3-031-09002-8_9

heterogeneity, it is essential to acquire several complimentary 3D MRI including T1-weighted sequence (T1), T1 weighted sequence enhanced sequence using gadolinium contrast agents (T1Gd), T2 weighted sequence (T2), and T2 fluid attenuated inversion recovery sequence (T2-FLAIR).

Multimodal brain tumor segmentation challenge (BraTS) has been held for 10 years, which provides a platform to evaluate the state-of-the-art methods for the segmentation of brain tumor sub-regions such as the enhancing tumor (ET), the tumor core (TC), and the whole tumor (WT) by providing a 3D MRI dataset with ground truth tumor segmentation labels annotated. BraTS 2021 [2–6] training dataset comprises 1251 cases for training and 219 for validation, each with for 3D MRI modalities (T1, T1Gd, T2 and T2 FLAIR) rigidly aligned, resampled to a uniform isotropic resolution ($1mm^3$). The input image size is $240 \times 240 \times 155$. There are 25 institutions contributed data to this challenge.

In this work, the semantic approach for 3D brain tumor segmentation from multimodal 3D MRIs of Andriy Myronenko [7] is implemented. In addition to this, CLARA training sdk workflow from NVIDIA is also utilized to reduce training time and inference time (Fig. 1).

2   Methods

In this work, the training pipeline is designed based on Segentation ResNet model [7] without VAE branch and Clara training sdk workflow from NVIDIA.

2.1   Network Architecture

This network followed the common encoder-decoder architecture for segmentation, with larger encoder to extract features and smaller decoder to reconstruct the image (Fig. 2).

Two main components in this network are the blue and green blocks. The blue block is a 3D convolution layer with kernel size 3 with stride and padding equaled 1. The green one is ResNet-like block which consisted of normalization and non linear activation (ReLU [8]), followed by 3D convolution layer. For normalization method, Group Norm [9] is used because of its better performance with small batch size.

In the encoder, at each stages, image size reduces 2 times while the number of filter simultaneously increases 2 times in order to increase the feature size. At each spatial level, there are 2 green blocks where the first block has stride = 1 and out_channel = in_channel and the second one has stride = 2 and out_channel = $2 \times$ in_channel. At the end, the final feature map is 8 times spatially smaller then the input image, produces the highest level of feature map.

Decoder architecture is similar to the encoder one, but with a single green block per spatial level. At each stages, 3D convolution layer with kernel size 1 is used to reduce the number of features, followed by 3D Upsample with trilinear interpolation to increase the image size. Moreover, a skip connection from encoder was fused with the decoder at the same spatial level. At the end of

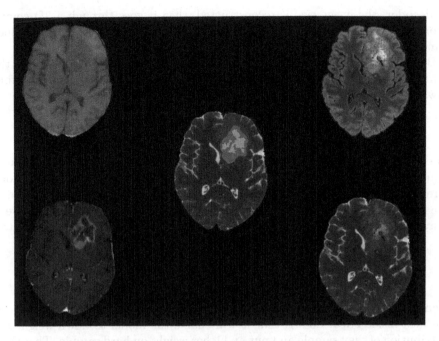

Fig. 1. Viusalization of an example in BraTS 2021 dataset. Upper left: FLAIR, Upper right: T1, Lower left: T1CE, Lower right: T2, Middle: T2 with labelmap overlay. In the Middle image, RED: Enhancing tumor (ET), GREEN: Tumor core (TC) and BLUE: whole tumor (WT).

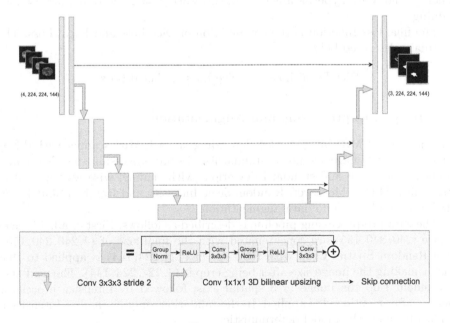

Fig. 2. Network architecture

the decoder, the image size is reconstructed, then it goes through a 3D convolution layer (kernel size 1, out_channel 3) and a sigmoid function to produce segmentation mask.

BraTS 2021 dataset contains 1251 images, and it is enough to train the network without VAE regularization. In the experiments, the proposed network shows higher result than the architecture in [7].

2.2 Dice Focal Loss

Dice Loss is the most common loss in semantic segmentation problem because it can capture the local and global information simultaneously and it has strong correlation with Dice Score (main metrics of semantic segmentation). Let y and $\hat{y}$ be the ground truth of segmentation and the prediction of model, respectively. To avoid NaN loss when $\hat{y} = y = 0$, ε is added into numerator and denominator.

$$\text{Dice Loss}\ (y, \hat{y}) = 1 - \frac{2\hat{y}y + \varepsilon}{\hat{y} + y + \varepsilon}.$$

Focal Loss [10] is as known as an variation of Binary Cross Entropy loss. The idea inside Focal Loss is that it will enable the model to down-weight the contribution of easy sample and put an higher weight on hard sample. Therefore, it works well with highly imbalance dataset.

$$\text{Focal Loss}\ (y, \hat{y}) = -\left(\alpha \cdot y \cdot \hat{y}^{\gamma} \log(1 - \hat{y}) + \alpha \cdot (1 - y)(1 - \hat{y})^{\gamma} \log(\hat{y}) \right).$$

Where γ and α are hyperparameters. In this work, $\gamma = 2$ and $\alpha = 1$ are used for training.

The final loss function is the combination of Dice Loss and Focal Loss. The formula is described below

$$\text{Dice Focal Loss}\ =\ \text{Dice Loss}\ +\ \text{Focal Loss}.$$

2.3 Image Pre-processing and Augmentation

The intensity of MRI image varied depending on each MRI scanner with different parameters, image should be standardize. In pre-processing step, Normalize Intensity (by mean and standard deviation) with channel wise was applied to solve this problem. Moreover, Random Scale Intensity and Random Shift Intensity are also added to do data augmentation.

The data pre-processing pipeline is described as follows. First of all, 4 images of size $(240, 240, 155)$ are concatenated with the final size of $(4, 240, 240, 155)$, then Random Spatial Crop with ROI size of $(224, 224, 144)$ is applied to that image, making the image size after being crop is $(4, 224, 224, 144)$. The next step is Random Flip the image in 3 spatial axis, followed by intensity processing method aforementioned is applied. In the validation, only Normalize Intensity is applied to make the model deterministic.

2.4   Training Details

In the training pipeline, five-fold cross-validation is used in order to utilize all of the data in training set while controlling model over-fitting or under-fitting. For monitoring purpose, Hausdorff distance (95 percentile) and Mean Dice Score are applied and calculated at each epoch. Simple Inference is used in the training step (the images went directly through the model and got the segmentation mask), while Sliding Window Inference is used in the validation, which increases the final dice score of models.

Adam optimization [11] is used for training purpose with the initial learning rate is 10^{-4} and CosineAnnealingLR is used as the learning rate scheduler associated with optimizer.

Float precision 16 (FP 16) is turned on, which enables the system to train efficiently on deep neural network, whereas the memory usage is reduced, thus lead to higher performance.

Clara training SDK[1] is used for end-to-end workflow: training, evaluation and inference time in order to accelerate deep learning model in various use cases, especially with optimized-pipeline and high-level API of many functions.

2.5   Ensemble Method and Post-processing

After 5-fold cross-validation training, ensemble is applied to increase the final performance on public and private test. In the ensemble phase, mean ensemble is used to leverage the final score, where weight of each fold is calculate based on their performance on our own test dataset.

Different ROI size of sliding window inference method are applied at each fold, for ensemble not only in each fold but also for the total validation phase. $(208, 208, 160)$, $(224, 224, 160)$, and $(240, 240, 160)$ are three different ROI size configurations for ensemble stages, where the ROI size of $(208, 208, 160)$ has the highest dice score of Enhancing Tumor (less false negative example), while achieving the same dice score over Tumor Core and Whole Tumor.

The result on the leaderboard shows there are a lot of false negative examples, which means there is no segmentation mask. Therefore, a threshold is applied to the Enhance Tumor mask. If the total number of pixels (in the final submission, 150 is chosen) are less than the threshold, that pixel becomes that pixel of tumor core. Although this method may lead to the fact that some tumor was ignore, the gain is outweighed the loss.

3   Results

3.1   Training Phase

1251 images from training are split: 800 for training, 200 for validation (5-fold) and 251 for testing. Testing is used for optimizing model and fine tuning. The

---

[1] https://docs.nvidia.com/clara/clara-train-sdk/pt/index.html.

Table 1a shows the average dice score of each fold while the Table 1b illustrates the testing one.

While fold 2, fold 3, fold 4 and fold 5 had the similar result on both validation and testing, fold 1 indicates its superior to the remaining fold, approximately 1% in validation and 0.5% in testing. Overall, the average dice score is consistent in each fold and in two tables.

Table 1. Evaluation on our own validation and testing

(a) Validation

	Validation		
	Mean	ET	TC	WT
Fold 1	0.9193	0.8960	0.9349	0.9304
Fold 2	0.9061	0.8817	0.9168	0.9277
Fold 3	0.9062	0.8801	0.9109	0.9281
Fold 4	0.9048	0.8767	0.9088	0.9305
Fold 5	0.9057	0.8840	0.9104	0.9257

(b) Testing

	Testing		
	Mean	ET	TC	WT
Fold 1	0.9202	0.8935	0.9269	0.9413
Fold 2	0.9161	0.8906	0.9206	0.9391
Fold 3	0.9163	0.8904	0.9206	0.9392
Fold 4	0.9164	0.8909	0.9235	0.9363
Fold 5	0.9175	0.8912	0.9234	0.9389

3.2   Online Validation Phase

Although the validation and testing of each fold have the similar results, the model performs not well in the online validation phase. This is mainly because the validation data contains many rare samples with the small region while in training data, there are not many samples with the small area, thus made the model not predict fairly well. Final result is showed in the Table 2 with the mean dice score of each fold and post pre-processing.

Post-processing shows the improvement in the dice score of Enhance Tumor a lot (about 3%) because almost false negative example which made the dice score equals to 0. Ensemble method also indicates better performance as it increase each tumor by more than 0.5%. Ensemble 3 ROI size has the similar result with the previous one in the online validation phase, while it outperformed the ensemble on the testing dataset by average 0.3% in term of dice score of each tumor.

The best performance on the validation phase for each type of tumor was: ET: **0.8451**, TC: **0.8785** and WT: **0.9244**.

Table 2. The result of online validation phase

	Validation phase		
	ET	TC	WT
Fold 1	0.7885	0.8668	0.9202
Fold 2	0.7974	0.8700	0.9178
Fold 3	0.8021	0.8696	0.9197
Fold 4	0.7965	0.8613	0.9172
Fold 5	0.7804	0.8713	0.9187
Fold 1 _ Post Process ET	0.8374	0.8668	0.9202
Fold 2 _ Post Process ET	0.8370	0.8700	0.9178
Fold 3 _ Post Process ET	0.8412	0.8696	0.9197
Fold 4 _ Post Process ET	0.8334	0.8613	0.9172
Fold 5 _ Post Process ET	0.8231	0.8713	0.9187
Ensemble 5 fold	0.8060	0.8785	0.9230
Ensemble 5 fold _ Post Process	**0.8451**	**0.8785**	0.9230
Ensemble 3 roi size	0.8421	0.8767	**0.9244**

Figure 3, 4 and 5 are the visualization of our model in online validation phase, which are best mean dice score, median mean dice score and worst mean dice score, respectively. It is worth noted that the image on the left was T1, while the middle is T2 and the last right image is T2 with segmentation overlay.

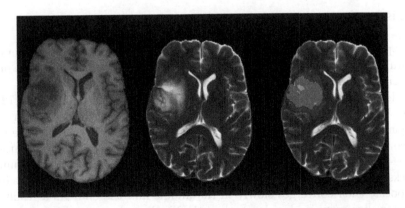

Fig. 3. ID 01793: Dice score: ET 0.9756 TC: 0.9885 WT: 0.9809. In the third image, RED: Enhancing tumor (ET), GREEN: tumor core (TC) and BLUE: whole tumor (WT).

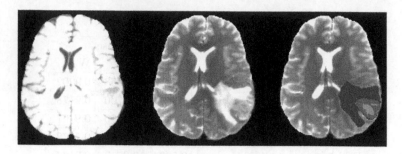

Fig. 4. ID 01766: Dice score: ET 0.8999 TC: 0.9368 WT: 0.9550. In the third image, RED: Enhancing tumor (ET), GREEN: tumor core (TC) and BLUE: whole tumor (WT).

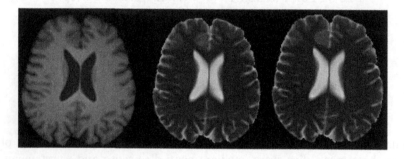

Fig. 5. ID 01743: dice score: ET 1.0 TC: 0.0 WT: 0.6849. In the third image, RED: enhancing tumor (ET), GREEN: Tumor core (TC) and BLUE: whole tumor (WT).

4   Discussion

The proposed solution to BraTS 2021 challenge is based on the training workflow of Clara training SDK from NVIDIA with small modifications and the model architecture from the winner of BraTS 2018 challenge [7].

Modern model achitecture like Unet with Transformer (UNETR [12]) is applied but does not perform well. It is gpu memory-consuming and training time consuming. However, the final result shows worse Dice Score, as the mean dice score of tumors converged at 88% in Dice Score (in our validation dataset).

Fine-tuning the model: increase number of filters and increase the number of blocks per spatial level. These modifications shows better performance on 50 first epochs, then converges slowly in the middle and the end. As a result, the final mean dice score is also slower than the baseline one.

References

1. Ronneberger, O., Fischer, P., Brox, T.: U-net: convolutional networks for biomedical image segmentation. In: Navab, N., Hornegger, J., Wells, W.M., Frangi, A.F. (eds.) MICCAI 2015. LNCS, vol. 9351, pp. 234–241. Springer, Cham (2015). https://doi.org/10.1007/978-3-319-24574-4_28
2. Baid, U., et al.: The RSNA-ASNR-MICCAI BraTS 2021 benchmark on brain tumor segmentation and Radiogenomic classification. In: CoRR abs/2107.02314 (2021). arXiv: 2107.02314. URL: https://arxiv.org/abs/2107.02314
3. Menze, B.H., et al.: The multimodal brain tumor image segmentation benchmark (BRATS). IEEE Trans. Med. Imaging **34**(10), 1993–2024 (2015). https://doi.org/10.1109/TMI.2014.2377694
4. Bakas, S., et al.: advancing the cancer genome atlas glioma MRI collections with expert segmentation labels and radiomic features. Sci. Data **4**(1), 1–13 (2017)
5. Bakas, S., et al.: Segmentation labels and radiomic features for the pre-operative scans of the TCGA-GBM collection. In: The Cancer Imaging Archive (2017). https://doi.org/10.7937/K9/TCIA.2017.KLXWJJ1Q
6. Bakas, S., et al.: Segmentation labels and radiomic features for the pre-operative scans of the TCGA-LGG collection. In: The Cancer Imaging Archive (2017). https://doi.org/10.7937/K9/TCIA.2017.GJQ7R0EF
7. Myronenko, A.: 3D MRI brain tumor segmentation using autoencoder regularization. In: CoRR abs/1810.11654 (2018). arXiv: 1810.11654, http://arxiv.org/abs/1810.11654
8. Agarap, A.F.: Deep learning using rectified linear units (ReLU). In: CoRR abs/1803.08375 (2018). arXiv: 1803.08375, http://arxiv.org/abs/1803.08375
9. Wu, Y., He, K.: Group Normalization. Int. J. Comput. Vis. **128**(3), 742–755 (2019). https://doi.org/10.1007/s11263-019-01198-w
10. Tsung-Yi, L., et al.: Focal Loss for Dense Object Detection. In: CoRR abs/1708.02002 (2017). arXiv: 1708.02002, http://arxiv.org/abs/1708.02002
11. Loshchilov, I., Hutter, F.: Fixing weight decay regularization in adam. In: CoRR abs/1711.05101 (2017). arXiv: 1711.05101, http://arxiv.org/abs/1711.05101
12. Hatamizadeh, A., et al.: UNETR: Transformers for 3D medical image segmentation (2021). arXiv: 2103.10504 [eess.IV]

HNF-Netv2 for Brain Tumor Segmentation Using Multi-modal MR Imaging

Haozhe Jia[1,2,4], Chao Bai[1,2], Weidong Cai[3], Heng Huang[4,5],
and Yong Xia[1,2(✉)]

[1] Research & Development Institute of Northwestern Polytechnical University
in Shenzhen, Shenzhen 518057, China
yxia@nwpu.edu.cn
[2] National Engineering Laboratory for Integrated Aero-Space-Ground-Ocean
Big Data Application Technology, School of Computer Science and Engineering,
Northwestern Polytechnical University, Xi'an 710072, China
[3] School of Computer Science, University of Sydney, Sydney, NSW 2006, Australia
[4] Department of Electrical and Computer Engineering, University of Pittsburgh,
Pittsburgh, PA 15261, USA
[5] JD Finance America Corporation, California, CA 94043, USA

Abstract. In our previous work, *i.e.*, HNF-Net, high-resolution feature representation and light-weight non-local self-attention mechanism are exploited for brain tumor segmentation using multi-modal MR imaging. In this paper, we extend our HNF-Net to HNF-Netv2 by adding inter-scale and intra-scale semantic discrimination enhancing blocks to further exploit global semantic discrimination for the obtained high-resolution features. We trained and evaluated our HNF-Netv2 on the multi-modal Brain Tumor Segmentation Challenge (BraTS) 2021 dataset. The result on the test set shows that our HNF-Netv2 achieved the average Dice scores of 0.878514, 0.872985, and 0.924919, as well as the Hausdorff distances (95%) of 8.9184, 16.2530, and 4.4895 for the enhancing tumor, tumor core, and whole tumor, respectively. Our method won the RSNA 2021 Brain Tumor AI Challenge Prize (Segmentation Task), which ranks 8th out of all 1250 submitted results.

Keywords: Brain tumor · Segmentation · HNF-Netv2 · Multi-scale fusion

1 Introduction

Brain gliomas are the most common primary brain malignancies, which generally contain heterogeneous histological sub-regions, i.e. edema/invasion, active tumor structures, cystic/necrotic components, and non-enhancing gross abnormality. Accurate and automated segmentation of these intrinsic sub-regions using multi-modal magnetic resonance (MR) imaging is critical for the potential diagnosis and treatment of this disease. To this end, the multi-modal brain tumor segmentation challenge (BraTS) has been held for many years, which provides a platform to evaluate the state-of-the-art methods for the segmentation of brain tumor sub-regions [2–5,13].

With deep learning being widely applied to medical image analysis, fully convolutional network (FCN) based methods have been designed for this segmentation task and have shown convincing performance in previous challenges. Kamnitsas *et al.*. [11] constructed a 3D dual pathway CNN, namely DeepMedic, which simultaneously processes the input image at multiple scales with a dual pathway architecture so as to exploit both local and global contextual information. DeepMedic also uses a 3D fully connected conditional random field to remove false positives. In [7], Isensee *et al.*. achieved outstanding segmentation performance using a 3D U-Net with instance normalization and leaky ReLU activation, in conjunction with a combination loss function and a region-based training strategy. In [14], Myronenko *et al.*. incorporated a variational auto-encoder (VAE) based reconstruction decoder into a 3D U-Net to regularize the shared encoder, and achieved the 1st place segmentation performance in BraTS 2018. In BraTS 2019, Jiang *et al.*. [10] proposed a two-stage cascaded U-Net to segment the brain tumor sub-regions from coarse to fine, where the second-stage model has more channel numbers and uses two decoders so as to boost performance. This method achieved the best performance in the BraTS 2019 segmentation task. In our previous work [9], we proposed a High-resolution and Non-local Feature Network (HNF-Net) to segment brain tumor in multi-modal MR images. The HNF-Net is constructed based mainly on the parallel multi-scale fusion (PMF) module, which can maintain strong high-resolution feature representation and aggregate multi-scale contextual information. The expectation-maximization attention (EMA) module is also introduced to the model to enhance the long-range dependent spatial contextual information at the cost of acceptable computational complexity. In BraTS 2020 challenge, we designed a two-stage cascaded HNF-Net and thereby constructed a Hybrid High-resolution and Non-local Feature Network (H^{2}NF-Net) [8], which uses the single and cascaded models to segment different brain tumor sub-regions. The proposed H^{2}NF-Net won the second place in the BraTS 2020 challenge segmentation task out of 78 ranked participants.

It is well recognized that the features in shallow stages tend to have more detailed spatial information while those in deep stages can obtain more semantic discrimination. Attributed to our PMF modules, the high-resolution features are well maintained in the original HNF-Net, however, the semantic discrimination of the obtained features might be insufficient due to the limited global context learning ability of the current network. To address these, in this paper, we further propose a HNF-Netv2 to improve the segmentation performance for this challenging task. Specifically, we extend the original HNF-Net by adding inter-scale and intra-scale semantic discrimination enhancing (inter-scale SDE and intra-scale SDE) blocks, which can exploit the global context and thereby enhance the current high-resolution features with semantic discrimination. We evaluated the proposed HNF-Netv2 on the BraTS 2021 challenge dataset and

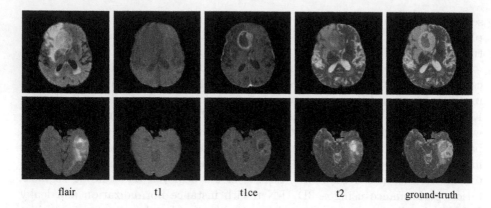

flair   t1   t1ce   t2   ground-truth

Fig. 1. Example scans with all modalities and attached corresponding ground-truths. The NCR/NET, ED, and ET regions are highlighted in red, green, and yellow, respectively.

the results on the validation set and test set indicate the superior segmentation performance of our method, while the ablation study on the training set demonstrates the effectiveness of the proposed intra-scale and inter-scale SDE blocks.

2   Dataset

This year, the BraTS challenge celebrates its 10th anniversary and is jointly organized by the Radiological Society of North America (RSNA), the American Society of Neuroradiology (ASNR), and the Medical Image Computing and Computer Assisted Interventions (MICCAI) society [1,3,3,4,13]. The BraTS21 dataset contains 2,000 multi-modal brain MR studies (8,000 mpMRI scans), including 1,521 training, 219 validation, and 260 test cases. Same to the data setting of challenge of previous years, each study has four MR images, including T1-weighted (T1), post-contrast T1-weighted (T1ce), T2-weighted (T2), and fluid attenuated inversion recovery (Flair) sequences, as shown in Fig. 1. All MR images have the same size of $240 \times 240 \times 155$ and the same voxel spacing of $1 \times 1 \times 1mm^3$. For each study, the enhancing tumor (ET), peritumoral edema (ED), and necrotic and non-enhancing tumor core (NCR/NET) were annotated on a voxel-by-voxel basis by experts. The annotations for training studies are publicly available, and the annotations for validation and test studies are withheld for online evaluation and final segmentation competition, respectively.

3   Method

In this section, we first review the original HNF-Net and its two key modules, *i.e.*, PMF module and EMA module. Then we give the structure of our HNF-Netv2 and provide the details of the newly proposed inter-scale and intra-scale SDE blocks.

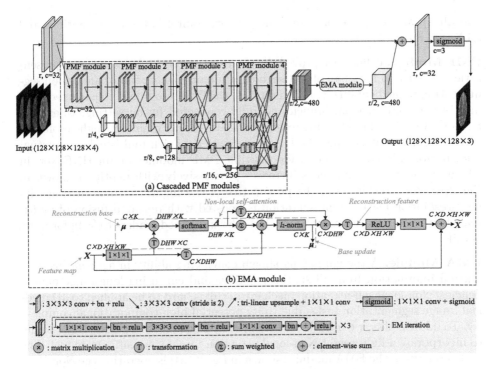

Fig. 2. Architecture of the original HNF-Net [8]. For each study, four multi-modal brain MR sequences are first concatenated to form a four-channel input and then processed at five scales. r denotes the original resolution and c denotes the channel number of feature maps. All downsample operations are achieved with 2-stride convolutions, and all upsample operations are achieved with joint $1 \times 1 \times 1$ convolutions and tri-linear interpolation. It is noted that, since it is inconvenient to show 4D feature maps $(C \times D \times H \times W)$ in the figure, we show all feature maps without depth information, and the thickness of each feature map reveals its channel number.

3.1   HNF-Net

The HNF-Net has an encoder-decoder structure with five scales, as shown in Fig. 2. At the original scale r, there are four convolutional blocks, two for encoding and the other two for decoding. At other four scales, four PMF modules are jointly used as a high-resolution and multi-scale aggregated feature extractor. At the end of the last PMF module, the output feature maps at four scales are first recovered to the $1/2r$ scale and then concatenated as mixed features. Next, the EMA module is used to efficiently capture long-range dependent contextual information and reduce the redundancy of the obtained mixed features. Finally, the output of the EMA module is recovered to original scale r and 32 channels via $1 \times 1 \times 1$ convolutions and upsampling and then added to the full-resolution feature map produced by the encoder for the dense prediction of voxel labels. All downsample operations are achieved with 2-stride convolutions, and all upsample operations are achieved with joint $1 \times 1 \times 1$ convolutions and tri-linear interpolation.

PMF Module. It has been proved that learning strong high-resolution representation is essential for small object segmentation tasks, *e.g.*, tumor and lesion segmentation in medical image. Based on this, the PMF module is constructed with multi-scale convolutional branch and fully connected fusion setting, where the former can fully exploit multi-resolution features but maintain high-resolution feature representation, and the latter can aggregate rich multi-scale contextual information. Moreover, we cascade multiple PMF modules in our HNF-Net, in which the number of branches increases progressively with depth, as shown in Fig. 2(a). As a result, from the perspective of the highest resolution stage, its high-resolution feature representation is boosted with repeated fusion of multi-scale low-resolution representations. We refer interested readers to [8,9] for more details.

EMA Module. Although having shown convincing ability in aggregating contextual information from all spatial positions and capturing long-range dependencies, Non-local self-attention mechanism [16] is hard to be applied to 3D medical image segmentation tasks, due to its potential high computational complexity. To address this, we introduce the EMA module [12] to our HNF-Net, aiming to incorporate a lightweight Non-local attention mechanism into our model. The main concept of the EMA module (shown in Fig. 2 (b)) is operating the Non-local attention on a set of feature reconstruction bases rather than directly achieving this on the high-resolution feature maps. Since the reconstruction bases have much less elements than the original feature maps, the computation cost of the Non-local attention can be significantly reduced. The details of EMA module can also be found in [8,9].

3.2 HNF-Netv2

In the proposed HNF-Netv2, we deploy inter-scale and intra-scale SDE blocks in the cascaded PMF modules. As shown in Fig. 3, we construct the intra-scale SDE block inside each convolutional branch of the PMF module. Meanwhile, to control the computational complexity cost, we only insert a inter-scale SDE block between the 3th PMF module and 4th PMF module. We now delve into the details of the these key components.

Intra-Scale and Inter-Scale SDE Blocks. The inter-scale SDE module is deployed following the fully connected fusion block of the PMF module with the structure shown in Fig. 4 (a). Specifically, we first apply a global average pooling (GAP) layer to the features of scale n (the branch with the smallest scale of the current PMF module) to obtain the global context with high semantic information. Then, we separately upsample the obtained features to the resolution of each branch of the PMF module. Considering the spatial information of the upsampled features is poor, we use a $1 \times 1 \times 1$ convolutional layer to reduce the channel number to 1 before concatenating them with the high-resolution

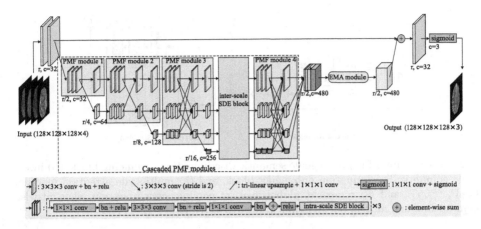

Fig. 3. Architecture of the HNF-Netv2. Similar to Fig. 2, r denotes the original resolution and c denotes the channel number of feature maps. Also we show all feature maps without depth information, and the thickness of each feature map reveals its channel number. Compared to the HNF-Net, we further add inter-scale and intra-scale SDE blocks in the cascaded PMF modules.

features. With this setting, we can add the global semantic discrimination to the high-resolution features but reduce the damage to the original spatial information. Different from the inter-scale SDE module, the intra-scale SDE block is constructed inside each convolutional branch of the PMF module with the structure shown in Fig. 4 (b). We also utilize a GAP layer to generate global contextual features and apply two $1 \times 1 \times 1$ convolutional layers to adjust the channel number. Similar to the prediction layer of the CNN-based classification network, the obtained global features gather the information from all spatial positions and thereby have strong semantic information. As a result, we can use these global features to re-weight the input high-resolution features so as to further enhance the global semantic discrimination. Following previous work [8,9], we finally concatenate the multi-scale boosted features as the input of the EMA module.

4   Experiments and Results

4.1   Implementation Details

Pre-processing. Following our previous work [9], we performed a set of pre-processing on each brain MR sequence independently, including brain stripping, clipping all brain voxel intensity with a window of [0.5%–99.5%], and normalizing them into zero mean and unit variance.

Training. In the training phase, we randomly cropped the input image into a fixed size of $128 \times 128 \times 128$ and concatenated four MR sequences along the channel dimension as the input of the model. The training iterations were set

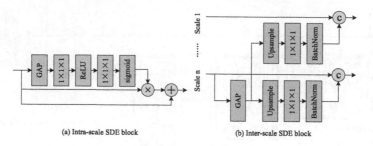

(a) Intra-scale SDE block   (b) Inter-scale SDE block

Fig. 4. Structures of (a) intra-scale semantic discrimination enhancing block, (b) inter-scale semantic discrimination enhancing block, and (c) multi-scale attention module. GAP, ©, ⊕, and ⊗ represent global average pooling, concatenation, element-wise summation, and matrix dot multiplication, respectively.

to 250 epochs with a linear warmup of the first 5 epochs. We trained the model using the Adam optimizer with a batch size of 4 and betas of (0.9, 0.999). The initial learning rate was set to 0.001 and decayed by multiplied with $(1 - \frac{current\_epoch}{max\_epoch})^{0.9}$. We also regularized the training with an l_2 weight decay of $1e - 5$. To reduce the potential overfitting, we further employed several online data augmentations, including random flipping (on all three planes independently), random rotation ($\pm 10°$ on all three planes independently), random per-channel intensity shift of $[\pm 0.1]$ and intensity scaling of $[0.9 - 1.1]$. Follow our previous work [8,9], we empirically set the base number $K = 256$ for the EMA module. We adopted a combination of generalized Dice loss [15] and binary cross-entropy loss as the loss function. All experiments were performed based on PyTorch 1.2.0 with 4 NVIDIA Tesla P40 GPUs.

Inference. In the inference phase, we first center cropped the original image with a size of $176 \times 224 \times 155$, which was determined based on the statistical analysis across the whole dataset to cover the whole brain area but with minimal redundant background voxels. Then, we segmented the cropped image with sliding patches instead of predicting the whole image at once, where the input patch size and sliding stride were set to $128 \times 128 \times 128$ and $32 \times 32 \times 27$, respectively. For each inference patch, we adopted test time augmentation (TTA) to further improve the segmentation performance, including 7 different flipping $((x), (y), (z), (x, y), (x, z), (y, z), (x, y, z)$, where x, y, z denotes three axes, respectively). Then, we averaged the predictions of the augmented and partly overlapped patches to generate the whole image segmentation result. At last, suggested by the previous work [7,9], we performed a post-processing by replacing enhancing tumor with NCR/NET when the volume of predicted enhancing tumor is less than the threshold which was empirically set to 200.

4.2   Results on the BraTS 2021 Challenge Dataset

To evaluate the effectiveness of the proposed SDE blocks in HNF-Netv2, we first give an ablation study on the training set using a five-fold cross-validation.

Table 1. Ablation study on the BraTS 2021 training set. Inter-SDE: inter-scale SDE block, Intra-SDE: intra-scale SDE block, DSC: dice similarity coefficient, HD95: Hausdorff distance (95%), WT: whole tumor, TC: tumor core, ET: enhancing tumor core.

Method	Benchmark		Params(M)	FLOPs(G)	Dice(%)		
	Intra-SDE	Inter-SDE			ET	TC	WT
3D UNet			**15.80**	1240.27	85.7795	87.4699	92.4132
HNF-Net			16.85	**436.59**	86.6906	89.5270	92.8332
HNF-Netv2	√		17.31	436.75	87.0310	89.9685	93.1362
HNF-Netv2	√	√	17.91	449.79	**87.7336**	**90.9558**	**93.4373**

Table 2. Segmentation performances of our method on the BraTS 2021 validation set. DSC: dice similarity coefficient, HD95: Hausdorff distance (95%), WT: whole tumor, TC: tumor core, ET: enhancing tumor core. Both mean and median scores of the segmentation results of all files are provided.

Method		Dice(%)			95%HD(mm)		
		ET	TC	WT	ET	TC	WT
HNF-Netv2	Mean scores	84.8032	87.9639	92.5352	14.1787	5.8626	3.4551
	Median scores	90.1445	94.0622	94.4855	1.4142	1.7321	2.2361

We chose 3D U-Net [6] as the baseline model. Besides, we successively tested the performance of the original HNF-Net [9], using intra-scale SDE block, and further using inter-scale SDE block (the proposed HNF-Netv2). As shown in Table 1, the segmentation performance was evaluated by the Dice score and 95% Hausdorff distance (%95HD), while the number of parameters and FLOPs of each method were also calculated. It shows that (1) compared to 3D U-Net [6], using our original HNF-Net [9] not only dramatically improves the Dice score by 0.9111% for ET, 2.0571% for TC, and 0.4200% for WT but also reduces the computations significantly with around 1/3 of the FLOPs, though having slightly increased parameters; (2) incorporating the intra-scale SDE block into HNF-Net further improves the Dice score by 0.3404% for ET, 0.4415% for TC, and 0.3030% for WT but only increases the parameters and FLOPs slightly; (3) Using the proposed HNF-Netv2 deployed with both intra-scale and inter-scale SDE blocks can achieve best segmentation performance, with the Dice score of 87.7336%, 90.9558%, and 93.4373% for ET, TC, and WT but also has acceptable computation cost.

Then, we evaluated the performance of our method on the validation set, with the results shown in Table 2. The segmentation was generated by an ensemble of all five models obtained in the ablation study. Here the results were directly obtained from the BraTS 2021 challenge platform and we can observe that our approach achieved the average Dice scores of 0.848032, 0.879639, and 0.925352, as well as the 95%HD of 14.1787, 5.8626, and 3.4551 for the enhancing tumor, tumor core, and whole tumor, respectively.

Table 3. Segmentation performances of our method on the BraTS 2021 test set. DSC: dice similarity coefficient, HD95: Hausdorff distance (95%), WT: whole tumor, TC: tumor core, ET: enhancing tumor core. The data was provided by the challenge organizers and both mean and median scores of the segmentation results of all files are listed.

Method		Dice(%)			95%HD(mm)		
		ET	TC	WT	ET	TC	WT
HNF-Netv2	Mean scores	87.8514	87.2985	92.4919	8.9184	16.2530	4.4895
	Median scores	93.6785	95.9990	95.6831	1	1.4142	1.7321

At last, we provide the results of the final submitted segmentation of the test set as shown in Table 3. our approach achieved the average Dice scores of 0.878514, 0.924919, and 0.872985, as well as the 95%HD of 8.9184, 4.4895, and 16.2530 for ET, WT, and TC, respectively, which ranks 8th out of all 1250 submitted results.

5   Conclusion

In this paper, we propose a HNF-Netv2 for brain tumor segmentation using multi-modal MR imaging, which extends the HNF-Net by adding inter-scale and intra-scale SDE blocks to enhance features with strong semantic discrimination. We evaluated our method on the BraTS 2021 Challenge Dataset and the convincing results suggest the effectiveness of the newly proposed key blocks and the HNF-Netv2.

Acknowledgement. Haozhe Jia, Chao Bai, and Yong Xia were partially supported by the Science and Technology Innovation Committee of Shenzhen Municipality, China under Grant JCYJ20180306171334997, the National Natural Science Foundation of China under Grant 61771397, and the Innovation Foundation for Doctor Dissertation of Northwestern Polytechnical University under Grant CX202042.

References

1. Baid, U., et al.: The rsna-asnr-miccai brats 2021 benchmark on brain tumor segmentation and radiogenomic classification. arXiv preprint arXiv:2107.02314 (2021)
2. Bakas, S., Akbari, H., Sotiras, A., et al.: Segmentation labels for the pre-operative scans of the tcga-gbm collection (2017)
3. Bakas, S., Akbari, H., Sotiras, A., Bilello, M., Rozycki, M., Kirby, J., Freymann, J., Farahani, K., Davatzikos, C.: Segmentation labels and radiomic features for the pre-operative scans of the tcga-lgg collection. The cancer imaging archive 286 (2017)
4. Bakas, S., et al.: Advancing the cancer genome atlas glioma MRI collections with expert segmentation labels and radiomic features. Sci. Data 4(1), 1–13 (2017)

5. Bakas, S., et al.: Identifying the best machine learning algorithms for brain tumor segmentation, progression assessment, and overall survival prediction in the BRATS challenge. arXiv preprint arXiv:1811.02629 (2018)
6. Çiçek, Ö., Abdulkadir, A., Lienkamp, S.S., Brox, T., Ronneberger, O.: 3D u-net: learning dense volumetric segmentation from sparse annotation. In: Ourselin, S., Joskowicz, L., Sabuncu, M.R., Unal, G., Wells, W. (eds.) MICCAI 2016. LNCS, vol. 9901, pp. 424–432. Springer, Cham (2016). https://doi.org/10.1007/978-3-319-46723-8_49
7. Isensee, F., Kickingereder, P., Wick, W., Bendszus, M., Maier-Hein, K.H.: No new-net. In: Crimi, A., Bakas, S., Kuijf, H., Keyvan, F., Reyes, M., van Walsum, T. (eds.) BrainLes 2018. LNCS, vol. 11384, pp. 234–244. Springer, Cham (2019). https://doi.org/10.1007/978-3-030-11726-9_21
8. Jia, H., Cai, W., Huang, H., Xia, Y.: H2nf-net for Brain Tumor Segmentation using Multimodal MR Imaging: 2nd Place Solution to Brats Challenge 2020 Segmentation Task (2020)
9. Jia, H., Xia, Y., Cai, W., Huang, H.: Learning high-resolution and efficient non-local features for brain glioma segmentation in MR images. In: Martel, A.L., Abolmaesumi, P., Stoyanov, D., Mateus, D., Zuluaga, M.A., Zhou, S.K., Racoceanu, D., Joskowicz, L. (eds.) MICCAI 2020. LNCS, vol. 12264, pp. 480–490. Springer, Cham (2020). https://doi.org/10.1007/978-3-030-59719-1_47
10. Jiang, Z., Ding, C., Liu, M., Tao, D.: Two-stage cascaded u-net: 1st place solution to BraTS challenge 2019 segmentation task. In: Crimi, A., Bakas, S. (eds.) BrainLes 2019. LNCS, vol. 11992, pp. 231–241. Springer, Cham (2020). https://doi.org/10.1007/978-3-030-46640-4_22
11. Kamnitsas, K., et al.: Efficient multi-scale 3D CNN with fully connected CRF for accurate brain lesion segmentation. Med. Image Anal. **36**, 61–78 (2017)
12. Li, X., Zhong, Z., Wu, J., Yang, Y., Lin, Z., Liu, H.: Expectation-maximization attention networks for semantic segmentation. In: Proceedings of the IEEE International Conference on Computer Vision, pp. 9167–9176 (2019)
13. Menze, B.H., et al.: The multimodal brain tumor image segmentation benchmark (brats). IEEE Trans. Med. Imaging **34**(10), 1993–2024 (2014)
14. Myronenko, A.: 3D MRI brain tumor segmentation using autoencoder regularization. In: Crimi, A., Bakas, S., Kuijf, H., Keyvan, F., Reyes, M., van Walsum, T. (eds.) BrainLes 2018. LNCS, vol. 11384, pp. 311–320. Springer, Cham (2019). https://doi.org/10.1007/978-3-030-11726-9_28
15. Sudre, C.H., Li, W., Vercauteren, T., Ourselin, S., Jorge Cardoso, M.: generalised dice overlap as a deep learning loss function for highly unbalanced segmentations. In: Cardoso, M.J., Arbel, T., Carneiro, G., Syeda-Mahmood, T., Tavares, J.M.R.S., Moradi, M., Bradley, A., Greenspan, H., Papa, J.P., Madabhushi, A., Nascimento, J.C., Cardoso, J.S., Belagiannis, V., Lu, Z. (eds.) DLMIA/ML-CDS -2017. LNCS, vol. 10553, pp. 240–248. Springer, Cham (2017). https://doi.org/10.1007/978-3-319-67558-9_28
16. Wang, X., Girshick, R., Gupta, A., He, K.: Non-local neural networks. In: Proceedings of the IEEE Conference on Computer Vision and Pattern Recognition, pp. 7794–7803 (2018)

Disparity Autoencoders for Multi-class Brain Tumor Segmentation

Chandan Ganesh Bangalore Yogananda[1]([✉]), Yudhajit Das[1], Benjamin C. Wagner[1], Sahil S. Nalawade[1], Divya Reddy[1], James Holcomb[1], Marco C. Pinho[1], Baowei Fei[2], Ananth J. Madhuranthakam[1], and Joseph A. Maldjian[1]

[1] Advanced Neuroscience Imaging Research Lab, Department of Radiology, University of Texas Southwestern Medical Center, Dallas, TX, USA
chandanganesh.bangaloreyogananda@utsouthwestern.edu
[2] Department of Bioengineering, University of Texas at Dallas, Dallas, TX, USA

Abstract. Multi-class brain tumor segmentation is important for predicting the aggressiveness and treatment response of gliomas. It has various applications including diagnosis, monitoring, and treatment planning of gliomas. The purpose of this work was to develop a fully automated deep learning framework for multi-class brain tumor segmentation. Brain tumor cases with multi-parametric MR Images from the RSNA-ASNR-MICCAI Brain Tumor Segmentation (BraTS) Challenge 2021 were used. Six Disparity Autoencoders (DAE) were developed including 2 DAEs to segment the whole-tumor (WT), 2 DAEs to segment the tumor-core (TC) and 2 DAEs to segment the enhancing-tumor (ET). The output segmentations of a particular label from their respective DAEs were ensembled and post-processed. The DAEs were tested on the BraTS2021 validation dataset. The networks achieved average dice-scores of 0.90, 0.80 and 0.79 for WT, TC and ET respectively on the validation dataset and 0.89, 0.82, 0.81 for WT, TC and ET respectively on the test dataset. This framework could be implemented as a robust tool to assist clinicians in primary brain tumor management and follow-up.

Keywords: Brain tumor segmentation · Glioma segmentation · Deep learning · BraTS · Autoencoders · MRI · Imaging features

1 Introduction

Gliomas, which account for the most common type of primary brain tumors, originate from glial cells [1]. Based on the varying degree of growth rate, cell-differentiation, immunohistochemistry, aggressive tendency, and genetic profile in their microscopic appearances, these tumors can be histologically classified into high-grade (HGG) and low-grade (LGG) lesions. Owing to differences in the physical properties of tissues, the tumor can be segmented into different sub-regions, including active tumor, enhancing tumor tissue, necrotic or edematous tissue. Each of these sub-regions/components can be segmented using MRI (Magnetic Resonance Imaging) T1, T1c (T1 with contrast agent), T2 (and FLAIR (Fluid Attenuation Inversion Recover) [2] images. While some tumors are well-differentiable and their sub-regions can be easily segmented, most tumors are diffuse with surrounding edema, heterogeneous contrast enhancement and can be anywhere in the brain with a variety of shapes and sizes [3, 4]. This not only makes manual brain tumor segmentation a challenging task, but also leads to significant intra and inter-rater variability, making fully automated procedures preferable [5–7].

Recently, several deep learning based fully automated brain-tumor segmentation algorithms/methods have outperformed traditional computer vision methods in their ability to reproduce segmentation accuracy for tumor analysis [8–13]. Our work proposes a robust Convolutional Neural Network (CNN) based Disparity Autoencoder, trained on the RSNA-ASNR-MICCAI BraTS 2021 dataset, for multi-class brain tumor segmentation from MR images.

2   Material and Methods

The Brain Tumor Segmentation (BraTS) challenge 2021 is jointly hosted by the Radiological Society of North America (RSNA), the American Society of Neuroradiology (ASNR), and the Medical Image Computing and Computer Assisted Interventions (MICCAI) society. The challenge utilizes multi-parametric MR images with the aim of evaluating state-of-the-art algorithms for (i) **Task 1:** segmenting the histologically distinct sub-regions of brain tumor (WT, TC and ET) and (ii) **Task 2:** focusing on classification of MGMT (O [6]-methyl guanine-DNA methyl transferase) promoter methylation status.

2.1   Data and Pre-processing

The BraTS 2021 dataset consists of 8000 multimodal, multi-institutional, and multiparametric 3D-MRI pre-operative scans of gliomas, with pathologically confirmed diagnosis from 2000 subjects (including training, validation, and testing cases) [14–18]. The training dataset includes MRI scans from 1251 subjects, each with four modalities (T1, T1c, T2, and FLAIR). Ground truth tumor segmentation labels for all subjects were manually delineated by expert neuroradiologists and includes three nested sub-regions: enhancing tumor, non-enhancing tumor including necrosis and edema.

Pre-processing steps included co-registration to a common anatomical template, resampling to 1 cubic-mm isotropic resolution and skull-stripping prior to image labelling. N4BiasCorrection to remove the RF inhomogeneity [19] and intensity normalization to zero-mean and unit variance were also performed. In this study we followed a double DAE architecture to extract deep image features from each of the three tumor sub-regions (WT, TC and EN) separately as a binary task.

2.2   Network Architecture

2.2.1   Related Work

The winner of the BraTS 2018 challenge (Myronenko [20]) developed a CNN based variational autoencoder (VAE). It consisted of a large asymmetrical encoder and 2 decoder branches. The encoder was used to extract the deep imaging features, and the VAE branch of the decoder was used to regularize the encoder. The winner of BraTS 2019, Jiang et al. [21], developed a two-stage cascaded U-net. The first stage of this architecture is a variant of Myronenko's [20] network. The second stage of the architecture has two decoders, one utilizing traditional deconvolutions, and another utilizing trilinear interpolations. Both stages of the architecture use the VAE branch to facilitate encoder regularization, proving the power of VAE regularization in brain tumor segmentation.

2.2.2   Network Architecture of Disparity Autoencoders

In this work, we propose a Disparity autoencoder. The developed autoencoder has a U-net architecture with one encoder and two decoder branches. The encoder and both branches of the decoder are made up of dense connections. These dense connections along with 1x1 convolution layers were used to diminish the vanishing gradient problem and to gather more spatial information. Additionally, high resolution information from the images were passed from the encoder only to the first branch of the decoder through skip connections. Both branches of the decoder segment the tumor. However, since the second branch of the decoder (VAE branch) has very minimal to no high-resolution information

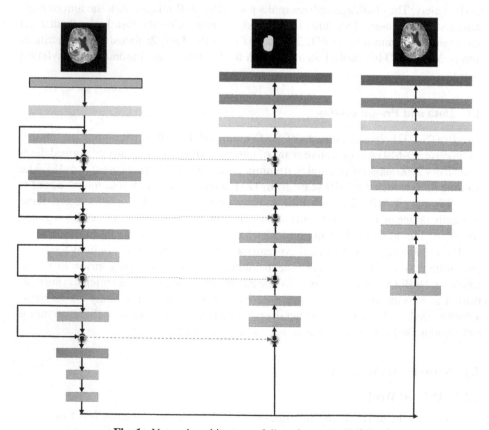

Fig. 1. Network architecture of disparity autoencoders

from the encoder, it is used only during training to regularize the encoder. To circumvent the problem of having higher numbers of convolution layers, (i) a bottleneck block was used to keep the convolutional layers to a smaller number and (ii) a compression factor was used to reduce the total number of feature maps after every block in the architecture. Additionally, due to a large number of high-resolution feature maps, a patch-based training and testing approach was implemented. The DAEs were designed to segment tumors and sub-components in multi-parametric brain MR images (Figs. 1 and 2).

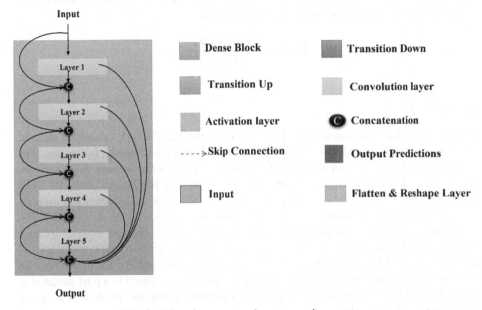

Fig. 2. Disparity autoencoders connection pattern

2.3 Training

Six Disparity Autoencoders (DAEs) were designed including 2 DAEs to segment the whole-tumor (WT), 2 DAEs to segment the tumor-core (TC) and 2 DAEs to segment the enhancing-tumor (ET). 1251 cases from the BraTS2021 dataset were used. The dataset was randomly shuffled and 70% (875 cases) was used for training and 30% (376 cases) for in-training validation. While the 875 cases were further split into 2 halves to train 2 DAEs for each tumor label, the in-training validation dataset remained the same for both the training sessions. 25% overlapping patches were extracted from the multi-parametric brain MR images that had at least 10% non-zero pixels on the corresponding ground truth patch. Data augmentation steps included horizontal and vertical flipping, random and translational rotation, height, width and shear shifting by 20% and, zooming in and out with a range of 20–50%. Data with simulated random and translational motion was also provided in the training step as an additional data augmentation step. To circumvent the problem of data leakage, no patch from the same subject was mixed between training and in-training validation [22, 23]. Networks were implemented using Keras python packages [24] and Tensorflow backend engine [25] with an adaptive moment estimation optimizer (Adam) [26]. The initial learning rate was set to 1e-4 with a batch size of 100 and maximal iterations of 100. The learning was scheduled to decline by a factor of 0.01 with a patience of 7. Additional parameters were chosen based on previous work with Dense-UNets using brain imaging data and semantic segmentation [27–29].

Dice loss: The Dice co-efficient was used as the training metrics.
The Dice co-efficient determines the amount of spatial overlap between the ground truth segmentation (X) and the network segmentation (Y)

$$dice\ loss = \frac{2|X_1 \cap Y_1|}{|X_1| + |Y_1|}$$

2.4   Testing

All the networks were tested on 219 cases from the BraTS2021 validation dataset. Patches of size 32x32x32 were extracted and provided to the networks for testing. The predicted patches were then reconstructed to a full segmentation volume. Each network was tested in 2 different ways including (a) non-overlapping patches and, (b) 25% overlapping patches. At the end of testing, each network produced 2 segmentation volumes for a particular label resulting in 4 segmentation volumes across the 2 networks. The exact same procedure was performed on whole tumor, tumor core and enhancing tumor labels. The 4 segmentation volumes were assigned with equal weights, averaged and thresholded at 0.5 for enhancing tumor, 0.5 for whole tumor and 0.5 for tumor core for every voxel. The thresholded outputs of WT, TC and ET were fused in a post-processing step that included 3D connected components algorithm to improve prediction accuracy by removing false positives.

3   Results

3.1   Brain Tumor Segmentation

The developed method achieved average dice scores of 0.92, 0.88 and 0.89, respectively on WT, TC and ET on the training dataset. It achieved average dice scores of (0.90, 0.80, 0.79), and Hausdorff distances of (5.22, 19.18, 19.99) mm for WT, TC and ET respectively on the BraTS2021 validation cases. The method also achieved average dice scores of (0.89, 0.82, 0.81), and Hausdorff distances of (7.85, 22.47, 19.44) mm for WT, TC and ET respectively on the BraTS2021 test dataset (Table 1 and Fig. 3).

Table 1. Mean dice scores on BraTS2021 datasets

	Whole Tumor	Tumor Core	Enhancing Tumor
BraTS2021 Training dataset	0.92	0.88	0.89
BraTS2021 Validation dataset	0.90	0.80	0.79
BraTS Testing dataset	0.89	0.82	0.81

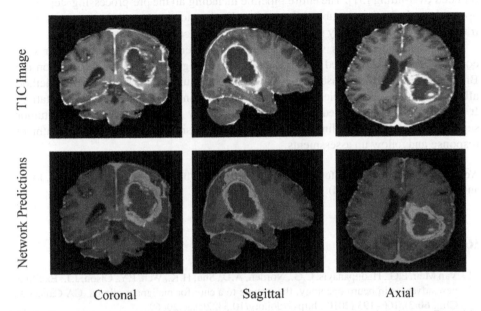

Fig. 3. Example segmentation result on a subject from BraTS2021 Validation dataset. Row (a) A post-contrast image. (b) Network predictions. Color Code: Red = Enhancing tumor, Blue = tumor core (Enhancing tumor + non-enhancing tumor + necrosis), Green = Edema, Whole tumor = Green + Blue + Red. (Color figure online)

4   Discussion and Conclusion

Reliable and accurate brain tumor segmentation algorithms have the potential to improve monitoring, and treatment response of GBM patients. Currently, various gross geometric measurements are used to evaluate treatment response of gliomas. Manual tumor segmentation is not just a tedious and time intensive task, but several quantitative evaluations of these segmentations have revealed substantial variations in Dice scores in the range 74%–85% [30]. To avoid such shortcomings, various machine learning algorithms have been developed to segment brain tumors [5, 6, 31]. Fully automated MRI-based deep learning algorithms have the potential to reduce subjectivity, provide accurate quantitative analysis for clinical decision making and improve patient outcomes. As a result, several challenges have been created to facilitate the progress of automated brain tumor segmentation. Although brain tumor segmentation can be expressed as a voxel-level classification, numerous semi- and fully automated algorithms have been developed. In this work, we developed a fully automated autoencoder-based deep learning method to segment brain tumors into subcomponents. This method was evaluated on 219 cases from the BraTS2021 validation dataset. A two-network (2DAEs for each of the 3 labels) framework was used, providing several advantages compared to the currently existing methods. Using six binary segmentation DAEs for segmenting the tumor into its sub-components allowed us to use a simpler network for each task [31]. As these are autoencoders with variational regularization, the networks were easier to train and reduced over-fitting [31]. The entire pipeline including all the pre-processing steps took approximately 3 min per subject for testing. Furthermore, since all the networks were trained separately for binary segmentation, misclassification was greatly reduced.

Fully automated DAEs were developed to segment brain tumors into their subcomponents. This developed method demonstrated high performance accuracy on the BraTS2021 validation dataset. High dice scores, accuracy and speed of this method allows for large scale application in research and clinical brain tumor segmentation. It can easily be implemented in the clinical workflow for reliable and accurate tumor segmentation to provide clinical guidance in diagnosis, surgical planning, treatment response and follow up assessments.

Acknowledgement. Support for this research was provided by NCI U01CA207091 (AJM, JAM) and NCI R01CA260705 (JAM).

References

1. Van Meir, E.G., Hadjipanayis, C.G., Norden, A.D., Shu, H.K., Wen, P.Y., Olson, J.J.: Exciting new advances in neuro-oncology: the avenue to a cure for malignant glioma. CA Cancer J. Clin. **60**(3), 166–193 (2010). https://doi.org/10.3322/caac.20069
2. Bakas, S., et al.: Advancing the cancer genome atlas glioma MRI collections with expert segmentation labels and radiomic features. Sci. Data **4**, 1–13 (2017)
3. Khosravanian, A., et al.: Fast level set method for glioma brain tumor segmentation based on superpixel fuzzy clustering and lattice boltzmann method. Comput. Methods Programs Biomed. **198**, 105809 (2021)
4. Tang, Z., et al.: Multi-atlas segmentation of MR tumor brain images using low-rank based image recovery. IEEE Trans. Med. Imaging **37**, 2224–2235 (2018)
5. Pei, L., et al.: Improved brain tumor segmentation by utilizing tumor growth model in longitudinal brain MRI. Proc. SPIE Int. Soc. Opt. Eng. 10134 (2017)
6. Kamnitsas, K., et al.: Ensembles of multiple models and architectures for robust brain tumour segmentation. BrainLes 2017, LNCS 10670, pp 450–462. https://doi.org/10.1007/978-3-319-75238-9_38 (2018)
7. Kamnitsas, K., et al.: Ensembles of multiple models and architectures for robust brain tumour segmentation. In: Crimi, A., Bakas, S., Kuijf, H., Menze, B., Reyes, M. (eds.) BrainLes 2017. LNCS, vol. 10670, pp. 450–462. Springer, Cham (2018). https://doi.org/10.1007/978-3-319-75238-9_38
8. Milletari, F., Navab, N., Ahmadi, S.-A.: V-net: fully convolutional neural networks for volumetric medical image segmentation. In: 2016 Fourth International Conference on 3D Vision (3DV). pp. 565–571. IEEE (2016)

9. Pereira, S., et al.: Brain tumor segmentation using convolutional neural networks in MRI images. IEEE Trans. Med. Imaging **35**, 1240–1251 (2016)

10. Havaei, M., et al.: Brain tumor segmentation with deep neural networks. Med. Image Anal. **35**, 18–31 (2017)

11. Zhuge, Y., et al.: Brain tumor segmentation using holistically nested neural networks in MRI images. Med. Phys. **44**, 5234–5243 (2017)

12. Zikic, D., et al.: Segmentation of brain tumor tissues with convolutional neural networks. Proc. MICCAI-BRATS **36**, 36–39 (2014)

13. Dvořák, P., Menze, B.: Local structure prediction with convolutional neural networks for multimodal brain tumor segmentation. In: Menze, B., Langs, G., Montillo, A., Kelm, M., Müller, H., Zhang, S., Cai, W., Metaxas, D. (eds.) MCV 2015. LNCS, vol. 9601, pp. 59–71. Springer, Cham (2016). https://doi.org/10.1007/978-3-319-42016-5_6

14. Baid, U., et al.: The RSNA-ASNR-MICCAI BraTS 2021 benchmark on brain tumor segmentation and radiogenomic classification. arXiv preprint arXiv:210702314 (2021)

15. Menze, B.H., et al.: The multimodal brain tumor image segmentation benchmark (BRATS). IEEE Trans. Med. Imaging **34**, 1993–2024 (2014)

16. Lloyd, C.T., Sorichetta, A., Tatem, A.J.: High resolution global gridded data for use in population studies. Sci. data **4**, 1–17 (2017)

17. Bakas, S., Akbari, H., Sotiras, A.: Segmentation labels for the pre-operative scans of the TCGA-GBM collection. The Cancer Imaging Archive (2017)

18. Bakas, S., et al.: Segmentation labels for the pre-operative scans of the TCGA-GBM collection (2017)

19. Tustison, N.J., et al.: Large-scale evaluation of ANTs and FreeSurfer cortical thickness measurements. Neuroimage **99**, 166–179 (2014)

20. Myronenko, A.: 3D MRI brain tumor segmentation using autoencoder regularization. In: Crimi, A., Bakas, S., Kuijf, H., Keyvan, F., Reyes, M., van Walsum, T. (eds.) BrainLes 2018. LNCS, vol. 11384, pp. 311–320. Springer, Cham (2019). https://doi.org/10.1007/978-3-030-11726-9_28

21. Jiang, Z., Ding, C., Liu, M., Tao, D.: Two-stage cascaded u-net: 1st place solution to brats challenge 2019 segmentation task. In: Crimi, A., Bakas, S. (eds.) BrainLes 2019. LNCS, vol. 11992, pp. 231–241. Springer, Cham (2020). https://doi.org/10.1007/978-3-030-46640-4_22

22. Wegmayr, V.A.S., Buhmann, J., Nicholas, P.: Classification of brain MRI with big data and deep 3D convolutional neural networks. In: Mori, K. (Ed) Published in SPIE Proceedings, Medical Imaging 2018: Computer-Aided Diagnosis, pp. 1057501 (2018)

23. Feng, X., Yang, J., Lipton, Z.C., Small, S.A., Provenzano, F.A.: Deep learning on MRI affirms the prominence of the hippocampal formation in Alzheimer's disease classification. bioRxiv 2018, 456277 (2018)

24. ea Chollet, F., Keras, C.P.: GitHub repository (2015)

25. Abadi, M., et al.: Tensorflow: a system for large-scale machine learning. In: 12th {USENIX} symposium on operating systems design and implementation ({OSDI} 16), pp. 265–283 (2016)

26. Kingma, D.P., Adam, B.J.: A method for stochastic optimization. arXiv preprint arXiv:141 26980 (2014)

27. Jégou, S., et al.: The one hundred layers tiramisu: fully convolutional densenets for semantic segmentation. In: Proceedings of the IEEE Conference on Computer Vision and Pattern Recognition workshops, pp. 11–19 (2017)

28. McKinley, R., Meier, R., Wiest, R.: Ensembles of densely-connected CNNs with label-uncertainty for brain tumor segmentation. In: Crimi, A., Bakas, S., Kuijf, H., Keyvan, F., Reyes, M., van Walsum, T. (eds.) BrainLes 2018. LNCS, vol. 11384, pp. 456–465. Springer, Cham (2019). https://doi.org/10.1007/978-3-030-11726-9_40

29. Bangalore Yogananda, C.G., et al.: A novel fully automated MRI-based deep-learning method for classification of IDH mutation status in brain gliomas. Neuro Oncol **22**, 402–411 (2020)
30. Menze, B.H., et al.: The Multimodal brain tumor image segmentation benchmark (BRATS). IEEE Trans. Med. Imaging **34**, 1993–2024 (2015)
31. Wang, G., Li, W., Ourselin, S., Vercauteren, T.: Automatic brain tumor segmentation using cascaded anisotropic convolutional neural networks. In: Crimi, A., Bakas, S., Kuijf, H., Menze, B., Reyes, M. (eds.) BrainLes 2017. LNCS, vol. 10670, pp. 178–190. Springer, Cham (2018). https://doi.org/10.1007/978-3-319-75238-9_16

Brain Tumor Segmentation in Multi-parametric Magnetic Resonance Imaging Using Model Ensembling and Super-resolution

Zhifan Jiang[1(✉)], Can Zhao[2], Xinyang Liu[1], and Marius George Linguraru[1,3]

[1] Sheikh Zayed Institute for Pediatric Surgical Innovation,
Children's National Hospital, Washington, DC, USA
zjiang@childrensnational.org
[2] NVIDIA, Bethesda, MD, USA
[3] School of Medicine and Health Sciences, George Washington University,
Washington, DC, USA

Abstract. Brain tumor segmentation in MRI offers critical quantitative imaging data to characterize and improve prognosis. The International Brain Tumor Segmentation (BraTS) Challenge provides a unique opportunity to encourage machine learning solutions to address this challenging task. This year, the 10th edition of BraTS collected a multi-institutional multi-parametric MRI dataset of 2040 cases with typical heterogeneity in large multi-domain imaging datasets. In this paper we present a strategy ensembling four parallelly-trained models to increase the stability and performance of our neural network-based tumor segmentation. Particularly, image intensity normalization and multi-parametric MRI super-resolution techniques are used in ensembled pipelines. The evaluation of our solution on 570 unseen testing cases resulted in Dice scores of 86.28, 87.12 and 92.10, and Hausdorff distance of 14.36, 17.48 and 5.37 mm for the enhancing tumor, tumor core and whole tumor, respectively.

Keywords: Brain tumor segmentation · Glioblastoma · Data homogenization · SegResNet · Super-resolution

1 Introduction

Glioblastoma multiform is an aggressive malignant tumor spreading rapidly through the brain. Multi-parametric magnetic resonance imaging (MRI) is widely used for diagnostic and prognosis of the disease. However, the quality of the prognosis remains low and variable in the clinical, human interpretation of MRI. The development of quantitative imaging techniques to assess this complex brain tumor can help improve the characterization and prognosis of patients

---

Z. Jiang and C. Zhao—These authors contributed equally.

A. Crimi and S. Bakas (Eds.): BrainLes 2021, LNCS 12963, pp. 125–137, 2022.
https://doi.org/10.1007/978-3-031-09002-8_12

with glioblastoma. For this purpose, accurate and automatic brain tumor segmentation in MRI is a critical step in the management of this condition.

The appearance, volume and shape of the glioblastoma vary significantly across affected individuals. Its heterogeneous nature that includes partly-enhancing areas, necrosis and edema makes the automatic annotation of tumor sub-regions in MRI an extremely challenging task. The International Brain Tumor Segmentation (BraTS) Challenge established in 2012 is in possession of a large, heterogeneous and continuously increasing collection of brain MRI, which assists in developing and evaluating machine learning solutions to the three-dimensional (3D) brain tumor segmentation.

In the BraTS challenge 2020, MRI scans of 660 cases were utilized for the competition. A modified nnU-Net model [11] took the first place in the competition with Dice scores of 82.03, 85.06 and 88.95, and Hausdorff distance of 17.805, 17.337 and 8.498 mm for enhancing tumor, tumor core and whole tumor, respectively. The nnU-Net is a deep learning framework that can be adapted to different datasets without manual tuning. Moreover, authors made BraTS-specific modification to further improve their results.

The BraTS Challenge 2021, as in the previous years, uses multi-institutional multi-parametric magnetic resonance images as training, validation and testing datasets. This year, the large and diverse cohort contains 2040 cases, among which 1251 cases with three ground truth labels are accessible for the training phase, and 219 cases with hidden ground truth are utilized for the validation phase. Finally, unseen testing data not available to the participants will be used for the final evaluation [1–4,17].

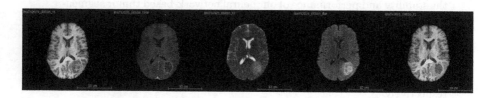

Fig. 1. An example of the BraTS multi-parametric MRI and associated annotation: (a) T1 (b) T1ce (c) T2 (d) T2-Flair (e) Segmentation labels (NCR-red, ED-green, ET-yellow).

Each case has five rigidly co-registered 3D volumes, of which four multi-parametric scans and one segmentation labels mask. The 3D MRI sequences are: 1) T1-weighted, 2) contrast enhanced T1-weighted (T1ce), 3) T2-weighted 4) T2 Fluid Attenuated Inversion Recovery (T2-Flair). In addition, manual segmentation of the tumor areas was created and approved by medical experts on all the cases. The segmentation labels correspond to three tumor parts: the necrotic area (NCR), peritumoral edematous/invaded tissue (ED) and enhancing tumor (ET). As shown in Fig. 1, the ET is highlighted by the T1ce sequence, while the ED is hyper-intense in T2-Flair. Combining lower intensity in T1ce and higher intensity in T2 helps identify the NCR. Based on the three labels, three tumor sub-regions are used to evaluate the performance of the segmentation methods: enhancing tumor (ET), tumor core (TC) and whole tumor (WT). The TC region includes NCR and ET except ED, and the WT region is the full extension of the annotated tumor (3-labeled areas).

All the data were pre-processed using a standard protocol before the ground truth was created. The pre-processing rigidly co-registered and resampled all the images to a template ($1 \times 1 \times 1$ mm^3 and $240 \times 240 \times 155$ voxels). In addition, all the MRI scans were skull-stripped.

Imaging techniques like MRI lack tissue value standardization. The BraTS MRI scans are acquired from multiple data contributors, using various clinical protocols and scanners, from all over the world. Thus, the variability in raw image intensity and resolution can affect training models. For example, Jacobsen et al. [12] demonstrated negative consequences of training a convolutional neural network on a multi-modality dataset. In order to address such data heterogeneity, the present paper uses additional processing methods to reduce the multi-domain effect before feeding training images to a deep neural network model. The main processing involves an image intensity normalization based on the histogram and a multi-sequence super-resolution technique. However, it is hard to generalize the positive effect on such a complex and diverse dataset. Therefore, we parallelly trained models with different pre-processing and then ensembled them to achieve a balanced and stable model. Moreover, experiments on the validation data showed a better predictive performance of the ensembled model than single models.

2   Methods

2.1   Training and Validation Strategy

We chose an approach based on deep neural networks. To optimally leverage the large training dataset, we implemented the following pre-processing processes before the network training:

- Normalization of image intensity to reduce the data heterogeneity;
- Unsupervised super-resolution of multi-sequence MRI to normalize the actual image resolution at acquisition;
- Data augmentation techniques to increase the amount and diversity of data.

We analyzed the predictive performance of the model with pre-processing on our self-produced validation dataset (1251 training cases were split into two groups of 1000 and 251) and on the online official validation dataset of the BraTS 2021 challenge (219 cases). We observed that these processes did not improve the performance on all the cases for such a complex and diverse collection of images. Even if a method had an overall better metric, it approximately improved 60% cases. Hence, instead of applying these pre-processing methods in a sequential way, we chose to use them in parallel, followed by separate training. As a consequence, our training and validation strategy consists in the ensemble of four models obtained by four parallel training pipelines (Fig. 2).

Model 1 Unprocessed input images + Training with data augmentation
Model 2 Normalized input images + Training without data augmentation
Model 3 Super-resolution input images + Training with data augmentation
Model 4 Three models fine-tuned from Model 1, optimized separately with the DSC of each label, using Unprocessed input images + Training with data augmentation

The data augmentation includes random flip of input images, and random scale and shift of image intensity.

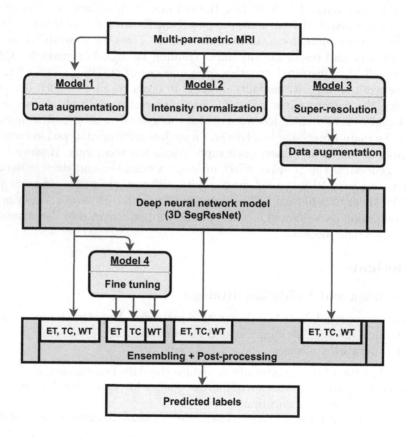

Fig. 2. Our training strategy.

2.2   Image Normalization

In the training pipeline of Model 2, an image intensity normalization process is applied to the original BraTS data using the method described by [19,24], which uses piecewise linear functions for histogram matching. Concretely, a shared standard histogram is learned across all the samples. First, landmarks are selected as intensity percentiles on each sample. Then, the standard histogram is computed by averaging the landmarks on the whole set of images. Finally, each image intensity is normalized by being rescaled piecewisely to the shared histogram. The advantages of this method are using the intensity information of the entire dataset, and not requiring time-consuming non-linear registration across subjects. We used the toolkit developed by Reinhold et al. [22] to normalize the 1470×4 MRI scans to the same intensity range, each modality independently. Figure 3 illustrates the change in individual histograms due to the normalization process.

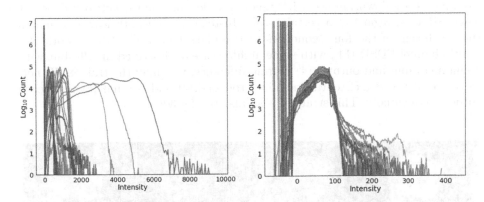

Fig. 3. Histogram of 24 randomly selected T1-weighted MRI sequences before (left) and after (right) intensity normalization.

2.3   Multi-sequence Super-resolution

Although BraTS data are resampled to $1mm^3$ voxel size, the actual resolutions at acquisition vary a lot. According to Table 1 in the BraTS 2018 report [5], T1 images are sagittal or axial acquisitions with slice thickness between 1–5 mm, T1ce images are axial 3D acquisition with unspecified slice thickness range, T2 images are axial 2D acquisitions with slice thickness between 2–4 mm, and T2 Flair images are axial or coronal or sagittal 2D acquisitions with unspecified slice thickness range. There has been research showing that super-resolution (SR) images can improve segmentation accuracy [8,10,13,16,20,23,27,30,31]. We therefore apply a multi-sequence unsupervised SR method in the training pipeline of Model 3 to normalize the actual resolution to $1mm^3$.

There are numerous SR algorithms developed for MRI, which predict high-resolution (HR) images from low-resolution (LR) images [6,7,15,21,28,29]. These SR methods require the actual acquired resolution of data to be known in order to generate LR training data and provide information to the network about the scale of SR. However, for the BraTS data, the biggest challenge is that the actual acquired resolution is unknown, which is uncommon in clinical practice. To overcome the challenge, we generate LR training data with random scale.

Our SR algorithm was implemented and tested using PyTorch and the PyTorch-based framework MONAI[1]. It follows these steps. (1) We manually selected nine training subjects that visually look HR in the axial plane for all the four sequences, i.e., T1, T1ce, T2, and T2 flair. We use the HR axial slices of the four sequences as HR training data for SR. (2) In each training iteration, to generate LR training data, we randomly pick three sequences and downsample their axial slices with random scale for each subject. (3) We train an SR network that predicts HR axial slices of four sequences from a HR axial slice of one sequence and LR axial slices from the other three sequences. Since the LR images are downsampled with random scale, the trained network does not learn SR with regard to a certain scale. Instead, the network learns to match the resolution of the four sequences to the highest one. The SR network is a multi-channel EDSR [14], with same architecture as described in [29], but with 4-channel input and output. (4) During inference, we apply the trained SR network to all the BraTS data, including the sagittal and coronal plane of each subject sequentially. This strategy is similar to [29,30].

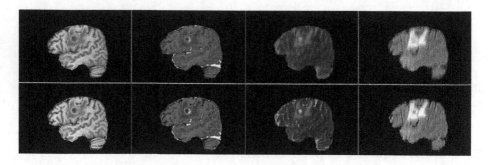

Fig. 4. Multi-sequence super-resolution. An example of BraTS data (case 01798, first row) and its super-resolution results (second row). From left to right: T1, T1ce, T2, T2 Flair. In this case, T1, T1ce images are acquired as high-resolution. The super-resolution algorithm enhanced the resolution of T2 and T2 Flair images, without damaging T1, T1ce images.

An example of SR results for subject 01798 is shown in Fig. 4. For this subject, we enhanced the resolution of the T2 and T2 Flair sequences. We noted artifacts around the edge of ET in T2 Flair because the network tried to transfer ET structures from other sequences to the T2 Flair image. However, as we train and test the segmentation network on SR results, so the artifacts do not introduce domain shift between training and testing data during segmentation. We believe the SR results can be further improved if the original acquired resolution is provided for all the data.

---

[1] https://monai.io.

2.4   Neural Network Model

The central component of the training models is a deep neural network called SegResNet, introduced and developed by Myronenko [18], the winner of BraTS 2018. SegResNet is a U-net style network with ResNet blocks. Compared with U-net, it has larger encoder but smaller decoder. For the training of the neural network dedicated to segmentation, we used the implementation in NVIDIA Clara Train framework[2], which is delivered as a docker container. The configurable existing model [18] was trained from scratch using only the permitted BraTS 2021 challenge data.

2.5   Post-processing

After investigating evaluations on the online validation dataset, we found that an important factor impacting the results is the definition of binary metrics (both Dice and Haussdorf distance (HD)) on cases with empty labeled mask of ET or TC. This typical issue has been mentioned by participants of previous editions of BraTS as well, such as in [11]. In fact, if the ground truth has no voxels attributed to ET, and an algorithm has a false positive prediction, the metrics are set to default values (Dice = 0, HD = 373.13 mm). On the contrary, if the same algorithm returns an empty mask too, the scores are switched to the best vaues (Dice = 1, HD = 0 mm). Thus, we included a post-processing step to eliminate some cases that have obviously no presence of ET or TC by defining a threshold on the predicted volume. However, the thresholding may also zero out some true positive predictions with very small volume, which penalizes the final scores.

3   Results

In our experiments, the training dataset was split into two subsets: 1000 cases for training and 251 validation cases with known ground truth for monitoring the training process.

In order to feed a 3D image into the UNet-like network model, a random spatial crop was applied to the 3D input image. The size of the region of interest was set to $240 \times 240 \times 144$ voxels. It has been suggested that a network trained on 3D volumes has better performance on segmentation [26], and increasing patch size provides more reliable segmentation results [9]. Therefore, we defined the size of the region of interest to be divisible by 16, which can cover the largest region of the whole 3D image. The numbers of input and output channels are 4 and 3, corresponding to the four MRI sequences and three labeled sub-regions.

---

[2] https://developer.nvidia.com/clara.

Table 1. Quantitative results on BraTS 2021 validation dataset (219 cases). The evaluation metrics are mean Dice coefficient and Hausdorff distance computed on all the validation cases, for enhancing tumor (ET), tumor core (TC) and whole tumor (WT) respectively. 'DA' refers to data augmentation.

Evaluated models	Dice (%)			Hausdorff (mm)		
	ET	TC	WT	ET	TC	WT
Model 1 (Baseline + DA)	79.86	87.22	92.13	25.03	8.26	3.95
Model 2 (Intensity normalization)	80.05	86.19	91.68	21.81	8.69	4.44
Model 3 (Super-resolution + DA)	78.26	86.38	91.07	26.97	8.30	5.24
Model 4 (Fine-tuned separately + DA)	79.81	87.35	92.18	25.44	8.29	**3.91**
4 Models ensembled	80.38	87.99	92.34	23.32	7.62	3.94
4 Models ensembled + post-processing	**84.37**	**87.99**	**92.34**	**16.06**	**7.62**	3.94

Training was performed on an NVIDIA RTX A6000 48G GPU. The batch size was set to 1 and the default number of epochs was set to 300. Approximately 200 epochs were sufficient for the algorithms to converge.

Table 2. Quantitative results on BraTS 2021 testing dataset (570 cases). The evaluated submission was the ensemble of 4 models with post-processing.

Testing dataset (n = 570)	Dice (%)			Hausdorff (mm)		
	ET	TC	WT	ET	TC	WT
Mean	86.28	87.12	92.10	14.36	17.48	5.37
StdDev	20.08	24.37	11.59	65.12	70.08	18.27
Median	92.81	95.87	95.49	1.00	1.41	1.73
25th percentile	85.06	91.18	91.45	1.00	1.00	1.00
75th percentile	96.59	97.98	97.47	2.00	3.00	4.12

Table 1 shows the overall evaluation of our models on the validation dataset provided by the BraTS challenge 2021. Among the three sub-regions, the ET was the most difficult to identify. The first observation is this tumor region generally has smaller volumes and the annotated voxels are sometimes sparse. Secondly, its detection strongly depends on the quality of the contrast enhanced T1-weighted images because ET is mainly highlighted by this sequence. Due to the diversity of data sources, low quality T1ce sequences were present in the validation dataset. Finally, as aforementioned, certain cases have empty annotation for the ET, and the binary metrics penalized a lot false positive predictions.

The comparison of different tested models in Table 1 revealed that the ensembled model provided more stable and better predictive performance on most metrics. The exception was the HD on ET (23.32 for model 2 v.s. 21.81 for the ensembled model), which is the result of the empty labels issue described above. The result of the ensembled model was improved by the proposed post-processing. The model fine-tuned on WT has a very similar HD. In addition, Fig. 5 illustrates qualitative results of the ensemble of 4 models with post-processing. Table 2 reports our quantitative results on 570 unseen testing cases.

25th percentile: BraTS2021_01715 ET=90.64 TC=78.75 WT=92.10

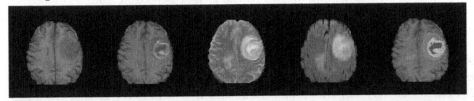

50th percentile: BraTS2021_01680 ET=89.57 TC=94.69 WT=90.90

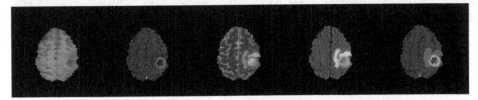

75th percentile: BraTS2021_01781 ET=94.66 TC=96.49 WT=95.36

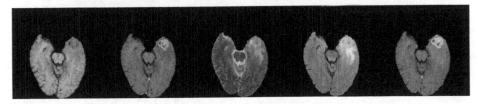

Fig. 5. Qualitative results on BraTS 2021 validation dataset. Among 219 cases, 3 cases were selected according to 25th percentile, median and and 75th percentile of the average Dice over 3 labels. From left to right: T1, T1ce, T2, T2-Flair and Segmentation labels shown on T1ce (NCR-red, ED-green, ET-yellow). (Color figure online)

4   Discussion

The 2021 BraTS challenge provides a much larger dataset than the previous 2020 edition (2040 cases compared to 660 cases). Preliminary results made public on the BraTS website have demonstrated an improved performance compared to last year. Effectively, using more training data helps build more robust machine learning algorithms.

Concerning the input data, the multi-sequence MRI increase also the chance of correctly identifying tumor sub-regions. However, as mentioned in Introduction, T1ce and T2-Flair sequences are more important than others to distinguish tumor regions within the brain tissue. A possible approach of improvement is to assign different weights for different modalities or randomly drop channels during the training process.

Because the large dataset is heterogeneous, data homogenization is a suitable pre-processing approach. However, the direct application of intensity normalization based on histogram to the whole dataset may not be sufficient. We are considering more sophisticated unsupervised learning algorithms to homogenized data optimal for segmentation, such as the idea presented in [25].

Finally, the correct prediction of empty volume on ET and TC plays a major role in the evaluation, as the binary change in the metrics can produce significant differences in mean values on a limited number of cases. While this observation is specific to the BraTS dataset, more generally, the segmentation of targets with small volumes is a challenging task. Figure 6 demonstrates on a validation set of 251 cases that very low Dice scores occur merely when the ET ground truth has small or zero volume. The scores presented in Table 2 suggested certain cases also have empty annotation for TC in the testing data, which penalized the Hausdorff metric.

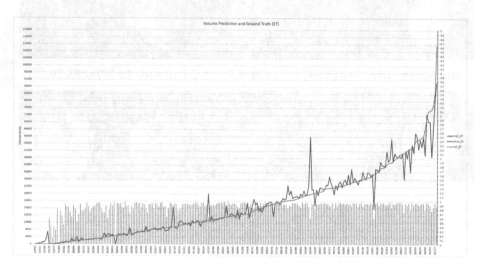

Fig. 6. Comparison of predicted volume and actual volume of ET sub-region. Analysis on our self-split validation set (251 cases with known ground truth). Actual volume-green, predicted volume-red, associated Dice score-blue.

In summary, more attention should be brought to deal with poorly contrasted images and small anatomical structures. As for the BraTS challenge, the design of a robust classification method to predict if one sub-region exists in the image will play an important role on the final performance of the models.

5   Conclusion

The BraTS challenge 2021 included twice more cases for the task of brain tumor segmentation than in 2020. To address this challenge task, we developed a strategy of combining multiple training models, each aimed to reduce a negative effect caused by the heterogeneity present in input images and labeled volumes. Better performance was achieved by the ensembled model compared to single models. Moreover, this opportunity allows us to investigate intensively how data affects predictive performance of a segmentation technique, and helps us to consider potential approaches of improvement.

Acknowledgements. The authors would like to thank Holger Roth from NVIDIA, Bethesda, MD, USA and Brendan Wang from Princeton University, NJ, USA for their contributions to this work. Partial support for this work was also provided by National Cancer Institute award UG3 CA236536.

References

1. Baid, U., et al.: The RSNA-ASNR-MICCAI brats 2021 benchmark on brain tumor segmentation and radiogenomic classification. CoRR abs/2107.02314 (2021), https://arxiv.org/abs/2107.02314
2. Bakas, S., Akbari, H., Sotiras, A., Bilello, M., Rozycki, M., Kirby, J.S., et al.: Advancing the cancer genome atlas glioma MRI collections with expert segmentation labels and radiomic features. Sci. Data **4**(1), 170117 (2017). https://doi.org/10.1038/sdata.2017.117
3. Bakas, S., Akbari, H., Sotiras, A., Bilello, M., Rozycki, M., Kirby, J.S., et al.: Segmentation labels and radiomic features for the pre-operative scans of the tcga-gbm collection. Cancer Imaging Arch. (2017). https://doi.org/10.7937/K9/TCIA.2017.KLXWJJ1Q
4. Bakas, S., Akbari, H., Sotiras, A., Bilello, M., Rozycki, M., Kirby, J.S., et al.: Segmentation labels and radiomic features for the pre-operative scans of the tcga-lgg collection. Cancer Imaging Arch. (2017). https://doi.org/10.7937/K9/TCIA.2017.GJQ7R0EF
5. Bakas, S., et al.: Identifying the best machine learning algorithms for brain tumor segmentation, progression assessment, and overall survival prediction in the brats challenge. arXiv preprint arXiv:1811.02629 (2018)
6. Chen, Y., Shi, F., Christodoulou, A.G., Xie, Y., Zhou, Z., Li, D.: Efficient and accurate MRI super-resolution using a generative adversarial network and 3D multi-level densely connected network. In: Medical Image Computing and Computer Assisted Intervention (MICCAI), vol. 2018, pp. 91–99 (2018)
7. Delannoy, Q., et al.: SegSRGAN: super-resolution and segmentation using generative adversarial networks–application to neonatal brain MRI. Comput. Biol. Med. **120**, 103755 (2020)
8. Gheshlaghi, S.H., Dehzangi, O., Dabouei, A., Amireskandari, A., Rezai, A., Nasrabadi, N.M.: Efficient OCT image segmentation using neural architecture search. In: 2020 IEEE International Conference on Image Processing (ICIP), pp. 428–432 (2020)

9. Hamwood, J., Alonso-Caneiro, D., Read, S.A., Vincent, S.J., Collins, M.J.: Effect of patch size and network architecture on a convolutional neural network approach for automatic segmentation of OCT retinal layers. Biomed. Opt. Exp. **9**(7), 3049–3066 (2018). https://doi.org/10.1364/BOE.9.003049, https://www.ncbi.nlm.nih.gov/pmc/articles/PMC6033561/

10. Hatvani, J., Horváth, A., Michetti, J., Basarab, A., Kouamé, D., Gyöngy, M.: Deep learning-based super-resolution applied to dental computed tomography. IEEE Trans. Radiat. Plasma Med. Sci. **3**(2), 120–128 (2019)

11. Isensee, F., Jäger, P.F., Full, P.M., Vollmuth, P., Maier-Hein, K.H.: nnU-net for brain tumor segmentation. In: Crimi, A., Bakas, S. (eds.) BrainLes 2020. LNCS, vol. 12659, pp. 118–132. Springer, Cham (2021). https://doi.org/10.1007/978-3-030-72087-2_11

12. Jacobsen, N., Deistung, A., Timmann, D., Goericke, S.L., Reichenbach, J.R., Güllmar, D.: Analysis of intensity normalization for optimal segmentation performance of a fully convolutional neural network. Zeitschrift Fur Medizinische Physik **29**(2) (2019). https://doi.org/10.1016/j.zemedi.2018.11.004

13. Kang, M., Cha, E., Kang, E., Ye, J.C., Her, N., Oh, J., Nam, D., Kim, M., Yang, S.: Accuracy improvement of quantification information using super-resolution with convolutional neural network for microscopy images. Biomed. Sig. Process. Control **58**, 101846 (2020)

14. Lim, B., Son, S., Kim, H., Nah, S., Mu Lee, K.: Enhanced deep residual networks for single image super-resolution. In: Proceedings of the IEEE Conference on Computer Vision and Pattern Recognition Workshops, pp. 136–144 (2017)

15. Lyu, Q., et al.: Multi-contrast super-resolution MRI through a progressive network. IEEE Trans. Med. Imaging **39**(9), 2738–2749 (2020)

16. Mahapatra, D., Bozorgtabar, B., Garnavi, R.: Image super-resolution using progressive generative adversarial networks for medical image analysis. Comput. Med. Imaging Graph. **71**, 30–39 (2019)

17. Menze, B.H., Jakab, A., Bauer, S., Kalpathy-Cramer, J., Farahani, K., Kirby, J., et al.: The multimodal brain tumor image segmentation benchmark (brats). IEEE Trans. Med. Imaging **34**(10), 1993–2024 (2015). https://doi.org/10.1109/TMI.2014.2377694

18. Myronenko, A.: 3d MRI brain tumor segmentation using autoencoder regularization. CoRR abs/1810.11654 (2018), http://arxiv.org/abs/1810.11654

19. Nyul, L., Udupa, J., Zhang, X.: New variants of a method of MRI scale standardization. IEEE Trans. Med. Imaging **19**(2), 143–150 (2000). https://doi.org/10.1109/42.836373

20. Oktay, O., et al.: Multi-input cardiac image super-resolution using convolutional neural networks. In: Ourselin, S., Joskowicz, L., Sabuncu, M.R., Unal, G., Wells, W. (eds.) MICCAI 2016. LNCS, vol. 9902, pp. 246–254. Springer, Cham (2016). https://doi.org/10.1007/978-3-319-46726-9_29

21. Pham, C., Ducournau, A., Fablet, R., Rousseau, F.: Brain MRI super-resolution using deep 3D convolutional networks. In: 2017 IEEE 14th International Symposium on Biomedical Imaging (ISBI 2017), pp. 197–200 (2017)

22. Reinhold, J.C., Dewey, B.E., Carass, A., Prince, J.L.: Evaluating the impact of intensity normalization on MR image synthesis. In: Medical Imaging 2019: Image Processing, vol. 10949, p. 109493H. International Society for Optics and Photonics (2019)

23. Sert, E., Özyurt, F., Doğantekin, A.: A new approach for brain tumor diagnosis system: single image super resolution based maximum fuzzy entropy segmentation and convolutional neural network. Med. Hypotheses **133**, 109413 (2019)

24. Shah, M., et al.: Evaluating intensity normalization on mris of human brain with multiple sclerosis. Med. Image Anal. **15**(2), 267–282 (2011). https://doi.org/10.1016/j.media.2010.12.003, https://www.sciencedirect.com/science/article/pii/S1361841510001337

25. Tor-Diez, C., Porras, A.R., Packer, R.J., Avery, R.A., Linguraru, M.G.: Unsupervised MRI homogenization: application to pediatric anterior visual pathway segmentation. In: Liu, M., Yan, P., Lian, C., Cao, X. (eds.) MLMI 2020. LNCS, vol. 12436, pp. 180–188. Springer, Cham (2020). https://doi.org/10.1007/978-3-030-59861-7_19

26. Yu, Q., Xia, Y., Xie, L., Fishman, E.K., Yuille, A.L.: Thickened 2d networks for 3d medical image segmentation. CoRR abs/1904.01150 (2019), http://arxiv.org/abs/1904.01150

27. Yun, H.R., J., M., Hong, H., Shim, K.W.: Super-resolution image generation for improvement of orbital thin bone segmentation. In: Lau, P.Y., Shobri, M. (eds.) International Workshop on Advanced Imaging Technology (IWAIT) 2020, vol. 11515, pp. 111–114 (2020)

28. Zeng, K., Zheng, H., Cai, C., Yang, Y., Zhang, K., Chen, Z.: Simultaneous single- and multi-contrast super-resolution for brain MRI images based on a convolutional neural network. Comput. Biol. Med. **99**, 133–141 (2018)

29. Zhao, C., Dewey, B.E., Pham, D.L., Calabresi, P.A., Reich, D.S., Prince, J.L.: Smore: a self-supervised anti-aliasing and super-resolution algorithm for MRI using deep learning. IEEE Trans. Med. Imaging **40**(3), 805–817 (2020)

30. Zhao, C., Shao, M., Carass, A., Li, H., Dewey, B.E., Ellingsen, L.M., Woo, J., Guttman, M.A., Blitz, A.M., Stone, M., et al.: Applications of a deep learning method for anti-aliasing and super-resolution in MRI. Magn. Reson. Imaging **64**, 132–141 (2019)

31. Özyurt, F., Sert, E., Avcı, D.: An expert system for brain tumor detection: fuzzy c-means with super resolution and convolutional neural network with extreme learning machine. Med. Hypotheses **134**, 109433 (2020)

An Ensemble Approach to Automatic Brain Tumor Segmentation

Yaying Shi[1]([envelope]), Christian Micklisch[1], Erum Mushtaq[2], Salman Avestimehr[2], Yonghong Yan[1], and Xiaodong Zhang[3]

[1] University of North Carolina at Charlotte, Charlotte, NC, USA
yshi10@uncc.edu
[2] University of Southern California, Los Angeles, CA, USA
[3] MD Anderson Cancer Center, Houston, TX, USA

Abstract. Medical image segmentation is the task of objective segmentation in medical field. 3D Tumor segmentation can help physicians efficiently diagnose cancer, track tumor change, and make treatment plans. With the development of machine learning (ML)/Deep Learning (DL) image segmentation methods, the performance of medical image segmentation has significantly improved especially in terms of accuracy and time efficiency. Performance of typical deep learning algorithms such as Fully Connection Networks, Unet, DeepLab varies with respect to different datasets, pre-processing and training parameter settings. In this paper, we propose a new architecture which utilizes the advantages of various models and aggregates their results. The original concept was inspired by Ensembles of Multiple Models and Architectures. In this paper, we train different sub-models separately. Then we train a gating network to credit the inference result from each individual model to get a better result.

Keywords: Medical image segmentation · BraTS challenge · Machine learning · Ensemble learning

1 Introduction

Brain Tumors spawn from abnormal cells which replicate in the brain without control. There are several different types of brain tumors [9]. Some are noncancerous tumors, others are cancerous or malignant tumors. Noncancerous tumors do not extend or transform to surrounding normal brain tissue and other tissue in the human body which means they can easily be distinguished from normal brain tissue. Cancerous tumors can originate in the brain or spread to the brain from other tissues in the body. Those types of tumors, cancerous, are difficult to discern from normal brain tissue. Magnetic resonance imaging (MRI) is an efficient tumor diagnostic imaging modality that generates a detailed image of human body tissues by using a magnetic field and computer generated radio waves. A typical 3D brain MRI can be categorized by T1 and T2 relaxation

A. Crimi and S. Bakas (Eds.): BrainLes 2021, LNCS 12963, pp. 138–148, 2022.
https://doi.org/10.1007/978-3-031-09002-8_13

time. T1 relaxation time is the time it takes the magnetic vector to return to the resting state. The T2 relaxation time is the time it takes the axial spin to return to resting state. A 3D T1-weighted brain tumor image is one of the modalities in MRI, which can show the differences between normal brain tissue and brain tumors with the help of T1 relaxation time. Similarly, a T2-Weighted brain tumor image is another modality based on T2 relaxation time which is important for long-term tumor tracking. T1 with contrast agent (T1-ce) and t2 Fluid Attenuation Inversion Recovery (FLAIR) are two modalities that highlight the position and shape of tumors relative to normal brain tissue.

Although these four 3D Brain MRIs (T1, T2, T1-CE, T2 FLAIR) aid physicians to locate, monitor, track, and treat the brain tumor, they're still a time consuming process that challenges physicians when manually segmenting a tumor from a 3D MRI. This is due to the complex structure of tumors. An automatic brain tumor segmentation method would help physicians save time by reducing the manual load of locating and segmenting a tumor, allowing them to focus more on the patients diagnosis and the treatment plan. Traditional segmentation methods, such as Markov random field (MRF) model [1], alter-based segmentation model [8], and Edge-Based Method [20], are based on the intensity image, image label and the clustering process [2]. With the success of ML/DL methods in computer vision tasks, Convolutional Neural Networks (CNN) show great potential and provide feasible solutions in automated brain tumor segmentation. RSNA-ASNR-MICCAI Brain Tumor Segmentation challenge (BraTS) is a segmentation competition to find the best state-of-art brain tumor segmentation algorithm [4]. BraTS challenge provides plenty of algorithm opportunity for medical image segmentation. Wang [27] proposed a triple cascaded framework for brain tumor segmentation, ranked second in the BraTS 2017 challenge. Three networks are proposed to hierarchically segment whole tumor (WNet), tumor core (TNet) and enhancing tumor core (ENet) sequentially and fuse them in different views. EMMA, ranked first in the BraTS 2017 challenge, introduced a novel ensemble of multiple models and architectures to get better result from several models [16]. The EMMA ensemble is composed of DeepMedic [17], FCN [19] and Unet [25] models and take the advantage of them to get a better segmentation result. No New-Net, ranked second in the BraTS 2018 challenge, uses U-net as baseline and is trained with different patch sizes and loss functions to improve performance [15]. Andriy [23] proposed a auto-encoder network with auto-encoder regularization and ranked first in the BraTS 2018 challenge.

In this work, we develop four different CNN networks and ensemble their inference output with a classifier network to get better segmentation results. Our approach was inspired by EMMA, but we use a different ensemble method which trains a new classifier model for the inference result from four base models. By using the ensemble method, we want to get a more stable and robust segmentation result for Brain Tumor Segmentation. We evaluate our approach through BraTS 2021 challenge validation submission.

The remainder of the paper is organized as follows: Sect. 2 presents each network structure and the ensemble method of our work. Section 3 includes evaluation of the models with BraTS 2021 Challenge datasets. Section 4 discusses related work and Sect. 5 discusses the result and future improvement of the our work.

2 Methods

In this section, we introduce the network architecture, each base network, training parameters and training details that we use in the validation stage of the challenge. As mentioned in the last paragraph, we used an ensemble approach on four different models to get a better segmentation result. We introduce each sub-Network with its training details in following subsections.

2.1 3D Unet

Unet is a well-known CNN architecture for biomedical image segmentation [25]. It has two parts: an encoder and a decoder, and they are connected at the bottom like a 'U'. The encoder part is a regular classification CNN which get the semantic information and reduce the spatial information [15]. The decoder part get the semantic information and deconvolve the feature maps to obtain higher resolution feature maps to restore both semantic and spatial information.

Our 3D Unet was developed based on the original Unet architecture and extended it to 3 dimensions. Due to the limitation of CUDA memory on our GPU, 3D Unet can only take batch size of two. The detailed network structure was shown as Fig. 1. The input is four channel resized 3D MRI image. Then the input go through a $3 \times 3 \times 3$ 3D convolution with a 32 filters. After convolution, we apply ReLU activation function, 3d batch Normalization and zero padding. The output has 4 channels which is same as input. Those 4 channels are background, whole tumor, tumor core, enhanced tumor respectively. After a sigmoid function, we get the segmentation result with three tumors.

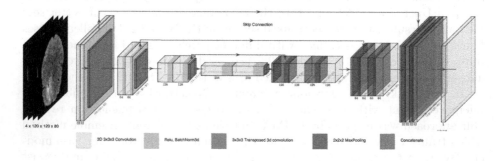

Fig. 1. Schematic visualization of 3D Unet Network architecture

For the training details, 3D Unet was trained by the input size $120 \times 120 \times 80$ with batch size 2. We used the Adam optimizer combined with Dice loss function and learning rate at 0.01. We also trained another 3D Unet model by SGD optimizer with cross entropy loss. We also set the learning rate at 0.01. Due to the time limit, we trained the model just in 200 epochs.

2.2 Residual 3D Unet

Residual 3D Unet has been used in the study of plant segmentation [29]. It was built upon the implementations of Çiçek et al.'s 3DUnet [13] and Lee et al.'s Residual UNet structure [18]. Each Encoder is structured as a Residual module whereby the output of the 1st Convolution module is skipped over to the pooling module is combined with the output of the third Convolution module passed to the ReLU. Due to GPU limitations, our Residual 3D net has been altered to accept the four 3D MRI images by decreasing the amount of levels to 4, as opposed to 5. We set an input of 4 channels at $120 \times 120 \times 80$ and 4 output channels for the segmentation classifications. Our Residual 3D Unet was trained on a batch size of 3. We used the Adam optimizer with the Cross Entropy loss function. The learning rate was set to 0.01 and was trained on 100 epochs (Figs. 2 and 3).

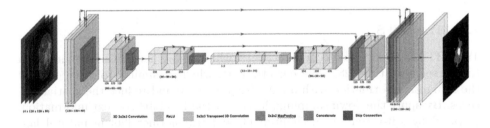

Fig. 2. Schematic visualization of residual 3D unet network architecture

2.3 3D Vnet

Vnet is a convolutional neural network that aims to segment MRI data by first compressing it to extract features and then decompressing it until original size of data is obtained [22]. The original Vnet work does not use all classes (4 channels/modality) data simultaneously. To adapt it to 3D, we apply a convolutional operation that takes 4 channel data as an input. Likewise, towards the end, instead of convolving 32 channels to reduce 2 channels as is done in the original work, we apply a filter to keep the output dimensions same as input dimensions ($4 \times 120 \times 120 \times 80$). We also skip the softmax operation that is used in the original Vnet for this 3D adaptation. Another change as compared to original Vnet work is that we reduce the length of compression path by one step and stop at 128 channels instead of 256 channels as it becomes infeasible to reduce the length and width of data $15 \times 15 \times 10$ by 2. For training, we use batch size 1 with Adam optimizer with Dice loss and learning rate 0.01 for 200 epochs.

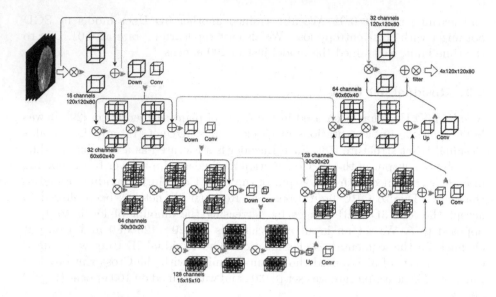

Fig. 3. Schematic visualization of 3D Vnet Network architecture

2.4   TransBTS

TransBTS is a encoder-decoder network which uses the transformer in brain tumor segmentation [28]. The encoder part, which is similar to Unet, extract the semantic information with a 3D CNN structure and reduce the spatial features. By apply the down sampling, it can get the local 3D context information. Inspired by self-attention mechanism [3] and transformer [26] in natural language processing, TransBTS add a transformer layer to the end of encoder part. This transformer layer saves the local context information to the transformer for global feature. The decoder part uses the feature from the transformer and do the up-sampling joint with the high resolution feature map to perform the tumor segmenting.

Our TransBTS sub-model was developed based on the original TransBTS architecture. We did minor modification on the TransBTS architecture. The original architecture is shown in Fig. 4. The input is still four channel random cropped 3D MRI with $3 \times 3 \times 3$ 3D convolution. After convolution, it apply ReLU activation function, 3D batch Normalization and padding set to 1, which means padding added to all four sides of the input. The decode part uses the pixel-level segmentation to restore the same dimension of original size of MRI.

For the training details, TransBTS was trained by input size $128 \times 128 \times 128$ with batch size 8. We used the Adam optimizer with dice loss functions. The initial learning rate is 1e−4 and reduce learning rate as the formula:

$$a = a * \left(1 - \frac{e}{es}\right)^{0.9} \tag{1}$$

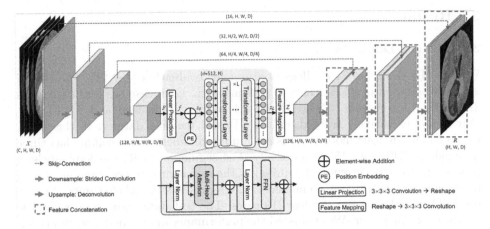

Fig. 4. Schematic visualization of TransBTS Network architecture [28]

where e is current epochs, es is total number of epochs. We use L2 norm regularization on the convolutional kernel parameters with a weight of 1e−5. The TransBTS was trained in total 1000 epochs.

2.5 Overview of Whole Architecture

After all four sub models (3D Unet, Residual 3D Unet, 3D Vnet, TransBTS) trained separately, we start to ensemble the inference result. Different from EMMA, we train a simple 3D classification model to integrate the result. The complete architecture is shown in Fig. 5. For the simple classifier, the input is stacked inference result we obtain from already trained models. This input is stacked with a 3D convolution layer. Then we flatten the output and pass it to the fully connected layer for a pixel level classification. Due to the time limit, we only trained it for 200 epochs.

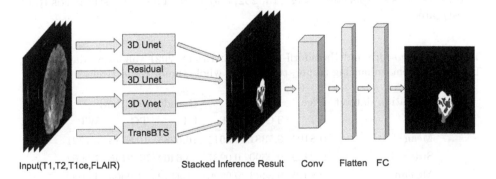

Fig. 5. Schematic visualization of whole architecture

3 Result

3.1 BraTS Datasets

We use the BraTS 2021 challenge dataset for evaluation [4–7,21]. The BraTS 2021 dataset contains 1251 cases in training data. Each case has four modalities 3D MRI, T1 weighted, T2 weighted, T1 contrast enhanced and T2 FLAIR. Our model exclusively trained with the BraTS training dataset. In this work, we consider our four modalities as four input channels. Each volume has three dimensions, 240, 240, 155 respectively. The segmented MRI has four labels: 0 represents the background, 4 represents the enhancing tumor, combined 1, 4 represents the tumor core, combined 1, 2, 4 represents the whole tumor, 3 is not used. The validation dataset has 219 cases. The test data wasn't release by the deadline of this paper. We evaluated the performance of our model on validation dataset for dice score, sensitivity, specificity and Hausdorff distances.

3.2 Preprocessing on Each Different Model

For different sub models, we apply different data augmentation. For 3D Unet, Residual 3D Unet, and Vnet we resized the image on different channels of the original 3D MRI. For TransBTS, we apply Z-score normalization of all modality 3D MRI with mean and standard deviation. After that, we applied linear normalization, random crop, random clip and random intensity shift.

3.3 Validation Phase Result

The performance of our model on BraTS 2021 validation data is shown in Table 1. Our model reached a dice score of 0.81, 0.74, 0.89 on ET, TC, WT respectively. From the deviation, we find that the enhancing tumor and tumor core has high variation. From the median and 25 quantile result, we observe that our model did not perform good in certain test cases. Our model's performance was low on several test cases especially cases 213, 252, and 1721. The cause still needs to be investigated.

Table 1. Dice score and Hausdorff distance on BraTS 2021 validation dataset. ET, TC, WT present enhancing tumor, tumor core, whole tumor respectively.

Validation dataset	Dice			Hausdorff95 (mm)		
	ET	TC	WT	ET	TC	WT
Mean	0.8194	0.7381	0.8915	16.6285	16.8743	5.7721
Stdev	0.2439	0.2590	0.0987	69.6464	35.9145	7.5963
Median	0.8915	0.8443	0.9220	1.4142	11.0000	4.0000
25quantile	0.8283	0.6793	0.8763	1.0000	6.8367	2.8284
75quantile	0.9465	0.9006	0.9475	2.9142	17.2612	6.0828

3.4 Test Phase Result

The performance of our model on BraTS 2021 test data is shown in Table 2. Our model reached a dice score of 0.86, 0.73, 0.58 on ET, WT, TC respectively. Compared with validation parse, the performance of WT reduce significantly. We will work on to improve the performance of WT in future work. Besides that, we observe that the standard deviation of whole tumor are higher than validation result. From the 25 quantile result, we found that our model performed bad in Tumor Core. From the median and 75 quantile result, our model had good performance on most test cases. The overall performance was hurt by some test cases. We will focus on those test cases in future work.

Table 2. Dice score and Hausdorff distance on BraTS 2021 Test dataset.ET, TC, WT present enhancing tumor, tumor core, whole tumor respectively.

Validation dataset	Dice			Hausdorff95 (mm)		
	ET	WT	TC	ET	WT	TC
Mean	0.8553	0.7302	0.5836	16.3118	39.0873	64.1392
Stdev	0.2113	0.3096	0.3552	70.1391	57.5957	82.7809
Median	0.9279	0.8958	0.7630	1.0000	4.6904	24.9198
25quantile	0.8463	0.5978	0.1948	1.0000	2.4495	12.3915
75quantile	0.9644	0.9416	0.8866	2.2361	57.8802	90.7419

4 Related Work

Brain tumor segmentation is a growing field of interest for researchers as it aims to automate previously used tedious manual segmentation and yield higher specificity and sensitivity. In literature, U-Net [25], an encoder-decoder based model, has served as a great baseline architecture to attain low level details and provide good performance on brain segmentation tasks. Its variants U-Net++ [31] and Res-UNet [30] have also been successful to further improve the performance. However, all these convolutional neural network (CNNs) based models were employed to perform segmentation for 2D data. Given the 3D nature of MRI brain scans, it becomes time-consuming process to perform segmentation channel by channel. In light of this, U-Net has been adapted to cater the volumetric brain data to perform segmentation [11,24]. In spite of its sophistication to extract low level details, it still suffered from capturing long-range dependency.

On the other hand, attention based architecture, vision transformer have achieved state of the art performance in classification tasks and have shown potential in capturing long range dependency [14]. TransUnet [12] is a recent network in this direction that combines UNet model as a local features extractor with transformer model to gather global level information. However, it still processes images on slice by slice fashion and focuses on retaining spatial correlation between image patches via transformer. Swin-Unet [10] is another network that combines two models, Unet and swin transformer, to enhance the performance of the segmentation model. Unfortunately it only supports 2D MRI images. To overcome this challenge TransBTS [28] combines UNet with transformer but process all slices simultaneously, and thus captures global information in a better way.

Our work exploits a different direction than these works. Instead of merging two different models in one, we consider each model as an expert. We pick four good representative models of 3D brain segmentation tasks and ensemble them using the Ensembles of Multiple Models and Architectures technique. Although this technique has been explored before for brain segmentation in the work [17], our work exploits it with advanced 3D models which are completely different and more challenging than the original work.

5 Discussion

In this work, we introduced a new ensemble model which take the advantages of several sub models to achieve a more promising segmentation result on multimodal 3D MRI. In the validation phase, we get an average good result on our model. By combining the sub models, we get a better segmentation output than each single model. We also introduced a new naive method to integrate the segmentation result from several models to get a more robust output.

However, there are several aspects we can improve after the end of BraTs 2021 challenge. In upcoming work, we can apply random crop, flip, intensity to all our sub models. In preprocessing of data, the 3D Unet uses resize method which results in loss of a lot of pixel value during the train. A bad performance sub model has limited contribution to the overall model. We will add more data augmentation techniques such as affine image transforms, random image rotation and so on. We also aim to add more data post-processing methods to generate a more stable and robust segmentation model. We will apply data parallel distributed training method or federated learning method to speed up the train period. We will work on the test cases which has significantly bad performance cases and investigate the cause of the performance. We will also apply the mix-precision to the code to speed up the training phase. We will also try to train the whole network in one big network instead of train them separately.

To summarize, we achieved 0.85, 0.90, 0.76 median dice score on ET, WT, TC respectively. We aim to further improve above mentioned approach for a better model for next years challenge.

Acknowledgment. This work was performed under the Grant 2015254 and gift by the National Science Foundation and Konica Minolta, respectively. We also acknowledge support from the University of Texas at Anderson Cancer Center, Texas Advanced Computing Center, and Oden Institute for Computational and Engineering Sciences initiative in Oncological Data and Computational Science.

References

1. Abdulbaqi, H.S., Jafri, M.Z.M., Omar, A.F., Mutter, K.N., Abood, L.K., Mustafa, I.S.B.: Segmentation and estimation of brain tumor volume in computed tomography scan images using hidden markov random field expectation maximization algorithm. In: 2015 IEEE Student Conference on Research and Development (SCOReD), pp. 55–60. IEEE (2015)
2. Angulakshmi, M., Lakshmi Priya, G.: Automated brain tumour segmentation techniques–a review. Int. J. Imaging Syst. Technol. **27**(1), 66–77 (2017)
3. Bahdanau, D., Cho, K., Bengio, Y.: Neural machine translation by jointly learning to align and translate. arXiv preprint arXiv:1409.0473 (2014)
4. Baid, U., et al.: The rsna-asnr-miccai brats 2021 benchmark on brain tumor segmentation and radiogenomic classification. arXiv preprint arXiv:2107.02314 (2021)
5. Bakas, S., et al.: Segmentation labels and radiomic features for the pre-operative scans of the tcga-gbm collection. the cancer imaging archive. Nat. Sci. Data **4**, 170117 (2017)
6. Bakas, S., et al.: Segmentation labels and radiomic features for the pre-operative scans of the tcga-lgg collection. The cancer imaging archive 286 (2017)
7. Bakas, S., et al.: Advancing the cancer genome atlas glioma MRI collections with expert segmentation labels and radiomic features. Sci. Data **4**(1), 1–13 (2017)
8. Bauer, S., Seiler, C., Bardyn, T., Buechler, P., Reyes, M.: Atlas-based segmentation of brain tumor images using a markov random field-based tumor growth model and non-rigid registration. In: 2010 Annual International Conference of the IEEE Engineering in Medicine and Biology, pp. 4080–4083. IEEE (2010)
9. Bousselham, A., Bouattane, O., Youssfi, M., Raihani, A.: Towards reinforced brain tumor segmentation on MRI images based on temperature changes on pathologic area. Int. J. Biomed. Imaging **2019** (2019)
10. Cao, H., et al.: Swin-unet: Unet-like pure transformer for medical image segmentation. arXiv preprint arXiv:2105.05537 (2021)
11. Chang, J., Zhang, X., Ye, M., Huang, D., Wang, P., Yao, C.: Brain tumor segmentation based on 3d unet with multi-class focal loss. In: 2018 11th International Congress on Image and Signal Processing, BioMedical Engineering and Informatics (CISP-BMEI), pp. 1–5. IEEE (2018)
12. Chen, J., et al.: Transunet: Transformers make strong encoders for medical image segmentation. arXiv preprint arXiv:2102.04306 (2021)
13. Çiçek, Ö., Abdulkadir, A., Lienkamp, S.S., Brox, T., Ronneberger, O.: 3D U-net: learning dense volumetric segmentation from sparse annotation. In: Ourselin, S., Joskowicz, L., Sabuncu, M.R., Unal, G., Wells, W. (eds.) MICCAI 2016. LNCS, vol. 9901, pp. 424–432. Springer, Cham (2016). https://doi.org/10.1007/978-3-319-46723-8_49
14. Dosovitskiy, A., et al.: An image is worth 16×16 words: Transformers for image recognition at scale. arXiv preprint arXiv:2010.11929 (2020)
15. Isensee, F., Kickingereder, P., Wick, W., Bendszus, M., Maier-Hein, K.H.: No new-net. In: Crimi, A., Bakas, S., Kuijf, H., Keyvan, F., Reyes, M., van Walsum, T. (eds.) BrainLes 2018. LNCS, vol. 11384, pp. 234–244. Springer, Cham (2019). https://doi.org/10.1007/978-3-030-11726-9_21
16. Kamnitsas, K., et al.: Ensembles of multiple models and architectures for robust brain tumour segmentation. In: Crimi, A., Bakas, S., Kuijf, H., Menze, B., Reyes, M. (eds.) BrainLes 2017. LNCS, vol. 10670, pp. 450–462. Springer, Cham (2018). https://doi.org/10.1007/978-3-319-75238-9_38

17. Kamnitsas, K., et al.: Deepmedic for brain tumor segmentation. In: Crimi, A., Menze, B., Maier, O., Reyes, M., Winzeck, S., Handels, H. (eds.) Brainlesion: Glioma, Multiple Sclerosis, Stroke and Traumatic Brain Injuries. BrainLes 2016. Lecture Notes in Computer Science(), vol. 10154, pp. 138–149. Springer, Cham (2016). https://doi.org/10.1007/978-3-319-55524-9_14

18. Lee, K., Zung, J., Li, P., Jain, V., Seung, H.S.: Superhuman accuracy on the snemi3d connectomics challenge. arXiv preprint arXiv:1706.00120 (2017)

19. Long, J., Shelhamer, E., Darrell, T.: Fully convolutional networks for semantic segmentation. In: Proceedings of the IEEE Conference on Computer Vision and Pattern Recognition, pp. 3431–3440 (2015)

20. Mathur, N., Mathur, S., Mathur, D.: A novel approach to improve sobel edge detector. Procedia Comput. Sci. **93**, 431–438 (2016)

21. Menze, B.H., et al.: The multimodal brain tumor image segmentation benchmark (brats). IEEE Trans. Med. Imaging **34**(10), 1993–2024 (2014)

22. Milletari, F., Navab, N., Ahmadi, S.A.: V-net: Fully convolutional neural networks for volumetric medical image segmentation. In: 2016 fourth International Conference on 3D Vision (3DV), pp. 565–571. IEEE (2016)

23. Myronenko, A.: 3D MRI brain tumor segmentation using autoencoder regularization. In: Crimi, A., Bakas, S., Kuijf, H., Keyvan, F., Reyes, M., van Walsum, T. (eds.) BrainLes 2018. LNCS, vol. 11384, pp. 311–320. Springer, Cham (2019). https://doi.org/10.1007/978-3-030-11726-9_28

24. Qamar, S., Jin, H., Zheng, R., Ahmad, P., Usama, M.: A variant form of 3d-unet for infant brain segmentation. Future Gener. Comput. Syst. **108**, 613–623 (2020)

25. Ronneberger, O., Fischer, P., Brox, T.: U-net: convolutional networks for biomedical image segmentation. In: Navab, N., Hornegger, J., Wells, W.M., Frangi, A.F. (eds.) MICCAI 2015. LNCS, vol. 9351, pp. 234–241. Springer, Cham (2015). https://doi.org/10.1007/978-3-319-24574-4_28

26. Vaswani, A., et al.: Attention is all you need. In: Advances in Neural Information Processing Systems, pp. 5998–6008 (2017)

27. Wang, G., Li, W., Ourselin, S., Vercauteren, T.: Automatic brain tumor segmentation using cascaded anisotropic convolutional neural networks. In: Crimi, A., Bakas, S., Kuijf, H., Menze, B., Reyes, M. (eds.) BrainLes 2017. LNCS, vol. 10670, pp. 178–190. Springer, Cham (2018). https://doi.org/10.1007/978-3-319-75238-9_16

28. Wang, W., Chen, C., Ding, M., Li, J., Yu, H., Zha, S.: Transbts: multimodal brain tumor segmentation using transformer. arXiv preprint arXiv:2103.04430 (2021)

29. Wolny, A., et al.: Accurate and versatile 3d segmentation of plant tissues at cellular resolution. eLife **9** (2020). https://doi.org/10.7554/elife.57613

30. Zhang, Z., Liu, Q., Wang, Y.: Road extraction by deep residual u-net. IEEE Geosci. Remote Sens. Lett. **15**(5), 749–753 (2018)

31. Zhou, Z., Rahman Siddiquee, M.M., Tajbakhsh, N., Liang, J.: UNet++: a nested u-net architecture for medical image segmentation. In: Stoyanov, D., et al. (eds.) DLMIA/ML-CDS -2018. LNCS, vol. 11045, pp. 3–11. Springer, Cham (2018). https://doi.org/10.1007/978-3-030-00889-5_1

Quality-Aware Model Ensemble for Brain Tumor Segmentation

Kang Wang[1,2], Haoran Wang[1,2], Zeyang Li[3], Mingyuan Pan[4],
Manning Wang[1,2(✉)], Shuo Wang[1,2(✉)], and Zhijian Song[1,2(✉)]

[1] Digital Medical Research Center, School of Basic Medical Sciences,
Fudan University, Shanghai, China
{mnwang,shuowang,zjsong}@fudan.edu.cn
[2] Shanghai Key Lab of Medical Image Computing and Computer
Assisted Intervention, Shanghai, China
[3] Department of Neurosurgery, Zhongshan Hospital,
Fudan University, Shanghai, China
[4] Radiation Oncology Center, Huashan Hospital, Fudan University, Shanghai, China

Abstract. Automatic segmentation of brain tumors is still a challenging task. To improve the segmentation performance and better ensemble all the candidate models with different architectures, we proposed a three-stage model with the quality-aware model ensemble. The first stage locates the tumor with coarse segmentation, while the second stage refines the coarse segmentation in the region of interest. The last stage performs the quality-aware model ensemble with a quality score prediction net to fuse the results from the multiple outputs of sub-networks. Besides, we warp a standard SRI24 brain template to the subject image, which is a strong prior of the brain structure and symmetry. Our method shows competitive performance on the BraTS 2021 online validation dataset, obtaining an average dice similarity coefficient (DSC) of 0.911, 0.850, 0.816, and average 95_{th} percentile of Hausdorff distance (HD95) of 4.58, 8.959, 10.400, for whole tumor, tumor core, and enhancing tumor, respectively.

Keywords: Brain tumor segmentation · Multi-stage segmentation · Quality prediction

1 Introduction

Glioblastoma (GBM) is the most common and aggressive type of tumor within the brain, which is usually treated with chemotherapy and radiotherapy after surgical resection [23]. The localization and delineation of glioma on medical images are of great importance for clinical diagnosis and treatment. Accurate delineation of glioma helps the surgical planning for maximum safe resection of glioblastoma with preservation of neurological function. Radiomics analysis

---

K. Wang, H. Wang—Equally contributed.

A. Crimi and S. Bakas (Eds.): BrainLes 2021, LNCS 12963, pp. 149–162, 2022.
https://doi.org/10.1007/978-3-031-09002-8_14

[4,18] of pre-operative images shows promising potentials in improving the prognostic modeling such as the prediction of overall survival (OS) and progression-free survival (PFS). Also, post-operative images provide the target delineation for precise radiotherapy. However, in the current clinical routine, the manual localization and delineation are tedious, time-consuming, and require expert knowledge. The development of accurate segmentation can significantly accelerate the process of personalized surgical planning, computer-assisted intervention, and tumor growth detection.

Glioblastoma is characterized by its intrinsic heterogeneity which poses specific technical challenges in the development of automatic segmentation. Multiple sub-regions such as necrosis (NCR), non-enhancing tumor (NET), enhancing tumor (ET) and peri-tumoral edema (ED) coexist within one single lesion. To depict the tumor micro-environment, multi-parametric magnetic resonance imaging (mpMRI) scans are often acquired for quantitative analysis. The complex distribution of these tumor sub-regions makes the clear boundary delineation difficult. Moreover, inter-tumor heterogeneity makes the development of a generic and robust automatic segmentation model of GBM more challenging.

The Brain Tumor Segmentation Challenge (BraTS) [1–4,20] is aimed at promoting the research of automatic segmentation for glioma and has established the most extensive multi-center multi-parameter Magnetic Resonance Imaging (MRI) scan dataset for glioma segmentation. In the BraTS 2021 challenge, organizers release the mpMRI data of more than 1,000 patients as well as expert annotation of tumor sub-regions. All mpMRI scans contained four different modalities: native (T1), post-contrast T1-weighted (T1Gd (Gadolinium)), T2-weighted (T2), and T2 Fluid Attenuated Inversion Recovery (T2FLAIR). All scans were acquired with different protocols and various scanners from multiple institutions. This provides a unique opportunity to the performance of automatic segmentation models of GBM and identifies the future directions.

We proposed a three-stage model with quality-aware ensemble. The first stage get the approximate localization of the tumor with coarse segmentation, while the second stage refined the coarse segmentation in cropped region of interest. The last stage performed quality-aware model ensemble with pair-wise ranking net to pick the best results from the multiple sub-networks' outputs. Besides, we registered a standard SRI24 brain template for every case to get brain map, which provides a strong prior of the brain structure and symmetry. Our method is tested on the BraTS 2021 online validation dataset, obtaining an average DSC of 0.911, 0.850, 0.816, and average Hausdorff Distance 95 of 4.58, 8.959, 10.400, for whole tumor, tumor core and enhancing tumor, respectively.

2   Related Works

In recent years, motivated by the successful application of deep learning in medical image analysis, deep learning-based methods dominated the BraTS challenge. Most of these methods adopted the encoder-decoder network architecture with skip connections like U-Net [25] and 3D U-Net [6]. Numerous improvements have been introduced to improve the segmentation performance for GBM, for example, residual connection [8,17], dense connection [9,30], attention mechanism [15,16], and dilated convolution [29] are integrated into the segmentation networks. Also, training with deep supervision was shown to boost up the segmentation performance [7,10].

Multiple solutions have been proposed to solve the class imbalance problem between the tumor and background voxels. The winning solution of BraTS 2018 [22] added a variational auto-encoder (VAE) based decoder to reconstruct the image itself in order to regularize the shared encoder. In BraTS 2019, Jiang et al. [17] used a decoder with trilinear interpolation to regularize the shared encoder. As for loss function, Dice Loss [21] and focal loss [19] were popular choices among BraTS participants' solutions.

Since the BraTS challenge evaluated segmentation performance on three sub-regions of Whole Tumor (WT, NCR/NET+ET+ED), Tumor Core (TC, NCR/NET+ET), and Enhancing Tumor (ET), optimizing the above three sub-regions using sigmoid function with binary cross-entropy loss, rather than the 3 label classes using softmax function with categorical cross-entropy loss, was considered to improve performance on BraTS challenge [11,15,17,22].

The multi-stage cascaded structure and multi-scale feature fusion obtained a more fine-grained tumor boundary. The 2nd solution in BraTS 2020 [15] introduced a parallel multi-scale fusion module and a cascaded network to refine the coarse segmentation. To better incorporate prior knowledge with a deep network, modality-pairing learning network [28] with two branches was proposed: one branch uses T2FLAIR and T2 to extract features of the whole tumor, and the other branch takes T1 and T1Gd to learn other useful information. For the model ensemble, Isensee et al. [11] used a 'rank and aggregate' approach to pick up the best model via comparing with all the candidate models.

3   Method

In clinical practice, the radiologists first screen the whole mpMRI volumes and identified the lesion region. Then attention is focused on the region of interest (ROI) to delineate the tumor boundaries and intra-tumor partitions. Finally, the radiologists took a second look across the whole image volumes to perform the quality control of segmentations. Inspired by the expert annotation, we propose a three-stage framework (Fig. 1) for brain tumor segmentation. Firstly, we develop a localization net to detect and propose a coarse segmentation. Secondly, in stage II, the refinement network modifies the coarse segmentation within the ROI with attentions on mpMRIs and brain templates. Finally, for different segmentations from various model architectures with various hyper-parameters and network architectures, we develop a quality control network to predict the quality metric of each segmentation and rank them to obtain the best-quality refined segmentation.

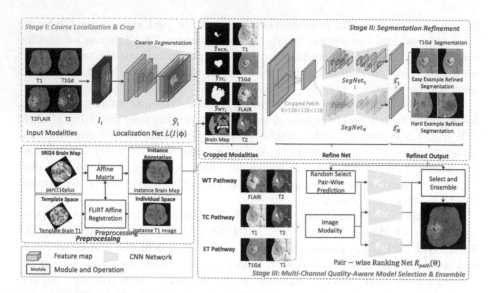

Fig. 1. Overview of the proposed three-stage framework for automatic brain tumor segmentation. Stage I is for coarse localization of brain tumor, Stage II refines the coarse segmentation in the cropped region of interest, while stage III picks the best prediction among all candidate models using a quality-aware ensemble scheme.

Brain Map. Under certain conditions, it's hard to learn efficient information only by using image information caused by low contrast and high local structural similarity in extreme cases. We stress it's important to fuse prior knowledge rather than get segmentation results depending only on image(or signal) information. We construct a symmetry brain atlas based on the standard brain atlas SRI24/TZO map [24] and registered to every case as a strong prior of the brain structure and symmetry to form additional information and help the network get a better performance not only by using the image information. For not all the data were registered to SRI24 standard space properly. Thus, we first use flirt [12,14] tool of FSL [13] to apply normal affine transformation ($DOF = 12$) between the standard atlas and individual patient (i.e. registered the standard atlas in standard space to individual space.), so that we can get a new modality to utilize prior knowledge to assist network to make decisions. As for the affine transformation, we set the search angle range $[-180°, 180°]$ for x and y axis, $[-90°, 90°]$ for z axis, and use corratio as registration cost function to get affine transform $M_{A_i}(\cdot)$ under the affine matrix A_i by using standard T2 image from SRI24 and T2 image from each patient. Affined coordinates y_i and brain map could represents as fellows $\mathbf{y}_i = A_i \cdot \mathbf{x}_i$, $I_{Affined_i} = M_{A_i}(I_{SRI24})$ the interpolation method is nearest interpolation.

Additionally, for the purpose of learning symmetric information of brain structure, we modify the origin asymmetric SRI24 atlas to get a simplified symmetric brain atlas following three steps. 1). Change odd (represent left hemisphere) areas to corresponding even area (right hemisphere); 2). Get continuous atlas by dividing 2; 3). Merge redundant subareas into a large area to get a simplified atlas and finally normalized into zero mean and 1 standard deviation atlas.

Localization Net. In the first stage, localization net $L(\mathbf{x} \mid \phi)$ was used to localize the approximate location and get coarse segmentation of the tumor by utilizing the image information. Considering the outstanding segmentation performance and feature extraction capacity of HR-Net [27], we use a 3D localization net similar with HR-Net and HNF-Net [15,16] combines high-resolution feature representation and lightweight non-local attention module, which could get better global information and maintain high resolutions.

As previously mentioned in related works, directly optimizing overlapping regions WT, TC and ET separately is more effective than optimizing the provided label classes. So, we use the sigmoid function as the final activation function to get separate prediction outputs of the three overlapping regions of WT, TC, and ET, and the binary cross-entropy loss as the pixel classification loss of segmentation. The loss function $\mathcal{L}_{Loc}$ of localization net $L(\mathbf{x} \mid \phi)$ is a linear combination of generalized dice loss $\mathcal{L}_{GDS}$ [26], binary cross-entropy loss $\mathcal{L}_{BCE}$ and dice loss $\mathcal{L}_{Dice}$ [21] (i.e. $\mathcal{L}_{Loc} = \mathcal{L}_{GDS} + \mathcal{L}_{BCE} + \mathcal{L}_{Dice}$).

In the training phase, input image I_i was cropped into small patches whose size is $4 \times 128 \times 128 \times 128$ (in the order of number of channels, width, height and depth). In inference time, the input image I_i was cropped into small patches with overlap $\mathcal{P} = \{p_i \mid p_i \in \mathbb{R}^{C_{in} \times 128 \times 128 \times 128}; i = 1, 2, \ldots, N\}$ by sliding window of multiple different position in original image. The step of sliding window is 32 voxel. After network inference and patch assemble, localization net finally output a coarse segmentation $\hat{\mathbf{y}}_i \in \mathbb{R}^{3 \times 240 \times 240 \times 155}$ which could split into $\hat{\mathbf{y}}_{NCR_i}$, $\hat{\mathbf{y}}_{TC_i}$, $\hat{\mathbf{y}}_{WT_i} \in \mathbb{R}^{1 \times 240 \times 240 \times 155}$ represents the coarse segmentation results of NCR/NET, TC and WT respectively. The above 3 independent channels will be used as auxiliary channels in the second stage. In the meantime, the coarse segmentation was used for lesion localization. The cropped ROI is centered on the segmentation center point with a bounding box of $128 \times 128 \times 128$ in each modality and used for refining segmentation. Cause the coarse segmentation was used to provide coarse localization and auxiliary information in the next stage, the small response or wrong prediction will be dealt in the latter procedure.

Refinement Nets. According to referential experiences [15,17], we focus on getting fine-grained results based on the coarse segmentation of the previous stage. Unlike previous works, we implement segmentation refinement in an ROI rather than in the entire image to accelerate the processing speed considering the highly time-consuming sliding window procedure of the entire image. Focusing on the most crucial part of the image is more effective.

According to previous studies, it's hard for a single network to get satisfied prediction results [17]. However, different CNN (Convolutional Neural Network) with different learning strategies and data distribution will get enough candidate predictions to be chosen as the final prediction and provide complementary information. From this point, we build different models to implement refining tasks in the second stage. To increase the diversity of the refined segmentation, we choose HNF-Net [15], and nnU-Net-like network [11] as alternative models and trained separately to provide candidate predictions. Training configuration of HNF-Net is the same with localization net. The nnU-Net-like network follows an encoder-decoder fashion, and downsampling was performed 5 times with stride convolutions while upsampling was performed with transposed convolutions. The loss function is a sum combination of Dice loss [21] and binary cross-entropy loss. Deep supervision is adopted for better performance [7,10], an $1 \times 1 \times 1$ convolution with trilinear upsampling is added to expand the decoder output to the same size with the groundtruth. Single alternative network was trained in the following strategies: 1) Split training set in the ratio of 4:1 and chose the best model in local validation; 2) Training by using full training set with an early stop strategy to avoid overfitting; 3) Using whole training set and pseudo label of validation set; 4) Training network only using the hard examples to improve potential performance for hard examples. Following these principles, we pick 4 models of each type to constitute alternative models. The refinement model $\{SegNet_i \mid i = 1, \ldots, N\}$ is an ensemble of several single model to provided candidate segmentation predictions. Considering time-consuming, we set $N = 7$ to meet the time limit.

As illustrate in Fig. 1, the input of Refinement $SegNet_i$ is a ROI region whose size is $8 \times 128 \times 128 \times 128$ including 8 modalities that is 4 raw modalities (T1, T1Gd, T2FLAIR, T2) provided by the cropped MRI scan, 4 additional information modalities contain 1 registered brain map mentioned above and 3 coarse segmentation prediction channels of $L(\mathbf{x} \mid \phi)$. The size of the ROI is $128 \times 128 \times 128$ and centering on tumor center according to coarse prediction. For each $SegNet_i$, the prediction output constitute a candidate set $\hat{S} = \{\hat{s}_i \mid \hat{s}_i \in \mathbb{R}^{3 \times 128 \times 128 \times 128}; i = 1, 2, \ldots, N\}$ which used in the following step.

Ranking Net. In previous BraTS challenges, ensemble methods had been widely used to improve segmentation performance. How to ensemble multiple segmentation models with different architectures and hyper-parameters is still a challenging task. The most intuitive way is via a voting mechanism that averages the pixel-level prediction. Assigning different voting weights according to the performance of each model would take the confidence into consideration. Nevertheless, these naive bagging methods do not consider the performance shifting among different samples, which means that one model could yield superior performance than another model in some patients but may fail in other patients.

In this work, we utilize a ranking network to predict the quality score(i.e. DSC) of segmentation. Then the segmentation generated by the model with the best quality score is selected. This selection method can be performed at the patient level or slice level.

In this stage, we construct 3 ranking models to implement quality-aware model selection for each target component (WT, TC, ET). Ranking models including R_{WT}, R_{TC}, R_{ET} are light-weighted twin network made up of two 3d ResNet-18 [8] pretrained in Kinetics-400 [5]. The input of each ranking net in each pathway including 2 image modalities and 2 pair-wise refined segmentation predictions. The image modality is chosen according to clinical practice to judge the corresponding areas. The pair-wise refined segmentation prediction $\hat{s}_i, \hat{s}_j$ is chosen from all the output of refined net $\hat{s}_i (i = 1, 2, \ldots, N)$ for ranking.

The twin quality prediction net takes the concatenation of image modality and single prediction of prediction pair as input of each branch. The output of the Ranking net is the predicted DSC of each prediction and the ranking range r_{WT}, r_{TC} and r_{ET} to sort the prediction list and get the best prediction of each pathway. For training the quality prediction network, the ranking loss $\mathcal{L}_{R_{WT}}, \mathcal{L}_{R_{TC}}, \mathcal{L}_{R_{ET}}$ are hybrid losses contain L1-loss between the prediction DSC and real DSC and margin ranking loss between two random segmentations corresponding to the same mpMRIs to be segmented. Ranking loss $\mathcal{L}_{Rank}$ is shown as below:

$$\mathcal{L}_{Rank} = \frac{1}{2} \times \mathcal{L}_{DSC1} + \frac{1}{2} \times \mathcal{L}_{DSC2} + \mathcal{L}_{MarginRankingLoss} \qquad (1)$$

where the regression loss of DSC prediction is a normal L1 loss, x is predicted DSC and y is the true DSC between prediction $\hat{s}_i$ and ground truth:

$$\mathcal{L}_{DSC}(x, y) = \|x - y\| \qquad (2)$$

The margin ranking loss is used to accelerate convergence and make the ranking net to get a better DSC prediction and get ranking score,

$$\mathcal{L}_{MarginRankingLoss}(x_1, x_2, y) = \max(0, -y * (x_1 - x_2) + \text{margin}) \qquad (3)$$

where x_1 and x_2 are DSC predictions of $\hat{s}_i$ and $\hat{s}_j$. y is the ranking ground truth. If $y = 1$, then it assumed the first input should be ranked higher (have a larger value) than the second input, and vice-versa for $y = -1$. margin is the distance set for discriminate and set as default 0 here. Albeit the predicted DSC may differ from the ground truth DSC, the ranking net only needs to predict relative high and low differences to achieve the pair-wise ranking task. After sorting all candidates, we could obtain the final prediction with a higher DSC score.

Optimization. The BraTS challenge evaluates segmentation performance on three sub-regions of WT, TC, and ET. Optimizing the above three sub-regions directly is shown to be beneficial for improvement. Our experiment results show that directly minimizing the loss of ET would create voids in areas that should be the necrotic tumor. We solved this problem by separately learning WT, TC, and necrotic areas for both HNF-Net and nnU-Net. Cosine learning rate decay is adopted in our training strategy. The learning rate η_t of t step is

$$\eta_t = \eta_{\min} + \frac{1}{2} (\eta_{\max} - \eta_{\min}) \left(1 + \cos \left(\frac{T_{\text{cur}}}{T_{\text{max}}} \pi \right) \right), \qquad (4)$$

where $\eta_{\max}$ and $\eta_{\min}$ are initial and final learning rate, T_{cur} are T_{max} current iteration steps and maximum iteration steps (Fig. 2).

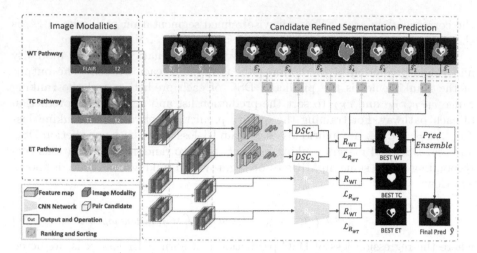

Fig. 2. Illustration of Pair-wise Ranking Net. For each pathway, we choose 2 image modalities according to clinical practice and two pair-wise refined segmentation to identify and choose the best prediction of the refined candidate segmentation. The Ranking Net of each pathway is a twin network made up of 3D ResNet-18, which output the DSC of individual predictions and choose the best prediction of a specific component (i.e., WT, TC, ET). All the best components will be assembled as the final prediction.

4   Experiments and Results

4.1   Dataset

The training set of BraTS 2021 consists of 1251 MRI scans. Each scan was annotated by experienced radiologists with three different subregions: Gd-enhancing tumor (ET – label 4), the peritumoral edematous/invaded tissue (ED – label 2), and the necrotic tumor core (NCR/NET - label 1).

4.2   Evaluation Metrics

The BraTS challenges provided four evaluation metrics: 'Dice' measures overlap between segmentation results and annotations in voxel space, 'Hausdorff distance (HD95)' measures the closet distances between segmentation surface and groundtruth surface, 'Sensitivity' and 'Specificity' shows the percentage of true positive or true negative voxels being correctly classified.

The Dice coefficient is an F1-oriented statistic used for estimation the similarity of two given sets. DSC coefficient is a typical 3D medical image segmentation voxel-related set similarity measurement function used to calculate the similarity between two samples of segmentation and gold standard:

$$DSC = \frac{2\left|\mathcal{V}_{\text{pred}} \cap \mathcal{V}_{gt}\right|}{\left|\mathcal{V}_{\text{pred}}\right| + \left|\mathcal{V}_{gt}\right|} = \frac{2TP}{2TP + FP + FN} \tag{5}$$

Hausdorff distance is a common distance measure based on the set of surface points, which generally measures the maximum surface difference between the prediction body and the gold standard.

$$HD\left(\mathcal{V}_{\mathrm{pred}},\mathcal{V}_{gt}\right) = \max\left\{\sup_{x\in\mathcal{V}_{\mathrm{pred}}} d\left(x,\mathcal{V}_{gt}\right), \sup_{y\in\mathcal{V}_{gt}} d\left(\mathcal{V}_{\mathrm{pred}},y\right)\right\} \quad (6)$$

In the formula, sup stands for upper certainty bound (supermum). HD distance is usually used in the form of 95 quantile rather than directly using the maximum value. (i.e. $HD_{95}(Vpred, Vgt)$).

4.3 Experimental Settings

For this study, based on a Linux platform with Intel® Xeon™ Gold 6133 (2.50 GHz x 16 CPUs), 64 GB of RAM, and NVIDIA Tesla V100 GPU (32 GB), we implemented all the models and experiments. The model is built primarily based on the Python deep learning framework Pytorch (version 1.7.0, CUDA 11.1).

Data Preprocessing. We first clipped the intensity of brain voxels with a window of [0.2%, 99.8%], then normalized the brain voxels of each modality by subtracting their mean and dividing their standard deviation. All the non-brain voxels remain zero.

Data Augmentation. To prevent overfitting, we randomly picked 4 from 8 data augmentations during training, including scaling of factors 0.6 to 1.6, random rotation of 90°, random rotation of 10°, random flip, random intensity change of shift 0.2, and scale 0.1, random noise and Gaussian blur.

Model Training. We trained our multi-stage models separately. For training iteration, Adam optimizer with a batch size of 12 is trained for 100 epochs. The initial learning rate is 1e−4 and decayed with cosine annealing. Weight decay of 1e-5 is also adopted for model regularization.

4.4 Experimental Results

Our method was tested on the BraTS 2021 validation dataset. As shown in Table 1, our method achieved an average DSC of 0.911, 0.850, 0.816, and average HD95 of 4.58, 8.959, 10.400, for whole tumor, tumor core, and enhancing tumor, respectively. Table 1 also provides standard deviation, median, 25 quantiles, and 75 quantiles of all the evaluation metrics.

Table 1. Performance on BraTS 2021 validation set (submission id: 9715220), std stands for standard deviation.

	DSC ET	DSC TC	DSC WT	HD95 ET	HD95 TC	HD95 WT
Mean	0.8164	0.8500	0.9108	10.400	8.959	4.582
std	0.2184	0.2117	0.1070	50.112	36.690	8.480
Median	0.8824	0.9289	0.9402	1.414	2.236	2.449
25 quantile	0.8139	0.8327	0.8981	1.000	1.000	1.414
75 quantile	0.9310	0.9592	0.9619	2.828	5.050	4.243

4.5 Ablation Study

Effect of Brain Map. To verify the effect of the brain map, we conduct a comparative trial in local validation data under the same condition. The local training data is split into local training data and local validation data randomly in a ratio of 4:1. The segmentation network is a 3D HR-Net with an expectation maximization attention module.

As shown in Table 2, We first use SRI24/STZO standard brain atlas as additional information that is normalized brain map into zero mean and 1 standard deviation and concatenate as the fifth channel of input images. The DSC score of 3 target areas was all get improved. Then we simplify the SRI24/STZO atlas and unify the odd and even area, which represents left and right hemisphere, into symmetry areas. Finally, we merge some small areas to get a simplified brain map and normalize them as the 5_{th} channel of the input image. The result shows the simplified symmetry brain map could further boost the segmentation net's performance in a further step (Fig. 3).

Table 2. Effect of brain map in local validation set. The init learning rate are both set as 1e−4 and under the same condition. ✗ means without that setting and ✓ means with that setting vice-versa. Asymmetry means using the origin SRI24/TZO atlas, while simplified and symmetry means using the modified simplified and symmetry brain map

Network	Asymmetry	Simplified	Symmetry	DSC ET	DSC TC	DSC WT	HD95 ET	HD95 TC	HD95 WT
HR-Net	✗	✗	✗	0.7949	0.8482	0.9147	6.178	**6.541**	8.190
HR-Net	✓	✗	✗	0.8044	0.8669	0.9202	5.903	6.557	7.123
HR-Net	✗	✓	✓	**0.8222**	**0.8833**	**0.9317**	15.29	8.030	**6.120**

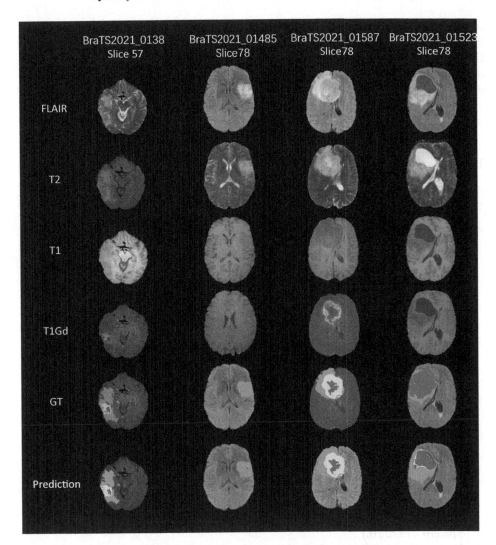

Fig. 3. Visualization of axial segmentation results from local valid set. Each column shows one typical case in the local valid set. Each row of first 4 rows displays 4 modalities (T2FLAIR, T2, T1, T1Gd) of the raw data. Last 2 rows show the ground truth (GT) and the segmentation result of the model (Prediction). Labels include enhancing tumor (yellow), edema (green), and necrotic and non-enhancing tumor (red). (Best viewed in color) (Color figure online)

5   Conclusion

Automatic segmentation of the brain tumor is an essential but challenging task. Here we propose a three-stage model with the quality-aware ensemble. Our method showed a multi-stage segmentation framework with a quality-aware model ensemble could get a competitive performance according to the BraTS 2021 leaderboard. Our method was tested on the BraTS 2021 online validation dataset, obtaining an average DSC score of 0.911, 0.850, 0.816, and HD95 distance of 4.58 mm, 8.959 mm, 10.400 mm, for whole tumor, tumor core, and enhancing tumor, respectively. The experiment result also shows the simplified symmetry brain map could further boost the segmentation net's performance in a further step.

References

1. Baid, U., et al.: The RSNA-ASNR-MICCAI BraTS 2021 benchmark on brain tumor segmentation and radiogenomic classification. arXiv e-prints arXiv:2107.02314, July 2021
2. Bakas, S., et al.: Segmentation labels and radiomic features for the pre-operative scans of the TCGA-GBM collection. Cancer Imaging Arch. (2017). https://doi.org/10.7937/K9/TCIA.2017.KLXWJJ1Q
3. Bakas, S., et al.: Segmentation labels and radiomic features for the pre-operative scans of the TCGA-LGG collection. Cancer Imaging Arch. (2017). https://doi.org/10.7937/K9/TCIA.2017.GJQ7R0EF
4. Bakas, S., et al.: Advancing the cancer genome atlas glioma MRI collections with expert segmentation labels and radiomic features. Sci. Data **4**(1), 170117 (2017). https://doi.org/10.1038/sdata.2017.117
5. Carreira, J., Noland, E., Banki-Horvath, A., Hillier, C., Zisserman, A.: A short note about kinetics-600. arXiv e-prints arXiv:1808.01340, August 2018
6. Çiçek, Ö., Abdulkadir, A., Lienkamp, S.S., Brox, T., Ronneberger, O.: 3D U-Net: learning dense volumetric segmentation from sparse annotation. In: Ourselin, S., Joskowicz, L., Sabuncu, M.R., Unal, G., Wells, W. (eds.) MICCAI 2016. LNCS, vol. 9901, pp. 424–432. Springer, Cham (2016). https://doi.org/10.1007/978-3-319-46723-8_49
7. Futrega, M., Milesi, A., Marcinkiewicz, M., Ribalta, P.: Optimized U-Net for brain tumor segmentation. arXiv preprint arXiv:2110.03352 (2021)
8. He, K., Zhang, X., Ren, S., Sun, J.: Deep residual learning for image recognition. In: Proceedings of the IEEE Conference on Computer Vision and Pattern Recognition, pp. 770–778 (2016)
9. Huang, G., Liu, Z., Van Der Maaten, L., Weinberger, K.Q.: Densely connected convolutional networks. In: Proceedings of the IEEE Conference on Computer Vision and Pattern Recognition, pp. 4700–4708 (2017)
10. Isensee, F., Jaeger, P.F., Kohl, S.A., Petersen, J., Maier-Hein, K.H.: nnU-Net: a self-configuring method for deep learning-based biomedical image segmentation. Nat. Methods **18**(2), 203–211 (2021)
11. Isensee, F., Jäger, P.F., Full, P.M., Vollmuth, P., Maier-Hein, K.H.: nnU-Net for brain tumor segmentation. In: Crimi, A., Bakas, S. (eds.) BrainLes 2020. LNCS, vol. 12659, pp. 118–132. Springer, Cham (2021). https://doi.org/10.1007/978-3-030-72087-2_11
12. Jenkinson, M., Bannister, P., Brady, M., Smith, S.: Improved optimization for the robust and accurate linear registration and motion correction of brain images. Neuroimage **17**(2), 825–841 (2002). https://doi.org/10.1006/nimg.2002.1132

13. Jenkinson, M., Beckmann, C.F., Behrens, T.E.J., Woolrich, M.W., Smith, S.M.: FSL. NeuroImage **62**(2), 782–790 (2012). https://doi.org/10.1016/j. neuroimage.2011.09.015.   https://www.sciencedirect.com/science/article/pii/ S1053811911010603

14. Jenkinson, M., Smith, S.: A global optimisation method for robust affine registration of brain images. Med. Image Anal. **5**(2), 143–156 (2001). https://doi.org/10. 1016/S1361-8415(01)00036-6

15. Jia, H., Cai, W., Huang, H., Xia, Y.: H^2NF-Net for brain tumor segmentation using multimodal MR imaging: 2nd place solution to BraTS challenge 2020 segmentation task. In: Crimi, A., Bakas, S. (eds.) BrainLes 2020. LNCS, vol. 12659, pp. 58–68. Springer, Cham (2021). https://doi.org/10.1007/978-3-030-72087-2_6

16. Jia, H., Xia, Y., Cai, W., Huang, H.: Learning high-resolution and efficient non-local features for brain glioma segmentation in MR images. In: Martel, A.L., et al. (eds.) MICCAI 2020. LNCS, vol. 12264, pp. 480–490. Springer, Cham (2020). https://doi.org/10.1007/978-3-030-59719-1_47

17. Jiang, Z., Ding, C., Liu, M., Tao, D.: Two-stage cascaded U-Net: 1st place solution to BraTS challenge 2019 segmentation task. In: Crimi, A., Bakas, S. (eds.) BrainLes 2019. LNCS, vol. 11992, pp. 231–241. Springer, Cham (2020). https://doi.org/10. 1007/978-3-030-46640-4_22

18. Li, C., et al.: Multi-parametric and multi-regional histogram analysis of MRI: modality integration reveals imaging phenotypes of glioblastoma. Eur. Radiol. **29**(9), 4718–4729 (2019). https://doi.org/10.1007/s00330-018-5984-z

19. Lin, T.Y., Goyal, P., Girshick, R., He, K., Dollár, P.: Focal loss for dense object detection. In: Proceedings of the IEEE International Conference on Computer Vision, pp. 2980–2988 (2017)

20. Menze, B.H., Jakab, A., Bauer, S., Kalpathy-Cramer, J., Farahani, K., Kirby, J., et al.: The multimodal brain tumor image segmentation benchmark (BRATS). IEEE Trans. Med. Imaging **34**(10), 1993–2024 (2015). https://doi.org/10.1109/ TMI.2014.2377694

21. Milletari, F., Navab, N., Ahmadi, S.A.: V-Net: fully convolutional neural networks for volumetric medical image segmentation. In: 2016 Fourth International Conference on 3D Vision (3DV), pp. 565–571. IEEE (2016)

22. Myronenko, A.: 3D MRI brain tumor segmentation using autoencoder regularization. In: Crimi, A., Bakas, S., Kuijf, H., Keyvan, F., Reyes, M., van Walsum, T. (eds.) BrainLes 2018. LNCS, vol. 11384, pp. 311–320. Springer, Cham (2019). https://doi.org/10.1007/978-3-030-11726-9_28

23. Ricard, D., Idbaih, A., Ducray, F., Lahutte, M., Hoang-Xuan, K., Delattre, J.Y.: Primary brain tumours in adults. Lancet **379**(9830), 1984–1996 (2012)

24. Rohlfing, T., Zahr, N.M., Sullivan, E.V., Pfefferbaum, A.: The SRI24 multichannel atlas of normal adult human brain structure. Hum. Brain Mapp. **31**(5), 798–819 (2010). https://doi.org/10.1002/hbm.20906

25. Ronneberger, O., Fischer, P., Brox, T.: U-Net: convolutional networks for biomedical image segmentation. In: Navab, N., Hornegger, J., Wells, W.M., Frangi, A.F. (eds.) MICCAI 2015. LNCS, vol. 9351, pp. 234–241. Springer, Cham (2015). https://doi.org/10.1007/978-3-319-24574-4_28

26. Sudre, C.H., Li, W., Vercauteren, T., Ourselin, S., Jorge Cardoso, M.: Generalised dice overlap as a deep learning loss function for highly unbalanced segmentations. In: Cardoso, M.J., et al. (eds.) DLMIA/ML-CDS -2017. LNCS, vol. 10553, pp. 240–248. Springer, Cham (2017). https://doi.org/10.1007/978-3-319-67558-9_28

27. Sun, K., et al.: High-resolution representations for labeling pixels and regions. arxiv 2019. arXiv preprint arXiv:1904.04514 (2019)

28. Wang, Y., et al.: Modality-pairing learning for brain tumor segmentation. arXiv preprint arXiv:2010.09277 (2020)
29. Zhang, J., Lv, X., Sun, Q., Zhang, Q., Wei, X., Liu, B.: SDResU-Net: separable and dilated residual U-Net for MRI brain tumor segmentation. Curr. Med. Imaging **16**(6), 720–728 (2020)
30. Zhao, Y.-X., Zhang, Y.-M., Liu, C.-L.: Bag of tricks for 3D MRI brain tumor segmentation. In: Crimi, A., Bakas, S. (eds.) BrainLes 2019. LNCS, vol. 11992, pp. 210–220. Springer, Cham (2020). https://doi.org/10.1007/978-3-030-46640-4_20

Redundancy Reduction in Semantic Segmentation of 3D Brain Tumor MRIs

Md Mahfuzur Rahman Siddiquee and Andriy Myronenko[⊠]

NVIDIA, Santa Clara, CA, USA
mrahmans@asu.edu, amyronenko@nvidia.com

Abstract. Another year of the multimodal brain tumor segmentation challenge (BraTS) 2021 provides an even larger dataset to facilitate collaboration and research of brain tumor segmentation methods, which are necessary for disease analysis and treatment planning. A large dataset size of BraTS 2021 and the advent of modern GPUs provide a better opportunity for deep-learning based approaches to learn tumor representation from the data. In this work, we maintained an encoder-decoder based segmentation network, but focused on a modification of network training process that minimizes redundancy under perturbations. Given a set trained networks, we further introduce a confidence based ensembling techniques to further improve the performance. We evaluated the method on BraTS 2021, and in terms of dice for enhanced tumor core, tumor core and whole tumor, we achieved 0.8600, 0.8868 and 0.9265 average dice for the validation set, and 0.8769, 0.8721, 0.9266 average dice for the testing set. Our team (NVAUTO) submission was the top performing in terms of ET and TC scores, and using the Brats ranking system (based on the dice and Hausdorff distance ranking per case) achieved the 2nd place on the validation set, and the 4th place on the testing set.

Keywords: Brats · Redundancy reduction · Brain · Tumor · 3D MRI

1 Introduction

This year, 2021 multimodal brain tumor segmentation challenge (BraTS) [2], boasts a large dataset of 2000 cases. Long gone the days of a modest couple of hundred image datasets [6,13]. With a large data size comes more confidence in the achieved solution to be better generalizible in clinical practice. The dataset includes data from the previous year challenges, which also implies that some cases might be very dated (of low image quality), but this can be considered a positive feature to ensure the robustness of the solution. A large data size, in theory, should lead to a more accurate solution, but also requires a large computational resource. Thankfully, modern GPUs, such as Nvidia A100 (RTX generation), have substantially improved over the last years in terms of speed, performance and GPU memory sizes. It is also interesting to note of the paradigm

A. Crimi and S. Bakas (Eds.): BrainLes 2021, LNCS 12963, pp. 163–172, 2022.
https://doi.org/10.1007/978-3-031-09002-8_15

change, that it is no longer necessary to motivate the necessity of deep learning based approach here, as every solution in this challenge is probably deep learning based.

Gliomas are primary brain tumors, which originate from brain cells, whereas secondary tumors metastasize into the brain from other organs. Gliomas can be of low-grade (LGG) and high-grade (HGG) subtypes. High grade gliomas are an aggressive type of malignant brain tumor that grow rapidly, usually require surgery and radiotherapy and have poor survival prognosis. Magnetic Resonance Imaging (MRI) is a key diagnostic tool for brain tumor analysis, monitoring and surgery planning. Usually, several complimentary 3D MRI modalities are acquired - such as T1, T1 with contrast agent (T1c), T2 and Fluid Attenuation Inversion Recover (FLAIR) - to emphasize different tissue properties and areas of tumor spread. For example the contrast agent, usually gadolinium, emphasizes hyperactive tumor subregions in T1c MRI modality.

Multimodal Brain Tumor Segmentation Challenge (BraTS) aims to evaluate state-of-the-art methods for the segmentation of brain tumors by providing a 3D MRI dataset with ground truth tumor segmentation labels annotated by physicians [3–6,11]. This year, BraTS 2021 training dataset included 1251 cases, each with four 3D MRI modalities (T1, T1c, T2 and FLAIR) rigidly aligned, resampled to $1 \times 1 \times 1$ mm isotropic resolution and skull-stripped. The input image size is $240 \times 240 \times 155$. The data were collected from multiple institutions, using various MRI scanners. Annotations include 3 tumor subregions: the enhancing tumor, the peritumoral edema, and the necrotic and non-enhancing tumor core. The annotations were combined into 3 nested subregions: whole tumor (WT), tumor core (TC) and enhancing tumor (ET), as shown in Fig. 1. Two additional datasets without the ground truth labels were provided for validation and testing. The validation dataset (219 cases) allowed multiple submissions and was designed for intermediate evaluations. The testing dataset (530 cases) will be analysed blindly using the docker submission, and is used to calculate the final challenge ranking.

In this work, we describe our approach for 3D brain tumor segmentation from multimodal 3D MRIs and participate in BraTS 2021 challenge.

2   Related Work

Previous years of BraTS challenge winners include our work in 2018 [13], using encoder-decoder based network with asymmetrically large encoder. In 2019, Jiang et al. [10] used a similar encoder-decoder architecture, but added a second network to refine the segmentation in a cascade fashion. In 2020, Isensee et al. [9] proposed modifications to their nnUnet work. The authors continue to demonstrate that a standard encoder-decoder based architecture can achieve state of the art results, given the best practices of all components of the segmentation workflow (pre-processing, normalization, augmentations, ensembling). Here, we generally follow our encoder-decoder based network from [13] as a backbone, but modify the training and ensembling strategies.

3   Methods

We used SegResNet from MONAI [1,13] with encoder-decoder based CNN architecture. We switched to Instance Normalization [14], as it has a lightly lower memory footprint compared to Group Normalization (GN) [15], for equivalent performance. Briefly speaking, the encoder part uses ResNet [8] blocks, where each block consists of two convolutions with normalization and ReLU, followed by additive identity skip connection. We progressively downsize image dimensions by 2 and simultaneously increase feature size by 2. Each decoder level begins with upsizing followed by an addition of encoder output of the equivalent spatial level. The end of the decoder has the same spatial size as the original image, and the number of features equal to the initial input feature size, followed by $1 \times 1 \times 1$ convolution into 3 channels and a sigmoid function. See Table 1 for the details.

Table 1. Backbone network structure, where IN stands for group normalization, Conv - $3 \times 3 \times 3$ convolution, AddId - addition of identity/skip connection.

Name	Ops	Repeat
InitConv	Conv	1
EncoderBlock0	IN, ReLU, Conv, IN, ReLU, Conv, AddId	1
EncoderDown1	Conv stride 2	1
EncoderBlock1	IN, ReLU, Conv, IN, ReLU, Conv, AddId	2
EncoderDown2	Conv stride 2	1
EncoderBlock2	IN, ReLU, Conv, IN, ReLU, Conv, AddId	2
EncoderDown3	Conv stride 2	1
EncoderBlock3	IN, ReLU, Conv, IN, ReLU, Conv, AddId	4
DecoderUp2	UpConv, +EncoderBlock2	1
DecoderBlock2	IN, ReLU, Conv, IN, ReLU, Conv, AddId	1
DecoderUp1	UpConv, +EncoderBlock1	1
DecoderBlock1	IN, ReLU, Conv, IN, ReLU, Conv, AddId	1
DecoderUp0	UpConv, +EncoderBlock0	1
DecoderBlock0	IN, ReLU, Conv, IN, ReLU, Conv, AddId	1
DecoderEnd	IN, ReLU, Conv1, Sigmoid	1

3.1   Redundancy Reduction

We would like to encourage structure on the learned feature representations of our network. Firstly, we want to enforce invariance of the result under perturbations. Generally, it is common to use image augmentations, such as intensity modifications or spatial transforms, to implicitly enforce network robustness to such image perturbations. However, this alone does not often lead to a similar feature representation under perturbations, even if the final segmentation masks are similar. In semi-supervised learning, people adopted such method as contrasting coding of SimCLR [7] to enforce consistency of learned features under perturbations. Contrastive coding requires large number of negative samples/batches, which is too computationally expensive for 3D images. Secondly, we also want another useful property of the learned image features: minimal redundancy. Loosely speaking, we want different samples to have different learned representation with minimal information overlap. For these reason, we adopted the loss term from Barlow Twins [16], which is:

$$\mathbf{L}_{BT} = \mathbf{L}_{invariance} + \mathbf{L}_{redundancy} \tag{1}$$

Unlike the original paper concerning classification, our adaptation is for the segmentation which requires some modifications. For example, when training with a 3D batch size of 1, we copy it and augment it each copy independently, forming a batch of 2. For augmentations we use, both intensity and spatial augmentations. We then attach a projection branch to the output feature dimension (one level before the final normalization). The projection branch first average pools the features by a factor of 16, for two reasons: the output features are of the original image size, and it's too computationally expensive to use them directly, secondly spatial augmentation transforms would produce geometrical image misalignment between the two images, and average pooling ensures that the pooled features are roughly of the same spatial content. After pooling the newly formed features are reshaped to form a large batch of 1D features. At the stage we proceed with the projection branch (3 layer MLP) and compute the empirical cross-correlation matrix C between all combinations of spatial regions [16]:

$$C_{ij} = \frac{\sum_b z_{b,i}^A z_{b,j}^B}{\sqrt{\sum_b (z_{b,i}^A)^2} \sqrt{\sum_b (z_{b,j}^B)^2}} \tag{2}$$

where b indexes batch samples and i,j index the vector dimension of the networks' outputs. C is a square matrix with size the dimensionality of the network's output, and with values comprised between -1 (i.e. perfect anti-correlation) and 1 (i.e. perfect correlation).

Unlike the original work, which uses a batch of many different 2D images, our cross-correlation matrix is based on the various regions of the same image under permutations. Based on the cross-correlation matrix, we can compute a differentiable loss:

$$\mathbf{L}_{BT} = \sum (1 - C_{ii})^2 + \lambda \sum_{i \neq j} C_{ij}^2 \tag{3}$$

where the first part enforces invariance of learned feature representations from the same spatial regions under perturbations, and second term reduces redundancy between different spatial regions. We used $\lambda = 0.005$ weight, to balance the parts, as proposed in the original paper. The projection branch is discarded during inference. We use this loss in additional to the main soft Dice loss [12]:

$$\mathbf{L}_{dice} = 1 - \frac{2 * \sum p_{true} * p_{pred}}{\sum p_{true}^2 + \sum p_{pred}^2 + \epsilon} \tag{4}$$

where p_{true} is a ground truth binary mask, and p_{pred} is the predicted probability (after sigmoid) per class.

3.2 Confidence Based Ensembling

Given a trained set of models, ensembling is a popular technique to boost the performance, typically by averaging the probabilities of predictions. Alternatively one can employ a geometrical mean (instead of standard mean) to combine the probabilities. We take it one step further and design a technique to adaptively average the probability maps.

Assuming we know the confidence of the solution/prediction result of each model for a given image, then we could use the subset of the probability maps with the top confidence for ensembling (or we can use the weight mean of all such maps). We found that using the top $N/2$ probabilities (with equal weights) generally gives the best performance, where N is the number of all maps before the ensembling.

Estimation of the confidence measure of the given segmentation probability map is non-trivial. We propose a heuristic for such estimate as the average probability value of the segmented region. Such heuristic is based on the observation that given two probability maps of the same final segmentation volume, the one with the highest average probability is usually more accurate. This assumption is not true when different models produce substantially different region sizes, or if the trained model were very different to compare directly. In our experiment, we found such heuristic consistently improves the ensembling performance.

3.3 Optimization

We use AdamW optimizer with initial learning rate of $\alpha_0 = 10^{-4}$ and progressively decrease it according to Cosine schedule. We use 10^{-5} weight decay and no dropout.

3.4 Prepossessing and Augmentation

We normalize all input images to have zero mean and unit std (based on nonzero voxels only). We also apply a random axis mirror flip (for all 3 axes) with a probability 0.5. After this we copy the image, and apply the intensity and spatial transforms.

4   Data

The BraTS dataset describes a retrospective collection of brain tumor mpMRI scans acquired from multiple different institutions under standard clinical conditions, but with different equipment and imaging protocols, resulting in a vastly heterogeneous image quality reflecting diverse clinical practice across different institutions. These data have been updated, since last year, increasing the total number of cases from 660 to 2000. Ground truth annotations of every tumor subregion were approved by expert neuroradiologists.

The mpMRI scans included in the BraTS 2021 challenge describe a) native (T1) and b) post-contrast T1-weighted (T1Gd(Gadolinium)), c) T2-weighted (T2), and d) T2 Fluid Attenuated Inversion Recovery (T2-FLAIR) volumes, acquired with different protocols and various scanners from multiple institutions. Standardized preprocessing has been applied to all the BraTS mpMRI scans, including conversion co-registration to the same anatomical template, resampling to a uniform isotropic resolution ($1\,mm^3$), and skull-stripping. The annotated tumor subregions are based upon known observations visible to the trained radiologist (VASARI features) and comprise the Gd-enhancing tumor (ET - label 4), the peritumoral edematous/invaded tissue (ED - label 2), and the necrotic tumor core (NCR - label 1). ET is the enhancing portion of the tumor, described by areas with both visually avid, as well as faint, enhancement on T1Gd MRI. NCR is the necrotic core of the tumor, the appearance of which is hypointense on T1Gd MRI. ED is the peritumoral edematous and infiltrated tissue, defined by the abnormal hyperintense signal envelope on the T2 FLAIR volumes, which includes the infiltrative non enhancing tumor, as well as vasogenic edema in the peritumoral region.

This year, the BraTS 2021 challenge continues its focus on the segmentation of glioma subregions, with a substantially larger dataset (2,000 glioma cases = 8,000 mpMRIscans). These additional exams were obtained as a collection of the pre-operative cases of the TCIA public collections of TCGA-GBM, TCGA-LGG, IvyGAP, CPTAC-GBM, and ACRIN-FMISO-Brain, as well as contributions from private institutional collections.

In an attempt to offer a standardized approach to assess and evaluate various tumor subregions, the BraTS initiative, after consultation with internationally recognized expert neuroradiologists, defined the various tumor subregions. For the BraTS 2021 challenge the regions considered are: i) the "enhancing tumor" (ET), ii) the "tumor core" (TC) and iii) the complete tumor extent also referred to as the "whole tumor" (WT). The ET is described by areas that show hyperintensity in T1Gd when compared to T1, but also when compared to "healthy" white matter in T1Gd. The TC describes the bulk of the tumor, which is what is typically considered for surgical excision. The TC entails the ET, as well as the necrotic (NCR) parts of the tumor, the appearance of which is typically hypointense in T1Gd when compared to T1. The WT describes the complete extent of the disease, as it entails the TC and the peritumoral edematous/invaded tissue (ED), which is typically depicted by the abnormal hyper-intense signal in the T2-FLAIR volume.

The volunteer neuroradiology expert annotators were provided with four mpMRI scans along with the fused automated segmentation volume to initiate the manual refinements. The ITK-SNAP software was used for making these refinements. Once the automated segmentations were refined by the annotators, two senior attending board-certified neuroradiologists with more than 15 years of experience each, reviewed the segmentations. Depending upon correctness, these segmentations were either approved or returned to the individual annotator for further refinements. This process was followed iteratively until the approvers found the refined tumor sub-region segmentations acceptable for public release and the challenge conduction.

Consistent with the configuration of previous BraTS challenges, the "Dice similarity coefficient", and the "Hausdorff distance (95%)" was used as a performance evaluation metrics. Expanding upon this evaluation scheme, we will also provide the metrics of "Sensitivity" and "Specificity", allowing to determine potential over- or under-segmentations of the tumor sub-regions by participating methods. The ranking scheme followed during the BraTS 2017–2020 comprised the ranking of each team relative to its competitors for each of the testing subjects, for each evaluated region (i.e., ET, TC, WT), and for each measure (i.e., Dice and Hausdorff).

5   Results

We implemented our network in MONAI[1] and trained it on 4 Nvidia V100 32 GB GPUs using 5-fold cross-validation. During training we used a random crop of size $192 \times 192 \times 144$, which ensures that most image content remains within the crop area. We concatenated 4 available 3D MRI modalities into the 4 channel image as an input. We train it on 4 GPU for 300 epochs in about 24 h. The output of the network is 3 nested tumor subregions (after the sigmoid).

Typically, the output result, even of a single model, is accurate as shown in Fig. 1, however several cases still remain segmented imprecisely. Figure 2 shows an example of an incorrectly over-segmented whole tumor (WT) region, which is spilled over on the right side of the brain, most likely because the underlying MRI (Flair) has substantially higher intensity values in that region. More variability in training examples might have helped to solve the issue, or integration of anatomical knowledge of e.g. "symmetrical highlights around ventricles are unlikely to be a tumor", but such information is rather complicated to put inside of the network.

We report the cross-validation results using our own 5-fold splits of the training portion of the data in Table 2 and the evaluated results of the BraTS 2021 validation set (219 cases) in Table 4. To get the validation results, we uploaded our segmentation masks to the BraTS 2021 server for evaluation, since the ground truth is not provided. Compared to the validation results, our own cross-validation per fold results are very similar, but 1–2% higher. A slight disagreement is normal, and due to a variability of data in the validation sets, and due

---

[1] https://github.com/Project-MONAI/MONAI.

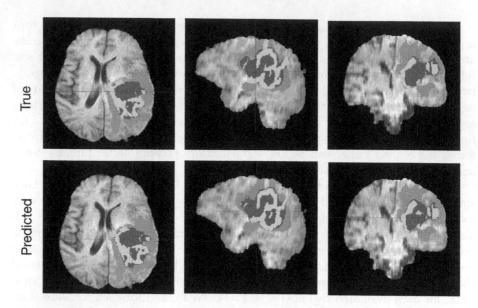

Fig. 1. A typical segmentation example with true and predicted labels overlaid over T1c MRI axial, sagittal and coronal slices. The whole tumor (WT) class includes all visible labels (a union of green, yellow and red labels), the tumor core (TC) class is a union of red and yellow, and the enhancing tumor core (ET) class is shown in yellow (a hyperactive tumor part). (Color figure online)

Table 2. 5-fold cross-validation results using our own random data splits on BraTS 2021 training dataset. Mean Dice: EN - enhancing tumor core, WT - whole tumor, TC - tumor core.

Fold	ET	TC	WT
0	0.8759 ± 0.007	0.9152 ± 0.009	0.9332 ± 0.011
1	0.8993 ± 0.012	0.9213 ± 0.007	0.9379 ± 0.005
2	0.8880 ± 0.006	0.9220 ± 0.013	0.9313 ± 0.014
3	0.8902 ± 0.008	0.9258 ± 0.007	0.9351 ± 0.008
4	0.8847 ± 0.011	0.9198 ± 0.013	0.9374 ± 0.005

Table 3. BraTS 2021 validation dataset results. Mean Dice and Hausdorff95 measurements of the proposed segmentation method. EN - enhancing tumor core, WT - whole tumor, TC - tumor core.

	Dice			Hausdorff95		
Validation dataset	ET	TC	WT	ET	TC	WT
Our result (NVAUTO)	0.8600	0.8868	0.9265	9.0541	5.8409	3.6009

Table 4. BraTS 2021 testing dataset results. Mean Dice and Hausdorff95 measurements of the proposed segmentation method. EN - enhancing tumor core, WT - whole tumor, TC - tumor core.

	Dice			Hausdorff95		
Testing dataset	ET	TC	WT	ET	TC	WT
Our result (NVAUTO)	0.8769	0.8721	0.9266	10.8938	16.8561	4.3925

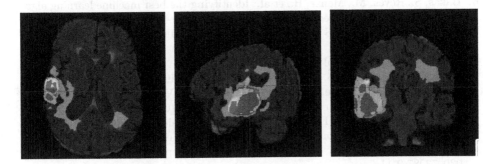

Fig. 2. An example of the incorrectly over-segmented result. The whole tumor (WT) in green is incorrectly spilled over on the right side of the brain, most likely because the underlying MRI (Flair modality) has high intensity regions which usually corresponds to the tumor.

to the fact that we are able to select the best checkpoint using our own 5-folds (Table 3).

6   Discussion and Conclusion

In this work, we described a semantic segmentation network for brain tumor segmentation from multimodal 3D MRIs for BraTS 2021 challenge. We have introduced redundancy reduction to enforce structure on the learned features, and demonstrated confidence based ensembling technique. Our team's (NVAUTO) BraTS 2021 final validation dataset results were 0.8600, 0.8868 and 0.9265 average dice for enhanced tumor core, tumor core and whole tumor, respectively, and were ranked as the 2nd place. Our testing dataset results were 0.8769, 0.8721, 0.9266 average dice for enhanced tumor core, tumor core and whole tumor, respectively, and ranked as the 4th place.

References

1. Project-monai/monai. https://doi.org/10.5281/zenodo.5083813
2. Baid, U., et al.: The RSNA-ASNR-MICCAI brats 2021 benchmark on brain tumor segmentation and radiogenomic classification. CoRR abs/2107.02314 (2021). https://arxiv.org/abs/2107.02314

3. Bakas, S., et al.: Segmentation labels and radiomic features for the pre-operative scans of the TCGA-GBM collection. Cancer Imaging Arch. (2017). https://doi.org/10.7937/K9/TCIA.2017.KLXWJJ1Q

4. Bakas, S., et al.: Segmentation labels and radiomic features for the pre-operative scans of the TCGA-LGG collection. Cancer Imaging Arch. (2017). https://doi.org/10.7937/K9/TCIA.2017.GJQ7R0EF

5. Bakas, S., et al.: Advancing the cancer genome atlas glioma MRI collections with expert segmentation labels and radiomic features. Sci. Data **4**, 1–13 (2017)

6. Bakas, S., Reyes, M., Menze, B., et al.: Identifying the best machine learning algorithms for brain tumor segmentation, progression assessment, and overall survival prediction in the BRATS challenge. arXiv:1811.02629 (2018)

7. Chen, T., Kornblith, S., Norouzi, M., Hinton, G.: A simple framework for contrastive learning of visual representations (2020)

8. He, K., Zhang, X., Ren, S., Sun, J.: Identity mappings in deep residual networks. In: Leibe, B., Matas, J., Sebe, N., Welling, M. (eds.) ECCV 2016. LNCS, vol. 9908, pp. 630–645. Springer, Cham (2016). https://doi.org/10.1007/978-3-319-46493-0_38

9. Isensee, F., Jäger, P.F., Full, P.M., Vollmuth, P., Maier-Hein, K.H.: nnU-Net for brain tumor segmentation. In: Crimi, A., Bakas, S. (eds.) BrainLes 2020. LNCS, vol. 12659, pp. 118–132. Springer, Cham (2021). https://doi.org/10.1007/978-3-030-72087-2_11

10. Jiang, Z., Ding, C., Liu, M., Tao, D.: Two-stage cascaded U-Net: 1st place solution to BraTS challenge 2019 segmentation task. In: Crimi, A., Bakas, S. (eds.) BrainLes 2019. LNCS, vol. 11992, pp. 231–241. Springer, Cham (2020). https://doi.org/10.1007/978-3-030-46640-4_22

11. Menze, B.H., et al.: The multimodal brain tumor image segmentation benchmark (BRATS). IEEE Trans. Med. Imaging **34**(10), 1993–2024 (2015)

12. Milletari, F., Navab, N., Ahmadi, S.A.: V-Net: fully convolutional neural networks for volumetric medical image segmentation. In: Fourth International Conference on 3D Vision (3DV) (2016)

13. Myronenko, A.: 3D MRI brain tumor segmentation using autoencoder regularization. In: Crimi, A., Bakas, S., Kuijf, H., Keyvan, F., Reyes, M., van Walsum, T. (eds.) BrainLes 2018. LNCS, vol. 11384, pp. 311–320. Springer, Cham (2019). https://doi.org/10.1007/978-3-030-11726-9_28. https://arxiv.org/abs/1810.11654

14. Ulyanov, D., Vedaldi, A., Lempitsky, V.S.: Instance normalization: the missing ingredient for fast stylization. In: CVPR (2016)

15. Wu, Y., He, K.: Group normalization. In: Ferrari, V., Hebert, M., Sminchisescu, C., Weiss, Y. (eds.) ECCV 2018. LNCS, vol. 11217, pp. 3–19. Springer, Cham (2018). https://doi.org/10.1007/978-3-030-01261-8_1

16. Zbontar, J., Jing, L., Misra, I., LeCun, Y., Deny, S.: Barlow twins: self-supervised learning via redundancy reduction. In: ICML (2021)

Extending nn-UNet for Brain Tumor Segmentation

Huan Minh Luu and Sung-Hong Park[✉]

Magnetic Resonance Imaging Laboratory, Department of Bio and Brain Engineering,
Korea Advanced Institute of Science and Technology, Daejeon, South Korea
{luuminhhuan,sunghongpark}@kaist.ac.kr

Abstract. Brain tumor segmentation is essential for the diagnosis and prognosis of patients with gliomas. The brain tumor segmentation challenge has provided an abundant and high-quality data source to develop automatic algorithms for the task. This paper describes our contribution to the 2021 competition. We developed our methods based on nn-UNet, the winning entry of last year's competition. We experimented with several modifications, including using a larger network, replacing batch normalization with group normalization and utilizing axial attention in the decoder. Internal 5-fold cross-validation and online evaluation from the organizers showed a minor improvement in quantitative metrics compared to the baseline. The proposed models won first place in the final ranking on unseen test data, achieving a dice score of 88.35%, 88.78%, 93.19% for the enhancing tumor, the tumor core, and the whole tumor, respectively. The codes, pretrained weights, and docker image for the winning submission are publicly available. (https://github.com/rixez/Brats21_KAIST_MRI_Lab https://hub.docker.com/r/rixez/brats21nnunet)

Keywords: Brain tumor segmentation · Deep learning · nn-UNet

1 Introduction

Brain tumor segmentation from magnetic resonance (MR) images is an essential procedure for brain tumor care, enabling clinicians to identify the tumors' location, extent, and types. This helps with the initial diagnosis and aids with administering and monitoring treatment progress. Given the importance of this task, precise delineation of the tumor and its sub-regions is typically performed manually by experienced neuro-radiologists. This tedious and time-consuming process demands significant effort and expertise, especially when the patient volume is high, the images are multi-parametric of different contrasts, and the tumors are heterogeneous. The labeling process is also subjected to inter and intra-rater variability [1], necessitating a consensus for determining the correct segmentation, adding an extra layer of complexity. Automatic or computer-aided segmentation algorithms can resolve these shortcomings as they can lower the

© The Author(s), under exclusive license to Springer Nature Switzerland AG 2022
A. Crimi and S. Bakas (Eds.): BrainLes 2021, LNCS 12963, pp. 173–186, 2022.
https://doi.org/10.1007/978-3-031-09002-8_16

labor-intensiveness of the labeling process and be consistent across different cases. However, sufficient annotated, high-quality data is needed to develop these algorithms with robustness suited for clinical purposes.

The Brain Tumor Segmentation Challenge (BraTS) [2,3,5–7] is an annual international competition that has been carried out since 2012. Participants are provided with a comprehensive dataset of fully-annotated, multi-institutional, multi-parametric MR images (mpMRI) of patients with varying degrees of gliomas. Since its inception, the dataset has grown from only 30 cases in 2012 to 2000 cases in 2021 [4]. In this year (2021) challenge, the participants can compete in two tasks. The first task is the usual brain tumor sub-region segmentation from mpMRI. The second task is novel and involves the prediction of MGMT (0[6]-methylguanine-DNA methyltransferase) promoter methylation status. MGMT is an important biomarker to determine the patients' response to cancer treatment. Noninvasive assessment of MGMT promoter methylation status through typical clinical MRI scans can have a tremendous impact on the treatment of patients. We participated only in the segmentation task, and this manuscript describes our entry in this part of the competition.

Initial attempts toward automatic segmentation of brain tumors have relied on hand-crafted features engineering with traditional machine learning methods such as Atlas-based [8], decision forest [9,10], conditional random field [11]. With the rising popularity of deep learning enabled by the improvement in computational capability of modern graphic processing units (GPU), the efficiency of algorithms, and the availability of training data, conventional methods have slowly been replaced by deep neural networks in several fields such as computer vision [12,13], natural language processing [14], or computational biology [15]. In the context of the BraTS competition, deep learning algorithms have been explored for tumor segmentation since 2014, and they were the algorithm of choice for most entries in recent years. Winners of the 4 most recent competitions all employed deep neural networks, testifying to the superior performance of this approach when more data is available. We summarized the main takeaways from these winning contributions. Kamnitsas et al. [16] proposed Ensemble of Multiple Models and Architecture (EMMA), combining the predictions from different 3D convolutional networks (DeepMedic [17,18], FCN [19], and U-Net [20]). Myronenko et al. [21] combined a 3D U-Net with an additional variational decoder branch to provide additional supervision and regularization to the encoder branch. Jiang et al. [22] trained a two-stage cascaded U-Net, the first stage was trained to produce coarse segmentation masks, and the second stage was trained to refine the output of the first stage. Isensee et al. [23] utilized nnU-Net [24], a self-configuring framework that automatically adapts U-Net to a particular dataset, and showed robust performance with minimal modifications to the conventional 3D U-Net by utilizing some BraTS-specific optimizations.

For our entry to the competition, we extended the nnU-Net framework proposed by last year winner by adding several components. Due to the ease of adapting nnU-Net to a new dataset as well as the fully open-source codes and models, nnU-Net serves as an excellent baseline for further experimentation. The modifications that we explored for this year competition are using group normalization instead of batch normalization, using an asymmetrically large encoder for the U-Net, and using axial attention in the decoder. Experimental results with cross-validation on the training dataset showed a minor improvement of the proposed modifications on performance. With our approach, We ranked fourth and first in the validation phase and the test phase leaderboard, respectively.

2 Methods

2.1 Data

Multi-parametric MRI scans from 2000 patients were used for BraTS2021, 1251 of which were provided with segmentation labels to the participants for developing their algorithms. 219 of which were used for the public leaderboard during the validation phase, and the remaining 530 cases were intended for the private leaderboard and the final ranking of the participants. 4 contrasts are available for the MRI scans: Native T1-weighted image, post-contrast T1-weighted (T1Gd), T2-weighted, and T2 Fluid Attenuated Inversion Recovery (T2-FLAIR). Annotation were manually performed by one to four raters, with final approval from experienced neuro-radiologists. The labels include regions of GD-enhancing tumor (ET), the peritumoral edematous/invaded tissue (ED), and the necrotic tumor core (NCR). All MRI scans were preprocessed by co-registration to the same anatomical template, interpolation to isotropic $1mm^3$ resolution, and skull-stripping. The image sizes of all MRI scans and associated labels are $240 \times 240 \times 155$. Figure 1 shows a representative slice of the four contrasts with segmentation. Further processing was done on the provided data before inputting it into the network. The volumes were cropped to non-zero voxels to reduce the computation. Since the intensity in MR images is qualitative, the voxels were normalized by their mean and standard deviation.

2.2 Model

In this section, the details of the models developed are described, starting from the strong baseline nnU-Net models that won last year's competition. Several modifications to this baseline and their rationales are then elaborated. All of these experiments were done with the excellent open-source nnU-Net framework[1].

Baseline nnU-Net. nnU-Net by Isensee *et al.* [23] was the winning entry for BraTS 2020. At its core is a 3D U-Net that operates on patches of size $128 \times 128 \times 128$. The network has the encoder-decoder structure with skip connections linking the two pathways. The encoder comprises five levels of same-resolution convolutional layers with strided convolution downsampling. The

---

[1] https://github.com/MIC-DKFZ/nnUNet.

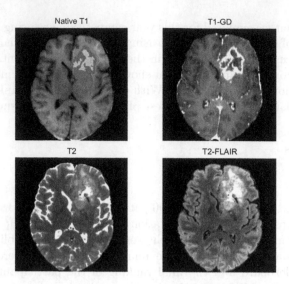

Fig. 1. Representative axial slice from one subject (BraTS2021_00001) showing the four different contrast with overlaid segmentation labels for the 3 tumor sub-regions on the T1 image. Green: peritumoral edematous/invaded tissue, red: necrotic tumor core, yellow: GD-enhancing tumor. (Color figure online)

decoder follows the same structure with transpose convolution upsampling and convolution operating on concatenated skip features from the encoder branch at the same level. Leaky ReLU (lReLU) with slope of 0.01 [25] and batch normalization [26] was applied after every convolution operations. The mpMRI volumes were concatenated and used as 4-channels input. nnU-Net employs region-based training: instead of predicting three mutually exclusive tumor sub-regions, as in the provided segmentation labels, the network predicts the three overlapping regions of enhancing tumor (ET, original region), tumor core or TC (ET + necrotic tumor), and whole tumor or WT (ET + NT + ED) instead. The softmax nonlinearity at the final layer of the network was replaced by a sigmoid activation, treating each voxel as a multi-class classification problem. This region-based training has been observed to improve the performance in previous competitions [21,23,27]. Except for the two lowest levels, additional sigmoid outputs were added to every resolution to apply deep supervision and improve gradient propagation to the earlier layers. The number of convolutional filters was initialized at 32 and doubled for every resolution reduction, up to a maximum of 320.

Largest Network and Group Normalization. The first modification we made was to increase the size of the network asymmetrically by doubling the number of filters in the encoder while maintaining the same filters in the decoder. The maximum number of filters was also increased to 512. The asymmetrically large encoder was utilized by Myronenko [21]. As the amount of training data is quadrupled compared to the previous year, increasing the network's capacity will help it model the more extensive data variety. The structure of the modified network is shown in Fig. 2. The second modification was to replace all batch normalization with group normalization [28]. 3D convolution networks demand significant GPU memories even with mixed-precision training, limiting the batch size used during training. Group normalization has been shown to work better than batch normalization for the low batch size regime and has also been adopted by previous winners of the competition [21, 22]. Unless specified otherwise, the number of groups was set at 32. The baseline nn-UNet model has 31.2M parameters and requires 8.2 GB of VRAM with batch size of 2 and mixed-precision training. The larger proposed model has 87.4M parameters and requires 14.4 GB of VRAM with the same settings.

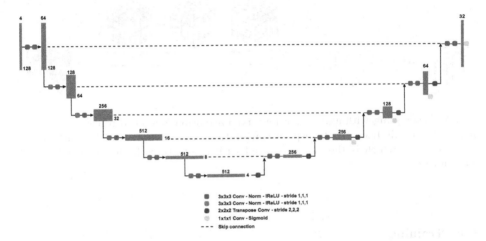

Fig. 2. Structure of the larger U-Net with asymmetric scaling on the encoder. The number at the top and bottom indicates the number of channels and the dimension of the features vectors, respectively.

Axial Attention Decoder. The final addition was using axial attention in the decoder. Self-attention or transformer [14] is a breakthrough idea that allows learning adaptive attention of an input sequence based only on its self. Originally conceived and popularized in the NLP literature [14,29,30], the self-attention mechanism has slowly been adopted by the computer vision research community [31]. One of the main obstacles when applying self-attention to vision problems is that the computational complexity of the attention mechanism scales quadratically with the input size, rendering it impossible to fit or train the network in a standard workstation setup. This limitation is even more of a problem when dealing with 3D data with the extra dimension. Axial attention [32,33] has recently been proposed as an efficient solution when applying attention to multi-dimensional data. By independently applying self-attention to each axis, the computation only scales linearly with image size, making it possible to integrate the attention mechanism even with 3D data. We applied axial attention to the decoder of the network by running it on the output of the transposed convolution upsampling and then summing them. Figure 3 showed an illustration of the axial attention decoder block. Even with more efficient attention, we found that applying the method to the highest resolution features ($128 \times 128 \times 128$) was not possible with our setup (RTX3090 24 GB VRAM) and opted for only the four lower resolutions. The number of attention heads and dimensions of each head was doubled for each resolution reduction, starting from 4 and 16 (at $64 \times 64 \times 64$ resolution), respectively.

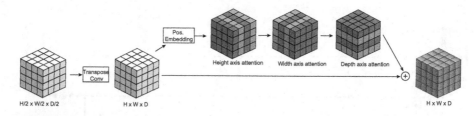

Fig. 3. Upsampling with axial attention: axial attention is applied to each axis of the upsampled result from the transpose convolution. The output is added back to the original input, which is then concatenated with the features from the encoder path (not shown).

2.3 Training

We followed the training methodology of nnU-Net for all networks. Each network was trained with 5-fold cross-validation. Data augmentation was applied on the fly during training to improve the generalization. Data augmentation consisted of random rotation and scaling, elastic deformation, additive brightness augmentation, and gamma scaling. The objective for optimization is the sum of the binary cross-entropy loss and the dice loss, calculated at the final full-resolution output and the auxiliary outputs with lower resolution. The batch version of the dice loss was used instead of the sample dice loss, computing the loss treating the whole batch as one sample instead of averaging dices from each sample in the minibatch. The batch dice helps stabilize the training by reducing the errors from samples with few annotated samples [23]. The networks were optimized with stochastic gradient descent with Nesterov momentum of 0.99. The initial learning rate was 0.01 and was decayed following a polynomial schedule

$$lr = 0.01 \times \left(1 - \frac{epoch}{1000}\right)^{0.9} \qquad (1)$$

Each training run lasted 1000 epochs, with 250 mini-batches per epoch. The dice score on the validation set of the current fold was used to monitor the training progress. All experiments were conducted with Pytorch 1.9 on NVIDIA RTX 3090 GPU with 24 GB VRAM. The following models were developed:

- **BL**: baseline nnUNet, batch normalization with batch size of 5
- **BL + L**: baseline with large Unet, batch size of 2, train on all training samples
- **BL + GN**: baseline with group normalization, batch size of 2
- **BL + AA**: baseline with axial attention, batch normalization, batch size of 2
- **BL + L + GN**: nnUNet with larger Unet, group normalization, batch size of 2 The baseline model with a batch size of 5 took around 400s per epoch or almost 5 days for 1000 epochs. Other models with batch size of 2 took roughly half as long. The **BL + L + GN** configuration, for example, took around 170s per epoch or 2 days for training one fold over 1000 epochs.

3 Results

3.1 Quantitative Results

Table 1 showed the dice scores for the three tumor sub-regions of the five models from the cross-validation. The model **BL + L** was trained on the whole training dataset (1 fold). Increasing the size of the U-Net yielded a minor improvement. Using group normalization instead of batch normalization did not improve the performance and even slightly harmed the dice metric. It is also worth noting that group normalization increases memory consumption modestly, which might cancel out the memory reduction when using a smaller batch size. Using the axial attention encoder did not improve the performance even at higher computation. Combining a large U-Net and group normalization increases the performance slightly for the tumor core and the whole tumor, with a significant increase in GPU memory usage.

Table 1. Dice metrics of the networks on 5-fold cross validation. ET: enhancing tumor, TC: tumor core, WT: whole tumor.

Model	ET	TC	WT	Average
BL	88.37	92.06	93.78	91.40
BL + L	89.82	94.03	94.58	92.81
BL + GN	88.17	92.11	93.66	91.30
BL + AA	87.23	91.88	93.21	90.77
BL + L + GN	88.23	92.35	93.83	91.47

Table 2 showed the Dice and 95% Hausdorff distance (HD95) computed by the competition organizers and displayed in the public leaderboard. A sliding window approach was used for inference. Segmentation was predicted for 8 sub-volumes, weighted with a 3D Gaussian, and reassembled for the whole volume segmentation. For test time augmentation (TTA), we applied axis mirroring for each of the 3 axes for each sub-volume. 64 (8 sub-volumes × 8 mirrorings) inferences were performed for each volume in the validation and test set, with an average latency of 20s per volume. All predicted segmentation labels were then ensembled from 5 folds by averaging the sigmoid probabilities, except for the **BL + L** configuration. The ensembled results were then post-processed by converting the enhancing tumor class into necrotic tumor if ET voxels were less than 200. The result for the axial attention model was not processed in time for the paper and was omitted. Incorporating the proposed changes led to a minor yet consistent improvement across all metrics compared to the baseline model. The **BL + L + GN** configuration's result was chosen for the validation leaderboard and got 4th place among the participants.

Table 2. Dice and 95% Hausdorff distance of the networks as computed by the online evaluation platform. ET: enhancing tumor, TC: tumor core, WT: whole tumor, HD95: 95% Hausdorff distance.

Model	Dice				HD95			
	ET	TC	WT	Average	ET	TC	WT	Average
BL	83.73	87.45	92.63	87.94	22.44	10.56	3.55	12.18
BL + L	83.28	86.53	92.51	87.44	22.50	12.75	3.71	12.99
BL + GN	84.09	87.85	92.77	88.24	22.41	9.20	3.42	11.68
BL + L + GN	84.51	87.81	92.75	88.36	20.73	7.623	3.47	10.61

We opted to include 5 baseline models in the ensemble for the unseen test evaluation considering the ranking metric for this phase. Instead of one ranking based on only the aggregated Dice or HD95 from all test cases, ranking is performed for each case, for each metric (Dice, HD95), and for each tumor region (ET, TC, and WT). In total, each participant receives N (number of cases) × 2 × 3 rankings. The final ranking is the average of these rankings normalized by the number of participants. Table 3 compares different ranking methods of the 4 models in Table 2 on the validation results. Even though the **BL + L + GN** model was the best performer for the average Dice or HD95 metrics, the baseline model consistently ranked first when the BraTS score was considered. For the final submission, 5 **BL + L + GN** and 5 **BL** models were ensembled following the same procedure described for the validation phase's submission. We took first place in the competition with this ensemble. The complete statistics of the ensemble's performance on the test dataset are shown in Table 4.

Table 3. Ranking of the 4 models with different ranking methods on the validation data.

Model	Dice	Rank	HD95	Rank	BraTS score	Rank
BL	87.94	3	12.18	3	0.488	1
BL + L	87.44	4	12.99	4	0.531	4
BL + GN	88.24	2	11.68	2	0.494	3
BL + L + GN	88.36	1	10.61	1	0.490	2

Table 4. Performance of our final submission on the test dataset.

Label	Dice			HD95			Sensitivity			Specificity		
	ET	WT	TC	ET	WT	TC	ET	WT	TC	ET	WT	TC
Mean	0.88	0.93	0.89	10.67	4.75	13.72	0.90	0.93	0.90	1.00	1.00	1.00
StdDev	0.18	0.09	0.23	55.56	17.33	61.43	0.19	0.10	0.21	0.00	0.00	0.00
Median	0.94	0.96	0.97	1.00	1.41	1.41	0.96	0.97	0.97	1.00	1.00	1.00
25th quantile	0.86	0.92	0.92	1.00	1.00	1.00	0.90	0.93	0.92	1.00	1.00	1.00
75th quantile	0.97	0.98	0.98	1.73	3.61	2.83	0.98	0.99	0.99	1.00	1.00	1.00

3.2 Qualitative Results

Figure 4 shows 2 representative examples of predictions from the **BL + L + GN** configuration. The network successfully identified all the tumor sub-regions for the first case with high accuracy. This accuracy can potentially be attributed to the quality of the scans, with well-defined contrasts for the tumor regions. For the second case, the network failed to segment the enhancing tumor and the tumor core while still performing decently for the whole extent of the tumor. The poor performance can also be explained by the quality of the MR scans: the T1 and T1-GD contrasts do not show a clear delineation of the tumor and even have visible artifacts and blurring. These two cases show the importance of ensuring data's quality for the proper operation of the network. It also indicates that this data integrity factor should be considered during development, either through more diverse data acquisition or more specific data augmentation to cover these edge cases.

BraTS2021_00174
ET: 97.78, TC: 98.93, WT: 98.66

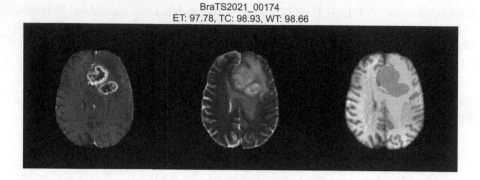

BraTS2021_01784
ET: 0, TC: 2.76, WT: 92.77

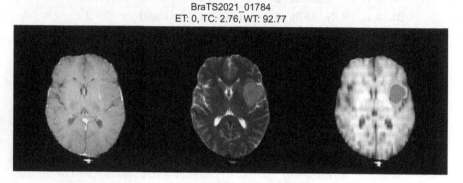

Fig. 4. Representative good and bad predictions from the validation set. T1-GD, T2, and T1 with prediction from the network for two cases with good and bad metrics. Green: necrotic tumor core, blue: GD-enhancing tumor, yellow: edematous tissues. (Color figure online)

4   Discussion

In this paper, we described our methodology for the BraTS 2021 competition. We extended the nn-UNet framework by using a larger network, replacing batch normalization with group normalization, and using axial attention decoder. These minor modifications slightly improved the baseline nn-UNet and won first place in the competition. As nn-UNet framework was extensively used for our method, we wanted to highlight the versatility, ease of use, and robustness of it. We were able to set up a solid baseline without much experimentation. The pretrained networks that were developed on last year's data still performed well on this year's validation data, showing the generalizability of the method.

With 3D data, any modifications need to be carefully balanced with the availability of the GPU memory to ensure training can run without memory problems. The larger U-Net and axial attention decoder we proposed can add a significant memory footprint to the model even with minor adjustments, so it should be tuned carefully. Group normalization somewhat alleviates this issue by enabling a smaller batch size without incurring significant performance degradation.

Recently, self-attention or transformer has become dominant in computer vision. We attempted to integrate this powerful mechanism as part of our network in the form of the axial attention decoder. Results from the 5-fold cross-validation indicate that it did not improve the performance. However, recent works for biomedical segmentation such as TransUNet [36], UNETR [34], and Swin-UNETR [35] have shown different results. Incorporating transformers into the network, such as the encoder in UNet, can improve the segmentation accuracy compared to the pure convolution counterparts. This is not surprising as transformers can learn global dependencies between features compared to more local representations of convolution. The property can be helpful for larger biological structures that do not fit in the receptive fields. In the context of the competition, some top-performing teams in the validation evaluation have experimented with transformer-based UNet models. However, most high-ranking teams in the final evaluation used conventional convolution networks. This does not necessarily mean that transformer-based models are less performant but rather how well-optimized convolution models are. Starting from its invention in 2015, UNet has been the dominant architecture for biomedical segmentation and has been highly optimized, especially for an annual competition like BraTS. We expect that with more widespread adoption and optimization of transformer models, future BraTS competitions will see a surge in popularity of these models, similar to the transition from hand-crafted features to deep learning in previous years.

It is essential to inspect the failure cases to understand the behavior of the models. Most cases with inaccurate segmentation are similar to the one shown in Fig. 4, with artifacts or quality issues in one of the contrasts. Other cases with bad Dice scores are due to the post-processing method, which favors the removal of small enhancing tumors. The reason behind this was explained in detail in ref [23]. For the short version, removing small enhancing tumors can improve the ranking on the leaderboard due to the dichotomy in the Dice and HD95 metrics when the ground truth segmentation does not have any enhancing tumor. We observed that this post-processing method improves the Dice score slightly but worsens the HD95 score significantly for the enhancing tumor. We suspect this is due to the addition of several scans with small enhancing tumors, which render the post-processing harmful for the HD95. We might need to consider more sophisticated post-processing methods to address those cases. Looking at the performance on the unseen data (Table 4), it is evident that while the model has almost perfect specificity, the sensitivity is much lower, which indicates that our model is quite conservative in predicting tumors. Lowering the threshold for detection can make the model more sensitive, which might be necessary for clinical usages. We did not investigate the effect of changing the detection threshold on the competition score. Selecting an appropriate value for each tumor region may improve the score significantly. As the ratio of the regions in the dataset is unbalanced, the networks have different confidence for each region and would benefit from optimizing the sensitivity-specificity tradeoffs.

Acknowledgements. We would like to acknowledge Fabian Isensee for his development of the nn-UNet framework and for sharing the models from last year competition.

References

1. Visser, M., et al.: Inter-rater agreement in glioma segmentations on longitudinal MRI. Neuroimage Clin. **22**, 101727 (2019)
2. Menze, B.H., et al.: The multimodal brain tumor image segmentation benchmark (BRATS). IEEE Trans. Med. Imaging **34**(10), 1993–2024 (2015). https://doi.org/10.1109/TMI.2014.2377694
3. Bakas, S., et al.: Identifying the best machine learning algorithms for brain tumor segmentation, progression assessment, and overall survival prediction in the brats challenge. arXiv preprint arXiv:1811.02629 (2018)
4. Baid, U., et al.: The RSNA-ASNR-MICCAI BraTS 2021 benchmark on brain tumor segmentation and radiogenomic classification. arXiv:2107.02314, 2021
5. Bakas, S., et al.: Segmentation labels and radiomic features for the pre-operative scans of the TCGA-GBM collection. Cancer Imaging Arch. (2017). https://doi.org/10.7937/K9/TCIA.2017.KLXWJJ1Q
6. Bakas, S., et al.: Segmentation labels and radiomic features for the pre-operative scans of the TCGA-LGG collection. Cancer Imaging Arch. (2017). https://doi.org/10.7937/K9/TCIA.2017.GJQ7R0EF
7. Bakas, S., et al.: Advancing the cancer genome atlas glioma MRI collections with expert segmentation labels and radiomic features. Nat. Sci. Data **4**, 170117 (2017). https://doi.org/10.1038/sdata.2017.117
8. Bauer, S., Seiler, C., Bardyn, T., Buechler, P., Reyes, M.: Atlas-based segmentation of brain tumor images using a Markov Random Field-based tumor growth model and non-rigid registration. In: 2010 Annual International Conference of the IEEE Engineering in Medicine and Biology, pp. 4080–4083 (2010)
9. Zikic, D.: Decision forests for tissue-specific segmentation of high-grade gliomas in multi-channel MR. Med Image Comput. Comput. Assist. Interv. **15**, 369–376 (2012)
10. Tustison, N., Wintermark, M., Durst, C., Avants, B.: ANTs and Àrboles. In: Proceedings of the NCI MICCAI-BRATS, vol. 1, pp. 47–50 (2013)
11. Wu, W., Chen, A.Y.C., Zhao, L., Corso, J.J.: Brain tumor detection and segmentation in a CRF (conditional random fields) framework with pixel-pairwise affinity and superpixel-level features. Int. J. Comput. Assist. Radiol. Surg. **9**(2), 241–253 (2013). https://doi.org/10.1007/s11548-013-0922-7
12. Krizhevsky, A., Sutskever, I., Hinton, G.E.: ImageNet classification with deep convolutional neural networks. In: Proceedings of the 25th International Conference on Neural Information Processing Systems - Volume 1, Lake Tahoe, Nevada, pp. 1097–1105. Curran Associates Inc. (2012)
13. He, K., Zhang, X., Ren, S., Sun, J.: Deep residual learning for image recognition. In: 2016 IEEE Conference on Computer Vision and Pattern Recognition (CVPR), pp. 770–778 (2016)
14. Vaswani, A., et al.: Attention is all you need. In: Proceedings of the 31st International Conference on Neural Information Processing Systems, Long Beach, California, USA, pp. 6000–6010. Curran Associates Inc. (2017)

15. Jumper, J., et al.: Highly accurate protein structure prediction with AlphaFold. Nature (2021)
16. Kamnitsas, K., et al.: Ensembles of multiple models and architectures for robust brain tumour segmentation. In: Crimi, A., Bakas, S., Kuijf, H., Menze, B., Reyes, M. (eds.) BrainLes 2017. LNCS, vol. 10670, pp. 450–462. Springer, Cham (2018). https://doi.org/10.1007/978-3-319-75238-9_38
17. Kamnitsas, K., Ledig, C., Newcombe, V.F., Simpson, J.P., Kane, A.D., Menon, D.K., Rueckert, D., Glocker, B.: Efficient multi-scale 3D CNN with fully connected CRF for accurate brain lesion segmentation. Med. Image Anal. **36**, 61–78 (2017)
18. Kamnitsas, K., Chen, L., Ledig, C., Rueckert, D., Glocker, B.: Multi-scale 3D convolutional neural networks for lesion segmentation in brain MRI. In: Proceedings of ISLES-MICCAI (2015)
19. Long, J., et al.: Fully convolutional networks for semantic segmentation. In: 2015 IEEE Conference on Computer Vision and Pattern Recognition (CVPR), pp. 3431–3440 (2015)
20. Ronneberger, O., Fischer, P., Brox, T.: U-Net: convolutional networks for biomedical image segmentation. In: Navab, N., Hornegger, J., Wells, W.M., Frangi, A.F. (eds.) MICCAI 2015. LNCS, vol. 9351, pp. 234–241. Springer, Cham (2015). https://doi.org/10.1007/978-3-319-24574-4_28
21. Myronenko, A.: 3D MRI brain tumor segmentation using autoencoder regularization. In: Crimi, A., Bakas, S., Kuijf, H., Keyvan, F., Reyes, M., van Walsum, T. (eds.) BrainLes 2018. LNCS, vol. 11384, pp. 311–320. Springer, Cham (2019). https://doi.org/10.1007/978-3-030-11726-9_28
22. Jiang, Z., Ding, C., Liu, M., Tao, D.: Two-stage cascaded U-Net: 1st place solution to BraTS challenge 2019 segmentation task. In: Crimi, A., Bakas, S. (eds.) BrainLes 2019. LNCS, vol. 11992, pp. 231–241. Springer, Cham (2020). https://doi.org/10.1007/978-3-030-46640-4_22
23. Isensee, F., Jäger, P.F., Full, P.M., Vollmuth, P., Maier-Hein, K.H.: nnU-Net for brain tumor segmentation. In: Crimi, A., Bakas, S. (eds.) BrainLes 2020. LNCS, vol. 12659, pp. 118–132. Springer, Cham (2021). https://doi.org/10.1007/978-3-030-72087-2_11
24. Isensee, F., Jaeger, P.F., Kohl, S.A.A., Petersen, J., Maier-Hein, K.H.: nnU-Net: a self-configuring method for deep learning-based biomedical image segmentation. Nat. Methods **18**, 203–211 (2021)
25. Maas, A.L., Hannun, A.Y., Ng, A.Y.: Rectifier nonlinearities improve neural network acoustic models. Proc. ICML **30**(1), 3 (2013)
26. Ioffe, S., Szegedy, C.: Batch normalization: accelerating deep network training by reducing internal covariate shift. In: ICML, pp. 448–456 (2015)
27. Zhao, Y.-X., Zhang, Y.-M., Liu, C.-L.: Bag of tricks for 3D MRI brain tumor segmentation. In: Crimi, A., Bakas, S. (eds.) BrainLes 2019. LNCS, vol. 11992, pp. 210–220. Springer, Cham (2020). https://doi.org/10.1007/978-3-030-46640-4_20
28. Wu, Y., He, K.: Group normalization. In: Ferrari, V., Hebert, M., Sminchisescu, C., Weiss, Y. (eds.) ECCV 2018. LNCS, vol. 11217, pp. 3–19. Springer, Cham (2018). https://doi.org/10.1007/978-3-030-01261-8_1
29. Devlin, J., Chang, M.-W., Lee, K., Toutanova, K.: BERT: pre-training of deep bidirectional transformers for language understanding. In: NAACL-HLT, pp. 4171–4186 (2019)
30. Brown, T., et al.: Language models are few-shot learners. In: NeurIPS, pp. 1877–1901. Curran Associates Inc (2020)
31. Dosovitskiy, A., et al.: An image is worth 16×16 words: transformers for image recognition at scale. In: ICLR (2021)

32. Ho, J., Kalchbrenner, N., Weissenborn, D., Salimans, T.: Axial attention in multi-dimensional transformers. arXiv preprint arXiv:1912.12180 (2019)
33. Wang, H., Zhu, Y., Green, B., Adam, H., Yuille, A., Chen, L.-C.: Axial-DeepLab: stand-alone axial-attention for panoptic segmentation. In: Vedaldi, A., Bischof, H., Brox, T., Frahm, J.-M. (eds.) ECCV 2020. LNCS, vol. 12349, pp. 108–126. Springer, Cham (2020). https://doi.org/10.1007/978-3-030-58548-8_7
34. Hatamizadeh, A., et al.: UNETR: transformers for 3D medical image segmentation. In: IEEE Winter Conference on Applications of Computer Vision (WACV) (2022)
35. Tang, Y., et al.: Self-supervised pre-training of swin transformers for 3D medical image analysis. arXiv preprint arXiv:2111.14791 (2021)
36. Chen, J., et al.: TransUNet: transformers make strong encoders for medical image segmentation. arXiv preprint arXiv:2102.04306 (2021)

Generalized Wasserstein Dice Loss, Test-Time Augmentation, and Transformers for the BraTS 2021 Challenge

Lucas Fidon[1]([✉]), Suprosanna Shit[2]([✉]), Ivan Ezhov[2], Johannes C. Paetzold[2], Sébastien Ourselin[1], and Tom Vercauteren[1]

[1] School of Biomedical Engineering and Imaging Sciences,
King's College London, London, UK
`lucas.fidon@kcl.ac.uk`
[2] Department of Informatics, Technical University of Munich, Munich, Germany
`suprosanna.shit@tum.de`

Abstract. Brain tumor segmentation from multiple Magnetic Resonance Imaging (MRI) modalities is a challenging task in medical image computation. The main challenges lie in the generalizability to a variety of scanners and imaging protocols. In this paper, we explore strategies to increase model robustness without increasing inference time. Towards this aim, we explore finding a robust ensemble from models trained using different losses, optimizers, and train-validation data split. Importantly, we explore the inclusion of a transformer in the bottleneck of the U-Net architecture. While we find transformer in the bottleneck performs slightly worse than the baseline U-Net in average, the generalized Wasserstein Dice loss consistently produces superior results. Further, we adopt an efficient test time augmentation strategy for faster and robust inference. Our final ensemble of seven 3D U-Nets with test-time augmentation produces an average dice score of 89.4% and an average Hausdorff 95% distance of 10.0 mm when evaluated on the BraTS 2021 testing dataset. Our code and trained models are publicly available at https://github.com/LucasFidon/TRABIT_BraTS2021.

Keywords: BraTS 2021 · Segmentation · Deep learning · Brain tumor · Transformers · Test-time augmentation

1 Introduction

Gliomas are the most common malignant brain tumors. Broadly, Gliomas are categorized into aggressive high-grade and slow-growing low-grade types. In both types of Gliomas, changes in tissues caused by tumor cells can be captured using multi-modality Magnetic Resonance Imaging (MRI). The commonly used modalities are T1, T2, contrast-enhanced T1 (ceT1), and FLAIR. These modalities are

A. Crimi and S. Bakas (Eds.): BrainLes 2021, LNCS 12963, pp. 187–196, 2022.
https://doi.org/10.1007/978-3-031-09002-8_17

the default choice for the radiologist to identify the tumor type and its progression stage. Towards this objective, accurate and automatic brain tumor segmentation based on multi-parametric MRI is an active field of research [23] and could support diagnosis, surgery planning [11,12], follow-up, and radiation therapy [1,2]. The BraTS 2021 challenge has offered an unique and unprecedented opportunity to machine learning researchers to develop a clinically deployable solution for Glioma multi-class segmentation.

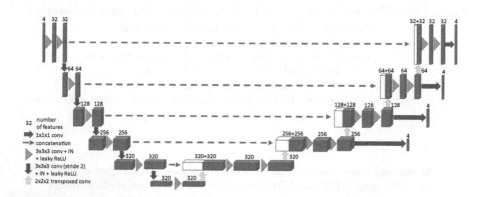

Fig. 1. Illustration of the 3D U-Net [10] **architecture used.** Blue boxes represent feature maps. IN stands for instance normalization [32]. The design of this 3D U-Net was determined using the heuristics of nnU-Net and our previous work [13,16,17,21]. (Color figure online)

Aiming for computational efficiency, we use 3D U-Net, and its recent transformer variation, TransUNet [9], as the primary models and focus on finding better learning schemes, such as, augmentation, loss function, optimizer, and efficient inference routine for ensemble model. Recently it has been shown that different loss function combinations may have a crucial impact on the resultant segmentation [24]. In our settings, we use the Generalized Wasserstein Dice loss [15] that has shown superior segmentation performance as compared to the mean Dice loss [26,28,30] in the BraTS 2020 challenge [16] and for other medical image segmentation tasks [8,31]. We investigate the effect of different state-of-the-art optimizers, such as, SGD, SGDP [20], ASAM [25]. Lastly, we use an efficient test-time ensemble approach for the final segmentation result.

2 Methods and Materials

2.1 Data

We have used the BraTS 2021 dataset[1] [3] in our experiments. No additional data were used. The dataset contains the same four MRI sequences (T1, ceT1,

---

[1] https://www.synapse.org/#!Synapse:syn25829067/wiki/610865.

T2, and FLAIR) for all cases, corresponding to patients with either a high-grade Gliomas [5] or a low-grade Gliomas [6]. All the cases were manually segmented for peritumoral edema, enhancing tumor, and non-enhancing tumor core using the same labeling protocol [3,4,7,27]. The training dataset contains 1251 cases, and the validation dataset contains 219 cases. MRI for training and validation datasets are publicly available, but only the manual segmentations for the training dataset are available. The evaluation on the validation dataset was performed using the BraTS 2021 challenge online evaluation platform[2]. For each case, the four MRI sequences are available after co-registration to the same anatomical template, interpolation to 1mm isotropic resolution, and skull stripping [27].

2.2 Deep Learning Pipeline

We used the DynU-Net of MONAI [29] to implement a baseline 3D U-Net with one input block, 4 down-sampling blocks, one bottleneck block, 5 upsampling blocks, 32 features in the first level, instance normalization [32], and leaky-ReLU with slope 0.01. An illustration of the architecture is provided in Fig. 1. We have used the same pipeline for our participation to the FeTA challenge 2021 [14].

Transformers have recently received attention in medical image computing for their multi-hop attention mechanism. As a second network architecture, we replace the bottleneck block of the U-Net with a vision transformer as proposed by [9]. We use the identical transformer architecture for our experiment as in [9]. A transformer in the bottleneck allows to accumulate the global context of the image and learn an anatomically consistent representation of the tumor classes.

Table 1. Network architecture specification

Network	No. of parameter	Avg. inference time
3D U-Net [10]	31.2M	6 s
TransUNet [9]	116.7M	10 s

Table 1 shows a comparison in terms of the number of parameters and inference time between 3D U-Net and transUNet. For both networks, we train using a patch size of $128 \times 192 \times 128$.

2.3 Loss Function

We have experimented with two loss functions: the sum of the cross-entropy loss and the mean-class Dice loss

$$\mathcal{L}_{DL+CE} = \mathcal{L}_{DL} + \mathcal{L}_{CE} \tag{1}$$

---

[2] https://www.synapse.org/#!Synapse:syn25829067/wiki/.

and the sum of the cross entropy loss and of the generalized Wasserstein Dice loss[3] [15,16].

$$\mathcal{L}_{GWDL+CE} = \mathcal{L}_{GWDL} + \mathcal{L}_{CE} \tag{2}$$

where $\mathcal{L}_{CE}$ is the cross entropy loss function

$$\mathcal{L}_{CE}(\hat{\mathbf{p}}, \mathbf{p}) = -\sum_{i=1}^{N} \sum_{l=1}^{L} p_{i,l} \log(\hat{p}_{i,l}) \tag{3}$$

with N the number of voxels, L the number of classes, i the index for voxels, l the index for classes, $\hat{\mathbf{p}} = (\hat{p}_{i,l})_{i,l}$ the predicted probability map, and $\mathbf{p} = (p_{i,l})_{i,l}$ the discrete ground-truth probability map.

$\mathcal{L}_{DL}$ is the mean-class Dice loss [26,30]

$$\mathcal{L}_{DL}(\hat{\mathbf{p}}, \mathbf{p}) = 1 - \frac{1}{L} \sum_{l=1}^{L} \frac{2 \sum_{i=1}^{N} p_{i,l} \hat{p}_{i,l}}{\sum_{i=1}^{N} p_{i,l} + \sum_{i=1}^{N} \hat{p}_{i,l}} \tag{4}$$

And $\mathcal{L}_{GWDL}$ is the generalized Wasserstein Dice loss [15]

$$\begin{cases} \mathcal{L}_{GWDL}(\hat{\mathbf{p}}, \mathbf{p}) = 1 - \dfrac{2 \sum_{l \neq b} \sum_i \mathbf{P}_{i,l}(1 - W^M(\hat{\mathbf{p}}_i, \mathbf{p}_i))}{2 \sum_{l \neq b}[\sum_i p_{i,l}(1 - W^M(\hat{\mathbf{p}}_i, \mathbf{p}_i))] + \sum_i W^M(\hat{\mathbf{p}}_i, \mathbf{p}_i)} \\ \forall i, \quad W^M(\hat{\mathbf{p}}_i, \mathbf{p}_i) = \sum_{l=1}^{L} p_{i,l} \left(\sum_{l'=1}^{L} M_{l,l'} \hat{p}_{i,l'} \right) \end{cases} \tag{5}$$

where $W^M(\hat{\mathbf{p}}_i, \mathbf{p}_i)$ is the Wasserstein distance between predicted $\hat{p}_i$ and ground truth $\mathbf{p}_i$ discrete probability distribution at voxel i. $M = (M_{l,l'})_{1 \leq l, l' \leq L}$ is a distances matrix between the BraTS 2021 labels, and b is the class number corresponding to the background. For the classes indices 0: *background*, 1: *enhancing tumor*, 2: *edema*, 3: *non-enhancing tumor*, we set

$$M = \begin{pmatrix} 0 & 1 & 1 & 1 \\ 1 & 0 & 0.7 & 0.5 \\ 1 & 0.7 & 0 & 0.6 \\ 1 & 0.5 & 0.6 & 0 \end{pmatrix} \tag{6}$$

The generalized Wasserstein Dice loss [15] is a generalization of the Dice Loss for multi-class segmentation that can take advantage of the hierarchical structure of the set of classes in BraTS. When the labeling of a voxel is ambiguous or too difficult for the neural network to predict it correctly, the generalized Wasserstein Dice loss and our matrix M are designed to favor mistakes that remain consistent with the sub-regions used in the evaluation of BraTS, i.e., core tumor and whole tumor.

---

[3] https://github.com/LucasFidon/GeneralizedWassersteinDiceLoss.

2.4 Optimization

Common Optimization Setting: For each network, the training dataset was split into 95% training and 5% validation at random. The random initialization of the weights was performed using He initialization [19] for all the deep neural network architectures. We used batch size 2. The CNN parameters used at inference corresponds to the last epoch. We used deep supervision with 4 levels during training. Training each 3D U-Net required 16GB of GPU memory.

SGD: SGD with Nesterov momentum. The initial learning rate was 0.02, and we used polynomial learning rate decay with power 0.9 for a total of 500 epochs.

ADAM [22]: For Adam, we used a linear warmup for 1000 iterations for the learning rate from 0 to 0.003 followed by a constant learning rate schedule at the value 0.003 for 500 epochs.

Adaptive Sharpness-Aware Minimization (ASAM) [18,25]: We have used SGD as the base optimizer with the initial learning rate set to 0.02 and we used polynomial learning rate decay with power 0.9 for a total of 500 epochs. We used the default hyperparameters of ASAM [25], $\rho = 0.5$, and $\eta = 0.1$. We have used the PyTorch implementation of the authors[4].

SGDP [20]: For SGD Projected (SGDP), we have used the exact same hyperparameter values as for SGD. We have used the PyTorch implementation of the authors[5].

2.5 Data Augmentation

We have used random zoom (zoom ratio range $[0.7, 1.5]$ drawn uniformly at random; probability of augmentation 0.3), random rotation (rotation angle range $[-15°, 15°]$ for all dimensions drawn uniformly at random; probability of augmentation 0.3), random additive Gaussian noise (mean 0, standard deviation 0.1; probability of augmentation 0.3), random Gaussian spatial smoothing (standard deviation range $[0.5, 1.5]$ in voxels for all dimensions drawn uniformly at random; probability of augmentation 0.2), random gamma augmentation (gamma range $[0.7, 1.5]$ drawn uniformly at random; probability of augmentation 0.3), and random right/left flip (probability of augmentation 0.5).

2.6 Inference

Single Models Inference: For the models evaluated and compared in Fig. 2, a patch-based approach is used. The input image is divided into overlapping patches of size $128 \times 192 \times 128$. The patches are chosen, so that neighboring patches have an overlap of at least half of their volume. The fusion of the patch

---

[4] https://github.com/SamsungLabs/ASAM.
[5] https://github.com/clovaai/AdamP.

prediction is performed using a weighted average of the patch predictions before the softmax operation. The weights are defined with respect to the distance of a voxel to the center of the patch using a Gaussian kernel standard deviation for each dimension equal to $0.125 \times$ patch-dimension. In addition, test-time augmentation [33] is used with right-left flip. The two softmax predictions obtained with and without right-left flip are merged by averaging.

Ensemble Inference: For the ensembles, the inference is performed in two steps. During the first step, a first segmentation is computed using only one model and the inference procedure for single models. In practice, we used the first model of the list and did not tune the choice of this model.

The first segmentation is used to estimate the center of gravity of the whole tumor. In the second step, we crop a patch of size $128 \times 192 \times 128$ with a center chosen as close as possible to the center of gravity of the tumor so that the patch fits in the image. The segmentation probability predictions of all the models of the ensemble are computed for this patch. The motivation for this two-step approach is to reduce the inference time as compared to using the patch-based approach described above for all the models of the ensemble. This strategy is based on the assumption that a patch of size $128 \times 192 \times 128$ is large enough to always contain the whole tumor. During the second step, test-time augmentations with right-left flip and zoom with a ratio of 1.125 are used. The four segmentation probability predictions obtained for the different augmentations (no flip - no zoom, flip - no zoom, no flip - zoom, and flip - zoom) are combined by averaging the softmax predictions. For the full image segmentation prediction, the voxels outside the patch centered on the tumor are set to the background.

3   Results

As a primary metric, we report the mean and the standard deviation of the Dice score and the Hausdorff distance for each class. Percentiles are common statistics for measuring the robustness of automatic segmentations [13]. To evaluate the robustness of the different models, we report the percentiles of the Dice score at 25% and 5% and the percentiles at 75% and 95% of the Hausdorff 95% distance. In Table 2, we report the validation scores of our individually trained models. In Table 3 we compare two ensemble strategies as described in the previous section. In the ensemble models, we don't include the TransUNet model as their individual performance is marginally worse than the 3D U-Net model.

4   Discussion

From Table 2, we see that 3D U-Net trained with generalized Wasserstein Dice loss performs consistently better than the one with Dice loss (baseline model). TransUNet does not offer any improvement over the baseline. Rather the performance deteriorates slightly. We hypothesize that over-parameterization can

Table 2. Segmentation results on the BraTS 2021 Validation dataset. The evaluation was performed on the BraTS online evaluation platform. ET: Enhancing Tumor, WT: Whole Tumor, TC: Tumor Core, Std: Standard deviation, p_x: Percentile x. The split number corresponds to the random seed that was used to split the training dataset into 95% training/5% validation at random.

Model	ROI	Dice score (%)				Hausdorff 95% (mm)			
		Mean	Std	p_{25}	p_5	Mean	Std	p_{75}	p_{95}
3D U-Net	ET	82.6	23.7	83.6	7.7	17.9	73.7	2.2	25.4
GWDL + CE SGD	TC	86.4	20.1	86.8	37.7	11.2	50.1	4.2	19.4
Split 1	WT	92.5	7.4	90.7	82.1	3.8	5.7	3.6	17.7
3D U-Net	ET	82.2	24.0	82.9	7.2	17.8	73.7	2.4	18.1
GWDL + CE SGD	TC	86.5	20.4	86.1	37.7	11.1	50.1	4.4	21.3
Split 2	WT	92.5	7.4	90.6	82.6	3.8	5.9	3.7	11.5
3D U-Net	ET	81.9	24.5	82.5	5.3	19.5	77.5	2.2	31.7
GWDL + CE SGD	TC	85.7	21.6	86.0	30.5	11.5	50.1	4.2	20.8
Split 27	WT	92.5	7.1	90.5	81.7	4.0	6.2	3.9	10.6
3D U-Net	ET	81.9	24.9	83.0	0.0	21.1	81.0	2.2	67.0
GWDL + CE SGD	TC	86.5	20.7	87.2	38.5	9.5	43.7	4.1	16.9
Split 1227	WT	92.5	7.3	90.6	81.1	3.8	5.8	3.7	11.7
3D U-Net	ET	82.4	24.4	83.2	2.9	19.5	77.5	2.4	30.3
GWDL + CE SGD	TC	85.8	21.7	86.3	27.6	11.5	50.1	4.6	23.0
Split 122712	WT	92.4	7.1	90.2	81.7	4.1	7.0	3.9	11.4
3D U-Net	ET	81.7	24.9	82.9	0.0	21.3	81.1	2.4	89.3
DL + CE SGD	TC	86.5	20.4	86.3	40.2	11.0	50.1	4.1	17.9
Split 1	WT	92.5	7.2	90.6	80.2	3.9	6.7	3.9	9.8
3D U-Net	ET	82.1	24.2	82.8	5.4	19.5	77.5	2.5	31.3
GWDL + CE SGDP	TC	86.3	20.5	86.4	40.4	9.7	43.7	4.1	20.2
Split 1	WT	92.6	7.4	90.5	82.0	3.8	5.9	3.7	11.0
3D U-Net	ET	80.0	25.7	81.5	0.0	23.4	84.5	3.0	373.1
GWDL + CE ASAM	TC	85.4	21.5	86.1	35.3	12.2	50.8	4.2	21.7
Split 1	WT	91.9	7.9	90.0	77.2	5.4	10.7	4.2	22.0
TransUNet	ET	79.7	25.3	80.1	0.0	22.4	81.0	3.0	113.4
GWDL + CE SGD	TC	84.5	22.0	84.5	36.5	8.7	36.5	4.9	24.9
Split 1	WT	91.8	7.3	90.2	77.2	4.4	7.6	4.1	12.7
TransUNet	ET	80.9	24.1	81.2	6.5	18.5	73.6	3.0	37.7
GWDL + CE ADAM	TC	84.8	21.9	84.7	36.44	10.3	43.8	4.6	24.6
Split 1	WT	91.9	7.8	90.0	80.1	4.1	6.5	4.1	14.9
TransUNet	ET	80.2	25.5	80.4	0.0	23.1	84.3	3.0	373.1
GWDL + CE SGDP	TC	85.2	21.9	85.6	27.6	11.45	50.0	4.5	19.9
Split 1	WT	92.0	7.4	90.1	79.7	4.7	9.1	4.0	18.0

Table 3. Segmentation results on the BraTS 2021 Validation dataset for ensembling and test-time augmentation. The evaluation was performed on the BraTS online evaluation platform. ET: Enhancing Tumor, WT: Whole Tumor, TC: Tumor Core, Std: Standard deviation, p_x: Percentile x. Best values are in **bold**.

Model	ROI	Dice score (%)				Hausdorff 95% (mm)			
		Mean	Std	p_{25}	p_5	Mean	Std	p_{75}	p_{95}
3D U-Net	ET	82.0	24.4	83.0	3.1	19.5	77.5	2.3	30.0
Ensemble	TC	86.6	20.2	86.5	39.2	9.5	43.7	4.1	20.1
	WT	92.6	7.2	90.6	82.0	3.9	6.3	3.6	12.8
3D U-Net	ET	**84.0**	**22.0**	**84.2**	**21.6**	**12.7**	**60.6**	**2.2**	**16.0**
Ensemble	TC	**87.0**	**20.0**	**86.8**	**43.1**	**11.0**	**50.1**	**4.1**	**18.7**
Zoom augmentation	WT	**92.7**	**7.2**	**90.6**	**82.1**	**3.9**	**6.3**	**3.6**	**12.6**

Table 4. Segmentation results on the BraTS 2021 Testing dataset using ensembling and test-time augmentation. The evaluation was performed by the BraTS 2021 challenge organizers using our docker submission. ET: Enhancing Tumor, WT: Whole Tumor, TC: Tumor Core, Std: Standard deviation, p_x: Percentile x.

Model	ROI	Dice score (%)			Hausdorff 95% (mm)		
		Mean	Std	p_{25}	Mean	Std	p_{75}
3D U-Net	ET	87.4	17.6	85.2	10.1	53.5	2.0
Ensemble	TC	87.8	23.6	91.3	15.8	66.7	3.0
Zoom augmentation	WT	92.9	9.0	91.6	4.1	7.3	3.7

be an issue in this case. The optimizer SGDP and ASAM perform similar to the baseline SGD. From Table 3, we see that ensemble strategy helps in increasing the robustness of the model. The best ensemble strategy turns out to be including zoom as a test time augmentation. This approach was submitted for evaluation on the BraTS 2021 testing dataset and the results can be found in Table 4. In conclusion, this paper proposes a detailed comparative study on the strategies to make a computationally efficient yet robust automatic brain tumor segmentation model. We have explored ensemble from multiple training configurations of different state-of-the-art loss functions and optimizers, and importantly, test-time augmentation. Future research will focus on further strategies on test-time augmentation and test-time hyper-parameter tuning.

Acknowledgments. This project has received funding from the European Union's Horizon 2020 research and innovation program under the Marie Skłodowska-Curie grant agreement TRABIT No 765148; Wellcome [203148/Z/16/Z; WT101957], EPSRC [NS/A000049/1; NS/A000027/1]. Tom Vercauteren is supported by a Medtronic/RAEng Research Chair [RCSRF1819\7\34]. Data used in this publication were obtained as part of the RSNA-ASNR-MICCAI Brain Tumor Segmentation (BraTS) Challenge project through Synapse ID (syn25829067).

References

1. Andres, E.A., et al.: Po-1002 pseudo computed tomography generation using 3D deep learning-application to brain radiotherapy. Radiother. Oncol. **133**, S553 (2019)
2. Andres, E.A., et al.: Dosimetry-driven quality measure of brain pseudo computed tomography generated from deep learning for MRI-only radiotherapy treatment planning. Int. J. Radiat. Oncol.* Biol.* Phys. **108**, 813–823 (2020)
3. Baid, U., et al.: The RSNA-ASNR-MICCAI BraTS 2021 benchmark on brain tumor segmentation and radiogenomic classification. arXiv preprint arXiv:2107.02314 (2021)
4. Bakas, S., et al.: Advancing the cancer genome atlas glioma MRI collections with expert segmentation labels and radiomic features. Sci. Data **4**, 170117 (2017)
5. Bakas, S., et al.: Segmentation labels and radiomic features for the pre-operative scans of the TCGA-GBM collection. Cancer Imaging Arch. (2017). https://doi.org/10.7937/K9/TCIA.2017.KLXWJJ1Q
6. Bakas, S., et al.: Segmentation labels and radiomic features for the pre-operative scans of the TCGA-LGG collection. Cancer Imaging Arch. (2017). https://doi.org/10.7937/K9/TCIA.2017.GJQ7R0EF
7. Bakas, S., et al.: Identifying the best machine learning algorithms for brain tumor segmentation, progression assessment, and overall survival prediction in the brats challenge. arXiv preprint arXiv:1811.02629 (2018)
8. Blanc-Durand, P., et al.: Prognostic value of anthropometric measures extracted from whole-body CT using deep learning in patients with non-small-cell lung cancer. Eur. Radiol. **30**(6), 3528–3537 (2020). https://doi.org/10.1007/s00330-019-06630-w
9. Chen, J., et al.: TransUNet: transformers make strong encoders for medical image segmentation. arXiv preprint arXiv:2102.04306 (2021)
10. Çiçek, Ö., Abdulkadir, A., Lienkamp, S.S., Brox, T., Ronneberger, O.: 3D U-Net: learning dense volumetric segmentation from sparse annotation. In: Ourselin, S., Joskowicz, L., Sabuncu, M.R., Unal, G., Wells, W. (eds.) MICCAI 2016. LNCS, vol. 9901, pp. 424–432. Springer, Cham (2016). https://doi.org/10.1007/978-3-319-46723-8_49
11. Ezhov, I., et al.: Neural parameters estimation for brain tumor growth modeling. In: MICCAI 2019. LNCS, vol. 11765, pp. 787–795. Springer, Cham (2019). https://doi.org/10.1007/978-3-030-32245-8_87
12. Ezhov, I., et al.: Geometry-aware neural solver for fast Bayesian calibration of brain tumor models. arXiv preprint arXiv:2009.04240 (2020)
13. Fidon, L., et al.: Distributionally robust segmentation of abnormal fetal brain 3D MRI. In: UNSURE/PIPPI -2021. LNCS, vol. 12959, pp. 263–273. Springer, Cham (2021). https://doi.org/10.1007/978-3-030-87735-4_25
14. Fidon, L., et al.: Partial supervision for the feta challenge 2021. arXiv preprint arXiv:2111.02408 (2021)
15. Fidon, L., et al.: Generalised Wasserstein dice score for imbalanced multi-class segmentation using holistic convolutional networks. In: Crimi, A., Bakas, S., Kuijf, H., Menze, B., Reyes, M. (eds.) BrainLes 2017. LNCS, vol. 10670, pp. 64–76. Springer, Cham (2018). https://doi.org/10.1007/978-3-319-75238-9_6
16. Fidon, L., Ourselin, S., Vercauteren, T.: Generalized Wasserstein dice score, distributionally robust deep learning, and ranger for brain tumor segmentation: Brats 2020 challenge. arXiv preprint arXiv:2011.01614 (2020)

17. Fidon, L., Ourselin, S., Vercauteren, T.: SGD with hardness weighted sampling for distributionally robust deep learning. arXiv preprint arXiv:2001.02658 (2020)
18. Foret, P., Kleiner, A., Mobahi, H., Neyshabur, B.: Sharpness-aware minimization for efficiently improving generalization. arXiv preprint arXiv:2010.01412 (2020)
19. He, K., Zhang, X., Ren, S., Sun, J.: Delving deep into rectifiers: surpassing human-level performance on ImageNet classification. In: Proceedings of the IEEE International Conference on Computer Vision, pp. 1026–1034 (2015)
20. Heo, B., et al.: AdamP: slowing down the slowdown for momentum optimizers on scale-invariant weights. arXiv preprint arXiv:2006.08217 (2020)
21. Isensee, F., Jäger, P.F., Kohl, S.A., Petersen, J., Maier-Hein, K.H.: Automated design of deep learning methods for biomedical image segmentation. arXiv preprint arXiv:1904.08128 (2020)
22. Kingma, D.P., Ba, J.: Adam: a method for stochastic optimization. arXiv preprint arXiv:1412.6980 (2014)
23. Kofler, F., Berger, C., Waldmannstetter, D., Lipkova, J., Ezhov, I., Tetteh, G., Kirschke, J., Zimmer, C., Wiestler, B., Menze, B.H.: Brats toolkit: translating brats brain tumor segmentation algorithms into clinical and scientific practice. Front. Neurosci. **14**, 125 (2020)
24. Kofler, F., et al.: Are we using appropriate segmentation metrics? Identifying correlates of human expert perception for CNN training beyond rolling the dice coefficient. arXiv preprint arXiv:2103.06205 (2021)
25. Kwon, J., Kim, J., Park, H., Choi, I.K.: ASAM: adaptive sharpness-aware minimization for scale-invariant learning of deep neural networks. arXiv preprint arXiv:2102.11600 (2021)
26. Li, W., Wang, G., Fidon, L., Ourselin, S., Cardoso, M.J., Vercauteren, T.: On the compactness, efficiency, and representation of 3D convolutional networks: brain parcellation as a pretext task. In: Niethammer, M., et al. (eds.) IPMI 2017. LNCS, vol. 10265, pp. 348–360. Springer, Cham (2017). https://doi.org/10.1007/978-3-319-59050-9_28
27. Menze, B.H., et al.: The multimodal brain tumor image segmentation benchmark (BRATS). IEEE Trans. Med. Imaging **34**(10), 1993–2024 (2014)
28. Milletari, F., Navab, N., Ahmadi, S.A.: V-Net: fully convolutional neural networks for volumetric medical image segmentation. In: 2016 Fourth International Conference on 3D Vision (3DV), pp. 565–571. IEEE (2016)
29. MONAI Consortium: MONAI: Medical open network for AI, March 2020. https://doi.org/10.5281/zenodo.4323058. https://github.com/Project-MONAI/MONAI
30. Sudre, C.H., Li, W., Vercauteren, T., Ourselin, S., Jorge Cardoso, M.: Generalised dice overlap as a deep learning loss function for highly unbalanced segmentations. In: Cardoso, M.J., et al. (eds.) DLMIA/ML-CDS -2017. LNCS, vol. 10553, pp. 240–248. Springer, Cham (2017). https://doi.org/10.1007/978-3-319-67558-9_28
31. Tilborghs, S., et al.: Comparative study of deep learning methods for the automatic segmentation of lung, lesion and lesion type in CT scans of COVID-19 patients. arXiv preprint arXiv:2007.15546 (2020)
32. Ulyanov, D., Vedaldi, A., Lempitsky, V.: Instance normalization: the missing ingredient for fast stylization. arXiv preprint arXiv:1607.08022 (2016)
33. Wang, G., Li, W., Aertsen, M., Deprest, J., Ourselin, S., Vercauteren, T.: Aleatoric uncertainty estimation with test-time augmentation for medical image segmentation with convolutional neural networks. Neurocomputing **338**, 34–45 (2019)

Coupling nnU-Nets with Expert Knowledge for Accurate Brain Tumor Segmentation from MRI

Krzysztof Kotowski[1], Szymon Adamski[1], Bartosz Machura[1], Lukasz Zarudzki[3], and Jakub Nalepa[1,2(✉)]

[1] Future Processing Healthcare, Gliwice, Poland
{kkotowski,sadamski,bmachura,jnalepa}@futureprocessinghealthcare.com
[2] Silesian University of Technology, Gliwice, Poland
jnalepa@ieee.org
[3] Maria Sklodowska-Curie Memorial Cancer Center and Institute of Oncology, Gliwice, Poland

Abstract. Accurate and reproducible segmentation of brain tumors from multi-modal magnetic resonance (MR) scans is a pivotal step in clinical practice, as MR imaging is the modality of choice in brain tumor diagnosis and assessment, and incorrectly delineated tumor areas may adversely affect the process of designing the treatment pathway. In this paper, we exploit an end-to-end 3D nnU-Net architecture for this task, and utilize an ensemble of five models using our custom stratification based on the distribution of the necrosis, enhancing tumor, and edema. To improve the segmentation, we benefit from the experience of a senior radiologist captured in a form of several post-processing routines. The experiments obtained for the BraTS'21 training and validation sets show that exploiting such expert knowledge can significantly improve the underlying models, delivering the average Dice score of 0.81977 (enhancing tumor), 0.87837 (tumor core), and 0.92723 (whole tumor). Finally, our algorithm allowed us to take the 6th place (out of 1600 participants) in the BraTS'21 Challenge, with the average Dice score over the test data of 0.86317, 0.87987, and 0.92838 for the enhancing tumor, tumor core and whole tumor, respectively.

Keywords: Brain tumor · Segmentation · Deep learning · U-Net · Expert knowledge

1 Introduction

Brain tumor segmentation from multi-modal MR scans is an important step in oncology care. Accurate delineation of tumorous tissue is pivotal for further diagnosis, prognosis and treatment, and it can directly affect the treatment pathway. Hence, ensuring the reproducibility, robustness, e.g., against different scanner types, and quality of an automated segmentation process are critical

A. Crimi and S. Bakas (Eds.): BrainLes 2021, LNCS 12963, pp. 197–209, 2022.
https://doi.org/10.1007/978-3-031-09002-8_18

to design personalized patient care and reliable patient monitoring. The state-of-the-art brain tumor segmentation algorithms are commonly divided into the *atlas-based, unsupervised, supervised,* and *hybrid* techniques. In the *atlas-based* algorithms, manually segmented atlases are used to elaborate the segmentation of unseen scans [22]. *Unsupervised* approaches elaborate intrinsic characteristics of the *unlabeled* data [7] with the use of clustering [13,23,25], Gaussian modeling [24], and other techniques [21]. Once the labeled data is available, we can utilize the *supervised* techniques [9,26,28]. Deep learning models for brain tumor segmentation are built upon various networks architectures [10,15,17,18], and they encompass holistically nested neural nets [27], ensembles of deep neural nets [14], U-Net-based architectures [12,20], autoencoder networks, convolutional encoder-decoder approaches [6], and more [8,19].

In this paper, we use a 3D nnU-Net architecture (Sect. 3) operating over multi-modal MR scans [11], in which brain tumors are segmented into the enhancing tumor (ET), peritumoral edema (ED), and necrotic core (NCR). To enhance the generalization abilities of our approach, we utilize five-fold ensembling with stratification based on the distribution of NCR, ET, and ED, alongside the post-processing routines that capture the expert knowledge of a senior radiologist. The experiments performed over the BraTS'21 training and validation datasets showed that our architecture delivers accurate multi-class segmentation, and the procedures that reflect expert knowledge may significantly improve the abilities of the underlying nnU-Nets (Sect. 4).

2   Data

The newest release of the Brain Tumor Segmentation (BraTS'21) dataset [1–4,16] includes MRI training data of 1251 patients with diagnosed gliomas. Each study was manually annotated by one to four experienced and trained readers. The data comes in four co-registered modalities: native pre-contrast (T1), post-contrast T1-weighted (T1Gd), T2-weighted (T2), and T2 Fluid Attenuated Inversion Recovery (T2-FLAIR). All pixels are labeled, and the following classes are considered: healthy tissue, Gd-enhancing tumor (ET), peritumoral edema/invaded tissue (ED) and the necrotic tumor core (NCR) [5].

The data was acquired with different protocols and scanners from multiple institutions. The studies were interpolated to the same shape ($240 \times 240 \times 155$, hence there are 155 images of 240×240 size, with voxel size of $1\,\mathrm{mm}^3$), and they were skull-stripped. Finally, there are 219 patients in the validation set V (see examples in Fig. 1), for which the manual annotations are not provided.

3   Methods

3.1   nnU-Net Architecture

We built upon an extremely successful nnU-Net [11], being a deep learning-based segmentation method that automatically configures itself, including pre-processing, basic post-processing, network architecture and training configurations. Here, we train the network over the BraTS'21 training data with the loss

T1	T1Gd	T2	T2-FLAIR

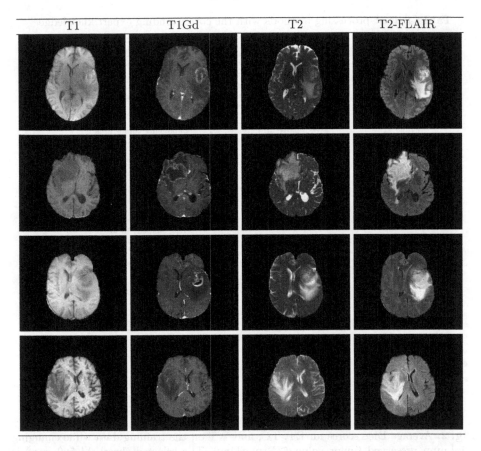

Fig. 1. Example scans of four patients (separate rows) included in the validation set.

function being the averaged cross-entropy and soft Dice, averaged across all target classes, hence do not utilize any previously trained and validated models. The generated network is a 3D U-Net consisting of an encoder and a decoder which are interconnected by skip connections. A patch size of $128 \times 128 \times 128$ with a batch size of 2 was selected.

3.2 Post-processing Using Expert Knowledge

We designed three post-processing methods (gathered in Table 1), in which we exploit the expert domain knowledge of the senior radiologist with 13 years of experience. First, we validated these post-processing methods in different combinations and ordering on our predictions for a complete training data. Then, we applied the most promising post-processing combinations to the predictions for the validation data. Here, we assume that a "good" post-processing pipeline should improve both training and validation predictions.

Table 1. Post-processing methods with the corresponding expert knowledge.

Method's short name	Algorithm	Expert knowledge
PruneTiny	We remove WT volumes smaller than 500 mm^3 from the predictions. The threshold was selected experimentally based on the training data (see Fig. 2)	Very small lesions are usually false positives. Gliomas should be compact volumes of significant size
PruneET	We remove all detected ET voxels that are not connected to ED (in 3D)	Enhancing tumor area is typically surrounded by edema
FillTC	Any voxels surrounded by TC in 2D in any slice on any plane are iteratively relabeled to NCR	Edema cannot be surrounded by necrosis only. Necrosis cannot have "holes" (tissue not labeled by model to any class) inside it. If enhancing tumor is "closed" (ring-shaped) in 2D everything inside it which is not enhancing has to be necrosis. Large tumors usually do not contain "holes" of healthy tissue

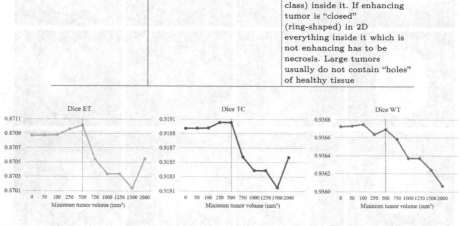

Fig. 2. Average Dice scores for ET, TC, and WT on the training data while changing minimum preserved tumor volume (PruneTiny). The selected threshold 500 mm^3 is marked with the dashed vertical line.

4 Experiments

4.1 Experimental Setup

The DNN models were implemented using `Python3` with `Keras` and `PyTorch`. The experiments were run on a high-performance computer equipped with an NVIDIA Tesla V100 GPU (32 GB) and 6 Intel Xeon E5-2680 (2.50 GHz) CPUs.

4.2 Training Process

The metric for training was a sum of the Dice score and cross-entropy. Training was performed on ET, ED, and NCR classes. Due to the limited time available, we decided to set the number of epochs to 500[1]. The optimizer was the stochastic

---

[1] Note that increasing the number of training epochs would likely improve the capabilities of the model even further.

gradient descent with the Nesterov momentum with the initial learning rate of 10^{-2}. The learning rate is decayed gradually to a value close to zero in the last epoch [11].

The training set was split into five non-overlapping stratified folds (each base model is trained over four folds, and one fold is used for validation during the training process; see Table 2). We stratify the dataset at the patient level with respect to the distribution of the size of the NCR, ED, and ET examples. The fold sizes were equal to 251, 253, 250, 248, and 249 patients.

Table 2. Characteristics of the folds (average volume of the corresponding tumor subregion in cm^3) used for training our model.

	WT vol.	NCR vol.	ED vol.	ET vol.
Fold 1	95.16	14.21	59.85	21.10
Fold 2	96.63	15.38	60.42	20.82
Fold 3	93.97	13.77	57.74	22.47
Fold 4	97.18	14.65	60.72	21.82
Fold 5	96.80	13.43	62.36	21.00

4.3   Experimental Results

In this section, we gather the results obtained for different post-processing pipelines over the BraTS'21 training and validation sets (as returned by the Synapse portal)[2]. The Dice and Hausdorff (95%) scores for predictions over training set are presented in Table 3, together with the p-values from one-sided Wilcoxon signed-rank tests for difference between the prediction without post-processing and each of the post-processing pipelines in Table 4. Altogether, we tested 15 combinations of the PruneTiny, FillTC, and PruneET routines.

All pipelines involving PruneET rule improve the average ET Dice from 0.8717 to over 0.8732, but surprisingly these methods have statistically significantly lower average ET Dice rank from one-sided Wilcoxon signed-rank test ($p < 1 \times 10^{-20}$). This is because of a couple of specific cases (without ET in ground truth, e.g., patients with ID: 1433 and 1435) with ET Dice fixed from 0 to 1. The average score is higher, but there are many studies with lower ET Dice after post-processing. On the other side, Hausdorff (95%) for ET for all these 11 pipelines has much worse average (12.3 instead of 11.8), but this difference is not statistically significant. In summary, post-processing with PruneET does not significantly improve the results for ET and is highly affected by very specific cases in the BraTS training data. Also, PruneET alone statistically significantly decreases Dice for TC and WT.

---

[2] Our team name is **Future Processing Healthcare**.

Table 3. The mean Dice and Hausdorff (95%) scores obtained over predictions for the BraTS'21 **training** set. Green/red cells denote results better/worse than without any post-processing. The best results for each metric are boldfaced.

	Pipeline	Dice ET	Dice TC	Dice WT	Haus. ET	Haus. TC	Haus. WT
1	PruneTiny	0.871840	0.919248	0.936692	11.735022	**5.093179**	5.733001
2	PruneTiny-FillTC	0.871840	0.919373	0.936745	11.735022	5.095544	5.725865
3	PruneTiny-FillTC-PruneET	**0.873301**	0.919238	0.936671	12.300442	5.097893	5.747066
4	PruneTiny-PruneET	0.873300	0.919113	0.936618	12.300540	5.101184	5.756955
5	PruneTiny-PruneET-FillTC	0.873300	0.919340	0.936721	12.300540	5.108197	5.732852
6	FillTC	0.871696	0.919291	**0.936775**	11.825262	5.141116	**5.287235**
7	FillTC-PruneTiny	0.871840	**0.919374**	0.936745	**11.734972**	5.095544	5.725865
8	FillTC-PruneTiny-PruneET	**0.873301**	0.919238	0.936671	12.300442	5.097918	5.747096
9	FillTC-PruneET	0.873260	0.919251	0.936723	12.342460	5.119635	5.334405
10	FillTC-PruneET-PruneTiny	**0.873301**	0.919238	0.936671	12.300442	5.111995	5.758140
11	PruneET	0.873260	0.919125	0.936670	12.342558	5.123232	5.345672
12	PruneET-PruneTiny	0.873300	0.919112	0.936618	12.300540	5.111352	5.765368
13	PruneET-PruneTiny-FillTC	0.873300	0.919340	0.936721	12.300540	5.118365	5.741265
14	PruneET-FillTC	0.873260	0.919353	0.936773	12.342558	5.129725	5.317099
15	PruneET-FillTC-PruneTiny	0.873300	0.919340	0.936721	12.300540	5.118365	5.741265
	No post-processing	0.871696	0.919165	0.936722	11.825262	5.139082	5.295796

Table 4. The p-values of one-sided Wilcoxon signed-rank tests for Dice and Hausdorff (95%) scores examined between the BraTS'21 **training** set prediction without post-processing and each of the post-processing pipelines. Green/red cells denotes statistically significant ($p < 0.001$) better/worse mean ranks. Dashes mean the results do not differ statistically ($p > 0.5$ for both sides).

	Pipeline	Dice ET	Dice TC	Dice WT	Haus. ET	Haus. TC	Haus. WT
1	PruneTiny	—	—	—	—	—	1.70E-05
2	PruneTiny-FillTC	—	5.86E-10	1.96E-10	—	—	1.60E-05
3	PruneTiny-FillTC-PruneET	2.48E-21	—	—	—	—	3.00E-06
4	PruneTiny-PruneET	2.45E-21	2.55E-67	2.57E-18	—	—	4.00E-06
5	PruneTiny-PruneET-FillTC	2.45E-21	5.96E-09	8.13E-09	—	—	2.00E-05
6	FillTC	—	5.43E-11	2.40E-29	—	—	—
7	FillTC-PruneTiny	—	5.09E-10	1.97E-10	—	—	1.60E-05
8	FillTC-PruneTiny-PruneET	2.48E-21	—	—	—	—	3.00E-06
9	FillTC-PruneET	1.88E-21	—	7.38E-06	—	—	—
10	FillTC-PruneET-PruneTiny	2.48E-21	—	—	—	—	3.00E-06
11	PruneET	1.86E-21	1.26E-67	2.46E-77	—	—	—
12	PruneET-PruneTiny	2.45E-21	2.55E-67	2.57E-18	—	—	4.00E-06
13	PruneET-PruneTiny-FillTC	2.45E-21	5.94E-09	8.13E-09	—	—	2.00E-05
14	PruneET-FillTC	1.86E-21	1.23E-09	3.52E-21	—	—	—
15	PruneET-FillTC-PruneTiny	2.45E-21	5.95E-09	8.13E-09	—	—	2.00E-05

All pipelines involving the PruneTiny rule significantly deteriorate the average Hausdorff (95%) for WT ($p < 0.0001$). PruneTiny alone slightly improves TC Dice, Hausdorff (95%) for ET and Hausdorff (95%) for TC, but the differences are not statistically significant. Thus, there are no strong advantages of using this post-processing method.

Finally, only the pipelines involving FillTC rule were able to significantly improve Dice of TC and WT ($p < 1 \times 10^{-8}$). Additionally, the best averages in most of the metrics (excluding Hausdorff (95%) for TC) were obtained for pipelines with FillTC. Moreover, using FillTC alone as a post-processing was the only way to avoid statistically significantly worse results in any other metric. Thus, FillTC is the most effective post-processing among all proposed methods.

Following the analysis on the training dataset, we selected four pipelines to test on the BraTS validation data: FillTC, FillTC-PruneTiny, PruneET-FillTC, and PruneTiny-PruneET-FillTC. The average metrics are presented in Table 5 together with p-values using the same tests as for training data in Table 6. All the pipelines gave statistically significantly better results for Dice obtained for TC and WT ($p < 0.005$), but only FillTC alone gives all the averages at least as good as without any post-processing. It confirms the observations from the training data. Thus, we selected FillTC as our final post-processing method.

Table 5. The mean Dice and Hausdorff (95%) scores obtained over predictions for the BraTS'21 **validation** set. Green/red cells denote results better/worse than without any post-processing. The best results for each metric are boldfaced.

	Pipeline	Dice ET	Dice TC	Dice WT	Haus. ET	Haus. TC	Haus. WT
5	PruneTiny-PruneET-FillTC	0.817469	0.878357	0.927241	21.766062	7.5977811	3.775022
6	FillTC	**0.819771**	**0.878375**	0.927235	**17.853337**	7.597125	**3.636371**
7	FillTC-PruneTiny	0.819760	0.878372	**0.927246**	**17.853337**	7.597793	3.775022
14	PruneET-FillTC	0.817480	0.878360	0.927230	21.766062	**7.597113**	**3.636371**
	No post-processing	**0.819771**	0.878174	0.927195	**17.853337**	7.602347	3.636563

Table 6. The p-values of one-sided Wilcoxon signed-rank tests for Dice and Hausdorff (95%) scores examined between the BraTS'21 **validation** set prediction without post-processing and each of the post-processing pipelines. Green/red cells denotes statistically significant ($p < 0.005$) better/worse mean ranks. Dashes mean the results do not differ statistically ($p > 0.5$ for both sides).

	Pipeline	Dice ET	Dice TC	Dice WT	Haus. ET	Haus. TC	Haus. WT
5	PruneTiny-PruneET-FillTC	9.77E-04	3.10E-05	6.34E-04	—	—	—
6	FillTC	—	1.00E-05	3.38E-04	—	—	—
7	FillTC-PruneTiny	—	1.40E-05	2.82E-04	—	—	—
14	PruneET-FillTC	1.32E-03	1.40E-05	1.33E-03	—	—	—

The detailed comparison of results for validation data between segmentations with and without FillTC post-processing is given in Table 7. All the statistics for all the metrics after FillTC are at least as good as without post-processing. All statistics for Dice for TC and WT, and sensitivity of TC are improved. For TC Dice the results are better for 108 studies and worse for 53 studies. The example of the patient with ID: 474 with the largest improvement in Dice TC (+0.017) is presented in Fig. 3. For WT Dice, the results are better for 66 studies and worse for 23 studies. Currently, our current research is focused on improving the aforementioned specific and difficult cases (see an example in Fig. 4), e.g., the patients with missing ET or TC in the predictions or the ground truth. This is reflected by much worse averages than medians, and much larger standard deviations for these classes.

Table 7. Segmentation performance quantified by Dice, sensitivity, specificity, and Hausdorff (95%) distance over the BraTS'21 **validation** set obtained using our model with and without FillTC post-processing (as returned by the **validation server**). The scores (average μ, standard deviation s, median m, and the 25 and 75 quantile) are presented for the whole tumor (WT), tumor core (TC), and enhancing tumor (ET). The best scores are boldfaced.

	Dice ET	Dice TC	Dice WT	Haus. ET	Haus. TC	Haus. WT	Sens. ET	Sens. TC	Sens. WT	Spec. ET	Spec. TC	Spec. WT
Without post-processing												
μ	0.81977	0.87817	0.92720	17.85334	7.60235	3.63656	0.82215	0.85880	0.92880	0.99979	0.99983	0.99938
s	0.24619	0.17872	0.07351	73.68160	36.04539	5.73161	0.26009	0.19935	0.07880	0.00038	0.00030	0.00082
m	0.89787	0.94090	0.94544	1.41421	1.73205	2.08262	0.91475	0.93676	0.95560	0.99991	0.99993	0.99964
25q	0.82421	0.87825	0.90319	1.00000	1.00000	1.41421	0.83038	0.85006	0.91154	0.99975	0.99983	0.99919
75q	0.95197	0.96853	0.96887	2.44949	3.87083	3.62106	0.96640	0.97241	0.97867	0.99997	0.99998	0.99985
With FillTC post-processing												
μ	0.81977	**0.87837**	**0.92723**	17.85334	**7.59712**	**3.63637**	0.82215	**0.85930**	**0.92890**	0.99979	0.99983	0.99938
s	0.24619	**0.17867**	**0.07349**	73.68160	**36.04532**	**5.72974**	0.26009	**0.19917**	**0.07878**	0.00038	0.00030	0.00082
m	0.89787	**0.94117**	**0.94569**	1.41421	1.73205	2.08262	0.91475	**0.93699**	**0.95565**	0.99991	0.99993	0.99964
25q	0.82421	**0.87840**	**0.90324**	1.00000	1.00000	1.41421	0.83038	**0.85134**	**0.91212**	0.99975	0.99983	0.99919
75q	0.95197	**0.96874**	**0.96890**	2.44949	3.87083	**3.62096**	0.96640	**0.97318**	0.97867	0.99997	0.99998	0.99985

In Table 8, we gather the results obtained over the test set using our final segmentation algorithm. We can appreciate that it delivers high-quality delineation and generalizes well in all tumor classes, indicating its potential clinical utility. Our model allowed us to take the 6th place in the BraTS'21 Challenge.

Without post-processing   **With** FillTC post-processing

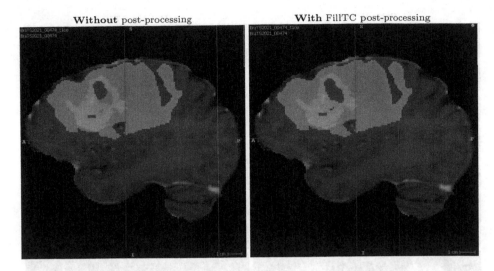

Fig. 3. The prediction for a patient with ID: 474 from BraTS'21 validation data for which the largest improvement of TC Dice was achieved after FillTC post-processing (green—ED, yellow—ET, red—NCR). (Color figure online)

Table 8. Segmentation performance quantified by Dice, sensitivity, specificity, and Hausdorff (95%) distance over the BraTS'21 **test** set obtained using our final model. The scores (average μ, standard deviation s, median m, and the 25 and 75 quantile) are presented for the whole tumor (WT), tumor core (TC), and enhancing tumor (ET).

	Dice ET	Dice TC	Dice WT	Haus. ET	Haus. TC	Haus. WT	Sens. ET	Sens. TC	Sens. WT	Spec. ET	Spec. TC	Spec. WT
μ	0.86317	0.87987	0.92838	13.08531	15.87305	4.77240	0.87607	0.88921	0.92916	0.99979	0.99973	0.99951
s	0.20375	0.23422	0.08992	61.45773	66.68659	17.01573	0.21473	0.21898	0.09462	0.00030	0.00083	0.00077
m	0.93506	0.96346	0.95725	1.00000	1.41421	1.73205	0.95226	0.96930	0.95837	0.99990	0.99992	0.99976
25q	0.85164	0.91752	0.91297	1.00000	1.00000	1.00000	0.88749	0.90947	0.91760	0.99973	0.99979	0.99947
75q	0.96600	0.98219	0.97765	2.00000	3.00000	4.00000	0.97877	0.98760	0.98119	0.99996	0.99997	0.99991

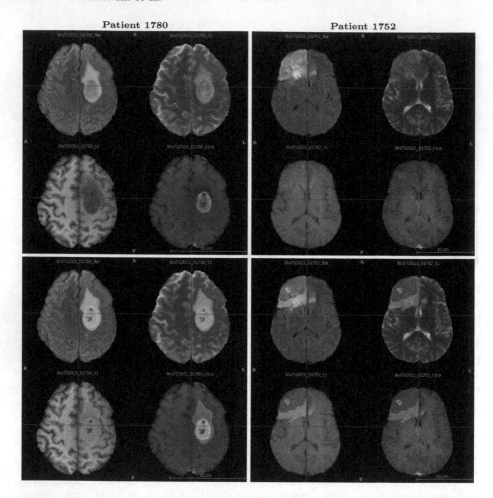

Fig. 4. Examples of high- and low-quality segmentations (patients with ID: 1780 and 1752, respectively) from the validation set (green—ED, yellow—ET, red—NCR). The Dice values amounted to 0.98990 (ET), 0.99232 (TC), and 0.98318 (WT) for patient 1780, and to 0.49577 (ET), 0.67378 (TC), and 0.78600 (WT) for patient 1752. (Color figure online)

5   Conclusion

In this paper, we utilized an ensemble of five nnU-Net models with our custom stratification based on the distribution of NCR, ET, and ED volumes for accurate brain tumor segmentation. Among the three different post-processing rules reflecting expert knowledge of a senior radiologist, the rule FillTC (filling the "holes" in TC with NCR) turned out to be the most effective one. It significantly improves TC and WT Dice, without deteriorating any other metric. It is robust to specific cases with missing classes in ground truth, because it extends the TC volume with additional voxels instead of removing any voxels, like methods PruneET or PruneTiny do. We recommend using this method as a post-processing step. Our algorithm allowed us to take the 6th place in the BraTS'21 Challenge over the hidden test data (out of 1600 participants).

The research undertaken in this paper constitutes an interesting departure point for further efforts. We currently focus on improving the segmentation quality of ET and TC by creating specialized models that could deal better with the aforementioned specific cases. Also, we believe that exploiting the expert knowledge which could be captured as various forms of pre- and post-processing routines (and also as the elements of the deep learning model's training strategies) could help us improve the segmentation quality even further.

Acknowledgment. JN was supported by the Silesian University of Technology funds through the grant for maintaining and developing research potential.

This paper is in memory of Dr. Grzegorz Nalepa, an extraordinary scientist and pediatric hematologist/oncologist at Riley Hospital for Children, Indianapolis, USA, who helped countless patients and their families through some of the most challenging moments of their lives.

References

1. Baid, U., et al.: The RSNA-ASNR-MICCAI BraTS 2021 benchmark on brain tumor segmentation and radiogenomic classification (2021)
2. Bakas, S., et al.: Advancing the cancer genome atlas glioma MRI collections with expert segmentation labels and radiomic features. Nat. Sci. Data **4**, 1–13 (2017). https://doi.org/10.1038/sdata.2017.117
3. Bakas, S., et al.: Segmentation labels and radiomic features for the pre-operative scans of the TCGA-GBM collection. Cancer Imaging Arch. (2017). https://doi.org/10.7937/K9/TCIA.2017.KLXWJJ1Q
4. Bakas, S., et al.: Segmentation labels and radiomic features for the pre-operative scans of the TCGA-LGG collection. Cancer Imaging Arch. (2017). https://doi.org/10.7937/K9/TCIA.2017.GJQ7R0EF
5. Bakas, S., et al.: Identifying the best machine learning algorithms for brain tumor segmentation, progression assessment, and overall survival prediction in the BRATS challenge. CoRR abs/1811.02629 (2018). http://arxiv.org/abs/1811.02629
6. Bontempi, D., Benini, S., Signoroni, A., Svanera, M., Muckli, L.: Cerebrum: a fast and fully-volumetric convolutional encoder-decoder for weakly-supervised segmentation of brain structures from out-of-the-scanner MRI. Med. Image Anal. **62**, 101688 (2020)
7. Chander, A., Chatterjee, A., Siarry, P.: A new social and momentum component adaptive PSO algorithm for image segmentation. Expert Syst. Appl. **38**(5), 4998–5004 (2011)
8. Estienne, T., et al.: Deep learning-based concurrent brain registration and tumor segmentation. Front. Comput. Neurosci. **14**, 17 (2020)
9. Geremia, E., Clatz, O., Menze, B.H., Konukoglu, E., Criminisi, A., Ayache, N.: Spatial decision forests for MS lesion segmentation in multi-channel magnetic resonance images. Neuroimage **57**(2), 378–390 (2011)

10. Ghafoorian, M., et al.: Transfer learning for domain adaptation in MRI: application in brain lesion segmentation. In: Descoteaux, M., Maier-Hein, L., Franz, A., Jannin, P., Collins, D.L., Duchesne, S. (eds.) MICCAI 2017. LNCS, vol. 10435, pp. 516–524. Springer, Cham (2017). https://doi.org/10.1007/978-3-319-66179-7_59

11. Isensee, F., Jaeger, P., Kohl, S., Petersen, J., Maier-Hein, K.: nnU-Net: a self-configuring method for deep learning-based biomedical image segmentation. Nat. Methods **18**, 1–9 (2021). https://doi.org/10.1038/s41592-020-01008-z

12. Isensee, F., Kickingereder, P., Wick, W., Bendszus, M., Maier-Hein, K.H.: No new-net. In: Crimi, A., Bakas, S., Kuijf, H., Keyvan, F., Reyes, M., van Walsum, T. (eds.) BrainLes 2018. LNCS, vol. 11384, pp. 234–244. Springer, Cham (2019). https://doi.org/10.1007/978-3-030-11726-9_21

13. Ji, S., Wei, B., Yu, Z., Yang, G., Yin, Y.: A new multistage medical segmentation method based on superpixel and fuzzy clustering. Comput. Math. Methods Med. **2014**, 747549:1–747549:13 (2014)

14. Kamnitsas, K., et al.: Ensembles of multiple models and architectures for robust brain tumour segmentation. In: Crimi, A., Bakas, S., Kuijf, H., Menze, B., Reyes, M. (eds.) BrainLes 2017. LNCS, vol. 10670, pp. 450–462. Springer, Cham (2018). https://doi.org/10.1007/978-3-319-75238-9_38

15. Korfiatis, P., Kline, T.L., Erickson, B.J.: Automated segmentation of hyperintense regions in FLAIR MRI using deep learning. Tomography J. Imaging Res. **2**(4), 334–340 (2016)

16. Menze, B.H., et al.: The multimodal brain tumor image segmentation benchmark (BRATS). IEEE Trans. Med. Imaging **34**(10), 1993–2024 (2015)

17. Moeskops, P., Viergever, M.A., Mendrik, A.M., de Vries, L.S., Benders, M.J.N.L., Isgum, I.: Automatic segmentation of MR brain images with a convolutional neural network. IEEE Trans. Med. Imaging **35**(5), 1252–1261 (2016)

18. Myronenko, A.: 3D MRI brain tumor segmentation using autoencoder regularization. In: Crimi, A., Bakas, S., Kuijf, H., Keyvan, F., Reyes, M., van Walsum, T. (eds.) BrainLes 2018. LNCS, vol. 11384, pp. 311–320. Springer, Cham (2019). https://doi.org/10.1007/978-3-030-11726-9_28

19. Nalepa, J., Marcinkiewicz, M., Kawulok, M.: Data augmentation for brain-tumor segmentation: a review. Front. Comput. Neurosci. **13**, 83 (2019)

20. Nalepa, J., et al.: Fully-automated deep learning-powered system for DCE-MRI analysis of brain tumors. Artif. Intell. Med. **102**, 101769 (2020)

21. Ouchicha, C., Ammor, O., Meknassi, M.: Unsupervised brain tumor segmentation from magnetic resonance images. In: Proceedings of the IEEE WINCOM, pp. 1–5 (2019)

22. Pipitone, J., et al.: Multi-atlas segmentation of the whole hippocampus and subfields using multiple automatically generated templates. Neuroimage **101**, 494–512 (2014)

23. Saha, S., Bandyopadhyay, S.: MRI brain image segmentation by fuzzy symmetry based genetic clustering technique. In: Proceedings of the IEEE CEC, pp. 4417–4424 (2007)

24. Simi, V., Joseph, J.: Segmentation of glioblastoma multiforme from MR images - a comprehensive review. Egyptian J. Radiol. Nuclear Med. **46**(4), 1105–1110 (2015)

25. Verma, N., Cowperthwaite, M.C., Markey, M.K.: Superpixels in brain MR image analysis. In: Proceedings of the IEEE EMBC, pp. 1077–1080 (2013)

26. Wu, W., Chen, A.Y.C., Zhao, L., Corso, J.J.: Brain tumor detection and segmentation in a CRF (conditional random fields) framework with pixel-pairwise affinity and superpixel-level features. Int. J. Comput. Assist. Radiol. Surg. **9**(2), 241–253 (2013). https://doi.org/10.1007/s11548-013-0922-7

27. Zhuge, Y., Krauze, A.V., Ning, H., Cheng, J.Y., Arora, B.C., Camphausen, K., Miller, R.W.: Brain tumor segmentation using holistically nested neural networks in MRI images. Med. Phys. **44**, 5234–5243 (2017)
28. Zikic, D., et al.: Decision forests for tissue-specific segmentation of high-grade gliomas in multi-channel MR. In: Ayache, N., Delingette, H., Golland, P., Mori, K. (eds.) MICCAI 2012. LNCS, vol. 7512, pp. 369–376. Springer, Heidelberg (2012). https://doi.org/10.1007/978-3-642-33454-2_46

Deep Learning Based Ensemble Approach for 3D MRI Brain Tumor Segmentation

Tien-Bach-Thanh Do[✉], Dang-Linh Trinh, Minh-Trieu Tran, Guee-Sang Lee[✉], Soo-Hyung Kim, and Hyung-Jeong Yang

Chonnam National University, Gwangju, South Korea
thanhdo.work@gmail.com, gslee@jnu.ac.kr

Abstract. Brain tumor segmentation has wide applications and important potential values for glioblastoma research. Because of the complexity of the structure of subtype tumors and the different visual scenes of multi modalities like T1, T1ce, T2, and FLAIR, most methods fail to segment the brain tumors with high accuracy. The sizes and shapes of tumors are very diverse in the wild. Another problem is that most recent algorithms ignore the multi-scale information of brain tumor features. To handle these problems, an ensemble method that utilizes the strength of dilated convolution in capturing larger receptive fields, which has more context information of brain image, also gets the ability of small tumor segmentation by using multiple tasks learning. Besides, we apply the generalized wasserstein dice loss function in training the model to solve the problem of imbalanced between multi-class segmentation. The experimental results demonstrate that the proposed ensemble method improves the accuracy in brain tumor segmentation, showing superiority to other recent segmentation methods.

Keywords: Brain tumor segmentation · Deep learning · MRI

1 Introduction

Glioma is one of the most primary brain tumors in the human brain, which cause most dead-on brain tumor patient. The glioma has some sub-regions structures, including peritumoral edema (ED), necrotic core (NCR), and enhancing tumor (ET). According to World Health Organization (WHO), glioma tumors are categorized into four levels based on their microscope images and tumor behaviors [1]. Four levels of glioma tumors are divided into two types: Low Grade Glioma (LGG) and High Grade Glioma (HGG). Grade I and Grade II are LGG, which are benign tumors and grow slowly. The precise treatment for LGG could extend the life of the patient more several years. Besides, HGG, which have Grade III and Grade IV, are aggressive and malignant tumors. The HGG tumor overgrows and requires surgery immediately. The patients are unable to survive more than 15 months for HGG tumors. Tumor removal is the typical treatment for gliomas patients, especially for HGG patients. Therefore, tumor segmentation plays an

A. Crimi and S. Bakas (Eds.): BrainLes 2021, LNCS 12963, pp. 210–221, 2022.
https://doi.org/10.1007/978-3-031-09002-8_19

essential role in gliomas diagnosis and treatment. Magnetic Resonance Imaging (MRI), a non-invasive method, is necessary for treatment planning and disease evaluation. The sequences of MRI are used for brain tumor segmentation, including T1-weighted, T2-weighted, contrast-enhanced T1-weighted (T1ce), and Fluid Attenuation Inversion Recovery (FLAIR). Each modality has its advantage for each tumor sub-region, such as FLAIR have a better view for the whole tumor, and T1 gives the better contrast on tumor core. The problem is that manual tumor segmentation causes time-consuming resources and expertise [2]. Furthermore, the manual segmentation results are unstable and slightly different because these are based on the experience of many clinical experts. Therefore, automatic segmentation saves time and improves the segmented tumor results because of the development of artificial intelligence. Recently, deep learning has been used in the medical segmentation field and has many advantages of accuracy and efficiency compared to conventional methods. However, brain tumor segmentation automatically from MRI modalities is one of the challenging tasks in medical image analysis. The MICCAI Brain Tumor Segmentation (BraTS) 2021 challenge provides sequences of MRI scans of glioma patients, the world's most common primary brain tumor. The aim of task 1 from this challenge is to boost and improve the performance of tumor segmentation, which helps clinical experts with treatment planning and disease assessment quickly. In previous BraTS challenges, many studies proposed medical segmentation architectures such as UNET and variants of UNET. These architectures are end-to-end networks, which have encoder parts and decoder parts. While the encoder extracts the features of input modalities, the decoder is expansive that feature maps are up-sampled to the original size of input modalities. Moreover, the ensemble approach is applied for robust segmentation results. Based on these, we propose the ensemble method that utilizes the strength of dilated convolution in capturing larger receptive fields, which has more context information of brain image, also gets the ability of small tumor segmentation by using multiple tasks learning.

2 Related Works

Convolution Neural Networks (CNN) for brain tumor segmentation have been using in a lot of research, with promising results. Havaei et al. [1] offer a two-pathway CNN architecture that predicts the label for each pixel using a sliding-window fashion input of a local image patch. Ronneberger et al. [2] create a U-Net which is developed based on a fully convolutional network (FCN) for dense prediction that processes the entire image. The network is trained fully to provide a full resolution segmentation and follows an encoder-decoder structure. Although these 2D CNN-based techniques have produced outstanding results, proven that most clinical imaging data is volumetric, such as 3D MR images, these models disregard essential 3D spatial context. Cricket et al. [3] expand the U-Net from 2D to 3D by researching 3D operations such as 3D convolution and 3D max pooling to better capture the 3D volumes of imaging data. Similarly, V-Net [4] processes MRI volumnes using volumetric convolutions, which results in more accurate segmentation than the 2D techniques. It has been demonstrated that reasoning volumetric structure with 3D convolutions in deep neural networks has good effective. However, because of the extra dimension, employing many layers of 3D convolutions has a higher computation cost than using ordinary 2D CNNs. Using light-weight network topologies, a few attempts have been made to solve this problem. 3D-ESPNet [5], for example, expands ESPNet, a quick and efficient network for 2D semantic segmentation based on point-wise convolution, to 3D medical image data. To decrease the number of learnable network parameters, SD-UNet [6] use separable 3D convolution, which separates each 3D convolution into three parallel branches. These efficient models, however, do not perform as well as state-of-the-art models. Multi-task learning has proven to be effective in a variety of deep learning applications, including brain tumor segmentation. Multi-task learning is a method of optimizing two or more tasks at the same time using a neural network. Auxiliary tasks are utilized in addition to the main task, which offers training for the network's intended function. The auxiliary task's goal is to increase the model's convergence or optimization for the primary task's benefit. These tasks are frequently connected and have similar characteristics. Multi-task learning has proven to be effective in a variety of deep learning applications, including image classification [7], video captioning [8], voice augmentation [9], and medical image segmentation [10,11]. With transformers, Wenxuan Want et al. [12] used multi-task learning to segment brain tumor. Despite the fact that this architecture works well for segmentation in general, their model demands a lot of memory and has a high computational cost. There has been a lot of application of brain tumor segmentation with boundary awareness. To increase performance, Haocheng Shen et al. [13] added boundary information into the loss function. Boundary loss is also used by Pablo Ribalta Lorenzo et al. [14] in their research. For brain tumor segmentation, they used two-step multi-modal UNet-based architecture with unsupervised pre-training and boundary loss components. However, their boundary information was only in 2D shape.

3   Proposed Method

The target segmentation framework of the proposed ensemble model is exhibited in Fig. 1, which is mainly composed of two parts, DMFNet [15], DKNet [16]. DMFNet is the model which employs the multi-fiber (MF) and dilated multi-fiber (DMF) units as the building blocks. The MF unit takes advantage of multiplexer for information routing. In MF unit, it combines 1 multiplexer and 3 convolutions $3 \times 3 \times 3$, and 3 convolutions $3 \times 3 \times 1$. The DMF unit with an daptive weighting scheme for different dilation rates. In DMF unit, it combines 1 multiplexer and 9 convolutions $3 \times 3 \times 3$ with 3 ADD operators and 3 convolutions $3 \times 3 \times 1$. This model is a variant of encoder-decoder network architecture. The input of DMFNet is four types of brain image such as T1, T1ce, T2, and FLAIR. Except for the first and last layers, all of the other layers in the model are controlled by a combination of DMF and MF units. To get the

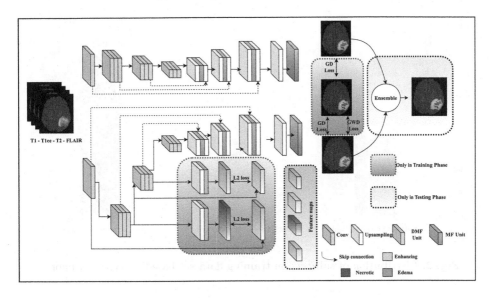

Fig. 1. The illustration of proposed method for brain tumor segmentation.

benefit of learning the multi-scale context of brain tumors in the encoding phase, the first six encoding units are generated based on DMF units. With the aim of preserving the information of features during learning, the model uses the concatenation operation between high-resolution features from the encoding path and the upsampled features. Note that trilinear interpolation has been used for the upsampling phase. The second network that we utilize in our method is DKNet which has been developed in [16]. This paper exploits the problem of segmentation in any size of brain tumors. DKNet is proposed to focus on accurate segmentation in small tumors. The second advantage of this model is the lightweight network, with the ability to learn multi-task. By applying the auxiliary task of feature reconstruction, this model can handle the problem of segmentation small size of brain tumors which is very usually observed in brain tumor analysis. Feature reconstruction is a procedure that maintain the information inside feature between convolution layers when downsampling. It aids in the better initialization of model parameters while preserving as many detailed features as feasible. Even if the resolution is diminished, this approach may be able to retain the characteristics of tiny tumors. DKNet uses multi-task learning, with brain tumor segmentation as the main goal and additional feature reconstruction as an auxiliary task. The model input for DMFNet with four MRI modalities is the same. There are two U-module feature reconstructions in DKNet architecture. The U-module is an auxiliary task that supports the model to retain as much relevant and useful information as possible.

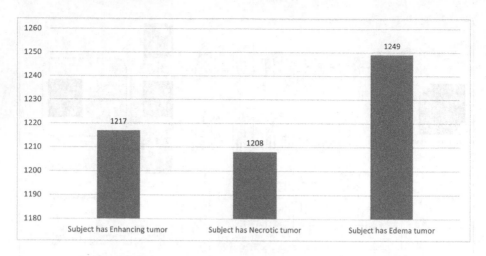

Fig. 2. Distribution of subjects on training data set based on type of tumors.

4 Loss Function

We used multiple kind of losses because each loss has its own advantages. Semantic relationships between classes are fully utilized while generalized dice loss tackled the severe class imbalance.

4.1 Generalized Dice Loss

The first loss function is the generalized dice loss (GDL). To overcome the problem of tiny region segmentation, the GDL is introduced. It can balance the contribution of each region to the loss and make the training more steady as compared to the common dice loss. The equation is below:

$$GDL = 1 - 2\left(\frac{\Sigma_{a=1}^{2}\beta_a\Sigma_m k_{am}b_{am}}{\Sigma_{a=1}^{2}\beta_a\Sigma_m k_{am} + b_{am}}\right) \tag{1}$$

which the k_{am} and b_{am} are the growth truth and the predicted result of a, respectively. The class weight β_a was employed to ensure that the different label set attributes were invariant.

4.2 Generalized Wasserstein Dice Loss

The Generalized Wasserstein Dice Loss (GWDL) is a loss function that can be used to train deep neural networks for multi-class segmentation in medical images. The GWDL is a generalization of the Dice loss and the Generalized Dice loss that can deal with hierarchical classes and take advantage of known class relationships. The equation is below:

$$GWDL_{(\hat{b},b)} = \frac{2\Sigma_{m\neq p}\Sigma_a b_{a,m}(1 - M^W(\hat{b}_a, b_a))}{2\Sigma_{m\neq p}\Sigma_a b_{a,m}(1 - M^W(\hat{b}_a, b_a) + \Sigma_a M^W(\hat{b}_a, b_a))} \tag{2}$$

where $M^W(\hat{b}_a, b_a)$ is the Wasserstein distance between the predicted $\hat{b}_a$ and the ground truth $b_a discrete$, the discrete probability distribution at voxel a. $W = (W_{m,m'})_{1 \leq m, m' \leq M}$ is the spacing matrix between the dataset labels and b is the class number corresponding to the background. The matrix W signals the loss of a generalized waterstone cube for relationships between classes. The following applies to two classes, indexes m and m'. The smaller the distance $W_{m,m'}$, the less penalties for confusing (ground truth) class m voxels with class m'. The matrix M is a distance matrix.

5 Experimental Results

5.1 Dataset

All of our experiments used the BraTS 2021 dataset without any additional data. The dataset includes four MRI sequences (T1, T1CE, T2 and FLAIR) for patients with gliomas. All the subjects are segmented for edema tumor, enhancing tumor and necrotic tumor with using the same labeling procedure [17]. During the challenge, there are total 1251 subjects in dataset for training. For validation phase, we are provided 219 subjects to evaluate our method by the challenge organizer. The images for training and validation are available for download from website, but only training set includes the segmentation map. To evaluate in validation set, we need to submit the segmentation results to challenge online Synapse evaluation platform. With each subject, four MRI images are the skull stripping [18] and interpolation to 1mm isotropic resolution. Figure 2 shows the distribution of number subjects on training dataset via type of tumors. Figure 3 shows the distribution of number subjects which have enhancing tumor based on size of tumors.

5.2 Training Implementation Details

Our approach is variant of the multi task learning model [16]. The code is modified from code which is publicly available at [19]. We set the maximum number of epochs as 2000. The batch size was set to 2 and the input patches were 128 × 128 × 128. We also used several augmentation techniques like random cropping of patch, random rotation, random zoom and gamma intensity augmentation. We used 2080 ti GPUs to train all the deep neural networks. The whole experiments are conducted using Pytorch. The learning rate is 1e-3. We applied Adam optimizer to optimize the model's parameters as well.

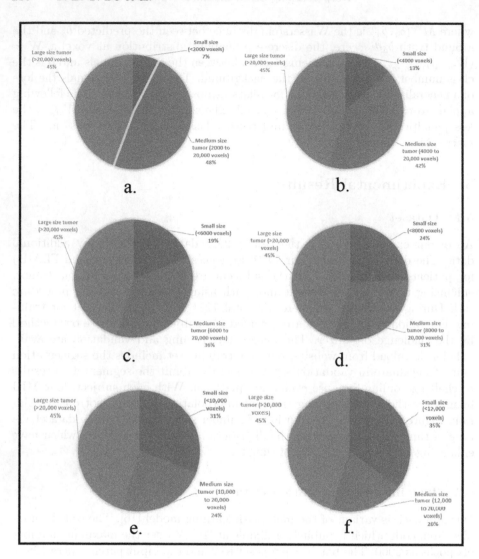

Fig. 3. Distribution of subjects have enhancing tumor based on size of tumors. We define the small size tumor with several thresholds of number of voxel. a) Threshold is set at 2000 voxels b) Threshold is set at 4000 voxels c) Threshold is set at 6000 voxels d) Threshold is set at 8000 voxels e) Threshold is set at 10000 voxels f) Threshold is set at 12000 voxels.

5.3   Small Tumor Segmentation Performance

To evaluate the proposed method's efficacy on small size augmenting tumors, we divided the training set into two parts: 80% for training and 20% for validation. As shown in Table 1, our method is effectiveness on small-sized enhancing tumors segmentation comparing to other methods. From the paper [16], we chose the

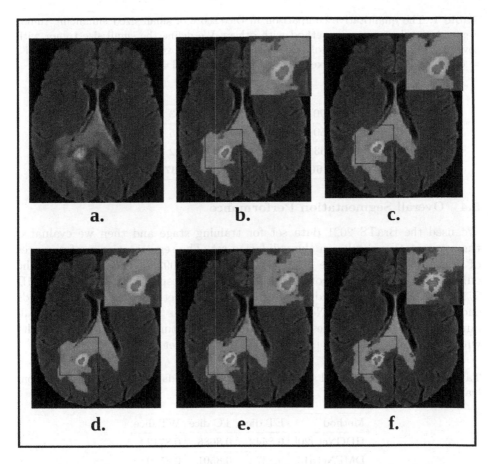

Fig. 4. The qualitative results comparison in brain tumor segmentation between our method with others. Green, yellow and red colors are the edema, enhancing and necrotic tumor, respectively. a) The input image b) output segmented result of DMFNet c) Output segmented result of DKNet d) Output segmented result of HDCNet e) Ours segmented result f) Ground truth of segmentation. (Color figure online)

same threshold for small size tumor with lower than 2000 voxels. Additionally, we added more threshold such as 4000, 6000, 8000, 10000, and 12000 voxels to see several levels of impact from small size enhancing tumor. Figure 4 introduces the comparison of qualitative results in brain tumor segmentation between our method with others.

Table 1. The quantitative comparison in Dice score of small-sized enhancing tumor segmentation between our method with others. We define the small size tumor with several thresholds of number of voxel such as T1 = 2000 voxels, T2 = 4000 voxels, T3 = 6000 voxels, T4 = 8000 voxels, T5 = 10000 voxels, T6 = 12000 voxels.

Method	T1	T2	T3	T4	T5	T6
HDCNet [20]	0.5790	0.6429	0.6951	0.7273	0.7645	0.7696
DMFNet [15]	0.5650	0.6266	0.6802	0.7155	0.7551	0.7603
DKNet [16]	0.5663	0.6248	0.6637	0.7032	0.7377	0.7446
Ours	**0.6260**	**0.6749**	**0.7268**	**0.7537**	**0.7852**	**0.7897**

5.4 Overall Segmentation Performance

We used the BraTS 2021 data set for training stage and then we evaluated the segmentation results on the validation set. The segmentation performances of our proposed model are 0.8274, 0.8312 and 0.9098 in Dice metric for the enhancing tumor, tumor core, and whole tumor respectively (Submission ID 9714784). We also compared the performance our method with others methods such as DMFNet [15], DKNet [16], HDCNet [20]. As shown in Tables 2 and 3, our method achieved the best results in all kind of tumor segmentation results when compare to DMFNet [15], DKNet [16], HDCNet [20].

Table 2. Segmentation results on the BraTS 2021 validation which split 20% from training dataset.

Method	ET dice	TC dice	WT dice
HDCNet [20]	0.8442	0.8686	0.8712
DMFNet [15]	0.8372	0.8501	0.8590
DKNet [16]	0.8284	0.8402	0.8559
Ours	**0.8554**	**0.8730**	**0.9052**

In the testing dataset, we got testing results with 0.8435, 0.8514 and 0.9017 in Dice metric and 15.4426, 19.0065 and 6.5218 in the Hausdorff 95 metric for the enhancing tumor, tumor core, and whole tumor respectively, as shown in Table 4.

Table 3. Segmentation results on the official BraTS 2021 validation dataset (submission ID 9714784).

Method	ET dice	TC dice	WT dice
HDCNet [20]	0.8258	0.8317	0.8965
DMFNet [15]	0.8223	0.8084	0.9051
DKNet [16]	0.8197	0.8131	0.8933
Ours	**0.8274**	**0.8312**	**0.9098**

Table 4. Segmentation results on the official BraTS 2021 testing dataset.(HD95: Hausdorff 95)

Method	ET dice	TC dice	WT dice	ET HD95	TC HD95	WT HD95
Ours	0.8435	0.8514	0.9017	15.4426	19.0065	6.5218

6 Conclusion

An ensemble method for small size enhancing brain tumor segmentation is proposed in this paper. The method exploits the multi-scale spatial context information and captures better characteristics of brain tumor features. The ability to segment small size enhancing brain tumors is a critical point inside our method. Because our method achieves the high performance in brain tumor segmentation, it can be more beneficial to apply in the area of automated brain tumor analysis.

Acknowledgement. This research was supported by Basic Science Research Program through the National Research Foundation of Korea(NRF) funded by the Ministry of Education (NRF-2018R1D1A3B05049058) and also by the Bio & Medical Technology Development Program of the National Research Foundation (NRF) & funded by the Korean government (MSIT) (NRF 2019M3E5D1A02067961).

References

1. Havaei, M., et al.: Brain tumor segmentation with deep neural networks. Med. Image Anal. **35**(2017), 18–31 (2017)
2. Ronneberger, O., Fischer, P., Brox, T.: U-Net: convolutional networks for biomedical image segmentation. In: Navab, N., Hornegger, J., Wells, W.M., Frangi, A.F. (eds.) MICCAI 2015. LNCS, vol. 9351, pp. 234–241. Springer, Cham (2015). https://doi.org/10.1007/978-3-319-24574-4_28
3. Çiçek, Ö., Abdulkadir, A., Lienkamp, S.S., Brox, T., Ronneberger, O.: 3D U-Net: learning dense volumetric segmentation from sparse annotation. In: Ourselin, S., Joskowicz, L., Sabuncu, M.R., Unal, G., Wells, W. (eds.) MICCAI 2016. LNCS, vol. 9901, pp. 424–432. Springer, Cham (2016). https://doi.org/10.1007/978-3-319-46723-8_49
4. Milletari, F., Navab, N., Ahmadi, S.-A.: V-Net: fully convolutional neural networks for volumetric medical image segmentation. In: 2016 Fourth International Conference on 3D Vision (3DV), pp. 565–571. IEEE (2016)
5. Nuechterlein, N., Mehta, S.: 3D-ESPNet with pyramidal refinement for volumetric brain tumor image segmentation. In: Crimi, A., Bakas, S., Kuijf, H., Keyvan, F., Reyes, M., van Walsum, T. (eds.) BrainLes 2018. LNCS, vol. 11384, pp. 245–253. Springer, Cham (2019). https://doi.org/10.1007/978-3-030-11726-9_22
6. Chen, W., Liu, B., Peng, S., Sun, J., Qiao, X.: S3D-UNet: separable 3D U-Net for brain tumor segmentation. In: Crimi, A., Bakas, S., Kuijf, H., Keyvan, F., Reyes, M., van Walsum, T. (eds.) BrainLes 2018. LNCS, vol. 11384, pp. 358–368. Springer, Cham (2019). https://doi.org/10.1007/978-3-030-11726-9_32

7. Kuang, Z., Li, Z., Zhao, T., Fan, J.: Deep multi-task learning for large-scale image classification. In: 2017 IEEE Third International Conference on Multimedia Big Data (BigMM), pp. 310–317. IEEE (2017)
8. Li, L., Gong, B.: End-to-end video captioning with multitask reinforcement learning. In: 2019 IEEE Winter Conference on Applications of Computer Vision (WACV), pp. 339–348. IEEE (2019)
9. Lee, G.W., Kim, H.K.: Multi-task learning U-Net for single-channel speech enhancement and mask-based voice activity detection. Appl. Sci. **10**(9), 3230 (2020)
10. He, T., Hu, J., Song, Y., Guo, J., Yi, Z.: Multi-task learning for the segmentation of organs at risk with label dependence. Med. Image Anal. **61**, 101666 (2020)
11. Imran, A.-A.-Z., Terzopoulos, D.: Semi-supervised multi-task learning with chest X-ray images. In: Suk, H.-I., Liu, M., Yan, P., Lian, C. (eds.) MLMI 2019. LNCS, vol. 11861, pp. 151–159. Springer, Cham (2019). https://doi.org/10.1007/978-3-030-32692-0_18
12. Wang, W., Chen, C., Ding, M., Li, J., Yu, H., Zha, S.: TransBTS: multimodal brain tumor segmentation using transformer. arXiv preprint arXiv:2103.04430 (2021)
13. Shen, H., Wang, R., Zhang, J., McKenna, S.J.: Boundary-aware fully convolutional network for brain tumor segmentation. In: Descoteaux, M., Maier-Hein, L., Franz, A., Jannin, P., Collins, D.L., Duchesne, S. (eds.) MICCAI 2017. LNCS, vol. 10434, pp. 433–441. Springer, Cham (2017). https://doi.org/10.1007/978-3-319-66185-8_49
14. Ribalta Lorenzo, P., Marcinkiewicz, M., Nalepa, J.: Multi-modal U-Nets with boundary loss and pre-training for brain tumor segmentation. In: Crimi, A., Bakas, S. (eds.) BrainLes 2019. LNCS, vol. 11993, pp. 135–147. Springer, Cham (2020). https://doi.org/10.1007/978-3-030-46643-5_13
15. Chen, C., Liu, X., Ding, M., Zheng, J., Li, J.: 3D dilated multi-fiber network for real-time brain tumor segmentation in MRI. In: Shen, D., et al. (eds.) MICCAI 2019. LNCS, vol. 11766, pp. 184–192. Springer, Cham (2019). https://doi.org/10.1007/978-3-030-32248-9_21
16. Ngo, D.-K., Tran, M.-T., Kim, S.-H., Yang, H.-J., Lee, G.-S.: Multi-task learning for small brain tumor segmentation from MRI. Appl. Sci. **10**, 7790 (2020). Multidisciplinary Digital Publishing Institute
17. Menze, B.H., et al.: The multimodal brain tumor image segmentation benchmark (BRATS). IEEE Trans. Med. Imaging **34**(10), 1993–2024 (2015). https://doi.org/10.1109/TMI.2014.2377694
18. Bakas, S., et al.: Advancing the cancer genome atlas glioma MRI collections with expert segmentation labels and radiomic features. Nat. Sci. Data **4**, 170117 (2017). https://doi.org/10.1038/sdata.2017.117
19. Bakas, S., et al.: Identifying the best machine learning algorithms for brain tumor segmentation, progression assessment, and overall survival prediction in the BRATS challenge. arXiv preprint arXiv:1811.02629 (2018)
20. Luo, Z., Jia, Z., Yuan, Z., Peng, J.: HDC-Net: hierarchical decoupled convolution network for brain tumor segmentation, pp. 737–745. IEEE (2020)
21. Baid, U., Ghodasara, S., Mohan, S., et al.: The RSNA-ASNR-MICCAI BraTS 2021 benchmark on brain tumor segmentation and radiogenomic classification. arXiv:2107.02314 (2021)

22. Bakas, S., et al.: Segmentation labels and radiomic features for the pre-operative scans of the TCGA-GBM collection. Cancer Imaging Arch. (2017). https://doi.org/10.7937/K9/TCIA.2017.KLXWJJ1Q
23. Bakas, S., et al.: Segmentation labels and radiomic features for the pre-operative scans of the TCGA-LGG collection. Cancer Imaging Arch. (2017). https://doi.org/10.7937/K9/TCIA.2017.GJQ7R0EF

Prediction of MGMT Methylation Status of Glioblastoma Using Radiomics and Latent Space Shape Features

Sveinn Pálsson[1(✉)], Stefano Cerri[1], and Koen Van Leemput[1,2]

[1] Department of Health Technology, Technical University of Denmark,
Lyngby, Denmark
svpa@dtu.dk

[2] Athinoula A. Martinos Center for Biomedical Imaging, Massachusetts General
Hospital, Harvard Medical School, Boston, USA

Abstract. In this paper we propose a method for predicting the status of MGMT promoter methylation in high-grade gliomas. From the available MR images, we segment the tumor using deep convolutional neural networks and extract both radiomic features and shape features learned by a variational autoencoder. We implemented a standard machine learning workflow to obtain predictions, consisting of feature selection followed by training of a random forest classification model. We trained and evaluated our method on the RSNA-ASNR-MICCAI BraTS 2021 challenge dataset and submitted our predictions to the challenge.

Keywords: MGMT prediction · Radiomics · Deep learning · Glioblastoma · Variational autoencoder

1 Introduction

Expression of O^6-methylguanine-DNA-methyltransferase (MGMT) in glioblastoma is of clinical importance as it has implications of the patient's overall survival [1,2]. The prognostic information of MGMT is believed to be due to resistance of tumors with unmethylated MGMT promoter to Temozolomide [3,4], a drug used in standard therapy [5]. Inference of the MGMT status in the clinic is done by histological analysis, as currently available non-invasive techniques are still too unreliable.

The RSNA-ASNR-MICCAI BraTS 2021 challenge [6–11] contains two tasks: tumor segmentation and MGMT methylation prediction from pre-operative magnetic resonance (MR) images. The challenge organizers have released a large dataset with the goal of facilitating comparison between methods and advancing state-of-the-art methods in these domains. In this paper we focus on the prediction task only.

Radiomics [12] is a method for extracting features from MR images. The features, called "radiomic" features are a variety of statistical, shape and texture

A. Crimi and S. Bakas (Eds.): BrainLes 2021, LNCS 12963, pp. 222–231, 2022.
https://doi.org/10.1007/978-3-031-09002-8_20

features, extracted from a target region within an MR image. Radiomics has gained much interest for prediction tasks related to brain tumors [13] and has been successfully applied to MGMT methylation prediction [14,15].

We propose a method for inference of the MGMT methylation that combines the use of radiomics with shape features learned by a variational autoencoder (VAE) [16]. VAE, implemented with deep neural networks, can learn high level features that are specific to the data structure it is trained on. By training the VAE on tumor segmentations, we may be able to extract complex tumor shape features that radiomics does not include. Combining hand-crafted features with a learned latent representation of medical images for classification has been previously studied [17], showing improved model classification performance.

The paper is structured as follows: In Sect. 2 we describe our methods in detail. In Sect. 3, we present our results and in Sect. 4 we discuss our results and conclude.

2 Methods

In this section we give a detailed description of our methods (illustrated in Fig. 1). We start by describing the datasets we use. We then describe our pre-processing pipeline, consisting of DICOM to NIFTI conversion, bias-correction and registration. Next, we describe how we obtain tumor segmentations, and how we use these segmentations to compute radiomics and latent shape features.

Finally, we describe the classification model.

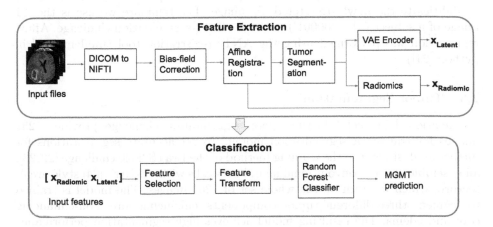

Fig. 1. Overview of our method. The figure shows the main components involved in going from input images to MGMT methylation prediction.

2.1   Data

The challenge data consists of pre-operative MR images of 2000 subjects, divided into training, validation and testing cohorts [6]. For the segmentation task, 1251 subjects are provided with ground truth labels for training segmentation models, whereas for the classification task, ground truth MGMT labels are provided for 585 of those subjects. Validation data for the classification task consists of image data for 87 subjects that are provided without ground truth labels but they can be used to evaluate model performance by submitting predictions to the challenge's online platform [18]. The testing cohort is kept private by the challenge organizers and is not included in this paper. This is because our code requires more processing time per subject than the platform allows.

For every subject, the available modalities are T1 weighted, post-contrast T1 weighted (Gadolinium), T2 weighted and T2-FLAIR (Fig. 2 (A-D)). A detailed description of the data and pre-processing applied to it by the challenge organizers is given in [6]. The segmentation task dataset has been registered to a standard template and is provided as NIFTI files while the classification data are not co-registered and are provided as DICOM files.

2.2   Pre-processing

Our pre-processing pipeline starts with conversion of the provided DICOM files to NIFTI (implemented in python [19]). Bias field correction is then performed using N4 bias field correction implemented in SimpleITK [20]. We then register the T1 image to a template T1 image and subsequently register the other modalities to the newly registered T1 image. The template we use is the T1 image of a subject (id = '00001') in the BraTS21 segmentation challenge. Affine registration was performed using the ANTs registration tool (implemented in python [21]).

2.3   Tumor Segmentation

As mentioned in Sect. 2.1, the tumor segmentation challenge provides 1251 images for training a segmentation model. To get accurate segmentations for further analysis, we use the winning method of the BraTS 2020 challenge [22,23], an ensemble of deep convolutional neural networks with "U-Net" [24] style architecture, which we train on the whole set of 1251 images. The model is trained to segment three different tumor components; enhancing core, non-enhancing core and edema. The resulting model achieves high segmentation performance (a representative sample is shown in Fig. 2 (F)). The resulting model is used to segment the images provided for the classification task.

2.4   Latent Shape Features

We obtain our latent shape features from a variational autoencoder (VAE) [16], implemented with 3D convolutional neural networks in tensorflow [25]. The VAE

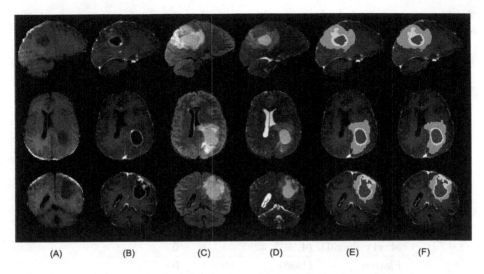

Fig. 2. The figure shows an example from the challenge dataset. From top to bottom: sagittal, axial and coronal view. Columns show (A) T1w, (B) T1c, (C) FLAIR, (D) T2w, (E) ground truth tumor segmentation, (F) automatic segmentation.

model consists of two networks; a decoder, designed to generate tumor segmentations from latent variables; and encoder, to infer latent variables when given tumor segmentations. The input to the encoder network is a segmentation with size (240,240,155,4) where the last dimension is a one-hot encoding of the tumor component (or background) present at each voxel. The encoder network consists of 3 convolutional network blocks, followed by two fully connected layers. Each block consists of 2 convolutional layers followed by a max pooling layer. The decoder network has a symmetrical architecture to the encoder, where the convolutional layers are replaced with deconvolutional layers [26]. After each convolutional layer in both networks, a leaky ReLU [27] activation is applied, except at the last layer of the decoder whose output is interpreted as logits. Tables 1 and 2, show the layer dimensions and parameter numbers for the encoder and decoder, respectively. The VAE is trained using the ADAM optimization algorithm [28].

We train the VAE on the 1251 available segmentations from the segmentation training dataset. To extract features from a given tumor segmentation, it is passed through the encoder network and its output is taken as the latent features. We set the number of latent features to 64, which we chose empirically by training the VAE with several different choices for the latent space dimension.

Table 1. Overview of the layers in the encoder network of the VAE. In total, the network has 551,808 parameters.

Layer	Output shape	Number of parameters
Input	(240, 240, 155, 4)	0
Conv3D	(120, 120, 78, 32)	3488
Conv3D	(60, 60, 39, 32)	27680
MaxPooling3D	(30, 30, 20, 32)	0
Conv3D	(15, 15, 10, 32)	27680
Conv3D	(15, 15, 10, 32)	27680
MaxPooling3D	(8, 8, 5, 32)	0
Conv3D	(8, 8, 5, 32)	27680
Conv3D	(8, 8, 5, 32)	27680
MaxPooling3D	(4, 4, 3, 32)	0
Flatten	(1536)	0
Dense	(256)	393472
Dense	(64)	16448

Table 2. Overview of the layers in the decoder network of the VAE. In total, the network has 600,420 parameters.

Layer	Output shape	Number of parameters
Input	(32)	0
Dense	(256)	8448
Dense	(1536)	394752
Reshape	(4, 4, 3, 32)	0
Conv3DTranspose	(4, 4, 3, 32)	27680
Conv3DTranspose	(4, 4, 3, 32)	27680
Conv3DTranspose	(8, 8, 6, 32)	27680
Conv3DTranspose	(16, 16, 12, 32)	27680
Conv3DTranspose	(32, 32, 24, 32)	27680
Conv3DTranspose	(64, 64, 48, 32)	27680
Conv3DTranspose	(128, 128, 96, 32)	27680
Conv3DTranspose	(240, 240, 155, 4)	3460

2.5   Radiomics

We extract radiomic features from three automatically segmented tumor regions and from each provided modality, resulting in a total of 1172 extracted radiomic features. The radiomic features comprise seven categories: first-order statistics, shape descriptors, gray level co-occurrence matrix (GLCM), gray level run length matrix (GLRLM), gray level size zone matrix (GLSZM), gray level dependece matrix (GLDM), and neighboring gray tone difference matrix (NGTDM). We use the PyRadiomics [29] python implementation of radiomics for the feature extraction.

The three tumor regions we consider is the whole tumor, enhancing core and non-enhancing core. The whole tumor is the union of all the three tumor components that are segmented.

2.6   Classification

After obtaining all of our features, in the next step we perform feature pre-processing to standardize feature values and feature selection to reduce dimensionality. We then train a random forest classifier on the selected features.

For each feature, we search for a threshold value that best splits the subjects in terms of the target variable. Specifically, for each candidate threshold value, we perform a Fisher's exact test [30], testing the hypothesis that the binomial distributions (over the target variable) of the two resulting groups are the same. The feature value resulting in the lowest P-value is chosen as the threshold for that feature. The features are subsequently transformed to binary variables according to which side of the threshold they land. Features are then selected if the P-value of the best threshold is $P < P_{\min}$, where $P_{\min}$ is experimentally chosen. The selected features and choice of $P_{\min}$ will be discussed further in Sect. 3.1.

We use a random forest [31] (implemented in python [32]) to obtain predictions of MGMT methylation status, given the input features we extracted. The model is trained on the 585 available subjects via K-fold cross validation, with K chosen such that in each fold, 5 subjects are held out while the remaining subjects are used to train a model ($K = 117$ in our case). In each fold, the model is trained on 580 subjects and predictions on the 5 held-out subjects are obtained. Once predictions are obtained for all subjects, a performance score is calculated. The performance score we use is the area under the receiver operating characteristic curve (AUC). Using grid search, we tune two hyperparameters of the model; the number of samples to split a node and maximum depth of trees. At test time, given an unseen subject, the 117 models are all used to predict the MGMT methylation status, each predicting either 0 or 1 for the unmethylated or methylated group, respectively. The average of the predictions is interpreted as the probability of belonging to the methylated group.

3   Results

3.1   Feature Selection

The number of features selected by the selection procedure described in Sect. 2.6 depends on our choice of $P_{\min}$, which we experimentally determine by searching a range of values and measuring model performance using the whole training cohort. We set $P_{min} = 5 \times 10^{-4}$ which leaves 23 features remaining; 16 of which are radiomic features and 7 latent shape features. The list of selected radiomic features is given in Table 3. We observe selected radiomic features from 6 out of 7 categories mentioned in Sect. 2.5, from 3 out of 4 modalities and from all 3 tumor regions.

Table 3. List of selected radiomic features.

Category	Feature name	Modality	Region
Shape	Maximum 3D Diameter	–	Enh-core
First order	Interquartile Range	T1-ce	Core
First order	Mean Absolute Deviation	T1-ce	Core
First order	Mean	T1-ce	Core
First order	Median	T1-ce	Core
First order	Median	T1-ce	Whole
First order	Variance	T1-ce	Core
First order	10Percentile	FLAIR	Core
GLRLM	Graylevel non-uniformity normalized	FLAIR	Whole
GLRLM	Graylevel variance	FLAIR	Whole
GLSZM	Small area emphasis	FLAIR	Whole
GLSZM	Small area high graylevel emphasis	FLAIR	Whole
GLSZM	Small area low graylevel emphasis	FLAIR	Whole
NGTDM	Busyness	FLAIR	Whole
GLSZM	Small area high graylevel emphasis	T2	Whole

3.2 Classification

We find the best hyperparameters for the random forest through grid search to be 2 samples to split a node and a maximum tree depth of 4 (we leave other parameters as default). The whole training cohort is used for the hyperparameter search.

To test the benefit of using the latent features in the model along with the radiomic features, we train the model on both feature sets separately and together and measure the AUC score. For a more accurate performance measure on the training dataset, we ran our cross validation 10 times (each time the dataset is shuffled) and in Table 4, we report the mean AUC score across the 10 iterations. The true labels of the validation dataset are unknown to us, but by submitting our predictions to the challenge platform, we obtain a validation AUC score reported in Table 4. We observe a substantial disagreement between the training and validation scores: the training results show improvement with the combination of feature sets, while the validation scores indicate that using radiomics alone is preferred and that the latent shape features have very low predictive value.

Table 4. Classification performance measured by AUC. For three feature sets, the table shows AUC score for both cross-validated training set predictions and predictions on the validation set.

Features	Training	Validation
Radiomics + Latent	0.603	0.598
Radiomics	0.582	0.632
Latent	0.568	0.488

4   Discussion

In this paper, we propose a method for MGMT methylation prediction that combines the use of radiomics with high level shape features learned by a variational autoencoder. We train a segmentation model to obtain tumor segmentations, and train a variational autoencoder on segmentations to learn high-level shape features of tumor. We use the tumor segmentation to compute radiomic features, and pass the segmentation to the encoder network of the variational autoencoder to obtain shape features from its latent space. We extracted these features from the training data provided by the RSNA-ASNR-MICCAI BraTS 2021 challenge and trained a random forest classifier. The method was submitted to the challenge and obtained a validation score (AUC) of 0.598.

As we discussed in Sect. 1, radiomic features have already been shown to be applicable to this prediction task while tumor shape has not been proven to predict MGMT methylation. Therefore, to test whether the feature set combination we propose performs better than simply using the radiomic features alone, we experiment with training the classifier on them separately. On our training data, we observe a performance benefit of using the shape features (cf. Table 4), but this is not reproduced on the validation set where the radiomic features alone achieve a score of 0.632 but the latent features only 0.488. This may be due to overfitting of our feature transform and hyperparameter selection to the training data or high uncertainty stemming from the small number of samples in the validation dataset. So far we are unable to run our methods on the testing data, as our code takes longer time to process subjects than facilitated by the online platform. Future work will involve applying our methods to the testing data if it becomes available.

Acknowledgement. This project was funded by the European Union's Horizon 2020 research and innovation program under the Marie Sklodowska-Curie project TRABIT (agreement No 765148) and NINDS (grant No R01NS112161).

References

1. Michaelsen, S.R., et al.: Clinical variables serve as prognostic factors in a model for survival from glioblastoma multiforme: an observational study of a cohort of consecutive non-selected patients from a single institution. BMC Cancer **13**(1), 402 (2013)
2. Gorlia, T., et al.: Nomograms for predicting survival of patients with newly diagnosed glioblastoma: prognostic factor analysis of EORTC and NCIC trial 26981–22981/ce 3. Lancet Oncol. **9**(1), 29–38 (2008)
3. Hegi, M.E., et al.: MGMT gene silencing and benefit from temozolomide in glioblastoma. New Engl. J. Med. **352**(10), 997–1003 (2005)
4. Kitange, G.J., et al.: Induction of MGMT expression is associated with temozolomide resistance in glioblastoma xenografts. Neuro Oncol. **11**(3), 281–291 (2009)
5. Stupp, R., et al.: Effects of radiotherapy with concomitant and adjuvant temozolomide versus radiotherapy alone on survival in glioblastoma in a randomised phase iii study: 5-year analysis of the eortc-ncic trial. Lancet Oncol. **10**(5), 459–466 (2009)
6. Baid, U., et al.: The RSNA-ASNR-MICCAI brats 2021 benchmark on brain tumor segmentation and radiogenomic classification. arXiv preprint arXiv:2107.02314 (2021)
7. Menze, B.H., et al.: The multimodal brain tumor image segmentation benchmark (brats). IEEE Trans. Med. Imaging **34**(10), 1993–2024 (2014)
8. Bakas, S., et al.: Identifying the best machine learning algorithms for brain tumor segmentation, progression assessment, and overall survival prediction in the brats challenge. arXiv preprint arXiv:1811.02629 (2018)
9. Bakas, S.: Advancing the cancer genome atlas glioma MRI collections with expert segmentation labels and radiomic features. Sci. Data **4**(1), 1–13 (2017)
10. Bakas, S., et al.: Segmentation labels and radiomic features for the pre-operative scans of the TCGA-LGG collection. The cancer imaging archive 286 (2017)
11. Bakas, S., et al.: Segmentation labels and radiomic features for the pre-operative scans of the TCGA-GBM collection. The cancer imaging archive. Nat. Sci. Data **4**, 170117 (2017)
12. Lambin, P., et al.: Radiomics: extracting more information from medical images using advanced feature analysis. Eur. J. Cancer **48**(4), 441–446 (2012)
13. Booth, T.C., Williams, M., Luis, A., Cardoso, J., Ashkan, K., Shuaib, H.: Machine learning and glioma imaging biomarkers. Clin. Radiol. **75**(1), 20–32 (2020)
14. Xi, Y., et al.: Radiomics signature: a potential biomarker for the prediction of MGMT promoter methylation in glioblastoma. J. Magn. Reson. Imaging **47**(5), 1380–1387 (2018)
15. Li, Z.-C., et al.: Multiregional radiomics features from multiparametric MRI for prediction of MGMT methylation status in glioblastoma multiforme: a multicentre study. Eur. Radiol. **28**(9), 3640–3650 (2018)
16. Kingma, D.P., Welling, M.: Auto-encoding variational Bayes. arXiv preprint arXiv:1312.6114 (2013)
17. Cui, S., Luo, Y., Tseng, H.-H., Ten Haken, R.K., El Naqa, I.: Combining handcrafted features with latent variables in machine learning for prediction of radiation-induced lung damage. Med. Phys. **46**(5), 2497–2511 (2019)
18. Rsna-miccai brain tumor radiogenomic classification challange. https://www.kaggle.com/c/rsna-miccai-brain-tumor-radiogenomic-classification/. Accessed 10 Aug 2021
19. dicom2nifti. https://github.com/icometrix/dicom2nifti. Accessed 10 Aug 2021

20. Beare, R., Lowekamp, B., Yaniv, Z.: Image segmentation, registration and characterization in r with simpleitk. J. Stat. Softw. **86**, 8 (2018)
21. Avants, B.B., Tustison, N., Song, G., et al.: Advanced normalization tools (ants). Insight J. **2**(365), 1–35 (2009)
22. Isensee, F., Jäger, P.F., Full, P.M., Vollmuth, P., Maier-Hein, K.H.: nnU-Net for brain tumor segmentation. In: Crimi, A., Bakas, S. (eds.) BrainLes 2020. LNCS, vol. 12659, pp. 118–132. Springer, Cham (2021). https://doi.org/10.1007/978-3-030-72087-2_11
23. Isensee, F., Jaeger, P.F., Kohl, S.A.A., Petersen, J., Maier-Hein, K.H.: nnU-Net: a self-configuring method for deep learning-based biomedical image segmentation. Nat. Methods **18**(2), 203–211 (2021)
24. Ronneberger, O., Fischer, P., Brox, T.: U-Net: convolutional networks for biomedical image segmentation. In: Navab, N., Hornegger, J., Wells, W.M., Frangi, A.F. (eds.) MICCAI 2015. LNCS, vol. 9351, pp. 234–241. Springer, Cham (2015). https://doi.org/10.1007/978-3-319-24574-4_28
25. Abadi, M., et al.: TensorFlow: large-scale machine learning on heterogeneous systems (2015). Software available from tensorflow.org
26. Dosovitskiy, A., Springenberg, J.T., Brox, T.: Learning to generate chairs with convolutional neural networks. In: Proceedings of the IEEE Conference on Computer Vision and Pattern Recognition (CVPR), June 2015
27. Nair, V., Hinton, G.E.: Rectified linear units improve restricted Boltzmann machines. In: ICML (2010)
28. Kingma, D.P., Ba, J.: Adam: a method for stochastic optimization. arXiv preprint arXiv:1412.6980 (2014)
29. Van Griethuysen, J.J.M.: Computational radiomics system to decode the radiographic phenotype. Can. Res. **77**(21), e104–e107 (2017)
30. Fisher, R.A.: On the interpretation of $\chi 2$ from contingency tables, and the calculation of p. J. Roy. Stat. Soc. **85**(1), 87–94 (1922)
31. Breiman, L.: Random forests. Mach. Learn. **45**(1), 5–32 (2001)
32. Pedregosa, F., et al.: Scikit-learn: machine learning in Python. J. Mach. Learn. Res. **12**, 2825–2830 (2011)

Combining CNNs with Transformer for Multimodal 3D MRI Brain Tumor Segmentation

Mariia Dobko[✉], Danylo-Ivan Kolinko, Ostap Viniavskyi, and Yurii Yelisieiev

The Machine Learning Lab at Ukrainian Catholic University, Lviv, Ukraine
{dobko_m,kolinko,viniavskyi,yelisieiev}@ucu.edu.ua

Abstract. We apply an ensemble of modified TransBTS, nnU-Net, and a combination of both for the segmentation task of the BraTS 2021 challenge. We change the original architecture of the TransBTS model by adding Squeeze-and-Excitation blocks, increasing the number of CNN layers, replacing positional encoding in the Transformer block with a learnable Multilayer Perceptron (MLP) embeddings, which makes Transformer adjustable to any input size during inference. With these modifications, we can improve TransBTS performance largely. Inspired by a nnU-Net framework, we decided to combine it with our modified TransBTS by changing the architecture inside nnU-Net to our custom model. On the Validation set of BraTS 2021, the ensemble of these approaches achieves 0.8496, 0.8698, 0.9256 Dice score and 15.72, 11.057, 3.374 HD95 for enhancing tumor, tumor core, and whole tumor, correspondingly. On test set we get Dice score 0.8789, 0.8759, 0.9279, and HD95: 10.426, 17.203, 4.93. Our code is publicly available. (Implementation is available at https://github.com/ucuapps/BraTS2021_Challenge).

Keywords: 3D Segmentation · Visual transformers · MRI · Self-supervised Pretraining · Ensembling

1 Introduction

Glioma is one of the most common types of brain tumors, and it can severely affect brain function and be life-threatening depending on its location and rate of growth. Fast, automated, and accurate segmentation of these tumors helps decrease doctors' time while also providing a second opinion to make a more confident clinical diagnosis. Magnetic Resonance Imaging (MRI) is a well-known scanning procedure for brain tumor analysis. It is usually acquired with several complementary modalities: T1-weighted and T2-weighted scans, Fluid Attenuation Inversion Recovery (FLAIR). T1-weighted images are produced using short

---

M. Dobko, D.-I. Kolinko, O. Viniavskyi and Y. Yelisieiev—These authors contributed equally to the work.

A. Crimi and S. Bakas (Eds.): BrainLes 2021, LNCS 12963, pp. 232–241, 2022.
https://doi.org/10.1007/978-3-031-09002-8_21

TE (echo time) and TR (repetition time) times; the T1 properties of tissue determine the contrast and brightness of the image. Sequence abnormalities remain bright in the Flair, but normal CSF fluid is attenuated and made dark; thus, Flair is sensitive to pathology. In general, all these modalities indicate different tissue properties and areas of tumor spread.

In this paper, we present our solution for The Brain Tumor Segmentation (BraTS) Challenge, which is held every year and aims to evaluate state-of-the-art methods for the segmentation of brain tumors. In 2021 it is jointly organized by the Radiological Society of North America (RSNA), the American Society of Neuroradiology (ASNR), and the Medical Image Computing and Computer-Assisted Interventions (MICCAI) society. The main task of this challenge is to develop a method for semantic segmentation of the different glioma sub-regions (the "enhancing tumor" (ET), peritumoral edematous/invaded tissue (ED), and the "necrotic" (NCR)) in mpMRI scans. All experiments in this work have been trained and evaluated on BraTS 2021 dataset [1–4,11].

Proposed method is inspired by two approaches: nnU-Net [8] and Trans-BTS [14] model. We incorporate several modifications to their architectures as well as the training process. For example, for TransBTS, we add Squeeze-and-Excitation blocks, change the positional encoding in Transformer, incorporate self-supervised pretraining. We also evaluated different postprocessing procedures to improve results and increase generalizability. For instance, we applied connected components, thresholding for noise filtering via class replacements, and Test Time Augmentations (TTA). We use our modified TransBTS to replace a model architecture inside a nnU-Net library, keeping the original preprocessing and training of nnU-Net while also including the useful features of the Transformer in combination with CNN.

2   Methods

Our solution is based on TransBTS architecture proposed by Wang et al. [14]. However, we also train nnU-Net [8] and combine both approaches using ensembling. We also tested the incorporation of our modified TransBTS inside nnU-Net, see Sect. 2.3.

In the following sections, we describe all of our custom components introduced for data preprocessing, training, and inference postprocessing including architecture modifications.

2.1   Data Preprocessing and Augmentations

We have different strategies for training each model that is used for the final ensemble, this includes alterations to data preprocessing.

Modified TransBTS: We combine all MRI modalities of a patient into one 4 channel 3D voxel for the input. The normalization used in our experiments is rescaling according to estimates of the mean and standard deviation of the variable per channel. Every scan is randomly cropped to the shape of

$128 \times 128 \times 128$. During training we also apply Random Flip for every dimension including depth and Random Intencity Shift according to this formulation:

$$scale\_factor = Uniform(1.0 - factor, 1.0 + factor)$$

$$shift\_factor = Uniform(-factor, factor)$$

$$image = image * scale\_factor + shift\_factor$$

where factor value was set to 0.1.

nnU-Net and Modified TransBTS: For this training, we use recommended by nnU-Net authors preprocessing which includes per-sample normalization and non-zero mask cropping. The augmentations that were applied during training include Elastic transformation, scaling with a range of 0.85 to 1.25, rotations for all dimensions, gamma correction with a range from 0.7 up to 1.5, mirroring for all axes.

2.2   Self-pretraining

Training deep architectures from scratch on 3D data is extremely time–consuming. Transfer learning allows the model to converge faster by incorporating knowledge (weights) acquired for one task to solve a related one. However, the use of any models pretrained on external datasets is forbidden in BraTS Challenge. This is why we perform self-pretraining on the same dataset, with the same model, but for a different task - image reconstruction. We train an autoencoder with an identical encoder from our segmentation model to reconstruct 3D scans. Mean absolute error (MAE) loss was used for this stage.

Since this step is mainly needed to ensure quicker convergence we train the model for 10 epochs. When segmentation starts we load pretrained weights for the encoder part of our TransBTS.

2.3   Models

TransBTS shows best or comparable results on both BraTS 2019, and BraTS 2020 datasets. The model is based on the encoder-decoder structure, where the encoder captures local information using 3D CNN, these inputs are then passed to Transformer, which learns global features and feeds them to a decoder for upsampling and segmentation prediction.

The idea behind this architecture is to use 3D CNN to generate compact feature maps capturing spatial and depth information while applying a Transformer following the encoder to handle long-distance dependency in a global space.

Our custom modifications (see Figure 1 and Figure 2 for comparison with original TransBTS):

– We add **Squeeze-and-Excitation** blocks [5] to every layer of an encoder. SE blocks help perform dynamic channel-wise feature recalibration.

- The **depth** of the model was increased compared to TransBTS by adding one layer in encoder and correspondingly in decoder.
- We also replaced **positional encoding** from TransBTS with a learnable MLP block, for more details please refer to Sect. 2.4.

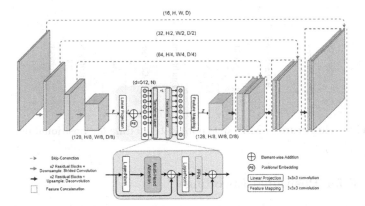

Fig. 1. Architecture of Original **TransBTS**, visualization inspired by [14]. Best viewed in color and zoomed in. (Color figure online)

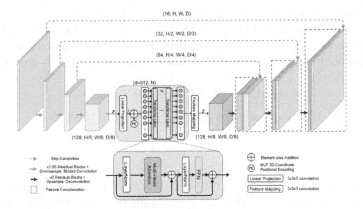

Fig. 2. Architecture of Our **Modified TransBTS**, visualization inspired by [14]. Best viewed in color and zoomed in. (Color figure online)

nnU-Net [8] proposes a robust and self-adapting framework based on three variations of UNet architecture, namely U-Net, 3D U-Net, and Cascade U-Net. The proposed method dynamically adapts to the dataset's image geometry and, more critically, emphasizes the stages that many researchers underestimate. At these stages, a model can get a significant increase in performance. These are the following steps: preprocessing (e.g., normalization), training (e.g., loss, optimizer setting, and data augmentation), inference (e.g., patch-based strategy and ensembling across test time augmentations), and a potential post-processing. It shows that non-model changes in the solution are just as important as model architecture. So we decided to exploit the nnU-Net pipeline to train modified TransBTS.

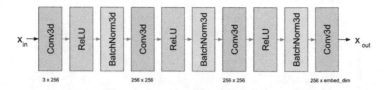

Fig. 3. The architecture of MLP 3D-coordinate module for positional embeddings.

2.4   MLP for Positional Encoding

In TransBTS, the learnable position embeddings, which introduce the location information, have fixed sizes. This results in limited input shape for inference since test images can not deviate in scale from the trained set when positional code is fixed. We include a data-driven positional encoding (PE) module in the form of Multilayer Perceptron (MLP) to address this issue. By directly using a 3D Convolution 1×1, we eliminate the problem with fixed resolution and add extra learnable parameters useful for positional embeddings. The MLP architecture consists of three consecutive blocks, where a single block has 3d convolution, relu activation followed by the batch norm. This operation is formulated as follows:

$$output = MLP(input) + input$$

where MLP block is displayed in Fig. 3.

2.5   Loss

Our training objective for the TransBTS model is the linear combination of Dice and cross-entropy (CE) losses [6,7] while the original TransBTS model was trained with solely softmax Dice loss. The loss operates on the three-class labels GD-enhancing tumor (ET - label 4), the peritumoral edematous/invaded tissue (ED - label 2), and the necrotic tumor core (NCR - label 1). The best weight between the two loss components was experimentally chosen to be 0.4 for Dice and 0.6 for cross-entropy.

When we combine nnU-Net with TransBTS architecture, we also use Dice with CE, but in this case, the weight for both of them is the same, so they have an equal contribution.

2.6   Optimization

We apply mixed-precision training [12], which enables both computational speedup and memory optimization. It is achieved by performing operations in half-precision format and requires two steps: setting the model to use the float16 data type where possible and adding loss scaling to keep small gradient values.

2.7   Postprocessing and Ensembling

First, to reduce memory consumption, we divide the original volume with shape $240 \times 240 \times 155$ into eight overlapping regions of $128 \times 128 \times 128$. After each part has gone through the model, we form our final prediction by combining all regions. There will be a prediction of the latter in places where areas intersect.

Secondly, we perform connected-component analysis (CCA) of predicted labels. The algorithm disassembles the segmentation mask into components according to the given connectivity. CCA can have 4-connected-neighborhood or 8-connected-neighborhood. Based on the ground truth labels on the whole training set, we chose a threshold of 15 voxels and removed components smaller than that. This postprocessing, however, didn't give any severe improvements, so we don't include it in final submissions.

We adopted the idea of another paper [15], which states that after analyzing the training set, authors noticed that some cases do not have an enhancing tumor class. Therefore, if the number of voxels of this class does not exceed the experimentally selected threshold of 300 pixels in our prediction, we replace it with necrosis; in our experiments, we label this procedure as Replacing.

To increase the performance and robustness of our solution, we create an ensemble of our trained models. One such submission included modified Trans-BTS trained for 700 epochs and nnU-Net with default configuration trained for 1,000 epochs, in Table 1 this experiment is named 'nnU-Net + Our TransBTS'. The weights for probabilities were selected separately for each class (the first coefficient corresponds to nnU-Net, while second to our custom TransBTS): 0.5 and 0.5 for NCR, 0.7 and 0.3 for ED, 0.6 and 0.4 for ET.

Our final solution is also an ensemble, which averages probabilities of three models: nnU-Net with default training, nnU-Net trained with our custom Trans-BTS, and our custom TransBTS trained independently for 700 epochs. The coefficients for these models (following the same order as they were named) are: 0.359, 0.347, 0.294 for NCR class, 0.253, 0.387, 0.36 for ED, 0.295, 0.353, 0.351 for ET class. The results can be viewed in Table 1 under the name 'Our Final Solution'.

3   Results

We evaluate our proposed method on the BraTS 2021 dataset and provide a short ablation study for our postprocessing customization. We compare several combinations of ensembling with training other approaches on the same data.

3.1 Metrics

This year's assessment follows the same configuration as previous BraTS challenges. Dice Similarity Coefficient and Hausdorff distance (95%) are used. A result of aggregation of all of these metrics per class determines the winners. The challenge leaderboard also shows Sensitivity and Specificity per each tumor class.

Table 1. Comparison of different methods on BraTS2021 validation set. Dice is computed per class, HD corresponds to Hausdorff Distance. nnU-Net + our TransBTS stands for an ensemble (averaging class probabilities) of both models trained separately (our for 700 epochs), 'Our TransBTS inside nnU-Net' is a proposed model based on TransBTS wrapped in nnU-Net training pipeline, lastly, Our Final Solution is an ensemble of three models: default nnU-Net, nnU-Net trained with custom TransBTS and our modified TransBTS.

Method	Dice ET	Dice TC	Dice WT	HD ET	HD TC	HD WT
Our TransBTS 500 epochs	0.78676	0.82102	0.8972	19.826	15.1904	6.7250
Our TransBTS 700 epochs	0.81912	0.82491	0.9008	15.858	16.7709	5.8139
nnU-Net default	0.81536	**0.8780**	0.9251	21.288	7.7604	3.6352
nnU-Net + our TransBTS	0.84565	0.87201	0.9239	17.364	7.7847	3.6339
Our TransBTS inside nnU-Net	0.79818	0.86844	0.9244	24.875	**7.7489**	3.6186
Our Final Solution	**0.8496**	0.86976	**0.9256**	**15.723**	11.0572	**3.3743**

3.2 Training Phase and Evaluation

We split training data into two sets: training (1,000 patients) and local validation (251 patients). We do this to have an opportunity to evaluate our customizations locally and see their impact before submitting to the challenge. Many of our additional modifications have shown negative or no effect locally, so we didn't use them in the final method. These include but are not limited to 2D segmentation model TransUNet [9], an ensemble of our 3D model and 2D TransUNet, gamma correction tta, etc.

To see which architecture or ensemble shows the best performance, we computed metrics locally and on BraTS2021 validation. On local validation, TransBTS trained for 500 epochs, for instance, shows 0.56284, 0.85408, 0.8382 Dice for NCR, ED, and ET correspondingly, and 21.858, 4.3625, 3.6681 HD score. While the model with our modifications trained for the same number of epochs enables us to achieve 0.7737, 0.8444, 0.8424 Dice and 5.017, 4.57, 3.125 HD. Comparison of our solution with other models is displayed in Table 1. We trained nnU-Net with default configurations to analyze our results and proposed model. We also tested the ensemble of our method together with nnU-Net.

For postprocessing, we applied different hyperparameters and evaluated them on local validation. Best configurations were also estimated on leaderboard validation data, refer to Table 3. We tested several tta combinations on the local validation set to determine the best fit, see results in Table 2.

We show some qualitative results of our segmentation predictions in Figure 4.

Our results on the challenge's closed test set are as follows: 0.8789 Dice ET, 0.8759 Dice TC, 0.9279 Dice WT, 10.4255 Hausdorff95 ET, 17.2033 Hausdorff95 TC, 4.9296 Hausdorff95 WT. With the sensitivity for enhancing tumor, tumor core, and whole tumor, correspondingly: 0.8892, 0.8804, 0.9259.

Table 2. Comparison of TTA techniques on local validation set using our modified TransBTS trained for 500 epochs with self-supervised pretraining. Dice is computed per class, HD corresponds to Hausdorff Distance, W/H/D signifies that three flips (width, height, depth) were used separately one dimension flip per TTA component.

TTA Type	Dice NCR	Dice ED	Dice ET
w/o TTA	0.75079	0.84068	0.82727
All flips & Rotation	0.72535	0.83284	0.81143
W/H/D flips & Rotation & Gamma	0.74752	**0.84871**	0.82896
W/H/D flips	0.75201	0.84297	0.82917
W/H/D flips & Rotation	**0.75230**	0.84518	**0.83033**

Table 3. Comparison of post processing techniques on challenge validation set. HD stands for Hausdorff Distance metric, while C.C is a removal of all, but the largest connected component. C.C per class - filtering with the largest connected component for each class separately.

Post Processing Type	Dice ET	Dice TC	Dice WT	HD ET	HD TC	HD WT
Original	0.78676	0.82102	0.89721	19.82	15.19	6.72
Replacing	0.81515	0.81868	0.89403	17.74	19.84	6.95
C.C + Replacing	0.81517	0.81869	0.89406	17.75	19.84	6.96
C.C per class + Replacing	0.81514	0.81868	0.89403	17.76	19.89	6.97

3.3 GPU Resources

We implemented our methods in PyTorch [13] and trained it on a single NVIDIA GeForce RTX 3090 GPU with 24GB graphics RAM size. We use one NVIDIA GeForce RTX 2080 Ti 11GB GPU at inference time. For a model input to fit in these memory constraints, we had to decrease the volume size, so we split the whole 3D sample with $240 \times 240 \times 155$ dimensionality into eight smaller overlapping voxels of approximately $128 \times 128 \times 128$ pixels and merged the output into one prediction.

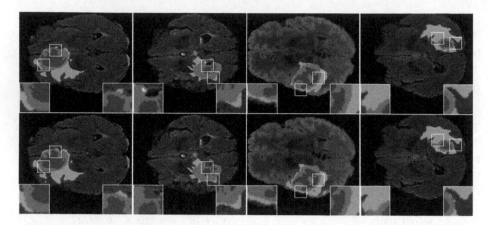

Fig. 4. Qualitative local validation set results. Upper row represents ground truth masks while lower row contains predictions from our custom TransBTS model trained for 700 epochs.

4   Discussion and Conclusion

Our proposed solution to the BraTS 2021 challenge includes aggregating predictions from several models and achieving better performance than any of those methods separately. We selected a CNN with Visual Transformer (based on TransBTS), added customization to its architecture, and incorporated it into the nnU-Net pipeline. This model was used in ensemble with default nnU-Net and our single modified TransBTS. There is still room for improvements in our method, and we discuss some ideas below.

In our solution, we didn't explore the data augmentations in depth. This creates a window of opportunity to improve current results for every model in the proposed ensemble. The easiest way to approach this would be to use augmentations described by winners from last-year challenge [7].

We also suggest experimenting with computing Hausdorff loss during training and optimizing it alongside Dice and Cross-entropy. This should also improve the Hausdorff distance metric and possibly overall performance on dice. However, this loss is very time-consuming and is usually implemented on CPU, so we recommended using the version based on applying morphological erosion on the difference between the actual and estimated segmentation maps [10], which saves computations.

The knowledge about labels combination into whole tumor and tumor core could be also used during training, perhaps even a separate model trained on most challenging class.

Acknowledgements. Authors thank Avenga, Eleks, and Ukrainian Catholic University for providing necessary computing resources. We also express gratitude to Marko Kostiv and Dmytro Fishman for their help and support in the last week of competition.

References

1. Baid, U., et al.: The RSNA-ASNR-MICCAI brats 2021 benchmark on brain tumor segmentation and radiogenomic classification. arXiv preprint arXiv:2107.02314 (2021)
2. Bakas, S., et al.: Segmentation labels for the pre-operative scans of the TCGA-GBM collection (2017). https://doi.org/10.7937/K9/TCIA.2017.KLXWJJ1Q, https://wiki.cancerimagingarchive.net/x/KoZyAQ
3. Bakas, S., et al.: Segmentation labels for the pre-operative scans of the TCGA-LGG collection (2017). https://doi.org/10.7937/K9/TCIA.2017.GJQ7R0EF, https://wiki.cancerimagingarchive.net/x/LIZyAQ
4. Bakas, S., et al.: Advancing the cancer genome atlas glioma MRI collections with expert segmentation labels and radiomic features. Nat. Sci. Data **4**(1) (2017). https://doi.org/10.1038/sdata.2017.117
5. Hu, J., Shen, L., Sun, G.: Squeeze-and-excitation networks. In: 2018 IEEE/CVF Conference on Computer Vision and Pattern Recognition. IEEE, June 2018. https://doi.org/10.1109/cvpr.2018.00745
6. Isensee, F., Jaeger, P.F., Kohl, S.A.A., Petersen, J., Maier-Hein, K.H.: nnU-net: a self-configuring method for deep learning-based biomedical image segmentation. Nature Methods **18**(2), 203–211 (2020). https://doi.org/10.1038/s41592-020-01008-z
7. Isensee, F., Jäger, P.F., Full, P.M., Vollmuth, P., Maier-Hein, K.H.: nnU-Net for brain tumor segmentation. In: Crimi, A., Bakas, S. (eds.) BrainLes 2020. LNCS, vol. 12659, pp. 118–132. Springer, Cham (2021). https://doi.org/10.1007/978-3-030-72087-2_11
8. Isensee, F., et al.: Abstract: nnU-Net: self-adapting framework for u-net-based medical image segmentation. In: Bildverarbeitung für die Medizin 2019. I, pp. 22–22. Springer, Wiesbaden (2019). https://doi.org/10.1007/978-3-658-25326-4_7
9. Jieneng, C., et al.: Transunet: transformers make strong encoders for medical image segmentation. arXiv preprint arXiv:2102.04306 (2021)
10. Karimi, D., Salcudean, S.E.: Reducing the hausdorff distance in medical image segmentation with convolutional neural networks. IEEE Trans. Med. Imaging **39**(2), 499–513 (2020). https://doi.org/10.1109/tmi.2019.2930068
11. Menze, B.H., et al.: The multimodal brain tumor image segmentation benchmark (BRATS). IEEE Trans. Med. Imaging **34**(10), 1993–2024 (2015). https://doi.org/10.1109/tmi.2014.2377694
12. Micikevicius, P., et al.: Mixed precision training. CoRR abs/1710.03740 (2017). http://arxiv.org/abs/1710.03740
13. Paszke, A., et al.: Pytorch: an imperative style, high-performance deep learning library, pp. 8024–8035 (2019). http://papers.neurips.cc/paper/9015-pytorch-an-imperative-style-high-performance-deep-learning-library.pdf
14. Wang, Wenxuan, Chen, Chen, Ding, Meng, Yu, Hong, Zha, Sen, Li, Jiangyun: TransBTS: multimodal brain tumor segmentation using transformer. In: de Bruijne, Marleen, et al. (eds.) MICCAI 2021. LNCS, vol. 12901, pp. 109–119. Springer, Cham (2021). https://doi.org/10.1007/978-3-030-87193-2_11
15. Wang, Y., et al.: Modality-pairing learning for brain tumor segmentation. In: Crimi, A., Bakas, S. (eds.) BrainLes 2020. LNCS, vol. 12658, pp. 230–240. Springer, Cham (2021). https://doi.org/10.1007/978-3-030-72084-1_21

Brain Tumor Segmentation Using Deep Infomax

Jitendra Marndi, Cailyn Craven, and Geena Kim$^{(\boxtimes)}$

University of Colorado, Boulder, CO 80309, USA
geena.kim@colorado.edu

Abstract. In this study, we apply Deep Infomax (DIM) loss to a U-Net variant model with DenseNet blocks (DenseUnet). Using DenseUnet as a baseline model, we compare performances when training with cross entropy loss alone versus training with DIM loss. From a pilot study on BraTS 2020 data, we observed improvements when training with DIM then retraining with cross entropy (DTC). The results from BraTS 2021 data also show slight improvements, however, a longer training epoch and further hyperparameter tuning are needed to achieve more effective results from DIM.

Keywords: Deep infomax · U-Net · Image segmentation

1 Introduction

Annually over 11,000 people in the United States are diagnosed with glioblastoma, a highly invasive brain glioma [1]. 3D MRI brain scans play an essential role in diagnosing brain tumors and longitudinal patient monitoring. To date, highly trained experts manually assess 3D MRI brain scans. The current process of labeling MRI scans is expensive, time-consuming, and assessment of the same 3D MRI scan can vary from expert to expert. A reliable automated method for brain tumor segmentation is desirable. The RSNA-ASNR-MICCAI BraTS 2021 challenge promotes research in this area. BraTS data has emerged as a benchmark dataset for the brain tumor segmentation problem, with the 2021 dataset growing to include 2,000 cases (8,000 mpMRI scans) [2–4].

Deep neural networks have been successfully applied in brain tumor segmentation, performing highly in the BraTS challenge [11]. Most models in the challenge employ supervised learning. Encoder-decoder architecture is the most common with segmentation loss computed from decoder output and actual labels.

Deep unsupervised learning attempts to learn useful representation of the data to overcome the scarce labels has gradually emerged as a promising alternative to supervised approaches for complex real-world problems. It often requires formulation of a surrogate task and can be used in conjunction with supervised learning. It could be particularly well-suited for medical imaging given the limitations of supervised methods to generalize. The Infomax optimization principle recommends maximizing the Mutual Information (MI) between the input and output of a neural network. MI between two distributions is the divergence between their joint probability distribution and the product of marginals.

Mutual Information Neural Estimator (MINE) algorithm [6] uses discriminative network to tackle tricky MI estimation task for continuous variables in deep neural network. During training, the discriminator network samples from the joint distribution and the product-of-marginals distribution to determine whether the input and output representation pair belong together, maximizing a lower bound to the MI. Inspired by the Infomax principle, Deep Infomax (DIM) [5] applied the MI maximization principle to deep unsupervised learning. In its simplest form, DIM [5] is a two-staged encoder. In the unsupervised setting, DIM's training maximizes the MI between outputs at each stage. The output of each stage is passed to an MI estimator network to maximize MI.

We apply the Deep InfoMax (DIM) approach to a U-Net variant model with Dense blocks [13] as a baseline model (DenseUnet). DenseUnet is a form of encoder-decoder architecture for image segmentation. We regularize its encoder similarly. We observed that appropriate formulation of loss function considering estimated MI and segmentation loss could improve the model's performance.

1.1   DIM

Hjelm et al. [5] applied the MI maximization principle in deep unsupervised learning to extract hidden codes which can be used in downstream tasks such as classification or image segmentation. It was reported that MI with emphasis on global information provides better results for image reconstruction tasks while local information is useful for downstream classification tasks.

The DIM model optimizes an objective that has three distinctive terms representing global information, local information, and prior enforcement. Two of the three terms represent global and local MI and the third is the regularization introduced by adversarial training to enforce a prior. E_ψ is the continuous differentiable parametric function with domain $\mathcal{X}$ and range $\mathcal{Y}$, $E_\psi : \mathcal{X} \to \mathcal{Y}$. $\mathbb{P}$ is the empirical distribution of training data, $X := \{x^{(i)} \in \mathcal{X}\}_{i=1}^N$. $\mathbb{U}_{\psi,\mathbb{P}}$ is the marginal distribution induced by pushing samples from $\mathbb{P}$ through E_ψ i.e. $\mathbb{U}_{\psi,\mathbb{P}}$ is the distribution over encodings $y \in \mathcal{Y}$ produced by the encoder E_ψ.

Global MI maximization is formulated as the maximization of neural information measure [6] between complete input and encodings:

$$(\hat{\omega}_g, \hat{\psi})_G = \underset{\omega_g, \psi}{\mathrm{argmax}} \; \hat{I}_{\omega_g}(X, E_\psi(X)) \tag{1}$$

Note that above formulation uses Donsker-Varadhan (DV) representation of KL divergence whereas other divergence measures can be used as well such as Jensen-Shannon divergence or InfoNCE [8] (based on Noise-contrastive estimation, [9]). For this project, only the global MI component of the loss function was considered along with the DV representation of KL divergence.

2   Methods

2.1   Data Preprocessing

The BraTS 2021 Train dataset contains co-registered and skull-stripped MR images from 1251 patients. We used the histogram-based preprocessing method as described in [10]. We also split the Train dataset into three subsets; train, validation and test subsets by tumor location and size pairs to evenly distribute the similar cases among those three subsets.

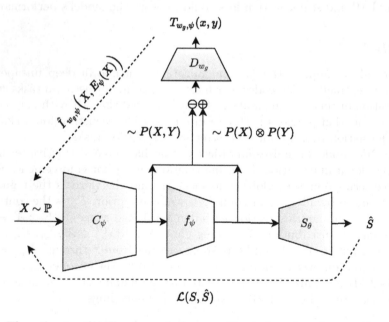

Fig. 1. The subnetworks C_ϕ, f_ϕ, and S_θ are collectively referred to as DenseUnet, the baseline model. The MI estimator D_{w_g} is the component used in MI regularization. Solid arrow indicates forward-pass, dashed arrow indicates back-propagation of gradient, all shaded quadrilaterals are neural networks.

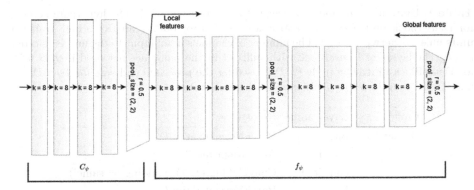

Fig. 2. The composition of Encoder in the terms of DenseBlock (rectangle) and Trans-Down (trapezoid) units.

2.2   Architecture

Figure 1 depicts a high-level overview of the main components adopted for the segmentation task with MI regularization. The C_ϕ and f_ϕ in Fig 1 constitutes the encoder and the sub-network S_θ is the decoder. The encoder extracts hidden codes which then the decoder uses to generate a segmentation map. This pair of encoder-decoder forms the baseline model, DenseUnet. The outputs of C_ϕ and f_ϕ are local and global features respectively. The local and global features are passed to a discriminator network D_{w_g} which acts as the MI estimator. The whole network is dubbed as DenseUnet-MI.

The baseline model, DenseUnet with cross entropy loss, is based on Model D in [10], and contains encoder and decoder sub-networks which are composed of DenseBlock, TransDown and TransUp units as listed in Table 1. The encoder subnetwork is constructed by repeating a group of four DenseBlock units and one TransUp unit three times. Similarly the decoder/segmentator network is obtained by repeating a group of four DenseBoock units and one TransDown unit three times. The final encoder output and the intermediate encoder output after first group is referred to as global features and local feature respectively (Fig. 2). To obtain the complete DenseUnet model, first the input is passed sequentially through encoder and decoder. The decoder output is then concatenated with the input to the model (not shown in Fig. 1 for simplicity) and then batch normalization and relu activation are applied. The final layer has 1×1 convolution layer to compress the channels to 3 output channels.

The model DenseUnet-MI is obtained by attaching MI estimator sub-network to DenseUnet. MI estimator is simple discriminative network containing a group of batch normalization, activation and dense layer repeated three times. First two groups use tanh activation after normalization and the dense layer contains 16 hidden units. Final group contains relu activation and one hidden/output unit in the dense layer. Three TransDown units, first two with $r = 0.5$ and the last one with $r = 1.0$, are applied to local features before flattening out and sending the output to MI estimator. Three TransDown units are also used for

Table 1. Units used in model DenseUnet and DenseUnet-MI. The hyperparameter k for DenseBlock unit is set to 8 and r is set to 0.5 for both TransDown and TransUp units unless otherwise stated. The number of channels in an input to the unit is referred as ch. The layers of DenseBlock with suffix _1 in the name are not used if $ch > 4 \cdot k$ for DenseBlock unit. The tuple $(2, 2)$ is used for the *pool_size* and *size* for TransDown and TransUp units respectively unless otherwise stated.

Unit	Layer name	Keras layer
DenseBlock	bn_1	BatchNormalization()
	relu_1	Activation('relu')
	conv2d_1	Conv2D(4·k, (1, 1), padding = 'same')
	bn_2	BatchNormalization()
	relu_2	Activation('relu')
	conv2d_2	Conv2D(k, (3, 3), padding= 'same')
	concat	Concatenate()
TransDown	bn	BatchNormalization()
	relu	Activation('relu')
	conv2d	Conv2D(r· ch, (1, 1), padding= 'same')
	ap2d	AveragePooling2D(pool_size)
TransUp	bn	BatchNormalization()
	relu	Activation('relu')
	conv2d	Conv2D(r·ch, (1, 1), padding= 'same')
	us2d	UpSampling2D(size)

global features but the last two units use *pool_size* $= (1, 1)$ and similar to local features, global features are flattened out as well before feeding the output to the MI estimator.

2.3   Training

To assess the effect of MI regularization on DenseUnet-MI, three training strategies were proposed, namely a) Cross entropy, b) DIM and cross entropy and, c) DIM then cross entropy.

Cross Entropy (CE). This is simply the training and evaluation of baseline model, DenseUnet. The MI estimator is removed from the DenseUnet-MI model. The segmentation/probability map $\hat{S} = S_\theta \circ f_\phi \circ C_\phi(X)$ is compared with actual probability labels, S, to get the categorical cross entropy loss $\mathcal{L}(S, \hat{S})$.

DIM and Cross Entropy (DAC). In this training strategy, the loss function has two components. One is the categorical cross entropy as described above. Another component is for MI regularization. The discriminator D_{w_g} is used to estimate MI between global features and local features. The order of magnitude of estimated MI can go up to 10^4. It's divided by 10^3 and tanh activation was applied to make its value comparable to categorical cross entropy loss.

DIM then Cross Entropy (DTC). Here the training epochs are divided into two halves. In the first half, the decoder is removed and (encoder and MI estimator) is trained to maximize MI. In the second half, the MI estimator is removed and DenseUnet-MI (encoder and decoder) is then trained to minimize categorical cross entropy loss.

A pilot study was conducted on BraTS 2020 training data with all the training strategies mentioned above. During the pilot study all experiments used either constant learning rate of 0.002, 0.0002 or triangular cyclic learning rate (Smith et al. [12]) with base learning rate 0.0002 and maximum learning rate 0.02. Extending upon the pilot study, experiments on BraTS 2021 data were conducted with constant learning rate of 0.005 with CE and DTC training strategies, as DTC method showed consistently better results than DAC method in the pilot study.

MI was incorporated to overall loss in three ways: (a) $tanh(-mi)$, (b) $tanh(-mi/10^3)$, and (c) $1+tanh(-mi/10^3)$. Dividing mi was by 10^3 also ensures sufficient gradient exists when mi has higher magnitude. Training strategy for the baseline model is cross entropy (CE) and only CCE is used as loss. Each of three losses from mi was added to CCE to get total loss during training using strategy DAC and DTC. One to four experiments were conducted for every valid combinations of loss functions and training strategies.

3 Results

Table 2 shows the results on BraTS 2021 data. The first three rows show the results when trained on 2D slices in a single view (sagittal, coronal and axial respectively), and the following two rows are from ensembling across those three views. Each row displays results (two sub-rows) from models trained with cross entropy (CE) and DIM-then-cross-entropy (DTC). The first set (column-wise) of results show the 3D Dice scores on the five labels (NCR, ED, ET, WT, TC) predicted on the set-a-side test subset from the BraTS 2021 Training dataset. The second set of results show the 3D Dice scores on three labels (ET, WT, TC) evaluated on the BraTS 2021 Validation dataset. In the single-view results on the Train data's set-aside test subset, all experiments were repeated 3–5 times to get average and standard deviation, whereas only the best model was used for evaluating on the Validation dataset. The ensemble A used voting for ensembling across the views, whereas the ensemble B used averaging the probability outputs from the three views then thresholding at 0.5 at each pixel to get labels. To reduce stochastic fluctuation, each view had three experiments, then the probabilities were averaged before applying the ensembling across the views. Evaluating on the test subset of the training data show little to no improvement from DIM (DIM-then-cross-entropy) on single view or ensemble results, except axial view. However, evaluation on Validation data show slight improvement by DIM for ensembled results for TC.

Table 2. Results Comparison of training strategies CE and DTC on BraTS 2021 data. For CE baseline, models were trained for 60 epochs. For DTC training models were trained with DIM loss for 30 epochs then switched to BCE loss for additional 30 epochs.

View	Loss	BRATS21 training data's test subset					BRATS21 validation data		
		NCR	ED	ET	WT	TC	ET	WT	TC
Sagittal	CE	0.667 ± 0.020	0.771 ± 0.011	0.753 ± 0.029	0.850 ± 0.002	0.788 ± 0.025	0.712	0.855	0.740
	DTC	0.654 ± 0.004	0.746 ± 0.026	0.761 ± 0.014	0.832 ± 0.021	0.788 ± 0.006	0.732	0.866	0.723
Coronal	CE	0.670 ± 0.008	0.779 ± 0.005	0.802 ± 0.012	0.863 ± 0.006	0.819 ± 0.004	0.736	0.861	0.744
	DTC	0.653 ± 0.016	0.772 ± 0.019	0.783 ± 0.008	0.852 ± 0.014	0.801 ± 0.010	0.717	0.855	0.715
Axial	CE	0.660 ± 0.014	0.784 ± 0.011	0.784 ± 0.015	0.865 ± 0.012	0.824 ± 0.015	0.715	0.879	0.772
	DTC	0.655 ± 0.017	0.781 ± 0.015	0.789 ± 0.006	0.864 ± 0.009	0.826 ± 0.006	0.720	0.877	0.773
Ensemble A	CE	0.693	0.816	0.808	0.878	0.827	0.776	0.879	0.745
	DTC	0.695	0.805	0.804	0.868	0.825	0.763	0.868	0.752
Ensemble B	CE	0.699	0.819	0.809	0.879	0.830	0.783	0.880	0.749
	DTC	0.697	0.808	0.806	0.870	0.827	0.769	0.870	0.756

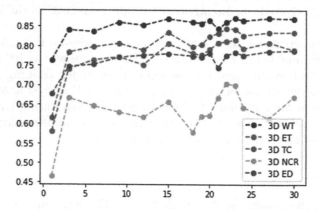

Fig. 3. Plot of Dice scores on tumor substructures as a function of epochs for continued training with CE loss after training with 30 epochs of DIM loss.

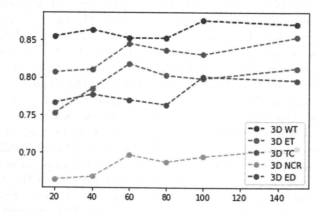

Fig. 4. Plot of Dice scores on tumor substructures as a function of epochs. In each experiment, a model was trained with DIM-then-cross-entropy method for the half of the total epochs.

Figure 3 shows the evaluation results using model checkpoints on Train's test subset at different training epochs with BCE loss after training with DIM loss for 30 epochs. The overall trends show that there is no sign of deterioration due to training with BCE for 30 epochs after training with DIM. Figure 4 shows a general trends of improved results from DTC approach as total epochs gets longer. It suggests that the training epochs can be longer. Also, a pilot study on BraTS 2020 data with 369 patients showed that longer training epochs (100–150 total epochs) may be needed to observe the effect of DIM.

Tables 3, 4, 5 and 6 show the test results on the BraTS21 Test dataset from the DTC ensemble B model. The model performed decently for median and above, but seems to do poorly on certain cases which makes big standard deviations. Some of the Dice score performances which the mean Dice score is less than the 25-quantile Dice score may mean there are a small number of failure cases where the model failed with big error.

Table 3. Dice scores of prediction on BraTS 2021 test data by ensemble B where the individual models were trained using DTC strategy

Label	Dice_ET	Dice_WT	Dice_TC
Mean	0.692	0.747	0.708
StdDev	0.359	0.335	0.379
Median	0.868	0.906	0.913
25 quantile	0.639	0.774	0.593
75 quantile	0.933	0.943	0.958

Table 4. Sensitivity scores of prediction on BraTS 2021 test data by ensemble B where the individual models were trained using DTC strategy

Label	Sensitivity_ET	Sensitivity_WT	Sensitivity_TC
Mean	0.681	0.723	0.682
StdDev	0.366	0.335	0.374
Median	0.866	0.881	0.886
25 quantile	0.552	0.708	0.470
75 quantile	0.937	0.935	0.950

Table 5. Specificity scores of prediction on BraTS 2021 test data by ensemble B where the individual models were trained using DTC strategy

Label	Specificity_ET	Specificity_WT	Specificity_TC
Mean	0.847	0.847	0.847
StdDev	0.360	0.359	0.360
Median	1.000	1.000	1.000
25 quantile	1.000	0.999	1.000
75 quantile	1.000	1.000	1.000

Table 6. Hausdorff95 scores of prediction on BraTS 2021 test data by ensemble B where the individual models were trained using DTC strategy

Label	Hausdorff95_ET	Hausdorff95_WT	Hausdorff95_TC
Mean	68.6086	62.9505	70.7106
StdDev	141.7708	132.2243	141.6636
Median	1.7321	5.6569	3.1623
25 quantile	1.0000	3.7417	2.0000
75 quantile	5.6547	10.4881	9.1515

4   Discussion

We have conducted experiments to show whether Infomax principle helps learning representations. We applied Deep Infomax (DIM) to our DenseUnet baseline model and compared on each single view and view ensembles. We used 30 epoch training on DIM then another 30 epochs with BCE loss, and observed a slight improvements on validation results. However, training on longer epochs may be needed to reach the performance saturation and observe the effect of Deep Infomax. Our demonstration of Deep Infomax uses local and global features with fixed sizes. More experimentation on those feature scale may be needed to optimize the efficacy of DIM approach. Also, exploring different surrogate tasks other than comparing local and global features may be helpful.

Acknowledgements. This work utilized resources from the University of Colorado Boulder Research Computing Group [14], which is supported by the National Science Foundation (awards ACI-1532235 and ACI-1532236), the University of Colorado Boulder, and Colorado State University.

This work used the Extreme Science and Engineering Discovery Environment (XSEDE) [15,16], which is supported by National Science Foundation grant number ACI-1548562, Comet-GPU through allocation TG-CIE170063.

References

1. Ostrom, Q.T., Gittleman, H., Truitt, G., Boscia, A., Kruchko, C., Barnholtz-Sloan, J.S.: CBTRUS statistical report: primary brain and other central nervous system tumors diagnosed in the United States in 2011–2015. Neuro Oncol. **20**, iv1–iv86 (2018). https://doi.org/10.1093/neuonc/noy131
2. Baid, U., et al.: The RSNA-ASNR-MICCAI BraTS 2021 Benchmark on Brain Tumor Segmentation and Radiogenomic Classification. arXiv:2107.02314 (2021)
3. Menze, B.H., et al.: The multimodal brain tumor image segmentation benchmark (BRATS). IEEE Trans. Med. Imaging **34**, 1993–2024 (2015). https://doi.org/10.1109/TMI.2014.2377694
4. Bakas, S., et al.: Advancing the Cancer Genome Atlas glioma MRI collections with expert segmentation labels and radiomic features. Sci. Data **4**, 170117 (2017). https://doi.org/10.1038/sdata.2017.117
5. Hjelm, R.D., et al.: Learning deep representations by mutual information estimation and maximization. arXiv arXiv:1808.06670 (2018)
6. Belghazi, M.I., et al.: MINE: Mutual Information Neural Estimation. arXiv arXiv:1801.04062 (2018)
7. Makhzani, A., Shlens, J., Jaitly, N., Goodfellow, I., Frey, B.: Adversarial Autoencoders. arXiv arXiv:1511.05644 (2015)
8. Oord, A. van den, Li, Y., Vinyals, O.: Representation learning with contrastive predictive coding. arXiv arXiv:1807.03748 (2018)
9. Gutmann, M., Hyvärinen, A.: Noise-contrastive estimation: A new estimation principle for unnormalized statistical models. In: Teh, Y.W. and Titterington, M. (eds.) Proceedings of the Thirteenth International Conference on Artificial Intelligence and Statistics. PMLR, Chia Laguna Resort, Sardinia, Italy, pp. 297–304 (2010)
10. Kim, G.: Brain Tumor Segmentation Using Deep Fully Convolutional Neural Networks. In: Crimi, A., Bakas, S., Kuijf, H., Menze, B., Reyes, M. (eds.) Brainlesion: Glioma, Multiple Sclerosis, Stroke and Traumatic Brain Injuries. BrainLes 2017. LNCS, vol. 10670, Springer, Cham (2018). https://doi.org/10.1007/978-3-319-75238-9_30
11. Bakas, S., et al.: Identifying the best machine learning algorithms for brain tumor segmentation, progression assessment, and overall survival prediction in the BRATS Challenge. arXiv arXiv:1811.02629 (2018)
12. Smith, L. N.: Cyclical learning rates for training neural networks. In: Computing Research Repository (2017). http://arxiv.org/abs/1506.01186
13. Huang, G., Liu, Z., van der Maaten, L., Weinberger, K.Q.: Densely connected convolutional networks. arXiv:1608.06993 [cs] (2018)
14. Anderson, J., Burns, P.J., Milroy, D., Ruprecht, P., Hauser, T., Siegel, H.J.: Deploying RMACC summit: an HPC resource for the rocky mountain region. In: Practice and Experience in Advanced Research Computing, New Orleans LA USA, PEARC17(7) (2017). https://doi.org/10.1145/3093338.3093379
15. Towns, J., et al.: Xsede: accelerating scientific discovery. Comput. Sci. Eng. **16**(5), 62–74 (2014). ISSN 1521–9615. https://doi.org/10.1109/MCSE.2014.80. doi.ieeecomputersociety.org/10.1109/MCSE.2014.80
16. Wilkins-Diehr, N., et al.: An overview of the XSEDE extended collaborative support program. In: Gitler, I., Klapp, J. (eds.) ISUM 2015. CCIS, vol. 595, pp. 3–13. Springer, Cham (2016). https://doi.org/10.1007/978-3-319-32243-8_1

17. Bakas, S., et al.: Segmentation labels and radiomic features for the pre-operative scans of the TCGA-GBM collection. Can. Imaging Archive (2017). https://doi.org/10.7937/K9/TCIA.2017.KLXWJJ1Q
18. Bakas, S., et al.: Segmentation labels and radiomic features for the pre-operative scans of the TCGA-LGG collection. Can. Imaging Archive (2017). https://doi.org/10.7937/K9/TCIA.2017.GJQ7R0EF

Automatic Brain Tumor Segmentation with a Bridge-Unet Deeply Supervised Enhanced with Downsampling Pooling Combination, Atrous Spatial Pyramid Pooling, Squeeze-and-Excitation and EvoNorm

Alexandre Carré⬤, Eric Deutsch⬤, and Charlotte Robert$^{(\boxtimes)}$⬤

Université Paris-Saclay, Institut Gustave Roussy, Inserm, Radiothérapie Moléculaire et Innovation Thérapeutique, 94800 Villejuif, France
ch.robert@gustaveroussy.fr

Abstract. Segmentation of brain tumors is a critical task for patient disease management. Since this task is time-consuming and subject to inter-expert delineation variation, automatic methods are of significant interest. The Multimodal Brain Tumor Segmentation Challenge (BraTS) has been in place for about a decade and provides a common platform to compare different automatic segmentation algorithms based on multiparametric magnetic resonance imaging (mpMRI) of gliomas. This year the challenge has taken a big step forward by multiplying the total data by approximately 3. We address the image segmentation challenge by developing a network based on a Bridge-Unet and improved with a concatenation of max and average pooling for downsampling, Squeeze-and-Excitation (SE) block, Atrous Spatial Pyramid Pooling (ASSP), and EvoNorm-S0. Our model was trained using the 1251 training cases from the BraTS 2021 challenge and achieved an average Dice similarity coefficient (DSC) of 0.92457, 0.87811 and 0.84094, as well as a 95% Hausdorff distance (HD) of 4.19442, 7.55256 and 14.13390 mm for the whole tumor, tumor core, and enhanced tumor, respectively on the online validation platform composed of 219 cases. Similarly, our solution achieved a DSC of 0.92548, 0.87628 and 0.87122, as well as HD95 of 4.30711, 17.84987 and 12.23361 mm on the test dataset composed of 530 cases. Overall, our approach yielded well balanced performance for each tumor subregion.

Keywords: Deep-learning · Brain tumor · Segmentation

1 Introduction

Glioma is the most frequent kind of tumor of the central nervous system (CNS) that arises from glial cells. These tumors infiltrate the surrounding brain tissue

A. Crimi and S. Bakas (Eds.): BrainLes 2021, LNCS 12963, pp. 253–266, 2022.
https://doi.org/10.1007/978-3-031-09002-8_23

and spread throughout the brain. They are divided into three types depending on the phenotypic features of the cells: astrocytomas, ependymomas, and oligodendrogliomas. Astrocytomas are the most frequent form of glioma, and they are the most deadly. The World Health Organization (WHO) grading system has recently classified glioma based on molecular markers that have been proven to have important predictive and therapeutic significance [21]. Depending on the degree of proliferation indicated by the mitotic index as well as the presence or absence of necrosis, gliomas are categorized into grades I to IV. Pilocytic astrocytomas are the least malignant brain tumors, whereas glioblastoma (GBM) is the most malignant tumor. GBM is the most agressive with a dismal prognosis and a median overall survival (OS) estimated between 12 and 18 months [35,40]. Magnetic resonance imaging (MRI) is the non-invasive imaging modality of choice in the investigation of patients with symptoms suggesting a brain tumor [6]. It enables the identification of the location, number and size of lesions and helps in tumor characterization. The conventional MRI protocol in the diagnosis of brain tumours includes multi-parametric magnetic resonance imaging (mpMRI) based at least on 4 sequences: T1-weighted sequence (T1w), T1-weighted contrast enhanced using gadolinium contrast agents (T1w-gd), T2-weighted (T2w), and a T2-sequence with suppression of the signal from fluids such as the fluid attenuated inversion recovery (FLAIR) sequence. Glioblastoma usually presents with a necrotic center, a heterogeneous and irregular contrasting peripheral annular region which reflects a rupture of the blood-brain barrier, and a peritumoral area in hypersignal on FLAIR sequences corresponding to either edema, tumor infiltration, or a combination of both. In several clinical applications, such as surgical planning, tumor development monitoring, and radiation therapy planning, accurate MRI brain tumor subregion boundary detection is critical. In a clinical setting, this procedure is mainly performed manually by neurosurgeons and radiation oncologists, making this task subjective, laborious, and error-prone. This highlights the tremendous challenge of developing high-throughput automated deterministic segmentation solutions that will significantly enhance and accelerate the procedures. For this purpose, the International Multimodal Brain Tumor Segmentation Challenge (BraTS), which has been held since 2012, serves as a platform for the evaluation of state-of-the-art machine learning (ML) methods for the segmentation of brain tumor subregions [1–5,30]. The year 2017 was a pivotal year because since this year only pre-operative imaging is considered with annotations reviewed by experts in the domain. This year BraTS celebrates its tenth anniversary and moves towards a new era. Indeed, until now the total number of collected cases was equal to 660 cases (2640 mpMRI scans). An important international work of collection and annotation of the data was carried out to reach 2000 cases (8000 mpMRI scans) for the 2021 edition. Thus, the BraTS challenge addresses a major stake in the development of artificial intelligence models, which is the difficulty of obtaining annotated data (ground truth) [23].

Due to the widespread use of deep learning in the computer vision field, particularly in medical imaging analysis, fully convolutional network (FCN) based methods are the most advanced solutions for this segmentation task. These techniques have shown impressive performance in the past challenges. In 2017, Kamnitsas et al. [24] won the challenge using an ensemble of multiple models and architectures for robust performance through prediction aggregation. Specifically, they employed 3 different architectures: i) Deepmedic which is a fully 3D, multi-scale convolutional neural network (CNN) [25], ii) three 3D FCNs [28], and iii) two 3D versions of the U-Net architecture [39]. In 2018, A. Myronenko [32] won through the adoption of a CNN architecture based on an encoder-decoder with an asymmetrically larger encoder to extract the image features and a smaller decoder to reconstruct the segmentation mask. The network was fed with very large patch size (160 × 192 × 128 voxels). Futhermore, due to the restricted amount of the training dataset, he also proposed the insertion of a variational auto-encoder (VAE) branch to reconstruct the input image itself in order to regularize the shared decoder and impose additional constraints on its layers. In 2019, Jiang et al. [22] won the first place by proposing a two-stage cascaded U-Net to segment the substructures of brain tumors from coarse to fine. Last year, Isensee et al. [17] won by applying the nnU-Net framework he developed. nnU-Net is a self adapting automatic segmentation framework able to cope with the diversity of datasets in the medical domain [16]. He thus proposed specific modifications to the BraTS task and realized an ensemble based on the three best models on the online validation determined by a re-implementation of the BraTS ranking. It is worth noting that the solutions he proposed in 2017 [18] and 2018 [19] ranked 2 and 3 respectively. Our work from the previous year [13] proposed two independent ensembles of models derived from two different training pipelines, each of which generated a brain tumor segmentation map. Afterwards, the two patient-based labeling maps were combined, taking into consideration the performance of each ensemble for specific tumor subregions. This solution allowed us to be placed fifth.

In this paper, we propose an ensemble of a Bridge-Unet enhanced with concatenation of max and average pooling for downsampling, Squeeze-and-Excitation (SE) block, Atrous Spatial Pyramid Pooling (ASSP), and EvoNorm-S0. In addition, we have improved the post-processing of the segmentation maps. We evaluated the method on the BraTS2021 validation and test datasets.

2   Material and Methods

2.1   Data

The data were collected from multiple institutions using various MRI scanners. BraTS 2021 training dataset included 1251 cases, each with four 3D MRI sequences (T1w, T1w-gd, T2w, and FLAIR). All mpMRI data followed a standard preprocessing with re-orientation to a common orientation system (i.e. Left, Posterior, Superior), co-registration to the same anatomical template (SRI24), resampling to a $1 \times 1 \times 1 \, mm^3$ isotropic voxel size and, skull-stripping. All image size was equal to 240 × 240 × 155. Annotations were approved by expert neuroradiologists and included 3 tumor subregions: the necrotic and non-enhancing tumor core (label 1), the peritumoral edema (label 2), and the enhancing tumor (label 4) (Fig. 1). These subregions were merged for evaluation into 3 volumes: the "enhancing tumor" (ET), the "tumor core" (TC), and the "whole tumor" (WT). ET shows a hyperintense signal on the T1w-gd sequence compared to the T1 sequence and the "healthy" white matter on the T1w-gd sequence. TC describes the tumor bulk usually removed during surgical resection. It includes the ET and the necrotic part (NCR). The NCR aspect is typically hypointense on T1w-gd compared to T1. The WT portrays the full extent of the disease, as it encompasses the TC and the peritumoral edematous/invaded tissue (ED), which is typically visualized by a hyperintense signal on FLAIR. One additional dataset of 219 cases without the ground truth labels is provided for validation. For this dataset, the participants had to upload the set of segments to be evaluated on the organization platform of the challenge which is synapse.org. The platform was limited to three submissions per participant per day and was intended for preliminary evaluations. The test dataset including 530 cases was kept hidden and used to calculate the final challenge ranking. The organization performed the evaluation after the submission of a Docker file.

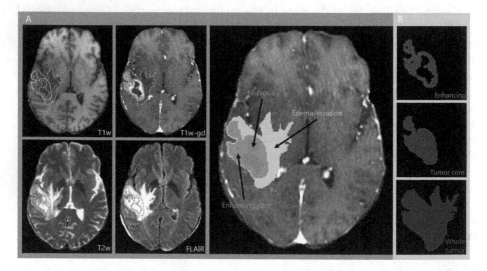

Fig. 1. Datas considered in the RSNA-ASNR-MICCAI BraTS 2021 challenge. (**A**) Different MRI sequences with associated clinical annotations. (**B**) Regions considered for the performance evaluation (Enhancing Tumor: ET, Tumor Core: TC, Whole Tumor: WT).

2.2 Neural Network Architecture

U-Net$_{V1}$. This architecture is the network leveraged in the BraTS 2020 Challenge, which ranked 5. It follows a 3D U-Net model [9] with minor modifications and consists of a four levels encoder-decoder with a pseudo-fifth level at the same spatial resolution as the fourth level that was interconnected by concatenations. The initial number of filters is 48, which is doubled at each downsampling. Downsampling was performed by a MaxPool layer with a kernel size of $2 \times 2 \times 2$ with stride 2, and Upsampling was performed using trilinear interpolation. The number of kernels in the decoder mirrors that of the encoder. ReLUs [33] are used as nonlinearities. Group normalization [42] with 8 groups is used for feature map normalization. The auxiliary segmentation outputs used for deep supervision during training branches out to all levels. The last convolutional layer used a $1 \times 1 \times 1$ kernel with three output channels and a sigmoid activation. The archicture is shown in Fig. 2.

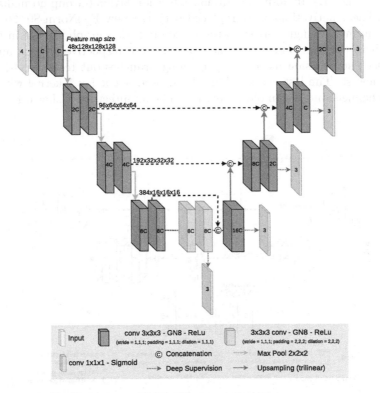

Fig. 2. U-Net$_{V1}$. Network architecture used in BraTS 2020. For training an input patch size of $128 \times 128 \times 128$ was selected. Features map size are displayed in the encoder part of the architecture. The letter in each block is the number of channels ($C = 48$).

U-Net$_{V2}$. Inspired by the state-of-the-art performance of the U-Net variants [17,34,38,39] and the successful results of last year's network, we have extended the architecture using several modules derived from the COPLE-Net [41]. The U-Net$_{V2}$ uses the same number of stages and filters per stage as the U-Net$_{V1}$. First, the downsampling performed by only max-pooling has been replaced by a concatenation of max-pooling and average-pooling, thanks to which the information loss is minimized. Second, a bridge layer (i.e., $1 \times 1 \times 1$ convolution) is used to map low-level encoder features to a lower dimension (i.e., the channel number is halved) before concatenating them with high-level decoder features to bridge the semantic gap between low-level and high-level features [36]. To match the output of the bridge layer, we construct each up-sampling layer in the decoder using a $1 \times 1 \times 1$ convolution layer followed by trilinear interpolation. Third, we include an Atrous Spatial Pyramid Pooling (ASPP) module [8] at the encoder-decoder bottleneck to better capture multi-scale information for segmentation of different lesion size. The ASSP is a simplified version with four dilations rates (1, 2, 4, 6) concatenated in a $1 \times 1 \times 1$ convolution (Fig. 4A). Fourth, after each convolutional block, we add a Squeeze-and-Excitation (SE) block [14] (Fig. 4B). In addition, all normalization layers (Group normalization) and non-linear activations were replaced with the new EvoNorm-S0 [26] which unify them into a single tensor-to-tensor computation graph, except in the SE block where the first and second activations were respectively ReLu and Sigmoid. Deep supervision used during training branches out to all levels, except the last lowest. The last convolutional layer used a $1 \times 1 \times 1$ kernel with three output channels and a sigmoid activation. The architecture is shown in Fig. 3.

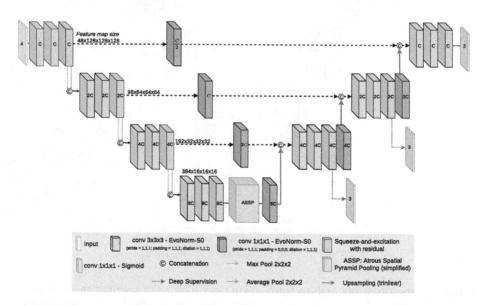

Fig. 3. U-Net$_{V2}$. Network architecture proposed in BraTS 2021. For training an input patch size of $128 \times 128 \times 128$ was selected. Features map size are displayed in the encoder part of the architecture. The letter in each block is the number of channels ($C = 48$). Max-pooling and average pooling were used to minimize downsampling information loss. Bridge layers were used to bridge the semantic gap between encoder and decoder features. ASPP block was utilized to better capture multi-scale information. EvoNorm-S0 replaced all normalization layers and non-linear activations in each convolution block.

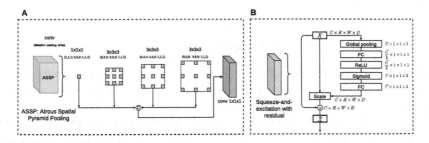

Fig. 4. Modules in U-Net$_{V2}$. (**A**) ASSP: Atrous Spatial Pyramid Pooling. ASSP exploits multi-scale features by employing multiple parallel filters with different rates. (**B**) Squeeze-and-Excitation with residual.

2.3 Generic Details for Training

On-the-Fly Preprocessing. mpMRI datas were converted into a 4-channel volume where each channel corresponded to an MRI sequence. Annotations labels (ET, NET-NCR, ED) were converted into a 3-channel volume where each channel corresponded to a region volume (TC, WT, ET). The 4-channel input image volumes were cropped to the minimum bounding box containing non-zeros voxels. Input images were then randomly cropped to the defined patch size of $128 \times 128 \times 128$ voxels. To avoid overfitting, augmentation techniques were applied as random rotation of $90°$ along the (x, z) plane (70% probability), random flip along all axes (70% probability), random shift of intensities (70% probability), random contrast intensities adjustment with gamma comprised between 0.5 and 4.5 (20% probability), random Gaussian noise using a centered normal distribution with a standard deviation of 0.1 (50% probability), random Gaussian smoothing (20% probability). Finally, z-score standardization was performed into the non-zeros voxels to each channel independently [7]. Outliers $> 3 \times std$ were clipped.

Optimization and Regularization. The Ranger 2020 optimizer was used [27, 44]. Ranger is a synergistic combination of RAdam + LookAhead. The initial learning rate was set to $\eta = 3e^{-4}$ and progressively decreased to 0 according to the cosine annealing strategy [12]:

$$\eta_t = \frac{1}{2}\left(1 + \cos\left(\frac{t\pi}{T}\right)\right)\eta \qquad (1)$$

where η_t is the learning rate at epoch t and T corresponds to the total numbers of epochs. The k parameters controlling the number of batchs before merging the LookAhead weights was set to 6. The *alpha* parameter controlling the percentage of the LookAhead difference to update was set to 0.5. Coefficients *betas* used for computing running averages of gradient and its square were set to (0.95, 0.99). L2 regularization was added with a weight of $1e^{-5}$.

Loss. The optimization was performed using the Dice Loss [31] computed batch-wise and channel-wise, without weighting, written as:

$$\mathcal{L}_{dice} = 1 - \frac{2 \times \sum_i^N p_i g_i + \epsilon}{\sum_i^N p_i^2 + \sum_i^N g_i^2 + \epsilon} \qquad (2)$$

where N is the number of voxels, p_i and g_i correspond to the predicted and ground truth labels per voxel respectively, and $\epsilon = 1e^{-5}$ is added to avoid zero division.

A variant which is the Jaccard Loss (soft intersection over union) has been used where the denominator $\sum_i^N p_i^2 + \sum_i^N g_i^2 + \epsilon$ in the Dice Loss was replaced with $2 \times (\sum_i^N p_i^2 + \sum_i^N g_i^2 - \sum_i^N p_i g_i) + \epsilon$.

Implementation and Scheme. The pytorch version 1.9.0 [37] and MONAI version 0.6.0 [29] for utilities were used. Automatic mixed precision training was used to reduce memory consumption, accelerated the training procedure, and gain a little extra performance [12]. Models were trained from scratch using a five-fold cross-validation procedure with fixed split. The validation set was only utilized to monitor the network's performance. The total number of epochs was set to 150, where one epoch represents a full pass on the train set. The batch size was set to 1. Every two epochs, a validation step was performed, and the models' weights were saved based on the consideration of a decrease in the value of the validation loss. Models were trained on a Nvidia Tesla V100 (16 GB memory).

2.4 Inference

Pre-processing. The initial 4-channel volume was cropped to the minimal brain extent, z-score standardized into the non-zero voxels to each channel independently with clipping of outliers $> 3 \times std$. Finally, the 4-channel volume was zero-padded, so that the matrices were divisible by 8.

Test-Time Augmentation (TTA). For each sample, TTA was adopted to further improve the segmentation performance, with 16 different augmentations. These augmentations have been made in 2 planes (axial and coronal) with 2 horizontal flips and 4 rotations (0°, 90°, 180°, 270°).

Ensembling. Each model gives 17 predictions (16TTA + 1). After cross-validation, we get 5 models, i.e. 85 predictions per sample ($5 \times (16 + 1)$). In order to obtain the binarized segmentation, all these predictions have been averaged, then thresholded at 0.5.

Post-processing. Voxels of the 3-channel volume (TC, WT, ET) potentially present in the background of the MRI images were removed. Then, the segmentation map was reconstructed into a 3D volume with the original labels (NCR/NET - label 1, ED - label 2, and, ET - label 4). Boolean operators were used for this purpose. Label 4 was left untouched, and label 1 was the TC excluding the ET, while label 2 was the WT excluding the TC. Then, isolated connected components under the threshold of 20 voxels were removed. As suggested by previous works [19,20,22], the ET label under the threshold of 300 voxels was replaced with its closest value in the axial plane (2D nearest interpolation).

2.5 Evaluation Metrics

The sub-regions considered for evaluation are the ET, TC, and WT. The two main metrics for the evaluation of segmentation performance in the medical domain are used. The first is the Dice similarity coefficient (DSC) [10], an overlap-based metric, defined as:

$$DSC = \frac{2\,|S_g \cap S_p|}{|S_g| + |S_p|} = \frac{2\,TP}{2\,TP + FP + FN} \tag{3}$$

where S_g is the ground truth segmentation and S_t the predicted segmentation. The DSC formula can also be written from the four basic cardinalities of the confusion matrix: true positives (TP), false positives (FP), true negatives (TN) and false negatives (FN). The best value is 1 and the lowest 0.

The second is the Hausdorff Distance (HD), a spatial distance-based metric. HD between two finite point sets A and B is defined by:

$$\mathrm{HD}(A, B) = \max(h(A, B), h(B, A)) \tag{4}$$

where $h(A, B)$ is called the directed Hausdorff distance and is given by:

$$h(A, B) = \max_{a \in A} \min_{b \in B} \|a - b\| \tag{5}$$

where $\|a - b\|$ is a norm, e.g. Euclidean distance. HD is usually sensitive to outliers. Given the prevalence of noise and outliers in medical segmentations, it is not advised to utilize HD directly [11,43]. A solution to remove outliers is to implement the percentile approach described by Huttenlocher et al. [15]. The 95th percentile is used in this assessment (HD95). The best value is 0 and the poorer value is the maximum euclidean distance of the image, that is 373.13 mm.

3 Results and Discussion

3.1 Online Validation Dataset

We evaluated the performance of our method on the provided validation set and reported the results given by the online evaluation platform for DSC and HD95 metrics. The results are presented in Table 1. The results reported were from models trained using the BraTS 2021 training set with 5-fold cross-validation and the usage of TTA during prediction. Here (*) and (**) denote models trained both using a 5-fold cross-validation but with different seeds. JL indicates the use of Jaccard Loss during training. For the same seed (*) used in the cross-validation, we can observe that the V1 network has the worst performance if we consider the average DSC for the three volumes with a value of 0.87326. However, even if the U-Net$_{V2}$ performs better in terms of DSC, results were contradictory for the HD95 metric for which the U-Net$_{V1}$ has an average value of 9.85108 mm compared to 10.84598 mm for the U-Net$_{V2}$. Using a different seed in the cross-validation for the U-Net$_{V2}$, the results are improved in terms

Table 1. Segmentation performances of our method on the BraTS 2021 validation set. DSC: dice similarity coefficient, HD95: Hausdorff distance (95%), WT: whole tumor, TC: tumor core, ET: enhancing tumor core. (*) indicates an ensembling of a fixed 5-fold cross-validation with a fixed seed. (**) indicates an ensembling of a fixed 5-fold cross-validation with a different fixed seed from (*). (*+**) indicates and ensembling of the two cross-validations with different seeds (i.e., 10 models). (*, JL) indicates the use of Jaccard loss in the cross-validation with seed from (*). (**+(*, JL)) indicates the ensembling of (**) and (*, JL), (i.e., 10 models). (*+**+(*, JL)) indicates the ensembling of (*), (**) and, (*, JL), (i.e., 15 models). The grey line corresponds to the model selected for the test.

Sub. ID	Method	DSC				HD95			
		WT	TC	ET	Mean	WT	TC	ET	Mean
9715210	U-Net$_{V1}$$^{(*)}$	0.91904	0.86616	0.83454	0.87326	4.40718	9.39596	15.75011	9.85108
9715055	U-Net$_{V2}$$^{(*)}$	0.92349	0.86827	0.83265	0.87475	**4.12874**	10.92845	17.48075	10.84598
9715112	U-Net$_{V2}$$^{(**)}$	0.92393	0.87063	0.83997	0.87782	4.61502	9.34665	15.80434	9.92200
9715113	U-Net$_{V2}$$^{(*+**)}$	0.92436	0.87168	0.84000	0.87868	4.49349	7.71372	14.15743	8.78821
9715160	U-Net$_{V2}$$^{(*, JL)}$	0.92462	0.87712	0.83994	0.88056	4.25690	9.21011	14.16697	9.21133
9715224	U-Net$_{V2}$$^{(**+(*, JL))}$	0.92457	**0.87811**	**0.84094**	**0.88121**	4.19442	7.55256	**14.13390**	**8.62696**
9715209	U-Net$_{V2}$$^{(*+**+(*, JL))}$	**0.92463**	0.87674	0.83916	0.88018	4.48539	**7.53955**	15.75771	9.26088

of DSC and HD95 with a mean value of 0.87782 and 9.92200 mm, respectively. The ensembling of the models from the two cross-validations (i.e., 10 models) has further improved the results for the U-Net$_{V2}$ for both DSC and HD95, with respectively a mean value of 0.87868 and 8.78821 mm. We also trained the model with the Jaccard loss from the cross-validation with the fixed split (*). This attempt gave the greatest improvement compared to all the previous ensemble strategies with an average DSC value of 0.88056, and an HD95 of 9.21133 mm. Assembling all the different cross-validation training of the U-Net$_{V2}$ (i.e., 15 models including the two different cross-validations with the Dice loss and the cross-validation with the Jaccard loss) did not improve the results (mean DSC: 0.88018, mean HD95: 9.26088 mm). The final model selected for testing (submission ID: 9715224) results from an ensemble of the V2 network trained with the cross-validation having given the best results with the Dice loss and the cross-validation using the Jaccard loss, whose performances in terms of mean value are respectively for the DSC and HD95, 0.88121 and 8.62696 mm.

We can see that the split of the data during training affects the performance of the models. This is probably due to noisy labels that we have reported on the discussion forum of the platform, but we did not have time to remove these patients and re-train models or use methods that would be less sensitive to noise. Moreover, it turns out that the Jaccard loss improves the results, but we could only train the models on one cross-validation due to lack of time. Furthermore, due to the limited number of three submissions per day to the online platform, it was not possible to consider a strategy for selecting the best models among the models resulting from cross-validation.

3.2   Test Dataset

Table 2 provides quantitative test set results. A significant discrepancy between validation and test datasets for the TC Hausdorff distance was noticeable, whereas all other measures showed a similar value. There was also an improvement in DSC for the enhanced tumor in the test dataset compared to the validation one.

Table 2. Quantitative test set results. Values were provided by the challenge organizers.

	DSC			HD95		
	WT	TC	ET	WT	TC	ET
Mean	0.92548	0.87628	0.87122	4.30711	17.84987	12.23361
StdDev	0.09898	0.23983	0.18204	8.45388	71.52831	59.54562
Median	0.95560	0.95975	0.93153	1.73205	1.41421	1.00000
25quantile	0.91378	0.91195	0.85409	1.00000	1.00000	1.00000
75quantile	0.97604	0.97916	0.95977	4.00000	3.00000	2.00000

4   Conclusion

In this work, we propose an ensemble of a Bridge-U-Net enhanced with a concatenation of max and average poolings for downsampling, Squeeze-and-Excitation (SE) block, Atrous Spatial Pyramid Pooling (ASSP), and EvoNorm-S0. This model reduces the gap between low and high-level features and captures the context at a multi-scale level. Compared to last year, this model allowed us to reduce the number of parameters from 23.2M (U-Net$_{V1}$) to 16.6M (U-Net$_{V2}$), which is helpful in the limited context of the challenge where the size limit of GPU for the evaluation was 12 Gb of memory. Given the limited timeline of the challenge, we did not have the time to leverage the network's potential and explore all parameters, such as modification of ASSP dilation rate, the addition of residual connection, modification of activation in SE block ... On the BraTS2021 online validation platform composed of 219 cases, the model selected for testing (submission ID: 9715224) which results from a U-Net$_{V2}$ ensemble trained on a cross-validation with a Dice loss and another with a Jaccard loss obtains an average DSC of 0.92457, 0.87811 and 0.84094, and a HD95 (in millimeters) of 4.19442, 7.55256 and 14.13390 for the WT, the TC and the ET respectively. Similarly, on the test dataset, results reached an average DSC of 0.92548, 0.87628 and 0.87122, and a HD95 (in millimeters) of 4.30711, 17.84987 and 12.23361. The source code for our submission is publicly available at https://github.com/Alxaline/BraTS21.

Acknowledgements. We would like to acknowledge Y. Boursin, M. Deloger, J.P. Larmarque and Gustave Roussy Cancer Campus DTNSI team for providing the infrastructure resources used in this work.

References

1. Baid, U., et al.: The RSNA-ASNR-MICCAI BraTS 2021 Benchmark on Brain Tumor Segmentation and Radiogenomic Classification. arXiv:2107.02314 [cs] (2021)
2. Bakas, S., et al..: Segmentation Labels for the Pre-operative Scans of the TCGA-GBM collection (2017). https://doi.org/10.7937/K9/TCIA.2017.KLXWJJ1Q
3. Bakas, S.: Segmentation Labels for the Pre-operative Scans of the TCGA-LGG collection (2017). https://doi.org/10.7937/K9/TCIA.2017.GJQ7R0EF
4. Bakas, S., et al.: Advancing The Cancer Genome Atlas glioma MRI collections with expert segmentation labels and radiomic features. Scientific Data 4(1), 170117 (2017). https://doi.org/10.1038/sdata.2017.117
5. Bakas, S., et al.: Identifying the best machine learning algorithms for brain tumor segmentation, progression assessment, and overall survival prediction in the BRATS challenge. arXiv:1811.02629 [cs, stat] (2019)
6. Benzakoun, J., et al.: Anatomical and functional MR imaging to define tumoral boundaries and characterize lesions in neuro-oncology. Cancer Radiotherapie: Journal De La Societe Francaise De Radiotherapie Oncologique 24(5), 453–462 (2020). https://doi.org/10.1016/j.canrad.2020.03.005
7. Carré, A., et al.: Standardization of brain MR images across machines and protocols: bridging the gap for MRI-based radiomics. Sci. Rep. 10(1), 12340 (2020). https://doi.org/10.1038/s41598-020-69298-z
8. Chen, L.C., Zhu, Y., Papandreou, G., Schroff, F., Adam, H.: Encoder-decoder with atrous separable convolution for semantic image segmentation. arXiv:1802.02611 [cs] (2018)
9. Çiçek, Ö., Abdulkadir, A., Lienkamp, S.S., Brox, T., Ronneberger, O.: 3D U-Net: learning dense volumetric segmentation from sparse annotation. arXiv:1606.06650 [cs] (2016)
10. Dice, L.R.: Measures of the amount of ecologic association between species. Ecology 26(3), 297–302 (1945). https://doi.org/10.2307/1932409
11. Gerig, G., Jomier, M., Chakos, M.: Valmet: a new validation tool for assessing and improving 3D Object segmentation. In: Niessen, W.J., Viergever, M.A. (eds.) MICCAI 2001. LNCS, vol. 2208, pp. 516–523. Springer, Heidelberg (2001). https://doi.org/10.1007/3-540-45468-3_62
12. He, T., Zhang, Z., Zhang, H., Zhang, Z., Xie, J., Li, M.: Bag of tricks for image classification with convolutional neural networks. arXiv:1812.01187 [cs] (2018)
13. Henry, T., et al.: Brain tumor segmentation with self-ensembled, deeply-supervised 3D U-Net neural networks: a BraTS 2020 challenge solution. In: Crimi, A., Bakas, S. (eds.) BrainLes 2020. LNCS, vol. 12658, pp. 327–339. Springer, Cham (2021). https://doi.org/10.1007/978-3-030-72084-1_30
14. Hu, J., Shen, L., Albanie, S., Sun, G., Wu, E.: Squeeze-and-Excitation Networks. arXiv:1709.01507 [cs] (2019)
15. Huttenlocher, D., Klanderman, G., Rucklidge, W.: Comparing images using the Hausdorff distance. IEEE Trans. Pattern Anal. Mach. Intell. 15(9), 850–863 (1993). https://doi.org/10.1109/34.232073

16. Isensee, F., Jaeger, P.F., Kohl, S.A.A., Petersen, J., Maier-Hein, K.H.: nnU-Net: a self-configuring method for deep learning-based biomedical image segmentation. Nat. Methods **18**(2), 203–211 (2021). https://doi.org/10.1038/s41592-020-01008-z

17. Isensee, F., Jäger, P.F., Full, P.M., Vollmuth, P., Maier-Hein, K.H.: nnU-net for brain tumor segmentation. In: Crimi, A., Bakas, S. (eds.) BrainLes 2020. LNCS, vol. 12659, pp. 118–132. Springer, Cham (2021). https://doi.org/10.1007/978-3-030-72087-2_11

18. Isensee, F., Kickingereder, P., Wick, W., Bendszus, M., Maier-Hein, K.H.: Brain tumor segmentation and radiomics survival prediction: contribution to the BRATS 2017 challenge. In: Crimi, A., Bakas, S., Kuijf, H., Menze, B., Reyes, M. (eds.) BrainLes 2017. LNCS, vol. 10670, pp. 287–297. Springer, Cham (2018). https://doi.org/10.1007/978-3-319-75238-9_25

19. Isensee, F., Kickingereder, P., Wick, W., Bendszus, M., Maier-Hein, K.H.: No new-net. In: Crimi, A., Bakas, S., Kuijf, H., Keyvan, F., Reyes, M., van Walsum, T. (eds.) BrainLes 2018. LNCS, vol. 11384, pp. 234–244. Springer, Cham (2019). https://doi.org/10.1007/978-3-030-11726-9_21

20. Jia, H., Cai, W., Huang, H., Xia, Y.: H2NF-net for brain tumor segmentation using multimodal MR imaging: 2nd place solution to BraTS challenge 2020 segmentation task. arXiv:2012.15318 [cs, eess] (2020)

21. Jiang, H., Cui, Y., Wang, J., Lin, S.: Impact of epidemiological characteristics of supratentorial gliomas in adults brought about by the 2016 world health organization classification of tumors of the central nervous system. Oncotarget **8**(12), 20354–20361 (2017). https://doi.org/10.18632/oncotarget.13555

22. Jiang, Z., Ding, C., Liu, M., Tao, D.: Two-stage cascaded U-Net: 1st place solution to BraTS challenge 2019 segmentation task. In: Crimi, A., Bakas, S. (eds.) BrainLes 2019. LNCS, vol. 11992, pp. 231–241. Springer, Cham (2020). https://doi.org/10.1007/978-3-030-46640-4_22

23. Jin, W., Fatehi, M., Abhishek, K., Mallya, M., Toyota, B., Hamarneh, G.: Artificial intelligence in glioma imaging: Challenges and advances. J. Neural Eng. **17**(2), 021002 (2020). https://doi.org/10.1088/1741-2552/ab8131

24. Kamnitsas, K., et al.: Ensembles of multiple models and architectures for robust brain tumour segmentation. In: Crimi, A., Bakas, S., Kuijf, H., Menze, B., Reyes, M. (eds.) BrainLes 2017. LNCS, vol. 10670, pp. 450–462. Springer, Cham (2018). https://doi.org/10.1007/978-3-319-75238-9_38

25. Kamnitsas, K., et al.: Efficient multi-scale 3D CNN with fully connected CRF for accurate brain lesion segmentation. Med. Image Anal. **36**, 61–78 (2017). https://doi.org/10.1016/j.media.2016.10.004

26. Liu, H., Brock, A., Simonyan, K., Le, Q.V.: Evolving normalization-activation layers. arXiv:2004.02967 [cs, stat] (2020)

27. Liu, L., et al.: On the variance of the adaptive learning rate and beyond. arXiv:1908.03265 [cs, stat] (2020)

28. Long, J., Shelhamer, E., Darrell, T.: Fully convolutional networks for semantic segmentation. arXiv:1411.4038 [cs] (2015)

29. Ma, N., et al.: Project-MONAI/MONAI: 0.6.0. Zenodo (2021). https://doi.org/10.5281/ZENODO.4323058

30. Menze, B.H., et al.: The multimodal brain tumor image segmentation benchmark (BRATS). IEEE Trans. Med. Imaging **34**(10), 1993–2024 (2015). https://doi.org/10.1109/TMI.2014.2377694

31. Milletari, F., Navab, N., Ahmadi, S.A.: V-Net: fully convolutional neural networks for volumetric medical image segmentation. In: 2016 Fourth International Conference on 3D Vision (3DV), Stanford, CA, USA, October 2016, pp. 565–571. IEEE (2016). https://doi.org/10.1109/3DV.2016.79

32. Myronenko, A.: 3D MRI brain tumor segmentation using autoencoder regularization. In: Crimi, A., Bakas, S., Kuijf, H., Keyvan, F., Reyes, M., van Walsum, T. (eds.) BrainLes 2018. LNCS, vol. 11384, pp. 311–320. Springer, Cham (2019). https://doi.org/10.1007/978-3-030-11726-9_28

33. Nair, V., Hinton, G.E.: Rectified linear units improve restricted Boltzmann machines. In: ICML, January 2010

34. Oktay, O., et al.: Attention U-Net: learning where to look for the pancreas. arXiv:1804.03999 [cs] (2018)

35. Ostrom, Q.T., Gittleman, H., Stetson, L., Virk, S.M., Barnholtz-Sloan, J.S.: Epidemiology of gliomas. In: Raizer, J., Parsa, A. (eds.) Current Understanding and Treatment of Gliomas. CTR, vol. 163, pp. 1–14. Springer, Cham (2015). https://doi.org/10.1007/978-3-319-12048-5_1

36. Pang, Y., Li, Y., Shen, J., Shao, L.: Towards bridging semantic gap to improve semantic segmentation. In: Proceedings of the IEEE/CVF International Conference on Computer Vision, pp. 4230–4239 (2019)

37. Paszke, A., et al.: PyTorch: an imperative style, high-performance deep learning library. arXiv:1912.01703 [cs, stat] (2019)

38. Qin, X., Zhang, Z., Huang, C., Dehghan, M., Zaiane, O.R., Jagersand, M.: U2-Net: Going deeper with nested U-structure for salient object detection. Pattern Recogn. **106**, 107404 (2020). https://doi.org/10.1016/j.patcog.2020.107404

39. Ronneberger, O., Fischer, P., Brox, T.: U-Net: convolutional networks for biomedical image segmentation. arXiv:1505.04597 [cs] (2015)

40. Tamimi, A.F., Juweid, M.: Epidemiology and outcome of glioblastoma. In: De Vleeschouwer, S. (ed.) Glioblastoma. Codon Publications, Brisbane (AU) (2017)

41. Wang, G., et al.: A noise-robust framework for automatic segmentation of COVID-19 pneumonia lesions from CT images. IEEE Trans. Med. Imaging **39**(8), 2653–2663 (2020). https://doi.org/10.1109/TMI.2020.3000314

42. Wu, Y., He, K.: Group normalization. arXiv:1803.08494 [cs] (2018)

43. Zhang, D., Lu, G.: Review of shape representation and description techniques. Pattern Recogn. **37**(1), 1–19 (2004). https://doi.org/10.1016/j.patcog.2003.07.008

44. Zhang, M.R., Lucas, J., Hinton, G., Ba, J.: Lookahead optimizer: K steps forward, 1 step back. arXiv:1907.08610 [cs, stat] (2019)

Brain Tumor Segmentation with Self-supervised Enhance Region Post-processing

Sergey Pnev[1], Vladimir Groza[1,4], Bair Tuchinov[1(✉)], Evgeniya Amelina[1], Evgeniy Pavlovskiy[1], Nikolay Tolstokulakov[1], Mihail Amelin[1,2], Sergey Golushko[1], and Andrey Letyagin[3]

[1] Novosibirsk State University, Novosibirsk, Russia
{s.pnev,n.tolstokulakov}@g.nsu.ru
{v.groza,bairt}@nsu.ru, vladimir.groza@mediantechnologies.com,
pavlovskiy@post.nsu.ru
[2] FSBI Federal Neurosurgical Center, Novosibirsk, Russia
letyaginay@bionet.nsc.ru
[3] Research Institute of Clinical and Experimental Lymphology, Branch of IC&G SB RAS, Novosibirsk, Russia
[4] Median Technologies, Valbonne, France

Abstract. In this paper, we extend the previous research works on the robust multi-sequences segmentation methods which allows to consider all available information from MRI scans by the composition of T1, T1C, T2 and T2-FLAIR sequences. It is based on the clinical radiology hypothesis and presents an efficient approach to combining and matching 3D methods to search for areas of comprised the GD-enhancing tumor in order to significantly improve the model's performance of the particular applied numerical problem of brain tumor segmentation.

Proposed in this paper method also demonstrates strong improvement on the segmentation problem. This conclusion was done with respect to Dice and Hausdorff metric, Sensitivity and Specificity compare to identical training/test procedure based only on any single sequence and regardless of the chosen neural network architecture. We achieved on the test set of 0.866, 0.921 and 0.869 for ET, WT, and TC Dice scores.

Obtained results demonstrate significant performance improvement while combining several 3D approaches for considered tasks of brain tumor segmentation. In this work we provide the comparison of various 3D and 2D approaches, pre-processing to self-supervised clean data, post-processing optimization methods and the different backbone architectures.

Keywords: Medical imaging · Deep learning · Neural network · Segmentation · Brain · MRI

The reported study was funded by RFBR according to the research project No 19-29-01103.

1   Introduction

MRI is the most common method of primary detection, non-invasive diagnostics and a source of recommendations for further treatment of brain diseases. The brain is a complex structure, different areas of which have different functional significance.

Structural and statistical analysis of brain lesions originates various associated problems and projects such as detection of the tumors, shape and specific sub-regions segmentation (i.e. necrotic part, (non-)enhanced part, edema), classification of the tumor presence and treatment follow up prognosis.

Recently, several methods and approaches aiming at the optimal usage of different neural networks were proposed. Usually the goal of these works is to improve the solutions stability, compensate for the lack of missing data and increase the model's explanatory ability. [1–4].

In the previous works we proposed and evaluated the data pre-processing method on the open and private datasets for brain tumor segmentation problems. [7,8]

The proposed approach is focused on the matching 3d methods search for areas comprising the GD-enhancing tumor and merging to generalized robust solution. Such methodology is explained by the currently used technique when the focused on the Enhance tumor Region for False Positive Predictions.

2   Dataset Analysis

BraTS 2021 dataset [9–13] consists of 2000 cases of gliomas including training (1251), validation (219), and testing parts. All available data is provided in the form of MRI scans describing a) native (T1) and b) post-contrast T1-weighted (T1C), c) T2-weighted (T2) and d) T2 Fluid Attenuated Inversion Recovery (T2-FLAIR) volumes.

Technically MRI multimodal volume scans are available as NIfTI files of the standardized shape of $155 \times 240 \times 240$ pixels. Accordingly, given details these scans were acquired with different clinical protocols and various scanners from multiple institutions. Also standardized pre-processing has been applied to all BraTS MRI scans including co-registration to the same anatomical template, resampling to a uniform isotropic resolution ($1\,\mathrm{mm}^3$) and skull-stripping [11].

As part of the presented work the authors of this paper performed an additional investigation and exploratory analysis on the provided dataset. As a result of this process some remarkable observations were made. There were multiple cases with the scans related to different MRI sequences that were performed in different directions and were not isovoxel-based. The interpolation performed during registration did not always result in high-quality images. Such significant mismatch in the data quality and visual representation made it difficult to compare various MRI sequences in order to make conclusions regarding the tumor's type, structure and correctness of the given segmentation GT. Mostly such difficulties were faced with the cases that required more than one sequence to be analyzed simultaneously (e.g., segmentation of the enhancing portion of the tumor).

All imaging volumes have been segmented using a number of machine learning algorithms, refined manually by volunteer neuroradiology experts, and were finally approved by experienced board-certified neuro-radiologists [11].

Provided within the RSNA-ASNR-MICCAI BraTS 2021 challenge ground truth (GT) segmentation annotations are given as multi-class segmentation masks with the following label values: the GD-enhancing tumor (ET - label 4), the peritumoral edematous/invaded tissue (ED - label 2) and the necrotic tumor core (NCR - label 1). The goal of the challenge comprises the metric evaluation based on the next sub-regions: 1) the "enhancing tumor" (ET), 2) the "tumor core" (TC) and 3) the "whole tumor" (WT) which are obtained directly from the initial annotation labels. According to the authors of the dataset, BraTS tumour visual features (sub-regions) are image-based and do not reflect strict biologic entities [11]. In accordance with the dataset description, this applies mainly to non-enhancing tumor, as it is difficult to distinguish from vasogenic edema. However in the given conditions TC region describes the bulk of the tumor, which is what is typically considered for surgical excision. The TC entails the ET, as well as the necrotic (NCR) parts of the tumor, the appearance of which is typically hypo-intense in T1Gd when compared to T1 [11].

Having encountered cases in the BraTS training sample where the TC volume was zero, we decided to exclude such items from our training set. Such a decision was made due to the fact that these images do not provide enough information (caused by various factors, and also possibly as the result of the original MRI scans quality) to identify the cancer process and do not help the competition's goal of segmenting brain *tumors*.

The features of the dataset listed above led us to make a pre-processing of the cases for the training dataset.

3   Methods

3.1   Pre-processing to Self-supervised Clean Data

This year, preliminary data partitioning was performed using the STAPLE [17] fusion of previous top-ranked BraTS algorithms namely, DeepScan [18], DeepMedic [19] and nnU-Net [20]. Radiologists then corrected and verified the cases. Our hypothesis was that many datasets contain complex and controversial cases. And these cases don't always give an increase in metrics on validation and test samples, but can worsen the grief. So we decided to split the training dataset into 5 training and validation subsamples, perform cross-validation and filter out unnecessary cases according to the metrics. We took nnU-Net as the baseline because of its ability to adapt to medical datasets and show strong results on them. We trained and ran 5 nnU-Net models on different folds of the training dataset. After running the inference on the corresponding validation subsamples, we obtained a description of the dataset and a list of cases suspected of being "bad". Next, we selected some thresholds for $DiceET$ and $DiceTC$ with the help of a specialist radiologist. All cases with metrics $DiceET < thr_1$ and $DiceTC < thr_2$ were removed from the training dataset. As a result, we filtered out 102 cases. We show the resulting metrics on the cleaned dataset in the Results section.

3.2   Initial 2D Approach

As the continuation of our previous research in this domain [5] we initially approached this problem with the use of well-proven methods. We considered both methods multi-class while optimizing the original GT labels and multi-label focused directly on the competition metrics ET/TC/WT.

To perform the segmentation of the brain tumors in head MRI scans, we used the *Encoder-Decoder* type neural networks. All exact models were originated from the *LinkNet* [14] pipelines with the pretrained encoder backbones, namely with the *se-resnext50_swsl* and *se-resnext101* [15] and corresponding decoders. Additionally we used Atrous Spatial Pyramid Pooling Module (ASPP) in the model bottleneck and Feature-pyramid network module (FPN) in the decoder.

Each block of the decoder consists of the 2D Convolution, Upsampling and another Convolution layer, each followed by the Batch Normalization and ReLU [16] activation function. In the last block of decoder we apply Softmax or Sigmoid activation (respectively for the multi-class and multi-label method).

We used only T1C, T1 and T2-FLAIR sequences as input for our models. We used the combination of these sequences to create the pseudo RGB-like images with three channels [6]. All Nifti volumes were processed to get 2D PNG images which were normalized to [0;1] range and resized from original size of 240×240 pixels to the common size of 256×256 pixels.

This 2D approach was tested using a 5-fold cross-validation scheme, strong data augmentations *on the fly* and simple ensemble averaging. Best obtained preliminary results on the local validation and Leader Board (LB) are given in the Table 1.

Table 1. Preliminary results on LB and local validation using 2D approach.

Validation	Dice_ET	Dice_TC	Dice_WT
Local 5-fold	0.72505	0.89408	0.79384
Leader Board	0.7763	0.8288	0.902

After in-depth analysis of obtained results, we concluded that the usage of described 2D methods is not consistent enough on this particular task due to the data-dependent specificity described in the Sect. 2 and will not lead to the strong performance. Such a conclusion routed our team to the use of more volume-specific and robust 3D methods.

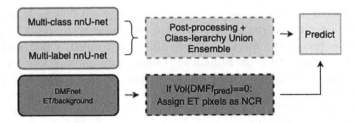

Fig. 1. Scheme of our final solution pipeline. We use an ensemble of 2 nnU-nets as a basic solution. DMFnet trained only on the ET-region acts as a classifier: if on the DMF predict, then translate all ET values on the ensemble predict into NCR.

3.3   NnU-Net

As a baseline 3D model, we took the winner BraTS2020 - 3d nnU-Net, without any modifications. It can automatically adapt itself to any given medical segmentation dataset. It is based on a standard encoder-decoder type architecture using skip-connection. The base unit consists of a Convolution 3×3, normalization as Instance Normalization and a Leaky ReLU activation function with a small negative slope of 0.01. Downsampling is done with Convolution with stride $= 2$ and Transposed Convolution for Upsampling. Deep supervision is performed on all decoder outputs except the 2 with the lowest resolution. The basic 3d nnU-Net uses the following hyperparameters: $patchsize = 128^3$, $batchsize = 2$, init number of convolution filters $= 32$, maximum number of convolution filters $= 320$.

It is known that training the model on classes used to evaluate the competition results allows to get a positive gain in metrics. In BraTS2021 the presented ground truth masks consist of classes: ED, ET, NCR. But metrics on validation are counted by the 3 overlapping regions: the "enhancing tumor" (ET), the "tumor core" (TC) and the "whole tumor" (WT). During the competition we tried optimization both for WT, TC, ET regions with sigmoid activation and training on the original classes NCR, ET, ED with softmax.

3.4   Post-processing

Enhance tumour is the most difficult class to segment because of its position and shape. When the ground truth mask for enhance tumor is empty, the BraTS score gives zero false positive predictions with a Dice score equal to 1, thus placing the corresponding algorithm in the (overall) first rank for this test case. Thus, by minimising the number of false positive predictions for enhance tumor, the Dice metric can be significantly improved, by about 1% for every 2 cases.

In past years, the main post-processing for the region of tumour accumulation was to replace enhance with necrosis if the enhance volume was below a certain threshold. This year, we did not find a clear correlation between the size of the contrasting part and whether or not enhancement would be false positive.

Having found false positives, we decided to help nnUNet look at it from a different perspective. In particular, to train the network to produce far fewer False Positive predicates for ET. To do this, we trained a fast and efficient DMFNet [21] architecture on Enhanced Tumor only, nulling loss for all other labels. We ended up with 3 DMF folds. Further, we selected 1 fold that gave the best results, both on training validation and on validation in the Synapse evaluation system. In Fig. 1 you can see a scheme of our final solution. Thus, the whole pipeline looks like this:

- predict the case with nnU-Net, get $pred_1$
- predict the case with DMFNet, get $pred_2$
- remove the really small ET regions on $pred_2$
- if tumor volume on $pred_2 = 0$, translate all enhance tumor voxels on $pred_1$ into necrosis.
- remove the really small WT and TC regions on $pred_1$

4   Results

In this work we present the segmentation performance as the main results, including the comparison of different various 3D and 2D approaches, pre-processing, post-processing optimization methods and several most commonly used architectures.

Calculating the mean Dice score with the consideration of the "empty" slices where Dice is assigned equal to 1 is a very common approach nevertheless not really fair. So, according to the BraTS challenge rules the mean Dice metric for each particular experiment was calculated only on the slices where ground truth (GT) or segmentation output is present at least for one of the given classes. All of our models were equally evaluated on the validation set of the BraTS 2021 challenge.

Table 2. The part of results Task 1 - Segmentation on the validation dataset.

Number of submit	Dice_ET	Dice_TC	Dice_WT
15_submit	0.7763	0.828	0.9020
70_submit	0.8498	0.8768	0.9229
73_submit	0.8474	0.8820	0.9242

In the Table 2 we presented 3 different submits just to highlight the improvement obtained regarding the modification and proposed hypothesis.

15_submit presents the initial 2D approach described above in the Methods section. 70_submit presents the solution based nn-Unet network with self-supervised clean data and post-processing for areas of the GD-enhancing tumor by DMF on ET. 73_submit stands for the merge two different nn-Unet networks with self-supervised clean data and post-processing for areas of the GD-enhancing tumor by DMF on ET.

All of our models were equally evaluated on the test set of the BraTS 2021 challenge. Detailed results can be observed below in the Tables 3 for the Multi-class Segmentation tracks respectively according to the official BraTS 2021 challenge metrics.

Table 3. Selected submission for the test set in Task 1 - Segmentation on the test dataset.

Label	Dice_ET	Dice_WT	Dice_TC	Hsdrf95_ET	Hsdrf95_WT	Hsdrf95_TC
Mean	0.86588	0.92067	0.86932	14.26795	5.63181	16.93973
StdDev	0.19707	0.10623	0.24502	65.09256	23.12064	68.40567
Median	0.93025	0.95320	0.95793	1	2	1.41421
25 quantile	0.85060	0.90773	0.91142	1	1	1
75 quantile	0.96357	0.97357	0.97958	2	4.18586	3.16228

We observe very strong stability of our results for both considered problems compared to the local and official validation with the constant increase of the metric values.

5 Conclusions

This work presents an efficient approach to combining and matching 3D methods to search for areas of the GD-enhancing tumor in order to significantly improve the model's performance of the particular applied numerical problem of brain tumor segmentation.

The proposed method also demonstrates significant improvement on the segmentation problem with respect to Dice and Hausdorff metrics compared to similar training/validation procedures based on any regardless of the chosen neural network architecture.

The stability and robustness of this method was confirmed with the various numerical experiments and with very high probability can be extended to many other applied problems. These particular results are very important from the clinical point of view and can strongly increase the quality of the computer-aided systems where similar solutions are deployed.

Acknowledgment. The reported study was funded by RFBR according to the research project No 19-29-01103.

References

1. Ge, C., Gu, I.Y., Store Jakola, A., Yang, J.: Cross-modality augmentation of brain MR images using a novel pairwise generative adversarial network for enhanced glioma classification In: 2019 IEEE International Conference on Image Processing (ICIP), pp. 559–563 (2019)
2. Havaei, M., Guizard, N., Chapados, N., Bengio, Y.: HeMIS: hetero-modal image segmentation. In: Ourselin, S., Joskowicz, L., Sabuncu, M.R., Unal, G., Wells, W. (eds.) MICCAI 2016. LNCS, vol. 9901, pp. 469–477. Springer, Cham (2016). https://doi.org/10.1007/978-3-319-46723-8_54
3. Varsavsky, T., Eaton-Rosen, Z., Sudre, C.H., Nachev, P., Cardoso, M.J.: PIMMS: permutation invariant multi-modal segmentation, CoRR, vol. abs/1807.06537 (2018). http://arxiv.org/abs/1807.06537
4. Dorent, R., Joutard, S., Modat, M., Ourselin, S., Vercauteren, T.: Hetero-modal variational encoder-decoder for joint modality completion and segmentation. arXiv:1907.11150 (2019)
5. Letyagin, A.Y., et al.: Artificial intelligence for imaging diagnostics in neurosurgery. In: 2019 International Multi-Conference on Engineering, Computer and Information Sciences (SIBIRCON), pp. 336–337. IEEE-Inst Electrical Electronics Engineers Inc. (2019)
6. Groza, V., et al.: Data preprocessing via multi-sequences MRI mixture to improve brain tumor segmentation. In: Rojas, I., Valenzuela, O., Rojas, F., Herrera, L.J., Ortuño, F. (eds.) IWBBIO 2020. LNCS, vol. 12108, pp. 695–704. Springer, Cham (2020). https://doi.org/10.1007/978-3-030-45385-5_62
7. Letyagin, A., et al.: Multi-class brain tumor segmentation via multi-sequences MRI mixture data preprocessing. In: 2020 Cognitive Sciences, Genomics and Bioinformatics (CSGB), Novosibirsk, Russia, pp. 185-189 (2020). https://doi.org/10.1109/CSGB51356.2020.9214645
8. Groza, V., et al.: Brain tumor segmentation and associated uncertainty evaluation using multi-sequences MRI mixture data preprocessing. In: Crimi, A., Bakas, S. (eds.) BrainLes 2020. LNCS, vol. 12659, pp. 148–157. Springer, Cham (2021). https://doi.org/10.1007/978-3-030-72087-2_13
9. Menze, B.H., Jakab, A., Bauer, S., Kalpathy-Cramer, J., Farahani, K., Kirby, J., et al.: The multimodal brain tumor image segmentation benchmark (BraTS). IEEE Trans. Med. Imaging 34(10), 1993–2024 (2015). https://doi.org/10.1109/TMI.2014.2377694
10. Bakas, S., Akbari, H., Sotiras, A., Bilello, M., Rozycki, M., Kirby, J.S., et al.: Advancing The Cancer Genome Atlas glioma MRI collections with expert segmentation labels and radiomic features. Nat. Sci. Data 4, 170117 (2017). https://doi.org/10.1038/sdata.2017.117
11. Baid, U., et al.: The RSNA-ASNR-MICCAI BraTS 2021 benchmark on brain tumor segmentation and radiogenomic classification. arXiv preprint arXiv:2107.02314 (2021)
12. Bakas, S., et al.: Segmentation labels and radiomic features for the pre-operative scans of the TCGA-GBM collection. Can. Imaging Archive (2017). https://doi.org/10.7937/K9/TCIA.2017.KLXWJJ1Q
13. Bakas, S., et al.: Segmentation labels and radiomic features for the pre-operative scans of the TCGA-LGG collection. Can. Imaging Archive (2017). https://doi.org/10.7937/K9/TCIA.2017.GJQ7R0EF

14. Chaurasia, A., Culurciello, E.: Linknet: exploiting encoder representations for efficient semantic segmentation. arXiv preprint arXiv:1707.03718 (2017)
15. Hu, J., Shen, L., Sun, G.: Squeeze-and-Excitation networks. arXiv preprint arXiv:1709.01507 (2017)
16. Agarap, A.F.: Deep learning using rectified linear units (ReLU). arXiv preprint arXiv:1803.08375 (2018)
17. Warfield, S.K., Zou, K.H., Wells, W.M.: Simultaneous truth and performance level estimation (staple): an algorithm for the validation of image segmentation. IEEE Trans. Med. Imaging **23**(7), 903–921 (2004)
18. McKinley, R., Meier, R., Wiest, R.: Ensembles of densely-connected CNNs with label-uncertainty for brain tumor segmentation. In: Crimi, A., Bakas, S., Kuijf, H., Keyvan, F., Reyes, M., van Walsum, T. (eds.) BrainLes 2018. LNCS, vol. 11384, pp. 456–465. Springer, Cham (2019). https://doi.org/10.1007/978-3-030-11726-9_40
19. Kamnitsas, K., et al.: Efficient multi-scale 3D CNN with fully connected CRF for accurate brain lesion segmentation. Med. Image Anal. **36**, 61–78 (2017)
20. Isensee, F., Jaeger, P.F., Kohl, S.A., Petersen, J., Maier-Hein, K.H.: nnU-Net: a self-configuring method for deep learning-based biomedical image segmentation. Nat. Methods **18**, 203–211 (2020)
21. Chen, C., Liu, X., Ding, M., Zheng, J., Li, J.: 3D dilated multi-fiber network for real-time brain tumor segmentation in MRI. In: Shen, D., et al. (eds.) MICCAI 2019. LNCS, vol. 11766, pp. 184–192. Springer, Cham (2019). https://doi.org/10.1007/978-3-030-32248-9_21

E_1D_3 U-Net for Brain Tumor Segmentation: Submission to the RSNA-ASNR-MICCAI BraTS 2021 challenge

Syed Talha Bukhari and Hassan Mohy-ud-Din$^{(\boxtimes)}$

Department of Electrical Engineering, Syed Babar Ali School of Science
and Engineering, LUMS,54792 Lahore, Pakistan
`hassan.mohyuddin@lums.edu.pk`

Abstract. Convolutional Neural Networks (CNNs) have demonstrated state-of-the-art performance in medical image segmentation tasks. A common feature in most top-performing CNNs is an encoder-decoder architecture inspired by the U-Net. For multi-region brain tumor segmentation, 3D U-Net architecture and its variants provide the most competitive segmentation performances. In this work, we propose an interesting extension of the standard 3D U-Net architecture, specialized for brain tumor segmentation. The proposed network, called E_1D_3 U-Net, is a one-encoder, three-decoder fully-convolutional neural network architecture where each decoder segments one of the hierarchical regions of interest: whole tumor, tumor core, and enhancing core. On the BraTS 2018 validation (unseen) dataset, E_1D_3 U-Net demonstrates single-prediction performance comparable with most state-of-the-art networks in brain tumor segmentation, with reasonable computational requirements and without ensembling. As a submission to the RSNA-ASNR-MICCAI BraTS 2021 challenge, we also evaluate our proposal on the BraTS 2021 dataset. E_1D_3 U-Net showcases the flexibility in the standard 3D U-Net architecture which we exploit for the task of brain tumor segmentation.

Keywords: U-Net · Segmentation · Brain tumors · MRI

1 Introduction

Accurate segmentation of brain tumor sub-regions is essential in the quantification of lesion burden, providing insight into the functional outcome of patients. In this regard, 3D multi-parametric magnetic resonance imaging (3D mpMRI) is widely used for non-invasive visualization and analysis of brain tumors. Different MRI sequences (such as T1, T1ce, T2, and FLAIR) are often used to provide

This work was supported by a grant from the Higher Education Commission of Pakistan as part of the National Center of Big Data and Cloud Computing and the Clinical and Translational Imaging Lab at LUMS.

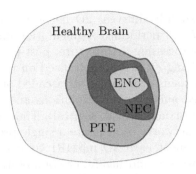

Fig. 1. The brain tumor region is usually considered as a hierarchical combination of three sub-regions: peritumoral edema (PTE), non-enhancing core (NEC), and enhancing core (ENC) [18]. The sub-regions are schematically shown here.

complementary information about different brain tumor sub-regions. The brain tumor region is usually categorized into three sub-regions: peritumoral edema (PTE), non-enhancing core (NEC), and enhancing core (ENC) [18], cf. Fig. 1. Alternatively, these sub-regions are usually considered in a hierarchical combination: Whole Tumor (WT: PTE ∪ NEC ∪ ENC), Tumor Core (TC: NEC ∪ ENC), and Enhancing Core (EN or ENC).

In the past decade, convolutional neural networks (CNNs) have achieved state-of-the-art performance in challenging medical image segmentation tasks. Among various CNN architectures, the U-Net [24] and its variants [6,8,16,20] stand out as the most promising architectures for medical image segmentation. However, segmentation of brain tumor and its sub-regions is challenging, even for deep neural networks, due to a number of reasons, including: (1) Scarcity of high quality imaging data, (2) presence of artifacts, (3) high class imbalance, and (4) large computational and memory requirements due to the volumetric nature of the data and its processing requirements when passed through the neural network.

In this paper, we presented an architecture comprising an encoder followed by three independent binary-output decoders (hence the name E₁D₃ U-Net), and fused the binary segmentations through standard image-processing techniques to generate a multi-class segmentation map. We made use of a reasonable computational budget to achieve competitive segmentation performance on the BraTS 2018 validation dataset, which we opted for since an extensive comparison with the state-of-the-art methods is readily available. Furthermore, as a submission to the RSNA-ASNR-MICCAI BraTS 2021 challenge, we also evaluated our proposal on the BraTS 2021 dataset.

2 Related Works

Previous work on brain tumor segmentation poses the problem from different perspectives: Pereira *et al.* [22] performed pixel-wise classification on small 2D segments through two slightly different 2D networks, one each for LGGs and HGGs. Kamnitsas *et al.* [13] performed segmentation on 3D segments through an efficient multi-scale processing architecture, post-processed by a 3D Conditional Random Field. Wang *et al.* [25] capitalized on the hierarchical structure of tumor sub-regions by using a hierarchical cascaded of networks: one for each sub-region. They utilized anisotropic convolutions and trained three such cascades, one for each view (axial, coronal, sagittal). Thus, the overall architecture requires 9 trained 2.5D networks to generate a single prediction. Dong *et al.* [8] used a 2D U-Net to segment each 3D mpMRI volume in slices. The method is fast in training and testing and has fewer computational requirements, but is massively over-parameterized ($\approx$ 35 million parameters) and does not capitalize on the 3D contextual information. Isensee *et al.* [11] used an ensemble of multiple 3D U-Nets trained on a large dataset, and focused on minor improvements to provide competitive segmentation performance. Myronenko [19] proposed an encoder-decoder architecture with an additional input reconstruction branch that guides and regularizes the encoder. The network stands out in terms of segmentation performance but is not implementable in a reasonable computational budget (the author mentions 32GB of GPU memory). Xu *et al.* [26] used an architecture composed of a common feature extractor which branches out to an attention-guided cascade of three relatively smaller 3D U-Nets to segment each hierarchical tumor sub-region. Each U-Net contains feature bridge modules, and the cascade is coupled by attention blocks to achieve a competitive segmentation performance.

Our proposed framework is independently developed from, but similar in essence to, the very recent work by Daza *et al.* [7]. The authors used a one-encoder, four-decoder architecture where three decoders perform binary segmentation (one for each hierarchical tumor sub-region) and the fourth decoder (arising from a *learned* linear combination of the learned parameters of the three binary decoders) performs the effective multi-class segmentation.

3   Methodology

3.1 E_1D_3 U-Net: One Encoder, Three Decoders

The *baseline* network in our study was based on the 3D No New-Net architecture [11] where we replaced max-pooling and tri-linear up-sampling layers with convolution-based up/down-sampling (as recommended in [12]). We refer to this baseline architecture as E_1D_1 U-Net, which is a variant of the original 3D U-Net [6], a fully-convolutional neural network consisting of a contracting path (encoder) and an expanding path (decoder). The encoder performs feature extraction through successive convolutions at different levels, and the decoder combines the encoded features with the semantic information at each level to produce the output segmentation map. Our proposed architecture, cf. Fig. 2, extends the baseline encoder-decoder architecture via a simple modification: Adding two additional decoders, similar in design to the original decoder. The resultant architecture consists of one encoder and three decoders, where

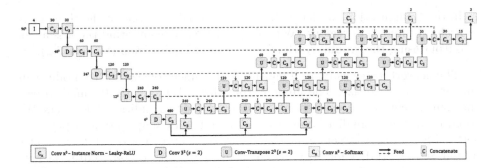

Fig. 2. The proposed E_1D_3 U-Net architecture is portrayed here. Each block denotes a *layer*, with the output spatial dimensions and number of feature maps noted beside it. The first layer $\boxed{I}$ denotes the input. All convolutional layers use zero-padding of $k-1$ (where k is the kernel-size) on both ends of each spatial dimension. Strided *Conv* layers (stride denoted by s) are used to down-sample the feature maps, while strided *Conv-Transpose* layers are used to up-sample the feature maps. *Copy and Concatenate* operation concatenates input feature maps with the corresponding output from the appropriate *Conv-Transpose* layer. Leaky-ReLU activation uses a *leakyness* parameter value of 0.01.

each decoder independently receives feature maps from the encoder to generate a segmentation at the output. We can write the overall functionality as:

$$\mathbf{z} = (\mathbf{z}_1, \mathbf{z}_2, \mathbf{z}_3, \mathbf{z}_4, \mathbf{z}_5) = E(\mathbf{x}) \tag{1}$$

$$\hat{\mathbf{y}}_r = D_r(\mathbf{z}), \quad r \in \{\text{WT}, \text{TC}, \text{EN}\} \tag{2}$$

where $E(.)$ and $D(.)$ respectively denote the Encoder and Decoder, $\mathbf{x}$ denotes the input sample/mini-batch, $\mathbf{z}$ is a tuple of feature maps obtained from each *level* of the encoder, and $\hat{\mathbf{y}}_r$ is the output binary mask of sub-region r from the decoder D_r. Note that E_1D_1 (standard U-Net) would simply be: $\hat{\mathbf{y}} = D(E(\mathbf{x}))$. The binary segmentation maps are fused to generate the final segmentation, cf. Sect. 3.3. In our proposed approach, we take inspiration from the following concepts:

1. *TreeNets* [15]: In these architectures, the network consists of multiple pathways that branch-off a common *stem*. This allows the network branches to share parameters at the earlier stages (where more generic features are anticipated during learning) while each branch has the freedom to specialize in a different task. Furthermore, parameters in the stem receive accumulated supervision from multiple sources (one per branch) which may favor learning robust low-level representations.

2. *Region-based Prediction* [25]: This concept proposes to organize the network in a way that it learns to optimize the hierarchical tumor regions, in contrast with segmenting each class independently. Such a configuration aims at directly optimizing the regions for which segmentation metrics are computed.

In our configuration, we let each decoder specialize in one of the three hierarchical tumor sub-regions (WT, TC, and EN) by computing the loss at its output using the ground truth of corresponding sub-region (cf. Sect. 3.2).

The network takes as input a multi-modal segment of size 96^3 to produce an output of the same size. The input/output size is kept relatively small to balance out the computational cost incurred by adding two additional decoders. We noted that using a smaller input size and more feature maps per layer performs better than using a larger input size and fewer feature maps per layer, under similar settings (GPU memory, batch size). In the latter case, a drop in performance is observed, more noticeably for TC and EN tumor sub-regions. Note that the architecture is still very simple and does not include many of the widely used components such as residual connections and deep supervision, which may significantly increase the memory requirements.

3.2   Training

Input to the network is a stack of 3D segments of shape 96^3 from each of the multi-parametric sequences. We extracted 3D segments at random from each subject volume within the whole-brain bounding box. Each extracted segment was subjected to *distortions* (with a 50% probability), which comprised of the following operations in sequence (each with a 50% probability): Random flipping along each axis, random affine transformation, random elastic deformation, and random gamma correction. We used a batch size of 2, the maximum allowable in our setup.

Parameters of all convolutional layers of the networks were initialized with He-normal weights. The networks were trained on the *mean* of the objective functions applied to the output from each *head* of the architecture. The overall objective function is therefore $\mathcal{L} = (\mathcal{L}_{WT} + \mathcal{L}_{TC} + \mathcal{L}_{EN})/3$, where each $\mathcal{L}_x$ is a non-weighted sum of the Soft Dice loss and the Cross-entropy loss functions, *i.e.* $\mathcal{L}_x = -\text{SoftDice} + \text{CrossEntropy}$. Stochastic Gradient Descent with Nesterov momentum (0.99), regularized by a weight decay of 10^{-6}, optimized the network. The learning rate was initially set to $\eta_0 = 10^{-2}$ and was modified at epoch-ends with a polynomial-decay policy $\eta_t = \eta_0(1 - t/t_{max})^{0.9}$, where $\eta(t)$ denotes the learning rate at the t-th epoch and t_{max} denotes the total number of epochs (500 in our setting).

3.3   Testing

During inference, segments of shape 96^3 (multi-parametric stack) were extracted from within the bounding box of the whole-brain region. Segments were extracted with a 50% overlap along each spatial axis, and *softmax* outputs from the network were averaged at all regions of overlap. The predicted hierarchical regions were fused to generate a multi-class segmentation map via a combination of morphological processing, cluster thresholding, and masking operations [25], cf. Fig. 3. The operations are ordered to impose the following constraints: (1)

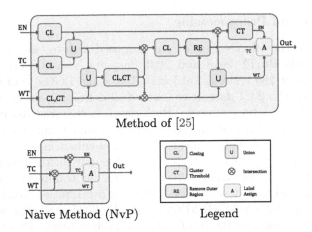

Method of [25]

Naïve Method (NvP)   Legend

Fig. 3. Label fusion procedure takes binary segmentation maps of WT, TC, EN regions and yields a multi-class segmentation map. *RE* block uses WT and TC binary maps to remove TC region that exists outside WT region. Refer to the code for implementation details.

The segmentations should be locally consistent and should not contain empty holes within the foreground (tumorous) region, (2) predicted tumor sub-regions in the segmentations should obey the hierarchical structure ($EN \subseteq TC \subseteq WT$), and (3) imposition of tumor hierarchy should not result in under-segmentation of tumor sub-regions.

In addition to raw segmentation results, we also present (where mentioned) results for test-time augmentation (TTA) [11,19] in which inference is performed on the original 3D mpMRI volume and its seven additional *transformed* versions. These transformations comprised of flipping along each of the three orthogonal axes (axial, coronal, and sagittal) individually as well as in combinations. The resulting probability maps were averaged (after un-flipping) to generate a unified probability map for each hierarchical region, before fusing the regions together to generate a multi-class segmentation map.

4 Experiments

4.1 System Specifications

For all experiments, we used open-source Python packages: NumPy [9], NiBabel [5], PyTorch [21], and TorchIO [23]. We used a computer system with 64 GB RAM and an NVIDIA RTX 2080Ti (11 GB) GPU. The source code for our method is made publicly available[1].

---

[1] https://github.com/Clinical-and-Translational-Imaging-Lab/brats-e1d3.

4.2   Dataset and Preprocessing

To demonstrate the effectiveness of our proposed architecture, we opt for the publicly available BraTS 2018 and 2021 datasets [1–4,18]. The BraTS 2018 dataset consists of 285 training subjects (HGGs and LGGs) and 66 validation subjects. The BraTS 2021 dataset consists of 1251 training subjects (HGGs and LGGs) and 219 validation subjects. Both datasets comprise 3D mpMRI scans (including T1, T1ce, T2, and FLAIR), with the manual segmentation of tumor sub-regions (comprising peritumoral edema, non-enhancing tumor, enhancing tumor, and healthy/background region) available only for the training subjects. For both BraTS 2018 and BraTS 2021 datasets, the training dataset was split into a training-fold and a validation-fold with a 9:1 ratio. Additionally, as a submission to the RSNA-ASNR-MICCAI BraTS 2021 challenge, we performed 5-fold cross validation over the BraTS 2021 training subjects. Predicted segmentations for each validation dataset are evaluated via the online portal provided by the organizers of the BraTS challenge[2]. We also provide scores on the BraTS 2021 testing dataset comprising 570 subjects (data and ground truth not provided), for which we provided the challenge organizers with a containerized inference routine of our method.

Before training/testing, we normalized each 3D MRI volume independently to zero-mean and unit-variance within the whole-brain region.

4.3   Segmentation Results

BraTS 2018: Evaluation results on the BraTS 2018 validation dataset are shown in Table 1. In terms of DSC, E_1D_3 (with as well as without TTA) performs competitively for the WT and TC regions, and outperforms most methods in the EN region. Coupled with test-time augmentation, E_1D_3 outperforms the best-performing ensemble of 3D VAE [19] in the whole tumor region, with only a fraction of the computational cost. E_1D_3 with single-prediction (without TTA) performs competitively with the ten-network ensemble of No New-Net [11]. These metrics show the efficacy of the proposed multi-decoder modification to the U-Net architecture, obviating the need for ensembles to obtain competitive performance. It must be noted that the No New-Net [11] architecture ensemble was trained on a larger training dataset (which the authors refer to as *co-training*) whereas we only make use of the BraTS 2018 training dataset. 3D VAE architecture and No New-Net architecture respectively bagged the top two positions in the BraTS 2018 challenge. The Anisotropic-RegCascade [25] uses a hierarchical cascade of three networks, one for each of the three tumor regions, and ensembles three different cascades, one trained for each 3D view. E_1D_3, with one trained network, outperformed the hierarchical cascaded networks in all three regions, in terms of DSC. The tumor core HD score achieved by E_1D_3 is better than all single-prediction and ensemble methods shown in Table 1.

---

[2] CBICA Image Processing Portal; https://ipp.cbica.upenn.edu/.

Table 1. Comparison of the state-of-the-art methods on the BraTS 2018 validation dataset. Mean of the Dice similarity coefficient (%) and 95-th percentile Hausdorff distance (mm) for each region were computed by uploading the predicted segmentations on the online evaluation portal of the BraTS challenge. '*' indicates the methods we implemented/evaluated on our system. For ensemble methods, (x) indicates an ensemble of x networks. Best scores for each section are in bold-face.

Method	Dice (%)			Hausdorff-95 (mm)		
	WT	TC	EN	WT	TC	EN
Ensemble Methods						
3D VAE$^{(10)}$ [19]	91.0	86.7	82.3	4.52	6.85	3.93
No New-Net$^{(10)}$ [11]	90.9	85.2	80.7	5.83	7.20	2.74
Kao et al.$^{(26)}$ [14]	90.5	81.3	78.8	4.32	7.56	3.81
Cerberus +TTA$^{(5)}$ [7]	89.5	83.5	79.7	7.77	10.30	4.22
Anisotropic-RegCascade$^{(3)}$ [25]	90.3 $\pm$5.7	85.4 $\pm$14.2	79.2 $\pm$23.3	5.38 $\pm$9.3	6.61 $\pm$8.6	3.34 $\pm$4.2
Single-prediction Methods						
3D VAE [19]	90.4	86.0	81.5	4.48	8.28	3.80
Cascaded-Attention-Net [26]	90.7	85.1	80.8	5.67	6.02	3.00
Cascaded V-Net [10]	90.5	83.6	77.7	5.18	6.28	3.51
3D-SE-Inception [27]	90.1	81.3	79.8	6.37	8.84	4.16
Cross-Modality GAN [28]	90.3	83.6	79.1	5.00	6.37	3.99
HDC-Net [17]	89.7	84.7	80.9	4.62	6.12	2.43
OMNet [29]	90.4	83.4	79.4	6.52	7.20	3.10
Proposed Method & Ablation Studies						
E_1D_3*	91.0 $\pm$5.4	86.0 $\pm$15.5	80.2 $\pm$22.9	6.56 $\pm$12.8	5.06 $\pm$6.8	3.02 $\pm$4.2
E_1D_3 +TTA*	91.2 $\pm$5.6	85.7 $\pm$16.6	80.7 $\pm$21.8	6.11 $\pm$12.1	5.54 $\pm$7.5	3.12 $\pm$4.1
E_1D_1 (Baseline)*	90.5 $\pm$6.4	84.0 $\pm$18.8	77.6 $\pm$25.6	6.44 $\pm$12.8	5.04 $\pm$6.0	3.67 $\pm$6.6
E_1D_1 (Baseline) +TTA*	90.8 $\pm$6.0	83.3 $\pm$20.6	78.4 $\pm$24.6	5.38 $\pm$9.8	6.13 $\pm$8.8	3.38 $\pm$6.2
E_1D_1-Wide*	89.6 $\pm$9.8	83.7 $\pm$19.4	77.7 $\pm$25.8	6.38 $\pm$12.2	6.02 $\pm$7.8	3.78 $\pm$7.6
E_1D_3-Br*	90.8 $\pm$6.0	85.4 $\pm$16.0	80.0 $\pm$22.1	7.02 $\pm$13.3	5.36 $\pm$5.9	3.13 $\pm$3.7
E_1D_3-Ens*	90.5 $\pm$6.4	84.0 $\pm$19.2	78.7 $\pm$24.5	6.10 $\pm$12.0	5.81 $\pm$6.5	2.75 $\pm$3.8
E_1D_3-NvP*	90.9 $\pm$5.6	85.8 $\pm$15.7	79.0 $\pm$25.0	6.83 $\pm$14.4	7.45 $\pm$15.6	3.09 $\pm$4.9

Since segmentation of the three hierarchical regions is not an independent task, we compare our E_1D_3 U-Net (with independent decoders) with a variant where the decoder for tumor core region branches-off the decoder for whole tumor region (after the first up-sampling stage), and the decoder for enhancing core region branches-off the decoder for tumor core region (also, after the first up-sampling stage). We refer to this variant as E_1D_3-Br. E_1D_3 performs slightly better than E_1D_3-Br and, therefore, advocates the use of three completely independent paths for WT, TC, and EN regions. One may also attribute the improvement in performance of E_1D_3 to greater expressivity arising from additional number of parameters added by two additional decoders. We therefore also compared E_1D_3 with E_1D_1-Wide, where the feature maps per layer were increased to match the parameter count of E_1D_3, and observed that this is not the case. To emphasize on the importance of specializing each decoder, we also trained E_1D_3-Ens, which is similar to E_1D_3 but with each decoder output being a multi-class probability map, which is averaged to generate the final prediction. In this case, we see slightly worse scores for WT region but larger differences in TC and EN sub-regions. Nevertheless, E_1D_3-Ens performs better overall compared to E_1D_1 (Baseline) and E_1D_1-Wide, reaffirming our intuition of TreeNets.

Table 2. Results for cross-validation on the BraTS 2021 training dataset (seen) and for evaluation on the BraTS 2021 validation and testing datasets (unseen) are presented. For the validation dataset, mean of the Dice similarity coefficient (%) and 95-th percentile Hausdorff distance (mm) for each tumor sub-region were computed by uploading the predicted segmentations on the online evaluation portal of the BraTS challenge. For the testing dataset, we uploaded a containerized inference routine to the online evaluation portal, which generated the segmentations and computed the corresponding metrics. For ensemble methods, (x) indicates an ensemble of x networks. Best scores for each section are in bold-face.

Method	Dice (%)			Hausdorff-95 (mm)		
	WT	TC	EN	WT	TC	EN
Training Dataset (cross-validation)						
E_1D_3	92.5 ±9.6	89.8 ±17.1	85.6 ±19.4	5.28 ±10.3	4.21 ±9.3	3.44 ±7.6
Validation Dataset (online)						
E_1D_3 (best fold)	91.9 ±7.7	86.5 ±19.1	82.0 ±23.4	4.13 ±5.6	7.51 ±35.5	16.61 ±69.6
E_1D_3+TTA (best fold)	92.3 ±7.5	86.6 ±20.1	82.6 ±22.9	3.99 ±5.7	8.23 ±36.2	18.14 ±73.6
$E_1D_3{}^{(5)}$	92.3 ±7.8	86.3 ±21.0	81.8 ±23.7	4.34 ±6.5	9.62 ±43.7	18.24 ±73.6
E_1D_3+TTA$^{(5)}$	92.4 ±7.6	86.5 ±20.8	82.2 ±23.4	4.23 ±6.4	9.61 ±43.7	19.73 ±77.4
Testing Dataset (online)						
E_1D_3+TTA (best fold)	91.8 ±10.2	86.7 ±24.3	86.5 ±17.2	5.68 ±17.7	17.36 ±68.4	9.51 ±48.9

To evaluate the impact of the employed post-processing pipeline of [25], we use a *Naïve* post-processing procedure, cf. Fig. 3, that simply imposes hierarchical constraints to generate the final segmentation map (termed as E_1D_3-NvP in Table 1). We observed that the network still produces DSC and HD scores comparable to top-performing methods, emphasizing that E_1D_3 by itself is well-designed, while the extensive post-processing method (comprising standard image-processing techniques) is recommended to yield better segmentations. To re-emphasize, we trained and tested all architectures mentioned under the *Proposed Method & Ablation Studies* heading of Table 1 using the same methodology (cf. Sects. 3.2 and 3.3), except for E_1D_1 (*training*: loss computed over single softmax output; *testing*: multi-class segmentation is readily obtained) and E_1D_3-Ens (*training*: loss averaged over each multi-class softmax output; *testing*: multi-class softmax outputs are averaged to yield final prediction). As stated previously, the difference between E_1D_3 and E_1D_3-NvP is only in the post-processing pipeline used in testing.

BraTS 2021: Results for five-fold cross-validation on the BraTS 2021 training dataset are presented along with inference results on the BraTS 2021 validation and testing datasets (unseen), cf. Table 2. E_1D_3 attained near-peak performance with single-model predictions only, as using an ensemble of five folds

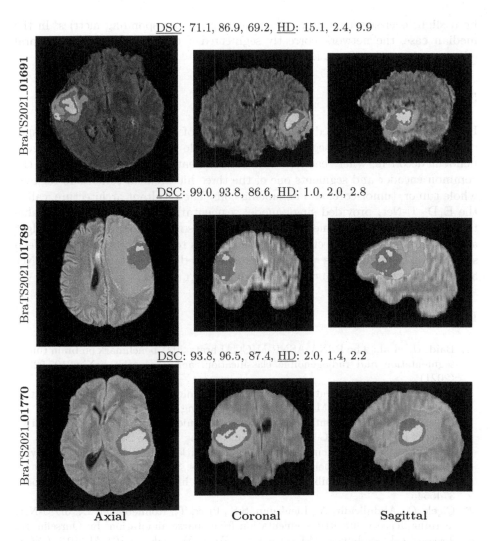

Fig. 4. Segmentations generated via E_1D_3+TTA for 25-th percentile (top), median (middle) and 75th-percentile (bottom) subjects from the BraTS 2021 validation dataset are shown alongside metrics, evaluated by the online portal, arranged as (WT, TC, EN). Label legend: Peritumoral Edema, Non-enhancing Core, Enhancing Core. (Ground truth is not publicly available.) (Color figure online)

did not improve significantly. One may attribute this to a well-designed architecture which extracts rich and useful features to achieve segmentations that are hard to improve further, without significant changes. Segmentation performance can be qualitatively judged through the segmentation maps shown in Fig. 4, where median, better and relatively worse cases are shown. In the worse case, we observe an isolated island of the peritumoral edema region, which may be a slight over-segmentation causing a drop in corresponding metrics. In the median case, the network correctly segmented a noticeably large peritumoral edema region, achieving a DSC of 99.0.

5   Conclusion

In this paper, we proposed a simple extension of the U-Net architecture specialized for brain tumor segmentation. We couple an encoder with three independent decoders, where each decoder receives features maps directly from the common encoder and segments one of the three hierarchical tumor sub-regions: whole tumor, tumor core, and enhancing core. The resultant architecture, called the E_1D_3 U-Net, provided single-model segmentation performance comparable to many state-of-the-art networks, within a reasonable computational budget and without major architectural novelties such as residual connections and deep supervision. Through this work, we demonstrated the flexibility of the U-Net architecture, which can be exploited for the task at hand.

References

1. Baid, U., et al.: The RSNA-ASNR-MICCAI brats 2021 benchmark on brain tumor segmentation and radiogenomic classification. arXiv preprint arXiv:2107.02314 (2021)
2. Bakas, S., et al.: Segmentation labels and radiomic features for the pre-operative scans of the TCGA-GBM collection. Can. Imaging Archive (2017)
3. Bakas, S., et al.: Segmentation labels and radiomic features for the pre-operative scans of the TCGA-LGG collection. Can. Imaging Archive 286 (2017)
4. Bakas, S., et al.: Advancing the cancer genome atlas glioma MRI collections with expert segmentation labels and radiomic features. Sci. Data **4**, 170117 (2017)
5. Brett, M., et al.: nipy/nibabel: 2.5.2, April 2020. https://doi.org/10.5281/zenodo. 3745545
6. Çiçek, Ö., Abdulkadir, A., Lienkamp, S.S., Brox, T., Ronneberger, O.: 3D U-Net: learning dense volumetric segmentation from sparse annotation. In: Ourselin, S., Joskowicz, L., Sabuncu, M.R., Unal, G., Wells, W. (eds.) MICCAI 2016. LNCS, vol. 9901, pp. 424–432. Springer, Cham (2016). https://doi.org/10.1007/978-3-319-46723-8_49
7. Daza, L., Gómez, C., Arbeláez, P.: Cerberus: a multi-headed network for brain tumor segmentation. In: Crimi, A., Bakas, S. (eds.) BrainLes 2020. LNCS, vol. 12659, pp. 342–351. Springer, Cham (2021). https://doi.org/10.1007/978-3-030-72087-2_30
8. Dong, H., Yang, G., Liu, F., Mo, Y., Guo, Y.: Automatic brain tumor detection and segmentation using U-Net based fully convolutional networks. In: Valdés Hernández, M., González-Castro, V. (eds.) MIUA 2017. CCIS, vol. 723, pp. 506–517. Springer, Cham (2017). https://doi.org/10.1007/978-3-319-60964-5_44
9. Harris, C.R., et al.: Array programming with NumPy. Nature **585**(7825), 357–362 (2020). https://doi.org/10.1038/s41586-020-2649-2

10. Hua, R., Huo, Q., Gao, Y., Sun, Yu., Shi, F.: Multimodal brain tumor segmentation using cascaded V-Nets. In: Crimi, A., Bakas, S., Kuijf, H., Keyvan, F., Reyes, M., van Walsum, T. (eds.) BrainLes 2018. LNCS, vol. 11384, pp. 49–60. Springer, Cham (2019). https://doi.org/10.1007/978-3-030-11726-9_5

11. Isensee, F., Kickingereder, P., Wick, W., Bendszus, M., Maier-Hein, K.H.: No new-net. In: Crimi, A., Bakas, S., Kuijf, H., Keyvan, F., Reyes, M., van Walsum, T. (eds.) BrainLes 2018. LNCS, vol. 11384, pp. 234–244. Springer, Cham (2019). https://doi.org/10.1007/978-3-030-11726-9_21

12. Isensee, F., Jäger, P.F., Full, P.M., Vollmuth, P., Maier-Hein, K.H.: nnU-Net for brain tumor segmentation. In: Crimi, A., Bakas, S. (eds.) BrainLes 2020. LNCS, vol. 12659, pp. 118–132. Springer, Cham (2021). https://doi.org/10.1007/978-3-030-72087-2_11

13. Kamnitsas, K., et al.: Efficient multi-scale 3D CNN with fully connected CRF for accurate brain lesion segmentation. Med. Image Anal. **36**, 61–78 (2017)

14. Kao, P.-Y., Ngo, T., Zhang, A., Chen, J.W., Manjunath, B.S.: Brain tumor segmentation and tractographic feature extraction from structural mr images for overall survival prediction. In: Crimi, A., Bakas, S., Kuijf, H., Keyvan, F., Reyes, M., van Walsum, T. (eds.) BrainLes 2018. LNCS, vol. 11384, pp. 128–141. Springer, Cham (2019). https://doi.org/10.1007/978-3-030-11726-9_12

15. Lee, S., Purushwalkam, S., Cogswell, M., Crandall, D., Batra, D.: Why m heads are better than one: training a diverse ensemble of deep networks. arXiv preprint arXiv:1511.06314 (2015)

16. Liu, Z., et al.: Liver CT sequence segmentation based with improved U-Net and graph cut. Expert Syst. Appl. **126**, 54–63 (2019)

17. Luo, Z., Jia, Z., Yuan, Z., Peng, J.: HDC-Net: hierarchical decoupled convolution network for brain tumor segmentation. IEEE J. Biomed. Health Inform. **25**(3), 737–745 (2020)

18. Menze, B.H., et al.: The multimodal brain tumor image segmentation benchmark (brats). IEEE Trans. Med. Imaging **34**(10), 1993–2024 (2014)

19. Myronenko, A.: 3D MRI brain tumor segmentation using autoencoder regularization. In: Crimi, A., Bakas, S., Kuijf, H., Keyvan, F., Reyes, M., van Walsum, T. (eds.) BrainLes 2018. LNCS, vol. 11384, pp. 311–320. Springer, Cham (2019). https://doi.org/10.1007/978-3-030-11726-9_28

20. Oktay, O., et al.: Attention u-net: learning where to look for the pancreas (2018)

21. Paszke, A., Gross, S., Massa, F., Lerer, A., et al.: Pytorch: An imperative style, high-performance deep learning library. In: Wallach, H., Larochelle, H., Beygelzimer, A., d'Alché-Buc, F., Fox, E., Garnett, R. (eds.) Advances in Neural Information Processing Systems 32, pp. 8024–8035. Curran Associates, Inc. (2019). http://papers.neurips.cc/paper/9015-pytorch-an-imperative-style-high-performance-deep-learning-library.pdf

22. Pereira, S., Pinto, A., Alves, V., Silva, C.A.: Brain tumor segmentation using convolutional neural networks in MRI images. IEEE Trans. Med. Imaging **35**(5), 1240–1251 (2016)

23. Pérez-García, F., Sparks, R., Ourselin, S.: TorchIO: a Python library for efficient loading, preprocessing, augmentation and patch-based sampling of medical images in deep learning. arXiv:2003.04696 [cs, eess, stat] (2020). http://arxiv.org/abs/2003.04696

24. Ronneberger, O., Fischer, P., Brox, T.: U-Net: convolutional networks for biomedical image segmentation. In: Navab, N., Hornegger, J., Wells, W.M., Frangi, A.F. (eds.) MICCAI 2015. LNCS, vol. 9351, pp. 234–241. Springer, Cham (2015). https://doi.org/10.1007/978-3-319-24574-4_28

25. Wang, G., Li, W., Vercauteren, T., Ourselin, S.: Automatic brain tumor segmentation based on cascaded convolutional neural networks with uncertainty estimation. Front. Comput. Neurosci. **13**, 56 (2019)
26. Xu, H., Xie, H., Liu, Y., Cheng, C., Niu, C., Zhang, Y.: Deep cascaded attention network for multi-task brain tumor segmentation. In: Shen, D., et al. (eds.) MICCAI 2019. LNCS, vol. 11766, pp. 420–428. Springer, Cham (2019). https://doi.org/10.1007/978-3-030-32248-9_47
27. Yao, H., Zhou, X., Zhang, X.: Automatic segmentation of brain tumor using 3D SE-inception networks with residual connections. In: Crimi, A., Bakas, S., Kuijf, H., Keyvan, F., Reyes, M., van Walsum, T. (eds.) BrainLes 2018. LNCS, vol. 11384, pp. 346–357. Springer, Cham (2019). https://doi.org/10.1007/978-3-030-11726-9_31
28. Zhang, D., Huang, G., Zhang, Q., Han, J., Han, J., Yu, Y.: Cross-modality deep feature learning for brain tumor segmentation. Pattern Recogn. **110**, 107562 (2021)
29. Zhou, C., Ding, C., Lu, Z., Wang, X., Tao, D.: One-Pass Multi-task Convolutional Neural Networks for Efficient Brain Tumor Segmentation. In: Frangi, A.F., Schnabel, J.A., Davatzikos, C., Alberola-López, C., Fichtinger, G. (eds.) MICCAI 2018. LNCS, vol. 11072, pp. 637–645. Springer, Cham (2018). https://doi.org/10.1007/978-3-030-00931-1_73

Brain Tumor Segmentation from Multiparametric MRI Using a Multi-encoder U-Net Architecture

Saruar Alam[1,2(✉)], Bharath Halandur[2,3], P. G. L. Porta Mana[2,4],
Dorota Goplen[5], Arvid Lundervold[1,2], and Alexander Selvikvåg Lundervold[2,4]

[1] Department of Biomedicine, University of Bergen, Bergen, Norway
saruar.alam@uib.no
[2] Mohn Medical Imaging and Visualization Centre (MMIV), Department
of Radiology, Haukeland University Hospital, Bergen, Norway
[3] Department of Clinical Science, University of Bergen, Bergen, Norway
[4] Department of Computer Science, Electrical Engineering and Mathematical
Sciences, Western Norway University of Applied Sciences, Bergen, Norway
[5] Department of Oncology, Haukeland University Hospital, Bergen, Norway

Abstract. This paper describes our submission to Task 1 of the RSNA-ASNR-MICCAI Brain Tumor Segmentation (BraTS) Challenge 2021, where the goal is to segment brain glioblastoma sub-regions in multiparametric MRI scans. Glioblastoma patients have a very high mortality rate; robust and precise segmentation of the whole tumor, tumor core, and enhancing tumor subregions plays a vital role in patient management. We design a novel multi-encoder, shared decoder U-Net architecture aimed at reducing the effect of signal artefacts that can appear in single channels of the MRI recordings. We train multiple such models on the training images made available from the challenge organizers, collected from 1251 subjects. The ensemble-model achieves Dice Scores of 0.9274 ± 0.0930, 0.8717 ± 0.2456, and 0.8750 ± 0.1798; and Hausdorff distances of 4.77 ± 17.05, 17.97 ± 71.54, and 10.66 ± 55.52; for whole tumor, tumor core, and enhancing tumor, respectively; on the 570 test subjects assessed by the organizer. We investigate the robustness of our automated segmentation system and discuss its possible relevance to existing and future clinical workflows for tumor evaluation and radiation therapy planning.

Keywords: Brain tumor segmentation · CNNs · BraTS 2021

1 Introduction

A primary brain tumor typically originates from glial cells, while a secondary (metastatic) brain tumor has its origin in another organ. Gliomas are the most

This work was supported by the Trond Mohn Research Foundation [grant number BFS2018TMT07]. Data used in this publication were obtained as part of the RSNA-ASNR-MICCAI Brain Tumor Segmentation (BraTS) Challenge project through Synapse ID (syn25829067).

common type of primary brain tumor. Based on their lethality they are classified into low-grade (LGG) and high-grade (HGG). LGGs are less malignant and grow slowly, whereas the more lethal HGGs are highly malignant and grow rapidly. Accurate characterization and localization of tumor-tissue types plays a key role in brain-tumor diagnosis and patient management. Neuroimaging methods, in particular magnetic resonance imaging (MRI), provide anatomical and pathophysiological information about brain tumors and can aid in diagnosis, treatment planning and follow-up of patients. Manual segmentation of tumor tissue is a tedious and time and resource consuming task, prone to inter and intra-rater variability.

The objective of the present work is to develop a model that can aid the clinicians in distinguishing between tumor and normal brain tissue. A reliable tumor segmentation system may have enormous impact both on preoperative tumor staging and planning of the resection extent and possibly increase/decrease the rate of gross tumor resection, the postoperative assessment of residual tumor, and on radiotherapy planning. Automatic segmentation may be applied for delineating the critical structures as well as residual tumor and risk zones. Such a system may contribute to more standardized treatment and limit the radiotherapy dose to critical structures.

Deep learning models most frequently used for image segmentation have encoder-decoder architectures based on convolutional neural networks [13]. A particular example is U-Net [20]. Its basic architecture has skip connections, but has recently been improved with several additional features such as residual blocks [7], attention mechanisms [17], and squeeze-and-excitation blocks [8]. Making such models sufficiently robust to signal artifacts present in MRI channels is an important and challenging goal. We propose a novel U-Net architecture with five encoders and a shared decoder with attention blocks. Our architectural modifications to the standard U-Net [20] are intended to reduce the impact of signal artifacts when segmenting brain tumor subregions.

2   Dataset

We use preprocessed multiparametric MRI recordings from the data collection provided by the Brain Tumor Segmentation challenge 2021 (BraTS 2021) [1–5]. This dataset contains 2000 multiparametric examinations, split into three sets: 1251 for training, 219 for validation, 530 for testing. Each subject's examination consists of four MRI sequences: T1w, T1cw, T2w, and FLAIR. All MRI recordings were preprocessed by the organizer through (i) DICOM to NIFTI file format conversion; (ii) re-orientation and co-registering to a fixed anatomical template (SRI24) [19] to obtain an isotropic spatial resolution of $1 \times 1 \times 1$ mm^3 and matrix size of $240 \times 240 \times 155$; (iii) skull-stripping.

Each subject has three mutually exclusive delineated regions: necrotic and non-enhancing tumor core (NCR/NET; intensity label 1), peritumoral edema (ED; intensity label 2), and enhancing tumor (ET; intensity label 4) stored in a 3D segmentation mask image (ground truth) with the same spatial resolution and matrix size as the corresponding channel images. The organizer consider three non-mutually-exclusive tumoral regions to standardize overall assessment and evaluation in the competition: (i) enhancing tumor (ET); (ii) tumor core (TC $=$ ET $\cup$ NCR), (iii) whole tumor (WT $=$ ET $\cup$ NCR $\cup$ ED). The three labeled regions ET, TC, WT are clinically relevant to patient management (e.g. treatment, prognosis). The organizer's annotation procedure followed two steps: (i) fusion of tumor regions of top-performing segmentation models of the previous editions of the challenge (DeepMedic [12], DeepScan [15], and nnUNet [9]), (ii) manual refinement of the fused tumor regions by a team of neuroradiologists.

The ground truth segmentations of the 1251 patient examinations used for training are available to the BraTS 2021 participants. The ground truths for the validation and testing subjects are withheld from the participants. For the validation data, the participants get access to the images without masks and are tasked with producing masks that can be uploaded to the competition's evaluation platform. For the test phase the participants do not get access to the test data, but must instead upload their algorithms to the evaluation platform. This prevents overfitting of the models to the test data that could be caused by multiple iterations of submission, evaluation and model development.

3 Methods

3.1 Data Splitting Approach

Gliomas are heterogeneous, varying in size, shape, volume, and location in the brain. Splitting the data at random into training and validation sets might lead to under- or over-representation of some volume subranges in either set, with a consequent bias in the model's learning and our estimate of its generalization performance. To avoid such a bias the data are first binned into equal ET-volume subranges, and a 75:25 random split is then performed bin-wise to construct a training set and a training-validation set of 923 and 328 subjects, respectively. We choose to use the ET volume for binning because this region is more difficult to detect than the WT and TC regions.

3.2 Normalization and Data Augmentation

The BraTS challenge's dataset is acquired from several institutions worldwide having different scanners and acquisition protocols. This heterogeneity may lead to a spurious non-uniform intensity distribution in the dataset (domain shift), to which a deep learning model may not be robust. To combat this we employ histogram standardization [16], i.e. the centering and standardization of the voxel intensity distribution, on each MRI scan of the training, training-validation, and validation sets.

Data augmentation, consisting in feeding the model with additional transformed views of the same image, is a crucial training step. It provides the model with some degree of invariance under particular natural transformations, improving its generalization ability. The following nine augmentation transforms are applied on the fly during training:

1. One of the following transforms two at each iteration are selected with a probability of 0.4:
   i) Affine transformation (scale range: 0.9 to 1.1; rotation range: −15 to +15) with a probability of 0.6
   ii) Elastic deformation (number of control points: 7; displacement: 0 to 7, in a coarse grid) with a probability of 0.4
2. Crop of the foreground area and then extraction of a 128 × 128 × 128 patch by considering a ratio of non-tumor and tumor region
3. Zoom with minimum factor 0.9 to maximum 1.2 with a probability of 0.15
4. Additive i.i.d. Gaussian $N(0, 0.01)$ noise with a probability of 0.15
5. Gaussian smoothing with $\sigma \in [0.5, 1.15]$ with a probability of 0.15
6. Shift of intensity with a factor of 0.3 with a probability of 0.15
7. Rescaling of intensity with a factor of 0.3 with a probability of 0.15
8. Addition of Gibbs noise with $\alpha \in [0.1, 0.5]$ with a probability of 0.15
9. Individual flip of each image axis with a probability of 0.5

For histogram standardization, affine transformation, and elastic deformation we use the implementations in the TorchIO library [18], while the remaining transforms are implemented using the MONAI library [14].

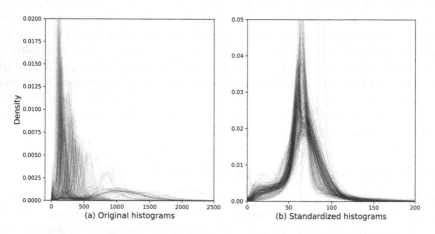

Fig. 1. (a) Original and (b) Standardized histograms of FLAIR images of the organizer's validation set (219 subjects). Note that the signal intensity distributions become more homogeneous across the standardized intensity range.

3.3 Multi-encoder U-Net Architecture

Our proposed architecture is based on an encoder-decoder U-Net, as illustrated in Fig. 2. The encoders reduce the spatial resolution of the feature map while increasing the number of channels at every step. The decoders increase the spatial resolution of the feature map while decreasing the number of channels.

Every encoder branch has five downsampling steps with filter sizes 16, 32, 64, 128, 160, 160. Each step has two consecutive $3 \times 3 \times 3$ convolution layers. Each convolution layer employs an Instance Normalization and a leaky ReLU activation (Conv3d-InstanceNorm3d-LReLU). At the first step of every encoder branch, we use stride size 1 for both convolutional layers. The resolution of the feature map therefore remains the same as the resolution of the input patch at the first step of the encoder. From the second step of the encoder branch to the bottleneck step, the first convolutional layer uses strided convolutions.

Every decoder branch has five upsampling steps, each with two consecutive $3 \times 3 \times 3$ convolution layers preceded by a $2 \times 2 \times 2$ transpose convolution, increasing feature map resolution and reducing channels. The feature map from the corresponding step of the encoder is concatenated with the feature map from the transpose convolution. The concatenated feature map is fed to the two convolutional layers. In the last n layers, a $1 \times 1 \times 1$ convolution finally maps the channels to three tumor regions for the decoder that has n deep-supervision heads (DS heads). The preceding $n\text{-}1$ DS heads are upsampled with nearest-neighbour interpolation to maintain the same resolution as n-th head. In other words, a model with n heads provides n feature maps having the same resolution as the input patch in training mode. While in inference mode, the model only considers the last layer (or head).

We use five encoders, each training a different MRI-image subset: {T1w, T1cw, T2w, FLAIR}, {T1w, T1cw, FLAIR}, {T1w, T1cw, T2w}, {T1w, T2w, FLAIR}, and {T1cw, T2w, FLAIR}. All encoders share a common decoder. In decoder steps, the feature maps from the corresponding steps of the encoders are concatenated to feed into channel attention blocks. The feature maps from channel attention blocks are concatenated with the feature map from the transpose convolution.

3.4 Training Variants of Multi-encoder U-Net

We employ two different pipelines to train our multiencoder U-Net (MEU-Net) model.

Pipeline A: The models are trained based on three consecutively inclusive BraTS-specific regions: ET $\subseteq$ TC $\subseteq$ WT. Earlier studies [9,10] found that such training increases the model's ability to segment the regions used to rank participants. This pipeline contains two model subtypes: (i) a MEU-Net with four DS heads; (ii) a MEU-Net with three DS heads. In *sub-type (i)*, all DS heads are jointly optimized with a weighted loss. The higher the layer is in the decoder, the larger the weights we assign to the head. We assign larger weights in the upper decoder layer to penalize the higher resolution feature map for achieving better

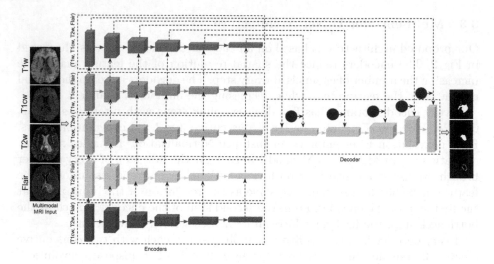

Fig. 2. Adopted multi-encoder-based U-Net architecture

spatial localization. In *sub-type (ii)*, the DS heads are optimized together with a weighted loss. The lower the layer is in the decoder, the larger the weight we provide to the head. Larger weights are provided in lower layers in the decoder to learn from the lower resolution feature map closer to the bottleneck layer, which contains compressed feature representations.

Pipeline B: A MEU-Net is trained on the mutually exclusive BraTS ground truth-specific regions: NCR/NET, ED, ET. The model has four DS heads, optimized with a weighted loss, with larger weights for the upsampling layer of the decoder. This pipeline also contains two model sub-types: (i) a MEU-Net containing encoders similar to the encoders of the models in pipeline A, (ii) a MEU-Net containing encoders with fewer filter set than that of *sub-type (i)*. The *sub-type (ii)* uses fewer filters than *sub-type (i)* to ensure that the model remains within the memory constraints when ensembling.

Pipelines A and B are trained with combined binary cross-entropy and dice loss to optimize each tumor region independently. We use the Ranger21 optimizer with an initial learning rate of $1e-03$ in both pipelines [21]. The Ranger21 combines the AdamW optimizer with various components such as adaptive gradient clipping, gradient centralization, stable weight decay, linear learning rate warm-up, a learning rate scheduler, and lookahead [21]. It has been shown to outperform the Adam optimizer in several benchmark datasets [21]. We observe that the Ranger21 achieves faster convergence and a smooth loss surface during the training phase. For the pipeline A and its subtypes, the MEU-Net is first trained for 120 epochs, using a single split (our training /training-validation set as described in Sect. 3.1). The models are thereafter fine-tuned on the entire training set. For the pipeline B and its subtypes, the MEU-Net is just fine-

tuned on the entire training set using the pre-trained weights from the models
of pipeline A.

We employ ensembling to increase the performance of the produced segmentation masks. For the inference on the BratTS validation set, three ensemble sets
are employed: (i) *ensemble-1*: the tumor regions WT, TC, ET are obtained by
averaging sigmoid outputs of two models available in pipeline A; (ii) *ensemble-2*:
the tumor sub-regions NCR/NET, ED, ET are obtained by averaging sigmoid
outputs of two models available in pipeline B; (iii) *ensemble-3*: ET is obtained by
averaging sigmoid outputs of ET from four different models of pipelines A and
B. NCR/NET is obtained by averaging the sigmoid outputs of the complement
of the intersection of TC and ET $((TC \cap ET)^C)$ from pipeline A, and NCR/NET
from pipeline B. Similarly, ED is obtained by averaging the sigmoids outputs of
$(WT \cap (ET \cup NCR/NET))^C$ from pipeline A, and ED from pipeline B.

During inference we perform post-processing to disjoin the overlapping
regions and convert them to unique NCR/NET, ED, ET regions in a single
multi-class image array, as the latter set is the one required by the competition's
evaluation platform. Small tumors are comparatively difficult to segment, and a
slight location variance in predicted tumor volume significantly reduces the performance metric. ET has in general a smaller volume than the other regions, and
it is particularly challenging to obtain precise segmentations. This also applies
to TC in cases where the TC volume is small. As part of our post-processing,
we therefore relabeled ET voxels in cases where they number <250 as necrosis
(to remain in the TC region).

4   Results

Table 1 shows the result (means, standard deviations, and quartiles of Dice
Scores and hausdorff95 distances) of models from pipeline A (PA), Dynamic
UNet (DynUNet) [9] and UNEt TRansformer (UNETR) [6]; validated on our
internal validation data set. Figure 3 compares the result of pipeline A with that
of DynUNet and UNETR (employed from MONAI library [14]). When calculating performance metrics, we provide a full reward (Dice Score = 1 & hausdorff95
distance = 0) to the model for each subject where the model does not predict
any tumor and the ground truth also doesn't contain any tumor. The *sub-type
(i)* of the pipeline A (MEU-Net(PA,4 Heads)) achieves average Dice Scores of
0.9325, 0.9082, and 0.8863; hausdorff95 distances (HD95) of 6.72, 4.40, and 3.28;
for whole tumor, tumor core, and enhancing tumor, respectively. The *sub-type
(ii)* of the same pipeline (MEU-Net(PA,3 Heads)) provides similar Dice Scores
across the tumor sub-regions. Both MEU-Net(PA,3 Heads) and MEU-Net(PA,4
Heads) perform better than that of DynUNet and UNETR.

Table 2 shows the results for three ensemble models validated on the organizer's validation set. For the WT, TC, ET regions: *ensemble-1* respectively
achieves Dice Scores 0.9249, 0.8607, 0.8419, and hausdorff95 distances (HD95)
4.042, 11.40, 17.71; *ensemble-2* achieves Dice Scores 0.9210, 0.8588, 0.8364,
and HD95 4.65, 9.96, 17.79; *ensemble-3* achieves Dice Scores 0.9244, 0.8600,

Table 1. Training-validation set results (328 subjects)

Models	Tumor regions	Dice Score					HD95				
		Mean	SD	Q1	Q2	Q3	Mean	SD	Q1	Q2	Q3
DynUNet (3 Heads) [9]	WT	0.9266	0.0774	0.9221	0.9549	0.9702	6.1161	10.2659	1.4142	2.4495	6.0411
	TC	0.9033	0.1621	0.9005	0.9608	0.9767	5.6188	10.1702	1.0000	2.0000	4.6095
	ET	0.8785	0.1576	0.8708	0.9280	0.9567	4.0873	7.5946	1.0000	1.4142	3.0000
UNETR [6]	WT	0.9118	0.1020	0.9085	0.9460	0.9648	8.0959	14.7898	1.7321	3.1177	7.2801
	TC	0.8578	0.1989	0.8690	0.9312	0.9604	7.1861	12.2032	1.6168	3.0000	6.8367
	ET	0.8434	0.1863	0.8366	0.9036	0.9426	5.2969	9.0289	1.0000	1.7321	4.2202
MEU-Net (PA,4 Heads)	WT	0.9325	0.0671	0.9242	0.9557	0.9735	6.7218	12.1481	1.4142	2.4495	5.8732
	TC	0.9082	0.1486	0.9119	0.9632	0.9784	4.4011	7.3866	1.0000	1.7321	3.3535
	ET	0.8863	0.1452	0.8759	0.9279	0.9598	3.2808	6.0803	1.0000	1.4142	2.4495
MEU-Net (PA,3 Heads)	WT	0.9365	0.0658	0.9285	0.9575	0.9750	5.2830	8.0237	1.4142	2.2361	5.1962
	TC	0.9075	0.1553	0.9100	0.9630	0.9785	4.3778	7.8173	1.0000	1.4142	3.3166
	ET	0.8863	0.1475	0.8782	0.9325	0.9589	3.2174	6.4322	1.0000	1.4142	2.2361

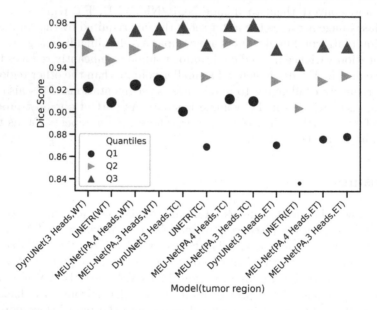

Fig. 3. Scatter plot comparing Dice Score quantiles of the models: MEU-Net (PA,4 Heads), MEU-Net (PA,4 Heads), DynUNet(3 Heads), and UNETR; on our internal validation-set

0.8445, and HD95 4.03, 10.16, 14.50. Ensemble-3 performs marginally better than ensemble-2 and is comparable to ensemble-1.

Table 3 shows the result (means, standard deviations, quartiles of Dice Scores and HD95) of the ensemble-3 assessed on the test set. Figure 5 compares the result of ensemble-3 assessed in the validation set and test set, and MEU-Net (PA, 4H) validated on the internal validation set. The ensemble-3 performs higher in the test set than the validation set for WT, TC, and ET.

Table 2. Validation-set results (219 subjects). *Ensemble-1, ensemble-2,* and *ensemble-3* are denoted by E-1, E-2, and E-1+E-2, respectively.

Ensemble models	Tumor regions	Dice Score					HD95				
		Mean	SD	Q1	Q2	Q3	Mean	SD	Q1	Q2	Q3
E-1	WT	0.9249	0.0749	0.9023	0.9434	0.9677	4.0403	6.4892	1.4142	2.2361	3.8708
	TC	0.8607	0.2102	0.8656	0.9411	0.9670	11.4049	50.1190	1.0000	1.7321	4.2500
	ET	0.8419	0.2194	0.8361	0.9002	0.9545	17.7092	73.6879	1.0000	1.4142	2.4495
E-2	WT	0.9210	0.0755	0.9005	0.9399	0.9669	4.6530	6.3841	1.7321	3.0000	4.8990
	TC	0.8588	0.2111	0.8572	0.9388	0.9663	9.9649	43.7501	1.0000	2.0000	4.2426
	ET	0.8364	0.2234	0.8325	0.9001	0.9531	17.7958	73.6651	1.0000	1.4142	2.4495
E-1+E-2	WT	0.9244	0.0748	0.9035	0.9433	0.9684	4.0345	6.4367	1.4142	2.2361	4.0000
	TC	0.8600	0.2078	0.8601	0.9385	0.9666	10.1635	44.0131	1.0000	2.0000	4.2426
	ET	0.8445	0.2100	0.8381	0.9012	0.9560	14.4990	65.3128	1.0000	1.4142	2.8284

Table 3. Test-set results (570 subjects). *Ensemble-3* is denoted by E-1+E-2

Ensemble models	Tumor regions	Dice Score					HD95				
		Mean	SD	Q1	Q2	Q3	Mean	SD	Q1	Q2	Q3
E-1+E-2	WT	0.9274	0.0930	0.9129	0.9562	0.9778	4.7680	17.0557	1.0000	1.7321	4.1108
	TC	0.8717	0.2456	0.9135	0.9607	0.9809	17.9765	71.5372	1.0000	1.4142	3.0000
	ET	0.8750	0.1798	0.8539	0.9314	0.9658	10.6618	55.5210	1.0000	1.0000	2.0000

5 Discussion

This work presents our modified U-Net architecture, denoted MEU-Net, incorporating multiple encoders and a shared decoder with attention blocks. We use it for the segmentation of three sub-regions of glioblastoma: whole tumor, tumor core, and enhancing tumor, from multi-parametric MRI scans. We trained multiple variations of the MEU-Net, as described in Sect. 3.4, on the 1251 training subjects of the BraTS challenge 2021. The models were evaluated on a separate validation set of 219 subjects provided by the organizers. Averaging the performance metrics across all tumor regions and all subjects, the three ensembles described above, *ensemble-1, ensemble-2, ensemble-3,* achieved Dice Scores of 0.8758, 0.8721, 0.8763, and HD95 distances of 11.05, 10.80, 9.56. *Ensemble-3* performs marginally better than *ensemble-2* and *ensemble-1* for the validation set. Also, *ensemble-3* performs better in the test set than the validation set. These findings signify that the ensembling of additional models increases robustness and generalizes well, as the ensemble model perhaps remains unaffected by the failure of a single model or a single independent CNN component [11]. The source code of experiments carried out, is available at https://github.com/MMIV-ML/brats2021.

A longer term aim is to evaluate a version of our segmentation pipeline integrated into the clinical workflow[1]. The goal is to provide a real-time clinically

---

[1] Using e.g. our research PACS setup at our local hospital region, https://mmiv.no/wiml/.

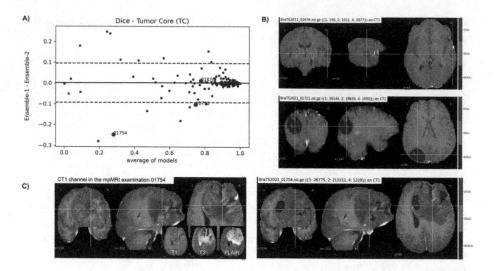

Fig. 4. A) Bland-Altman (BA) plot comparing Dice Scores for TC of *ensemble-1* and *ensemble-2* models, for the 219 subjects in the BraTS2021 validation dataset. The larger red dots with annotated ids refer to the two subjects in B) and the subject in C). **B**) Segmentation results from subjects 01676 and 01721 overlayed the mpMRI CT1 channel using the ensemble-1 model. **C**) Results from subject 01754. Here our model failed severely, with Dice Scores {MEU-Net segmentation vs. GT} of WT: 0.8320, TC: 0.1561, ET: 0.1194. Note the large and highly heterogeneous tumor mass seen in the CT1 channel without segmentation overlay, and the substantial variation in image quality among the four channels (small inserts depicts axial T1, T2 and FLAIR). Volumes of subregions NCR (red 1), ED (yellow 2) and ET (blue 4) are given in µL. The BA plot shows a difference in Dice Scores for TC between *ensemble-1* and *ensemble-2*, which prompts us to adopt *ensemble-3* using *ensemble-1&2* (as described in Sect. 3.4) aimed at achieving better generalization. (Color figure online)

relevant system that may be applied both in diagnostics and treatment planning. It can in principle be applied in the preliminary work up to define the tumor extent into the normal brain tissue and involvement of critical structures that might compromise resection. In the postoperative setting, the delineation of residual tumor is important for further therapy planning. However, the most interesting application is perhaps radiotherapy planning. The pipeline may be used for gross tumor volume delineation and contribute to more accurate delivery of irradiation. This may be particularly important for particle radiotherapy that allows limited irradiation to non-target tissue.

To be evaluated as a possible aid in established clinical workflows, it is especially important that the system is robust to naturally occurring variations in the input data. Currently, our model can completely fail in some cases (cf. Fig. 4C), with outputs that differ a lot from the "ground truth" segmentations produced by radiologists. Several factors may contribute to the problem, such as signal artifacts in MRI recordings, distribution shift, and that the models are trained

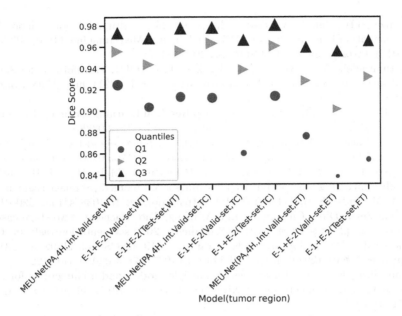

Fig. 5. Scatter plot comparing Dice Score quantiles of the models: MEU-Net (PA,4 Heads) on our internal validation-set(Int.Valid-set); E-1+E-2 on the organizer's validation-set(Valid-set); E-1+E-2 on the organizer's test-set. *Ensemble-1, ensemble-2, and ensemble-3* are denoted by E-1, E-2, and E-1+E-2, respectively. *n*H. denotes *n* deep supervision heads.

on limited data with too narrow diversity. We aim to tackle this by using various multi-pronged supervised and semi-supervised strategies, including more tailored augmentations and model architectures, and putting the human-in-the-loop. A crucial limitation of the current setup based on the BraTS challenge is the unavailability of clinical and radiological history for the BraTS subjects. Having all available MRI recordings for a given case available would enable sequential, longitudinal tumor analysis.

References

1. Baid, U., et al.: The RSNA-ASNR-MICCAI BraTS 2021 Benchmark on Brain Tumor Segmentation and Radiogenomic Classification. arXiv:2107.02314 [cs] (2021). http://arxiv.org/abs/2107.02314
2. Bakas, S., et al.: Segmentation labels and radiomic features for the pre-operative scans of the TCGA-GBM collection. Can. Imaging Archive (2017). https://doi.org/10.7937/K9/TCIA.2017.KLXWJJ1Q
3. Bakas, S., et al.: Segmentation labels and radiomic features for the pre-operative scans of the TCGA-LGG collection. Can. Imaging Archive (2017). https://doi.org/10.7937/K9/TCIA.2017.GJQ7R0EF
4. Bakas, S., et al.: Advancing The Cancer Genome Atlas glioma MRI collections with expert segmentation labels and radiomic features. Sci. Data **4**, 170117 (2017). https://doi.org/10.1038/sdata.2017.117

5. Menze, B.H., Jakab, A., Bauer, S., et al.: The multimodal brain tumor image segmentation benchmark (BRATS). IEEE Trans. Med. Imaging **34**(10), 1993–2024 (2015). https://doi.org/10.1109/TMI.2014.2377694

6. Hatamizadeh, A., Yang, D., Roth, H., Xu, D.: UNETR: Transformers for 3D medical image segmentation. arXiv:2103.10504 [cs, eess] (2021), http://arxiv.org/abs/2103.10504

7. He, K., Zhang, X., Ren, S., Sun, J.: Deep Residual Learning for Image Recognition. arXiv:1512.03385 [cs] (2015). http://arxiv.org/abs/1512.03385

8. Hu, J., Shen, L., Albanie, S., Sun, G., Wu, E.: Squeeze-and-Excitation Networks. arXiv:1709.01507 [cs] (2019). http://arxiv.org/abs/1709.01507. version: 4

9. Isensee, F., Jaeger, P.F., Kohl, S.A.A., Petersen, J., Maier-Hein, K.H.: nnU-Net: a self-configuring method for deep learning-based biomedical image segmentation. Nat. Methods **18**(2), 203–211 (2021). https://doi.org/10.1038/s41592-020-01008-z

10. Jiang, Zeyu, Ding, Changxing, Liu, Minfeng, Tao, Dacheng: Two-stage cascaded U-Net: 1st place solution to BraTS challenge 2019 segmentation task. In: Crimi, Alessandro, Bakas, Spyridon (eds.) BrainLes 2019. LNCS, vol. 11992, pp. 231–241. Springer, Cham (2020). https://doi.org/10.1007/978-3-030-46640-4_22

11. Kamnitsas, K., et al.: Ensembles of multiple models and architectures for robust brain tumour segmentation. arXiv:1711.01468 [cs] (2017). http://arxiv.org/abs/1711.01468

12. Kamnitsas, K., et al.: Efficient multi-scale 3D CNN with fully connected CRF for accurate brain lesion segmentation. Med. Image Anal. **36**, 61–78 (2017). https://doi.org/10.1016/j.media.2016.10.004, https://www.sciencedirect.com/science/article/pii/S1361841516301839

13. Lundervold, A.S., Lundervold, A.: An overview of deep learning in medical imaging focusing on MRI. Zeitschrift für Medizinische Physik **29**(2), 102–127 (2019). https://doi.org/10.1016/j.zemedi.2018.11.002, https://www.sciencedirect.com/science/article/pii/S0939388918301181

14. Ma, N., Li, W., Brown, R., Wang, Y., et al.: Project-MONAI/MONAI: 0.6.0 (2021). https://doi.org/10.5281/zenodo.5083813, https://zenodo.org/record/5083813

15. McKinley, Richard, Meier, Raphael, Wiest, Roland: Ensembles of densely-connected CNNs with label-uncertainty for brain tumor segmentation. In: Crimi, Alessandro, Bakas, Spyridon, Kuijf, Hugo, Keyvan, Farahani, Reyes, Mauricio, van Walsum, Theo (eds.) BrainLes 2018. LNCS, vol. 11384, pp. 456–465. Springer, Cham (2019). https://doi.org/10.1007/978-3-030-11726-9_40

16. Nyul, L., Udupa, J., Zhang, X.: New variants of a method of MRI scale standardization. IEEE Trans. Med. Imaging **19**(2), 143–150 (2000). https://doi.org/10.1109/42.836373, conference Name: IEEE Transactions on Medical Imaging

17. Oktay, O., et al.: Attention U-Net: Learning Where to Look for the Pancreas. arXiv:1804.03999 [cs] (2018). http://arxiv.org/abs/1804.03999

18. Pérez-García, F., Sparks, R., Ourselin, S.: TorchIO: a Python library for efficient loading, preprocessing, augmentation and patch-based sampling of medical images in deep learning. Comput. Methods Prog. Biomed. **208**, 106236 (2021). https://doi.org/10.1016/j.cmpb.2021.106236, https://www.sciencedirect.com/science/article/pii/S0169260721003102

19. Rohlfing, T., Zahr, N.M., Sullivan, E.V., Pfefferbaum, A.: The SRI24 multichannel atlas of normal adult human brain structure. Hum. Brain Mapping **31**(5), 798–819 (2009). https://doi.org/10.1002/hbm.20906, https://www.ncbi.nlm.nih.gov/pmc/articles/PMC2915788/

20. Ronneberger, Olaf, Fischer, Philipp, Brox, Thomas: U-Net: convolutional networks for biomedical image segmentation. In: Navab, Nassir, Hornegger, Joachim, Wells, William M.., Frangi, Alejandro F.. (eds.) MICCAI 2015. LNCS, vol. 9351, pp. 234–241. Springer, Cham (2015). https://doi.org/10.1007/978-3-319-24574-4_28
21. Wright, L., Demeure, N.: Ranger21: a synergistic deep learning optimizer. arXiv:2106.13731 [cs] (2021), http://arxiv.org/abs/2106.13731

AttU-NET: Attention U-Net for Brain Tumor Segmentation

Sihan Wang[1], Lei Li[2], and Xiahai Zhuang[1(✉)]

[1] School of Data Science, Fudan University, Shanghai, China
zxh@fudan.edu.cn
[2] School of Biomedical Engineering, Shanghai Jiao Tong University, Shanghai, China

Abstract. Tumor delineation is critical for the precise diagnosis and treatment of glioma patients. Since manual segmentation is time-consuming and tedious, automatic segmentation is desired. With the advent of convolution neural network (CNN), tremendous CNN models have been proposed for medical image segmentation. However, the small size of kernel limits the shape of the receptive view, omitting the global information. To utilize the intrinsic features of brain anatomical structure, we propose a modified U-Net with an attention block (AttU-Net) to tract the complementary information from the whole image. The proposed attention block can be easily added to any segmentation backbones, which improved the Dice score by 5%. We evaluated our approach on the dataset of BraTS 2021 challenge and achieved promising performance on this dataset. The Dice scores of enhancing tumor, tumor core, and whole tumor segmentation are 0.793, 0.819, and 0.879, respectively.

Keywords: Attention map · Brain tumor · Multi-scale supervision

1 Introduction

Glioma is the most common tumor of the central nerves system in adults and glioblatoma is the most aggressive one, with nonspecific signs and symptoms. Early diagnosis and promote therapy are main determinants of prognosis. Magnetic resonance images (MRI) is wildly utilized in clinical practice for tumor localization, diagnosis, risk stratification and precise resection.

Therefore, tumor delineation is quite important but manual segmentation is rather time-consuming. Automatic and precise tumor segmentation is desired. This year, the Brain Tumor Segmentation (BraTS) challenge is held to encourage the development of brain tumor segmentation [2,3]. Consistent with clinical practice, four common MRI sequences, a native pre-contrast (T1), a post-contrast T1-weighted (T1Gd), a T2-weighted (T2) and a T2 Fluid Attenuated Inversion Recovery (T2-FLAIR), are provided for segmentation. Figure 1 shows an example of image set. The tumor tissue shown in MRI could be categorized into 3 sub-regions, i.e., the enhancing tumor (ET), the tumor core (TC) and the whole tumor (WT). The TC entails the ET and the necrotic (NCR), while the whole tumor (WT) describes the whole tumor region, consisting TC and the peritumoral edematous/invaded tissue (ED) [4,5,15]. There is an intersection between ET, TC and WT, for prediction convenience, the independent regions, NCR, ED and ET, are set to segmentation labels. As shown in the Fig. 1, there is clear inclusion relation between target labels, i.e., $ED \notin$ ET, NCR.

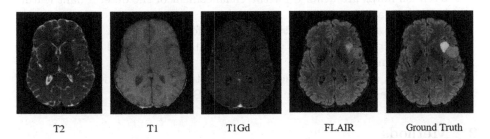

| T2 | T1 | T1Gd | FLAIR | Ground Truth |

Fig. 1. An example image set. Four sequences are provided. Ground Truth is tumor manual segmentation results, where red presents NCR (the smallest sub-region), green refers to ED and yellow is ET. Red plus yellow region is tumor core and all the three region together is WT. (Color figure online)

Recently, tremendous deep learning approaches for brain tumor segmentation have been proposed. U-Net [16] is a prevailing backbone in medical image segmentation, with symmetric encoder and decoder structure. Kayalibay et al. proposed a successful U-Net variant for BraTS 2015, and achieved state of art results that year [12]. Later, Fabian et al. enhanced the U-Net's skip-connection strategy, which was added after convolution layer in each encode and decode stage, to maintain previous extracted feature, and achieve promising performance in BraTS 2017 [10]. Moreover, Isensee et al. proposed a compositive and automatic segmentation framework with preprocessing, network and post-processing, which could automatically configures itself and suit for the most of tasks [8], and this network achieved top performance in BraTS2020 [9].

However, there are intrinsic drawbacks lying behind CNN. For brain datasets, its symmetric anatomical structure information would dramatically facilitate the pathology segmentation, i.e., doctors will highly concern about the asymmetric structure. Whereas, the size of CNN kernel is rather small, generally 3×3, leading to local receptive view and omitting global information while extracting feature [1,18]. In this way, the introduction of attention mechanism for global relation extraction, could alleviate the aforementioned drawback. Attention mechanism was first proposed for natural language processing task to perceive context [17]. Its promising performance boosted mass related research in the filed of computer vision [6,14]. Hu et al. first combined attention mechanism with CNN for classification. The attention map weighted the feature map, as the output of the attention block [7]. In [13], a lightweight attention mechanism were proposed, which applied to the feature maps of decoder, for retinal vessel image segmentation.

Inspired by the aforementioned works, we proposed a 3D attention U-Net, namely AttU-Net for brain tumor segmentation. The contribution of our approach can be summarized as follows.

1) We propose a segmentation model which could segment pathology with complementary information from the intrinsic anatomical brain structure. The attention maps are utilized for the enhancement of the determinant feature for segmentation.
2) We modify a light-weight attention block for volume data and combine it with U-Net organically. The proposed attention block could easily adapt for any common backbone.
3) We propose a fully automatic 3D segmentation framework for brain tumor, and validate it with a public dataset from BraTS 2021.

2   Methods

The overall structure of AttU-Net consists five components, i.e., an encoder, a symmetric decoder, attention blocks, multi-scale supervision and skip-connection strategy, shown in Fig. 2. We will formulate the backbone first in the Sect. 2.1 and then elaborate the structure of the attention block in Sect. 2.2.

2.1   Network Architecture

The backbone is modified from the typical U-Net [16]. The encoder is composed of five convolution blocks, connected by the maximum pooling layer. Each of convolution block consists of three $3 \times 3 \times 3$ convolution layers with stride 2 to reduce feature resolution, and followed by a Leaky-ReLu Activation Layer. The decoding process is symmetric with encoder, also with five block but connected by up-sampling layer. The shape of feature map in each encoder convolution blocks are 16, 32, 64, 128 and 256, while the order in decoder is opposite. The attention blocks (named A) are added to encoding process, to track feature correlation, which will be elaborated later. The last convolution layer in decoder is a $1 \times 1 \times 1$ convolution, and the number of output channel is 4, representing background, NCR, ET and ED. Moreover, we leverage multi-scale supervision for details segmentation. The output of each stage will go over a $1 \times 1 \times 1$ convolution layer to predict multi-scale segmentation map, followed by up-sampling. The reshaped predicted map will be added to the final segmentation map (Fig. 3).

2.2   Attention Block

As stated previously, the anatomic structure of brain is intrinsic symmetric. We assume that the region which is heterogeneous compared with the other side has higher probability to be tumor [11]. In order to extract global feature, we adopt a pixel-wise attention block to weight the middle layer feature map. We propose a slice-self attention block, to extract the asymmetric regions, which can indicate areas at risk.

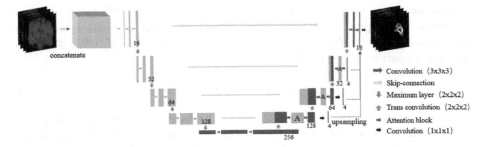

Fig. 2. The network structure of AttU-Net, which consists of an encoder, a symmetric decoder, skip-connection strategy, attention blocks and multi-scale supervision. A stands for attention block. The depths of feature map are signed above.

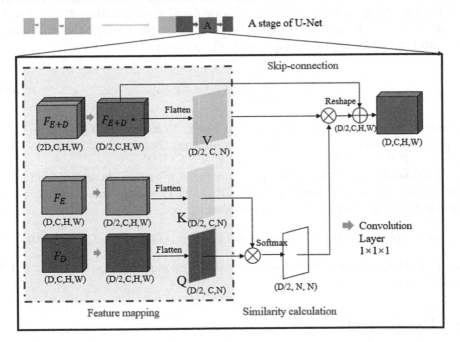

Fig. 3. The structure of attention block, which consists of feature mapping, similarity calculation and skip-connection. F_E, F_D and F_{E+D} present the feature from encoder, the feature from decoder in the same stage and concatenated feature, respectively.

An attention block consists three stages, feature mapping, similarity calculation and skip-connection. Feature mapping stage is to map the three origin feature map to the space K, Q, V for following calculation. K, Q are calculated from feature of decoder (F_D) and the feature from encoder in the same stage (F_E), respectively, while V are calculated from the feature after skip-connection (F_{D+E}). The target feature are first go over a convolution layer with $1 \times 1 \times 1$ kernel, to reduce dimension. F_D and $F_E \in R^{D \times C \times H \times W}$ while $F_{D+E} \in R^{D \times C \times H \times W}$, and the outputs of the convolution layer are all $\in R^{D/2 \times C \times H \times W}$. Since it's more convenient to compute similarity matrix in two dimension, we flatten the feature map from $D/2 \times C \times H \times W$ to $D/2 \times C \times N$, where $N = H \times W$. Then, we compute attention map with K and Q, using

$$A = K^T Q, \tag{1}$$

where A presents attention map $\in R^{D/2 \times N \times N}$. Since similarity matrix is a coefficient matrix whose value should be within [0,1], so we apply softmax on the previous result. As mentioned before, the attention map indicates the pixel-wide similarity, the a_{ji} represents the similarity between k_j and q_i. Since we compute the feature with encoder feature and decoder feature, the attention map highlights model attention, where is determinant to segmentation results. Then we utilize the attention map to weight V, calculated it by function $f(\cdot) = V \cdot A$, $\in R^{D/2 \times C \times N}$. Finally, we reshape the previous result to $D/2 \times C \times N$, and concatenate which with original feature F_{D+E}, using

$$Y_i = \lambda(\sum_{i=1}^{N}(a_{ij}V_j)) + F_{E+D_j^*}, \tag{2}$$

where Y represents output of attention block, X stands for F_{D+E} after first convolutional layer and λ is a hyper parameter. The input of attention map $F_{D+E} \in R^{2D \times C \times H \times W}$ while the output $\in R^{D \times C \times H \times W}$.

The Dice loss is utilized as loss function. Since, it's a four classes segmentation task, while training, we noticed that NCR (label 1) was the most difficult part. Hence we utilized weighted Dice score, that is,

$$Loss = \lambda_1 L_{Dice}(Lab1) + \lambda_2 L_{Dice}(Lab2) + \lambda_3 L_{Dice}(Lab3)) + \lambda_0 L_{Dice}(Lab0), \tag{3}$$

where Lab0 means value equal to 0, etc. Based on experiments, we set $\lambda_1 = 1.2$ while $others = 1$.

3   Experiments

3.1   Dataset

The proposed model was evaluated in the BraTS2021 challenge dataset which contains 1000 training instances and 216 validation instances, each of which consists four sequence, i.e., T1, T2, T1-Gd and FLAIR. The training sets is consisted of labeled image for supervised learning. The depth, width and length of 3D brain MR images are 155, 240, 240, respectively.

Table 1. The quantitative results of the proposed on test dataset.

Teams	Dice			Hausdorff Distance (mm)		
	ET	TC	WT	ET	TC	WT
Mean	0.793 ± 0.253	0.819 ± 0.267	0.879 ± 0.146	23.0 ± 80.3	20.7 ± 71.5	7.80 ± 14.2
Median	0.886	0.925	0.930	1.72	3.16	2.83

3.2 Pre-processing

To reduce the modeling difficulty, we omitted noisy information from original image, by cropping the image into $128 \times 128 \times 128$ size. Later, data augmentation techniques, including random crop, flipping, rotation, were utilized to improve model generalization ability. Four sequences were concatenated into four channel and the shape of input was $128 \times 128 \times 128$.

3.3 Implementations

We treated brain MRI as volume data with the depth, width and length were 155, 240, 240, respectively. Four sequences would be concatenated as four dimensions data, [4, 155, 240, 240], as a whole input. The origin images have been cropped into [4, 128, 128, 128], which could roughly contain all the brain tissue. The training process adopted the batch iteration method, with the batch size as 8, 1000 epochs performed. The model was implemented in Pytorch and optimized by the Adam algorithm. The initial learning rate was set to 0.004, and decay with epoch growing, updated by the equation,

$$lr = \frac{1}{8} * lr_{init} * (\frac{1 - epoch}{epoch_{max}})^{0.9}. \tag{4}$$

The all model was performed on four NVIDIA GTX 3080Ti grahics cards. Training time was about 12 h per model using 4 GPUs.

Table 2. Sensitivity and specificity results of the proposed model on test dataset.

Teams	Sensitivity			Specificity		
	ET	TC	WT	ET	TC	WT
Mean	0.814	0.872	0.828	1.000	0.999	1.000
Median	0.251	0.155	0.259	0.000	0.001	0.001

308   S. Wang et al.

Table 3. The quantitative results of the abaltion study on validation dataset. The AttU-NET represents the proposed model, while the U-Net has the same backbone as AttU-Net but without attention blocks. U-NET* is the structure without multi-scale strategy.

Teams	Dice			Hausdorff Distance (mm)		
	ET	TC	WT	ET	TC	WT
U-NET*	0.745 ± 0.294	0.752 ± 0.320	0.863 ± 0.159	29.2 ± 90.7	20.6 ± 66.1	8.54± 14.8
U-NET	0.748 ± 0.290	0.767 ± 0.302	0.871 ± 0.136	30.8 ± 93.5	18.2 ± 61.0	6.99 ± 9.82
AttU-NET*	0.782 ± 0.257	0.774 ± 0.301	0.895 ± 0.098	21.5 ± 77.4	**17.1 ± 60.8**	6.85 ± 12.1
AttU-NET	**0.808 ± 0.242**	**0.818 ± 0.276**	**0.912 ± 0.092**	**18.7 ± 73.7**	17.6 ± 65.6	**4.60±8.48**

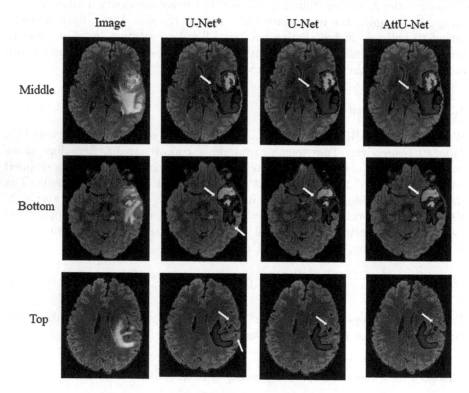

Fig. 4. The segmentation results. Three Prediction samples for randomly were selected slices from middle, top and bottom, respectively. AttU-Net obtained more precise prediction, especially on the edge and tiny regions, than U-Net. The predicited edge of AttU-Net is smoother and suit for origin image, represented by arrows.

3.4   Results

Our approach achieves final Dice score (on the testing dataset) 0.793, 0.879, 0.819 and Hausdorff Distance (HD) 23.1 mm, 7.80 mm and 20.7 mm on label ET, WT and TC respectively, as shown in Table 1. The sensitivity and specificity are also presented in Table 2. In general, the performance of the delineation of WT is much better than the other two labels. The reason for dramatic gap between the performance among labels may lie in the different size among them. Generally, the size of the of ET is dramatically smaller than WT region and with more variant shape, which would be more challenging for automatic segmentation.

In order to compare the performance of different strategies, we also present the quantitative results of ablation study on the validation dataset, shown in the Table 3, since the ground-truth of test dataset is not public.

The proposed network achieved the best value in almost every metrics, except for HD of TC. The performance of attention block can be clearly indicated by the metrics value's gap between Att-UNet and baseline U-Net. The baseline U-Net shares the same convolution backbone, but without attention block, achieving 0.748, 0.767 and 0.871 Dice scores on label ET, TC and WT, respectively. Attention block strategy improved the segmentation results by nearly 5%. Moreover, the multi-scale segmentation strategy could dramatically benefit the prediction, especially for edge and tiny regions, shown in Fig. 4.

The predicted results are presented in Fig. 4. Our algorithm is capable to detect large tumor regions as well as small details. The predicted edge of Att-Unet is smoother than baseline U-Net. However, there are drawback of segmenting the slices near top. Since the proposed model did not consider spatial information. We tried to flatten the last dimension (C, H, W) to calculate spatial similarity, but the results was under desired and additional computing consumption was introduced. It may be due to the lose of position after flatten.

3.5 Conclusion

In this paper, we designed an AttU-Net for the BraTS2021 challenge. We leveraged attention blocks to extract symmetric shape information. Moveover, we modified segmentation backbone from U-Net, adapting for volume datasets. On the validation set, we achieved Dice score 0.808, 0.818 and 0.913 on label ET, TC and WT, respectively. Due to the time limits, we omitted the number of architectural variants. As mentioned before, there were some outliers prediction on the slices near the top of brain. It may be due to the lacks of spatial information, since it just calculates the similarity within one slice. Moreover, there are intrinsic relation between targets regions, we could constrains the prediction using prior relation in the future.

Acknowledgement. This work was funded by the National Natural Science Foundation of China (grant no. 61971142, 62111530195 and 62011540404), the development fund for Shanghai talents (no. 2020015) and the Fujian Province Joint Funds for the Innovation of Science and Technology (2019Y9070).

References

1. Albawi, S., Mohammed, T.A., Al-Zawi, S.: Understanding of a convolutional neural network. In: 2017 International Conference on Engineering and Technology (ICET), pp. 1–6. IEEE (2017)
2. Baid, U., et al.: The rsna-asnr-miccai brats 2021 benchmark on brain tumor segmentation and radiogenomic classification. arXiv preprint arXiv:2107.02314 (2021)
3. Bakas, S., et al.: Segmentation labels and radiomic features for the pre-operative scans of the tcga-gbm collection. the cancer imaging archive. Nat. Sci. Data **4**, 170117 (2017)
4. Bakas, S., et al.: Segmentation labels and radiomic features for the pre-operative scans of the tcga-lgg collection. The cancer imaging archive 286 (2017)
5. Bakas, S., Akbari, H., Sotiras, A., Bilello, M., Rozycki, M., Kirby, J.S., Freymann, J.B., Farahani, K., Davatzikos, C.: Advancing the cancer genome atlas glioma MRI collections with expert segmentation labels and radiomic features. Sci. Data **4**(1), 1–13 (2017)
6. Chen, J., et al.: Transunet: transformers make strong encoders for medical image segmentation. arXiv preprint arXiv:2102.04306 (2021)
7. Hu, J., Shen, L., Sun, G.: Squeeze-and-excitation networks. In: Proceedings of the IEEE Conference on Computer Vision and Pattern Recognition, pp. 7132–7141 (2018)
8. Isensee, F., Jaeger, P.F., Kohl, S.A., Petersen, J., Maier-Hein, K.H.: nnu-net: a self-configuring method for deep learning-based biomedical image segmentation. Nat. Methods **18**(2), 203–211 (2021)
9. Isensee, F., Jäger, P.F., Full, P.M., Vollmuth, P., Maier-Hein, K.H.: nnU-Net for brain tumor segmentation. In: Crimi, A., Bakas, S. (eds.) BrainLes 2020. LNCS, vol. 12659, pp. 118–132. Springer, Cham (2021). https://doi.org/10.1007/978-3-030-72087-2_11
10. Isensee, F., Kickingereder, P., Wick, W., Bendszus, M., Maier-Hein, K.H.: Brain tumor segmentation and radiomics survival prediction: contribution to the BRATS 2017 challenge. In: Crimi, A., Bakas, S., Kuijf, H., Menze, B., Reyes, M. (eds.) BrainLes 2017. LNCS, vol. 10670, pp. 287–297. Springer, Cham (2018). https://doi.org/10.1007/978-3-319-75238-9_25
11. Kalavathi, P., Senthamilselvi, M., Prasath, V.: Review of computational methods on brain symmetric and asymmetric analysis from neuroimaging techniques. Technologies **5**(2), 16 (2017)
12. Kayalibay, B., Jensen, G., van der Smagt, P.: CNN-based segmentation of medical imaging data. arXiv preprint arXiv:1701.03056 (2017)
13. Li, X., Jiang, Y., Li, M., Yin, S.: Lightweight attention convolutional neural network for retinal vessel image segmentation. IEEE Trans. Industr. Inf. **17**(3), 1958–1967 (2020)
14. Liang, J., Homayounfar, N., Ma, W.C., Xiong, Y., Hu, R., Urtasun, R.: Polytransform: deep polygon transformer for instance segmentation. In: Proceedings of the IEEE/CVF Conference on Computer Vision and Pattern Recognition, pp. 9131–9140 (2020)
15. Menze, B.H., Jakab, A., Bauer, S., Kalpathy-Cramer, J., Farahani, K., Kirby, J., Burren, Y., Porz, N., Slotboom, J., Wiest, R., et al.: The multimodal brain tumor image segmentation benchmark (brats). IEEE Trans. Med. Imaging **34**(10), 1993–2024 (2014)

16. Ronneberger, O., Fischer, P., Brox, T.: U-Net: convolutional networks for biomedical image segmentation. In: Navab, N., Hornegger, J., Wells, W.M., Frangi, A.F. (eds.) MICCAI 2015. LNCS, vol. 9351, pp. 234–241. Springer, Cham (2015). https://doi.org/10.1007/978-3-319-24574-4_28
17. Vaswani, A., et al.: Attention is all you need. In: Advances in Neural Information Processing Systems, pp. 5998–6008 (2017)
18. Zheng, H., Fu, J., Mei, T., Luo, J.: Learning multi-attention convolutional neural network for fine-grained image recognition. In: Proceedings of the IEEE International Conference on Computer Vision, pp. 5209–5217 (2017)

Brain Tumor Segmentation in mpMRI Scans (BraTS-2021) Using Models Based on U-Net Architecture

Satyajit Maurya[1], Virendra Kumar Yadav[1], Sumeet Agarwal[1,2],
and Anup Singh[1,2,3](✉)

[1] Indian Institute of Technology, Delhi, India
anupsm@iitd.ac.in
[2] School of Artificial Intelligence, Indian Institute of Technology, Delhi, India
[3] All India Institute of Medical Science, Delhi, India

Abstract. Accurate segmentation of brain tumors from MR images has important clinical relevance. To overcome the limitations of manual segmentation, a semi-automatic or automatic approach is desirable. The current study mainly focused on task-1 defined in the BraTS'21 challenge, i.e., segmenting glioblastoma into sub-regions (the "enhancing tumor" (ET), the "tumor core" (TC), and the "whole tumor" (WT)). In the current study, deep learning models based upon UNet architecture were developed for producing tumor segmentation labels from 3D multi-parametric MRI (mpMRI) scans. During the segmentation process, the output mask resulting from the first developed Model (WT) was used to develop segmentation models for the remaining subregions. Optimizations were carried out to develop robust models, reduce computation time, and achieve high accuracy. Developed models showed high accuracy for the segmentation of tumor sub-regions on training as well as validation data.

Keywords: Brain tumor segmentation · Convolutional neural network · Magnetic resonance imaging · Enhancing tumor · Tumor core · Whole tumor

1 Introduction

Glioma is considered to be one of the most frequently occurring primary brain tumors [1]. Fact sheets of Globocan 2020 report that there are 3,08,102 new brain tumor cases, including both sexes and all age groups [2]. There are 2,51,329 deaths reported due to brain tumors across the globe in 2020 [2]. As per the WHO classification system, gliomas are divided into four grades. Grade I and Grade II gliomas are less malignant and grouped as low-grade gliomas. Grade III and Grade IV gliomas are more malignant in comparison to low-grade gliomas and grouped as high-grade gliomas [3, 11]. The median overall survival rate of patients suffering from glioblastoma is nearly equal to 12–18 months with standard clinical care [3, 4]. Current medical standard treatment involves safe

---

[1] Authors share equal contribution.

A. Crimi and S. Bakas (Eds.): BrainLes 2021, LNCS 12963, pp. 312–323, 2022.
https://doi.org/10.1007/978-3-031-09002-8_28

surgical resection followed by radiotherapy and chemotherapy or a combination of any of these procedures. Magnetic Resonance Imaging (MRI) is considered the first choice amongst clinicians for brain tumor detection and its characterization. The reason is, MRI is a non-invasive imaging technique and offers better soft-tissue contrast in comparison to other imaging modalities [4, 11, 13]. In order to plan or evaluate the effectiveness of the clinical procedure, precise segmentation of the lesion area is indispensable [4]. Manual segmentation of lesions from MR images is time-consuming and may contain inter and intraobserver variability. Segmenting brain glioblastoma into three subregions, i.e., whole tumor (WT), enhancing tumor (ET), and tumor core (TC) in multi-parametric MRI scans, were considered as task-1 in the BraTS'21 challenge.

Multiple methods have been proposed by experts across the different fields for the segmentation of tissues. Most of the recently available literature used the concept of the convolutional neural network, its different variants, and an ensemble of different models to produce their reported results. Zhao et al. [5] and Havaei et al. [14] used the Deep Neural Network for carrying out the 3D brain tumor segmentation. Jiang et al. [6] used the cascading U-Net concept for carrying out the segmentation task. As per their findings, progressive cascading U-Net improves the prediction results [6]. Islam et al. [7] used the attention CNN for carrying out the segmentation task. Authors reported that 3D attention U-net resulted in better accuracy for the tumor core in comparison to 3D UNet [8]. Sahayam et al. [8] used voxel-based classification for carrying out segmentation tasks. Voxels were classified with the help of a dense artificial neural network. Feng et al. [9] used the ensemble of 3D UNets for carrying out segmentation tasks. The six developed networks that were trained and used in segmentation contained different patch sizes and encoding/decoding blocks. Feng et al. [9] also reported that if a greater number of networks were used in the ensemble, the results produced would be better in comparison to what they have reported in their work. Guo et al. [10], in their segmentation work, used global context (GC) CNN. GC block improved the segmentation accuracy as it captures the long-range dependency information. Agravat et al. [11] and Liu et al. [12], in their carried-out segmentation work, used the concept of a fully convolutional neural network. Ranjbarzadeh et al. [13] used the cascade CNN along with the novel Distance-Wise Attention (DWA) method to segment the tumor subregions. DWA approach improved the segmentation accuracy as it takes account of the location of the tumor. Ramya et al. [15] used the ensemble of different clustering approaches to carry out the segmentation task. To improve their segmentation accuracy, Huang et al. [16] introduced the concept of group-cross channel attention residuals in UNet architecture. A detailed recovering (DT) path is also added to capture the fine details of the tumor from MR images. Huang et al. [17], in their carried-out work, used the concept of gamma correction neural network. The adaptive gamma correction (AGC) concept helps the network in finding significant regions. Multiple former participating teams used the U-Net architecture or ensemble with other algorithms [22–24]. Wang et al., in their presented work [22], used UNet for brain tumor segmentation and for predicting the survival rates. Chen M et al., in their presented work, used 3D-UNet for producing multiscale predictions [23]. Kim et al. used ensemble 2D UNets to generate ensemble maps [24]. Once maps were generated, these were fed into 3D UNets to produce the tumor subregions.

In the current study, a UNet based approach was proposed for producing segmentation labels for glioblastoma sub-regions from 3D mpMRI scans as described in the BraTS'21 challenge. The four models based on U-Net architecture were developed. As described in the next section, the first Model (Model-1) locates the tumor region on FLAIR images. The output region predicted from Model-1 was dilated. This dilated region was used by three other developed models for predicting labels, i.e., refined WT, ET, and necrotic region (NCR). Optimizations were also carried out for developing a robust Model, time reduction, and accurate segmentation.

2   Materials and Pre-processing

2.1   Dataset

The training data set (task-1), which was provided in the BraTS'21 challenge, contains 1251 subjects' mpMRI scans [18–20, 25–28]. Validation data which was provided afterward contains 219 subjects mpMRI scans. For every subject, the data set contains native T_1-weighted (W), post-contrast T_1-W, T_2-W, T_2 Fluid Attenuated Inversion Recovery (T_2 FLAIR) images covering the whole brain. Every subject provided in the training data set contains the tumor sub-region masks that were manually delineated and verified by the clinical neuro-radiologists (Fig. 1). Each patient data was already skull stripped, bias-corrected, denoised, and co-registered. Each patient's data in the training data set contains the tumor subregion segmented ground truth while ground truth of validation and testing datasets were not made available by the BraTS organizers.

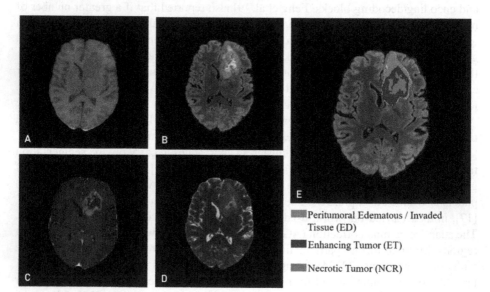

Peritumoral Edematous / Invaded Tissue (ED)

Enhancing Tumor (ET)

Necrotic Tumor (NCR)

Fig. 1. Show example images from the BraTS'21 training data set. (A) Native T_1-W image, (B) T_2-FLAIR image, (C) Post-contrast T_1-W image, (D) T_2-W image, (E) Segmented tumor sub-region mask image overlaid on T_2 FLAIR image.

2.2 Pre-processing

Although the MR images provided were skull stripped, bias-corrected, denoised, and co-registered, it contains variations in the dynamic range of signal intensity for different subjects. These variations may degrade the performance of developed models. To reduce the effect of such variations, images were normalized with their corresponding median value (only brain pixels).

3 Methods

UNet is an architecture widely used for semantic segmentation developed by Olaf Ronneberger [21] (Fig. 2). It contains two paths: contraction path (encoder) and expanding path (decoder). The contraction path consists of a stack of convolutional and max-pooling layers which capture the context in the input images. The symmetric expanding path decoder uses transpose convolutions for precise localization.

Figure 2 shows the proposed framework. In the current study, four UNet based models were developed to achieve the tumor subregion segmentation task as specified in the BraTS'21 challenge (Fig. 3). Model-1 was trained over FLAIR images and corresponding masks for initial WT segmentation. Before feeding masks into the Model-1, all labels were set equal to one (say mask-1). Model-1 helps in locating the tumor region. The output resulting from Model-1 was dilated (name it mask-2). Next, mask-2 was multiplied with corresponding FLAIR images. Model-2 was trained over this cropped FLAIR region. The output of Model-2 results in the final WT mask. The morphological operation such as hole-fill was applied to the resulting WT mask to improve the prediction accuracy. Next, Model-3 was trained over images obtained after multiplying post-contrast T_1 images with mask-2 and Msk^2. Msk^2 was developed by considering the enhancing label only from the ground truth provided. The developed Model-3 will result in the ET mask. Next, the Model-4 was trained over images obtained after multiplying post-contrast T_1 images with mask-2 and Msk^3. Msk^3 was developed by considering the necrotic tumor label only from the ground truth provided. The developed Model-4 will result in the NCR mask. The output mask resulted from Model-3 and Model-4 clubbed together to produce the tumor core, i.e., TC followed by hole filling. Edematous/invaded tissue (ED) masks were generated when TC masks were subtracted from the WT mask. Although Model-4 resulted in NCR but computed dice w.r.t ground truth was found to be less. So, an alternate approach was followed for computing the final NCR mask, i.e., subtracting ET from TC resulted in NCR. This approach resulted in an improved dice similarity coefficient (DSC) for the NCR mask. Following metrics were also considered for evaluating the performance of the models: Hausdorff distance (HD), Sensitivity, Specificity.

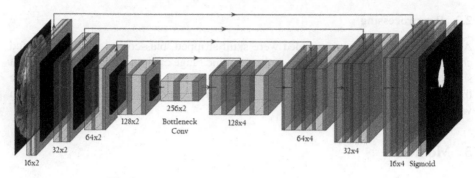

Fig. 2. Showing UNet architecture, adapted from [21]

In the current study, processing was performed using a desktop computer and Google Colab Pro version subscription, access to T4 and P100 GPUs. The models were developed on these T4 and P100 GPUs with a batch size equal to 16. Image generator was used for loading the training images as it helps in creating batches. Also, it overcomes the limitation of memory fit. The early stopping (with patience = 3) approach was used to overcome the limitations of too many epochs (resulting in overfitting) vs. few epochs (resulting in underfitting). Adaptive Moment Estimation (Adam) was used for optimization. Binary Cross Entropy was chosen for calculating the loss. Initially, models were

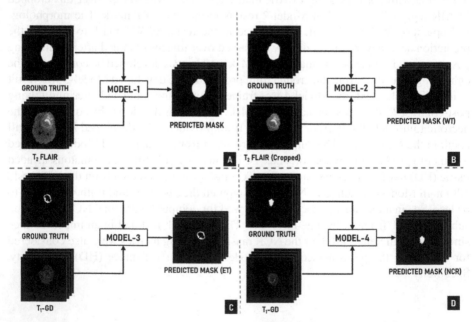

Fig. 3. Show the systematic approach to develop the (a) Model-1 (for locating tumor region), (b) Model-2 (for predicting label: WT), (c) Model-3 (for predicting label: ET), (d) Model-4 (for predicting label: NCR). The developed models were based on the U-Net architecture.

trained on the resampled training images. Images were resampled to (240 x 240 x 77) from the original dimension (240 x 240 x 155), and the results were recorded. Models were also trained on the original dimension MR scan volumes, and the results were recorded. The training dataset was divided into training, testing, and validation sets in the ratio of 80:10:10, respectively. The different labels of tumor subregions were predicted for validation data provided and submitted for online evaluation on the Synapse platform.

4 Results

Table 1 shows the results obtained from the test set created from the training data when the scan volumes were downsampled to a shape (240 x 240 x 77). The predictions of the validation data from the developed models trained on the downsampled data were evaluated online on the Synapse platform. The results obtained are shown in Table 2. Models were also trained using the original dataset size without resampling. A similar splitting ratio was considered for dividing the training data into train, validation, and test set. The result obtained on the test set made from the training data is shown in Table 3. Table 4 shows the predictions for the validation data from the models developed using the original dimension dataset (240 x 240 x 155), evaluated online on the Synapse platform. The developed models are also compared with the previous year's top-performing team's results evaluated on the validation dataset (Table 5). Figure 4 shows the visual comparison of the predicted mask with the actual ground truth provided in the BraTS dataset. Table 6 shows the results provided by the BraTS'21 organizers, containing mean values of DSC, HD, Sensitivity & Specificity on the BraTS'21 test data set. Table 7 shows the results provided by the BraTS'21 organizers, containing median values of DSC, HD, Sensitivity & Specificity on the BraTS'21 test data set.

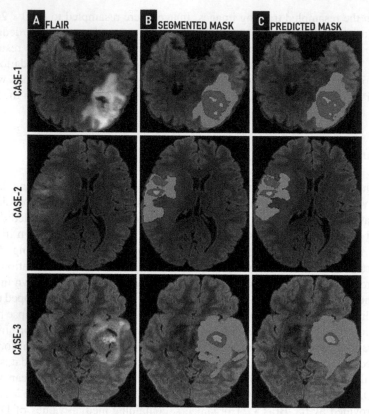

Fig. 4. Show example images from BraTS'21 training data set showing three different slices from three different cases (A) T_2-FLAIR images, (B) Ground truth mask overlaid on T_2-FLAIR images, (C) Predicted mask overlaid on T_2-FLAIR images.

Table 1. Shows produced DSC results on the test set made from the BraTS'21 training data when the models were trained on the resampled images (i.e., 240 x 240 x 77).

	ET	TC	WT
DSC (Testing Set)	0.799	0.843	0.881

* Abbreviation- DSC: Dice similarity coefficient

Table 2. Shows results obtained from the online evaluation portal, containing DSC, HD, Sensitivity & Specificity results on BraTS'21 validation data set when models were trained on the resampled images (i.e., 240 x 240 x 77).

	ET	TC	WT
DSC	0.694	0.736	0.880
HD	31.45	14.86	6.40
Sensitivity	0.7966	0.7644	0.9044
Specificity	0.9993	0.9995	0.9985

* Abbreviations- DSC: Dice similarity coefficient; HD: Hausdorff distance; ET: Enhancing Tumor; TC: Tumor Core; WT: Whole Tumor

Table 3. Shows produced DSC results on the test set made from the BraTS'21 training data provided without resampling the dataset.

	ET	TC	WT
DSC (Testing Set)	0.848	0.892	0.906

* Abbreviations- DSC: Dice similarity coefficient;

Table 4. Shows results obtained from the online evaluation portal, containing DSC, HD, Sensitivity & Specificity results on BraTS'21 validation data set when models were trained without resampling of the dataset.

	ET	TC	WT
DSC	0.761	0.781	0.888
HD	23.88	13.36	7.51
Sensitivity	0.770	0.753	0.886
Specificity	0.9996	0.9997	0.9990

* Abbreviations- DSC: Dice similarity coefficient; HD: Hausdorff distance; ET: Enhancing Tumor; TC: Tumor Core; WT: Whole Tumor

Table 5. Shows performance comparison of the proposed model with previous year BraTS'20 top-performing team's results

	Dice similarity coefficient			Hausdorff distance		
	WT	TC	ET	WT	TC	ET
Zhao et al. [5]	0.910	0.835	0.754	4.56	5.58	3.84
Jiang et al. [6]	0.909	0.864	0.802	4.26	5.43	3.14
Islam et al. [7]	0.898	0.792	0.704	6.29	8.76	7.05
Proposed Model	0.888	0.781	0.761	7.51	13.36	23.88

* Abbreviations- DSC: Dice similarity coefficient; HD: Hausdorff distance; ET: Enhancing Tumor; TC: Tumor Core; WT: Whole Tumor

Table 6. Shows the results provided by the BraTS'21 organizers, containing mean values of DSC, HD, Sensitivity & Specificity on the BraTS'21 test data set

	ET	TC	WT
DSC	0.664	0.689	0.745
Hausdorff95	73.57	73.79	64.59
Sensitivity	0.673	0.686	0.745
Specificity	0.8470	0.8470	0.8466

Table 7. Shows the results provided by the BraTS'21 organizers, containing median values of DSC, HD, Sensitivity & Specificity on the BraTS'21 test data set

	ET	TC	WT
DSC	0.839	0.894	0.901
Hausdorff95	73.57	73.79	64.59
Sensitivity	0.862	0.888	0.909
Specificity	0.9997	0.9998	0.9992

5 Discussions

Segmentation of brain tumors in MR images involves challenges due to its highly hetero-geneous appearance and shape. Deep learning models based on the U-Net architecture were developed on the BraTS'21 training dataset to classify the brain glioblastoma into three different subregions, i.e., ET, TC, and WT, as described in the BraTS'21 task-1 challenge. We obtained dice scores (for ET, TC, and WT) of 0.848, 0.892, and 0.906 on the test set made out from the training data and values of 0.761, 0.781, and 0.888 on the BraTS'21 validation data.

In the current study, volumes were also down-sampled to a shape (240 x 240 x 77) for evaluating its effect on segmentation accuracy. Downsampling was performed to reduce the dataset size and the computation cost associated with training the model. The dice scores produced, mentioned in the results section, were found lower in comparison to the model when trained without resampling. During the downsampling process for segmented labels, interpolation may result in values other than 0, 1, 2, and 4. Reassigning the erroneous valued labels to one of the classes may produce the wrong results. To overcome this limitation, resampling was not performed on the training dataset.

The final approach we adopted, and as discussed in the Methods section, was used to reduce the training data size by only using the cropped images for the training purpose. There was a ten-fold reduction in the training data size for the other three developed models.

One of the limitations of the proposed approach, i.e., by individually predicting the different class labels and then combining them, was that there might be unassigned pixels or overlaps in the predicted labels at some pixel locations during the combination process. This creates a need for designing methods to reassign the overlapped pixel regions to the correct class. To overcome this limitation, two approaches were tried out. The first one involved checking the mean intensity values of the different classes and assigning the unassigned pixels to that class whose intensity difference from a particular class's mean intensity is the least. However, there were no substantial improvements in the dice scores when this method was employed. The other method involved assigning the values of the unassigned pixel regions to one of the two possible adjacent classes to that pixel location in which it could fall in. Of the two classes, the pixel region was assigned the value of the class, which produced higher dice scores for their respective class predictions evaluated during the training process.

Dice scores were relatively high when computed on the test set made from the training data compared to that computed on the validation data obtained from the online validation portal and on the test data provided by the BraTS'21 organizers. Data biasness can be thought of as a contributing factor for this difference in the recorded dice scores.

The advantage of using the output of Model-1 as input to the other three models results in computational efficiency. Instead of training the other three models on whole-brain images, only the dilated tumor region is required.

In conclusion, proposed U-Net architecture-based segmentation models provided segmentation of brain glioblastoma sub-regions with high accuracy. The proposed model can be further improved by incorporating data augmentation as well as by including more data from multi-center studies.

Acknowledgments. The authors acknowledge funding support from the Science and Engineering Research Board, Department of Science and Technology project: CRG/2019/005032.

References

1. Hamghalam, M., Lei, B., Wang, T.: Brain Tumor Synthetic Segmentation in 3D Multimodal MRI Scans. In: Crimi, A., Bakas, S. (eds.) BrainLes 2019. LNCS, vol. 11992, pp. 153–162. Springer, Cham (2020). https://doi.org/10.1007/978-3-030-46640-4_15
2. Cancer today (2020). https://gco.iarc.fr/today/fact-sheets-cancers. Accessed 2 Aug 2021
3. Bush, N.A.O., Chang, S.M., Berger, M.S.: Current and future strategies for treatment of glioma. Neurosurg. Rev. **40**(1), 1–14 (2016). https://doi.org/10.1007/s10143-016-0709-8
4. Li, X., Luo, G., Wang, K.: Multi-step Cascaded Networks for Brain Tumor Segmentation. In: Crimi, A., Bakas, S. (eds.) BrainLes 2019. LNCS, vol. 11992, pp. 163–173. Springer, Cham (2020). https://doi.org/10.1007/978-3-030-46640-4_16
5. Zhao, Y.-X., Zhang, Y.-M., Liu, C.-L.: Bag of Tricks for 3D MRI Brain Tumor Segmentation. In: Crimi, A., Bakas, S. (eds.) BrainLes 2019. LNCS, vol. 11992, pp. 210–220. Springer, Cham (2020). https://doi.org/10.1007/978-3-030-46640-4_20
6. Jiang, Z., Ding, C., Liu, M., Tao, D.: Two-Stage Cascaded U-Net: 1st Place Solution to BraTS Challenge 2019 Segmentation Task. In: Crimi, A., Bakas, S. (eds.) BrainLes 2019. LNCS, vol. 11992, pp. 231–241. Springer, Cham (2020). https://doi.org/10.1007/978-3-030-46640-4_22
7. Islam, M., Vibashan, V.S., Jose, V.J.M., Wijethilake, N., Utkarsh, U., Ren, H.: Brain Tumor Segmentation and Survival Prediction Using 3D Attention UNet. In: Crimi, A., Bakas, S. (eds.) BrainLes 2019. LNCS, vol. 11992, pp. 262–272. Springer, Cham (2020). https://doi.org/10.1007/978-3-030-46640-4_25

8. Sahayam, S., Krishna, N.H., Jayaraman, U.: Brain Tumour Segmentation on MRI Images by Voxel Classification Using Neural Networks, and Patient Survival Prediction. In: Crimi, A., Bakas, S. (eds.) BrainLes 2019. LNCS, vol. 11992, pp. 284–294. Springer, Cham (2020). https://doi.org/10.1007/978-3-030-46640-4_27

9. Feng, X., Dou, Q., Tustison, N., Meyer, C.: Brain Tumor Segmentation with Uncertainty Estimation and Overall Survival Prediction. In: Crimi, A., Bakas, S. (eds.) BrainLes 2019. LNCS, vol. 11992, pp. 304–314. Springer, Cham (2020). https://doi.org/10.1007/978-3-030-46640-4_29

10. Guo, D., Wang, L., Song, T., Wang, G.: Cascaded Global Context Convolutional Neural Network for Brain Tumor Segmentation. In: Crimi, A., Bakas, S. (eds.) BrainLes 2019. LNCS, vol. 11992, pp. 315–326. Springer, Cham (2020). https://doi.org/10.1007/978-3-030-46640-4_30

11. Agravat, R.R., Raval, M.S.: Brain Tumor Segmentation and Survival Prediction. In: Crimi, A., Bakas, S. (eds.) BrainLes 2019. LNCS, vol. 11992, pp. 338–348. Springer, Cham (2020). https://doi.org/10.1007/978-3-030-46640-4_32

12. Liu, S., Guo, X.: Improving Brain Tumor Segmentation with Multi-direction Fusion and Fine Class Prediction. In: Crimi, A., Bakas, S. (eds.) BrainLes 2019. LNCS, vol. 11992, pp. 349–358. Springer, Cham (2020). https://doi.org/10.1007/978-3-030-46640-4_33

13. Ranjbarzadeh, R., et al.: Brain tumor segmentation based on deep learning and an attention mechanism using MRI multi-modalities brain images. Sci Rep 11, 10930 (2021). https://doi.org/10.1038/s41598-021-90428-8

14. Havaei, M., et al.: Brain tumor segmentation with Deep Neural Networks. Med Image Anal. 35, 18–31 (2017). https://doi.org/10.1016/j.media.2016.05.004. Epub 2016 May 19 PMID: 27310171 Jan

15. Ramya, P., Thanabal, M.S., Dharmaraja, C.: Brain tumor segmentation using cluster ensemble and deep super learner for classification of MRI. J. Ambient. Intell. Humaniz. Comput. 12(10), 9939–9952 (2021). https://doi.org/10.1007/s12652-021-03390-8

16. Huang, Z., Zhao, Y., Liu, Y., Song, G.: GCAUNet: a group cross-channel attention residual UNet for slice based brain tumor segmentation. Biomedical Signal Processing and Control 70, 102958 (2021). ISSN 1746–8094. https://doi.org/10.1016/j.bspc.2021.102958. (https://www.sciencedirect.com/science/article/pii/S1746809421005553)

17. Huang, Z., Liu, Y., Song, G., Zhao, Y.: GammaNet: an intensity-invariance deep neural network for computer-aided brain tumor segmentation. Optik 243, 167441 (2021). ISSN 0030–4026. https://doi.org/10.1016/j.ijleo.2021.167441. (https://www.sciencedirect.com/science/article/pii/S0030402621010706)

18. Baid, U., et al.: The RSNA-ASNR-MICCAI BraTS 2021 Benchmark on Brain Tumor Segmentation and Radiogenomic Classification (2021). arXiv:2107.02314

19. Menze, B.H., et al.: The Multimodal Brain Tumor Image Segmentation Benchmark (BRATS). IEEE Trans. Med. Imaging 34(10), 1993–2024 (2015). https://doi.org/10.1109/TMI.2014.2377694

20. Bakas, S., et al.: Advancing the cancer genome atlas glioma MRI collections with expert segmentation labels and radiomic features. Nature Scientific Data 4, 170117 (2017). https://doi.org/10.1038/sdata.2017.117

21. Ronneberger, O., Fischer, P., Brox, T., U-Net: Convolutional Networks for Biomedical Image Segmentation (2021). [online] arXiv.org. Available at: https://arxiv.org/abs/1505.04597. Accessed 16 July 2021

22. Wang, F., Jiang, R., Zheng, L., Meng, C., Biswal, B.: 3D U-Net Based Brain Tumor Segmentation and Survival Days Prediction. In: Crimi, A., Bakas, S. (eds.) BrainLes 2019. LNCS, vol. 11992, pp. 131–141. Springer, Cham (2020). https://doi.org/10.1007/978-3-030-46640-4_13

23. Chen, M., Wu, Y., Wu, J.: Aggregating Multi-scale Prediction Based on 3D U-Net in Brain Tumor Segmentation. In: Crimi, A., Bakas, S. (eds.) BrainLes 2019. LNCS, vol. 11992, pp. 142–152. Springer, Cham (2020). https://doi.org/10.1007/978-3-030-46640-4_14

24. Kim, S., Luna, M., Chikontwe, P., Park, S.H.: Two-Step U-Nets for Brain Tumor Segmentation and Random Forest with Radiomics for Survival Time Prediction. In: Crimi, A., Bakas, S. (eds.) BrainLes 2019. LNCS, vol. 11992, pp. 200–209. Springer, Cham (2020). https://doi.org/10.1007/978-3-030-46640-4_19

25. Bakas, S., et al.: Segmentation labels and radiomic features for the Pre-operative scans of the TCGA-GBM collection. The Cancer Imaging Archive (2017). https://doi.org/10.7937/K9/TCIA.2017.KLXWJJ1Q

26. Bakas, S., et al.: Segmentation labels and radiomic features for the pre-operative scans of the TCGA-LGG collection. The Cancer Imaging Archive (2017). https://doi.org/10.7937/K9/TCIA.2017.GJQ7R0EF

27. Braintumorsegmentation.org: MICCAI BRATS - The Multimodal Brain Tumor Segmentation Challenge (2022). [online] Available at: <http://braintumorsegmentation.org/>. Accessed 13 Oct 2021

28. Sage Bionetworks: i. Synapse | Sage Bionetworks (2022). [online] Synapse.org. Available at: <https://www.synapse.org/#!Synapse:syn25829067/wiki/610865>. Accessed 13 October 2021

29. Braintumorsegmentation.org: MICCAI BRATS - The Multimodal Brain Tumor Segmentation Challenge (2022). [online] Available at: <http://braintumorsegmentation.org/>. Accessed 13 Oct 2021.

Neural Network Based Brain Tumor Segmentation

Darshat Shah(ID), Avishek Biswas(ID), Pranali Sonpatki(ID),
Sunder Chakravarty(ID), and Nameeta Shah(✉)(ID)

Mazumdar Shaw Medical Foundation, Bangalore, India
nameeta.shah@gmail.com
http://www.msctr.org/

Abstract. Glioblastoma is the most common and lethal primary brain tumor in adults. Magnetic resonance imaging (MRI) is a critical diagnostic tool for glioblastoma. Besides MRI, histopathology features and molecular subtypes like MGMT methylation, IDH mutation, 1p19q codeletion, etc. are used for prognosis. Accurate tumor segmentation is a step towards fully utilizing the MRI data for radiogenomics that will allow use of MRI to predict genomic features of glioblastoma. With accurate tumor segmentation, we can get precise quantitative information about the 3D tumor volumetric features. We have developed an inference model for brain tumor segmentation using neural network algorithm with Resnet50 as an encoding layer. Major feature of our algorithm is the use of composite image generated from T1, T2, T1ce and FLAIR series. We report average Dice scores of 0.88716 for the whole tumor, 0.79052 for the necrotic core, and 0.72760 for the contrast-enhancing tumor on the validation set of BraTS 2021 Task1 challenge. For the final unseen test data, we report average Dice scores of 0.89656 for the whole tumor, 0.83734 for the necrotic core, and 0.81162 for the contrast-enhancing tumor.

Keywords: Glioma · Segmentation · Machine learning · Convolution neural network · U-Net

1 Introduction

Gliomas are the most common tumors of the central nervous system (CNS), and account for nearly 80% of all malignant primary brain tumors. Glioblastoma multiforme (GBM) is https://www.keybr.comthe most common primary malignant brain tumor, and accounts for more than 60% of all adult gliomas [12]. GBM is characterised by poor patient prognosis, and extreme intrinsic heterogeneity. Standard treatment of GBM includes surgical resection followed by radiation and concurrent adjuvant temozolomide (TMZ) therapy [13].

Radiologic analysis of GBM typically involves contrast-enhanced magnetic resonance imaging (MRI), specifically T1-weighted (T1), T1-weighted contrast enhanced (T1ce), T2-weighted (T2) and T2 fluid attenuated inversion recovery

(T2-FLAIR). However owing to GBM's heterogeneity, tumor margins may be irregular or poorly defined.

Prior studies have shown the significance of aggressive surgical resection when possible, with an improved progression free survival (PFS) and overall survival (OS) [12]. Improved identification of tumor boundaries and sub-sections can aid pre-operative planning and maximise surgical resection.

The RSNA-ASNR-MICCAI Brain Tumor Segmentation (BraTS) Challenge provides multi-parametric MRI (mpMRI) scans with manual expert annotations for over 1000 patients, with the aim of improving automated tumor segmentation.

Neural Networks are a powerful tool for the task of image segmentation. They are increasingly used for biomedical image segmentation. Here we describe an approach that uses the U-Net architecture for prediction of brain tumor segmentation using a composite pseudo RGBA images generated from the four aforementioned MRI image series; T1, T2, T1ce and T2-FLAIR. We report results with different encoders, and loss functions.

Since it was introduced by Ronneberger et al. [6] in 2015, U-Net has become the starting point for numerous approaches for biomedical image segmentation. For 3D input such as MRI scans, many approaches have modified U-Net with 3D convolutions keeping basic architecture the same [14,15]. However MRI scans are characterized by inputs that are not only 3D but also multi-modal. Very few approaches in past have utilized all the 4 modalities viz. T1, T2, T1CE, and Flair to enhance the semantic representation and segmentation of Brain Tumors. In this study, we present an innovative approach that utilizes all four modalities. We also utilize the Resnet-50 encoder (trained on ImageNet) in the encoding path of the U-Net. The segmentation is done in 2D along axial planes. This simple architecture still gave us very competitive results compared with more complex approaches that utilize Attention, cascaded U-Nets, full/partial 3D convolutions, etc.

2   Methods

The BraTS 2021 Task1 challenge dataset was used for the training [1–5]. We use the U-Net convolution neural network architecture [6] with the ResNet50 [7] as an encoding layer to compute segmentation of every slice in the 3D volume, followed by stacking the segmented output [8].

2.1   Input Image Mapping

For training purposes, we divided the axial view of each NIfTI image type (T1, T2, T1ce, FLAIR) into 155 slices, with corresponding slice from the segmented image as the ground truth. The annotations in the segmented image consist of the GD-enhancing tumor (ET—label 4), the peritumoral edematous/invaded tissue (ED—label 2), and the necrotic tumor core (NCR—label 1). We noted that between the axial, sagittal and coronal view, the axial view generally had better focus and less noise. For each image type (T1, T2, T1ce, FLAIR) the following steps were performed:

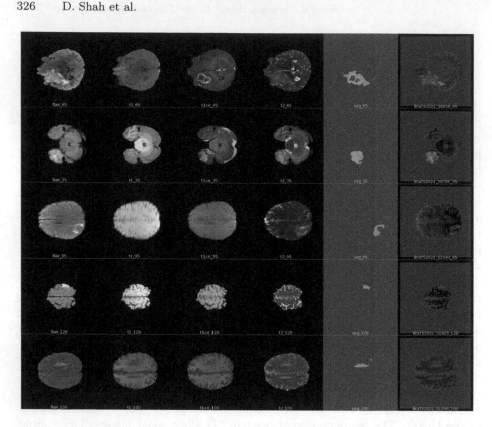

Fig. 1. Examples of pseudo RGB input constructed from T1, T2, T1ce, and FLAIR input. From top to bottom, these are axial plane slices 65, 35, 95, 128, and 100 of BraTS2021 00059, 01296, 00781, 01544, 01415, and 01296 inputs. From left to right - FLAIR, T1, T1ce, T2, segmentation, and pseudo RGB images. For segmentation image, the label colors are: 0-Red, 1-green, 2-purple, 4-blue

1. Z-score normalized each slice using mean/sd of the entire volume
2. Mapped the z-score normalized volume data to 0,255 range. We used non local means algorithm (in opencv, with searchwindow=25) to remove gaussian noise.
3. From this denoised, normalized input, we constructed a pseudo RGB image as follows:

Table 1. Pseudo RGB channel mapping

Channel	Input mapping
R	FLAIR
G	T1ce
B	T2 + (127-T1)*

*Here the idea was to brighten T2 further with darker areas of T1 (if any). Since T1 captures wavy CSF channels, and T2 mostly captures fat, the intent of this composite image was to create maximum contrast with FLAIR tumor areas. FLAIR sometimes captured CSF areas too, in addition to the tumor volume. We expected that the NN layers will learn and exploit the difference between T2 and FLAIR.

4. Finally, we cropped this RGB image to 224×224 and used as input to the neural network (NN). Cropping reduced the 8 pixel boundary around the image, and avoided use of a resize algorithm to create 224×224 image from 240×240 image (see Fig. 1).

2.2 Training

Given 1252 patients, with 155 training images from each, we did a train:validation:test split as 60:20:20 to get approximately 113k training images plus corresponding ground truth and 40k images for validation and test each. Data was randomly augmented with horizontal and vertical flips as well as gamma-based contrast variations using imgaug lib. Input shape for U-Net encoder was 224×224, and output shape in the upsampling path was also 224×224. Output was then inserted at the right position in an image of size 240×240. Each slice was segmented and stacked, thus resulting in 3D output volume.

2.3 U-Net Configuration

We used a standard U-Net with encoding layers of Resnet50 algorithm, and initialized with weights from Imagenet (https://image-net.org/). Two changes were made to the U-Net architecture: - since upsampling path ends at half of

original resolution using Resnet-50 encoder, we added an extra upsampling layer
followed by a convolution layer that resulted in 4 channel output, corresponding
to background plus 3 labels.

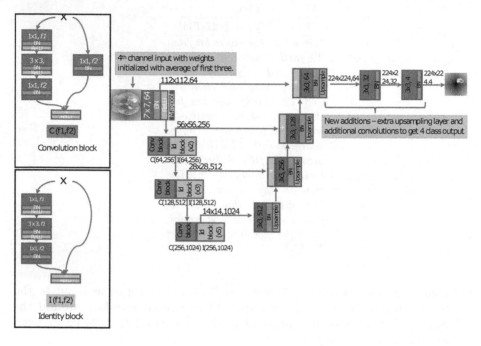

Fig. 2. U-Net with Resnet-50 based encoder. The architecture was left intact. In order
to accommodate 4 input channels, a new channel was added on input. Output was
upsampled as part of the decoder to learn weights versus a resize operation.

We experimented with different loss functions - multicategory cross entropy,
focal loss with custom alpha, averaged dice loss [9], and Tversky loss [10] with
custom alpha. Adam optimizer was used with different learning rates –0.01 for
cross entropy and focal loss; 0.001 to 0.0005 for averaged dice and Tversky loss.
Results from different models using VGG16 [11] and Resnet50 are listed in Table
For the submitted model we used the following

- Dice loss (1 - dice coefficient) averaged across the 4 classes.
- Label 4 was temporarily converted to 3 to satisfy an NN implementation constraint of contiguous label values
- Dice coefficient as metric to plot the train/validation performance, and pick point on the loss graph. We picked epoch 12.
- Learning rate set to 0.001 with decay rate as 1/10th of original every two epochs.

2.4 Post-processing

We further process the predicted 3D volume to removing artifacts. A volume based post-processing was performed as follows:

1. With a binary array of the 3D volume, find all connected components
2. Remove any components smaller than 10 voxels. If greater, remove any components with a convex hull volume less than 500, or with any of the height, width and length less than 8 pixels.
3. For components that remain, apply a minimum filter of (8,8,8) and remove any components that become 0. This is to remove all volumes thinner than 8 pixels.
4. Regain original labels by multiplying the resulting binary matrix with the image.

2.5 Updates for Unseen Test Data

The following changes were made before running on the final unseen test data:

- Pseudo RGB images were replaced by pseudo RGBA image mapping:
- Added an extra upsampling layer and additional convolutions in the UNet to get a 4 class output.
- Removed post-processing step.

Table 2. Pseudo RGBA channel mapping

Channel	Input mapping
R	FLAIR
G	T1ce
B	T2
A	T1

2.6 System Configuration

All analysis was performed on the following system configuration of OS: Ubuntu 18.04.5 LTS x86_64, CPU: Intel Xeon E5-2630 v4 (40) @ 3., GPU: NVIDIA Corporation Device - 2080Ti, and Memory: 63310 MiB.

3 Results

3.1 Challenge Test Data

For different models we ran inference on 240 to 720 scans from the test data. Performance of different models are shown in Table 3. Resnet50 with Traversky loss performed the best, however we were not able to submit it for validation testing. The model with Resnet50 and averaged multiclass dice loss was submitted for validation and is highlighted in bold in the table. All further results are described for this model with some examples shown in Fig. 3.

Table 3. Performance of Neural Network models with different parameter settings using multi-class Dice loss. The model used for validation is highlighted in boldface.

Encoder	Loss function	Additional information	Number of MRI scans	Label 0 (background)	Label 1 (TC)	Label 2	Label 4 (ET)
vgg16	cross categorical entropy	batchsize 64, steps per epoch 200, train data size 37k, learning rate 0.01	240	0.99701368	0.88008051	0.70369906	0.76246457
0.74082 for the necrotic core, and 0.72760 for the contrast-enhancing tumor vgg16	focal loss	batchsize 64, steps per epoch 590, train data size 37k, Alpha=0.25, gamma defaults for focal loss	240	0.99750082	0.85201288	0.60124781	0.75680203
vgg16	focal loss	batchsize 64, steps per epoch 775, train data size 49k, Alpha=0.25,0.5,0.8, gamma defaults for focal loss	720	0.99769684	0.85800296	0.70371188	0.74883617
resnet50	focal loss	batchsize 64, steps per epoch 775, train data size 49k, Alpha=[0.25,1,1,1], gamma default for focal loss	720	0.99773022	0.85767896	0.68001624	0.73863021
resnet50(biblname)	**averaged multiclass dice loss**	**batchsize 64, steps per epoch 1784, train data size 117k, Alpha=[0.25,0.5,0.5,0.5], gamma default for focal loss**	**120**	**0.99992675**	**0.84946028**	**0.66450874**	**0.68517122**
resnet50	tcversky loss	batchsize 64, steps per epoch 1784, train data size 117k, Alpha 0.7	720	0.99817137	0.65520948	0.73026171	0.80049994

Dice loss outperformed multi category cross entropy and custom weighted focal loss. The sensitivity for class 1 (NCR) has been a challenge and by averaging the dice score, generally all metrics have improved compared to earlier methods. From a computation perspective, each inference took about 1 min 15 s, with majority of time spent in noise removal routine. Since the gains from this are uncertain, we plan to baseline the numbers with and without this.

3.2 Validation Data

Table 4 shows the scores of our model on the validation data. Our model produced an average Dice score of 0.8872 for the whole tumor, 0.79052 for the necrotic core, and 0.72760 for the contrast-enhancing tumor.

Table 4. Scores on validation data from submission ID: 9715178

scan_id	Dice_ET	Dice_TC	Dice_WT	Hausdorff95_ET	Hausdorff95_TC	Hausdorff95_WT	Sensitivity_ET	Sensitivity_TC	Sensitivity_WT	Specificity_ET	Specificity_TC	Specificity_WT
mean	0.7276	0.7905	0.8872	31.2841	14.5532	4.6821	0.7482	0.7670	0.8665	0.9996	0.9997	0.9993
sd	0.2691	0.2510	0.0964	96.2005	55.3922	5.4839	0.2845	0.2719	0.1229	0.0005	0.0004	0.0007
median	0.8298	0.8973	0.9171	2.2361	3.0000	3.0000	0.8599	0.8877	0.9069	0.9997	0.9998	0.9995
25quantile	0.7410	0.7788	0.8741	1.4142	1.7320	2.0000	0.7213	0.6952	0.8269	0.9995	0.9997	0.9991
75quantile	0.8823	0.9327	0.9397	4.1231	7.0478	4.5826	0.9168	0.9434	0.9408	0.9999	0.9999	0.9997

3.3 Unseen Test Data

Table 5 shows the scores of our model on the final unseen test data. Our updated model produced an average Dice scores of 0.89656 for the whole tumor, 0.83734 for the necrotic core, and 0.81162 for the contrast-enhancing tumor.

The updated model performed better on the Hausdorff distance metric as well. The reported Hausdorff distance is low till the 75th percentile, but the average Hausdorff is raised by outliers. Improving the model's performance on small tumors would likely trim these outliers.

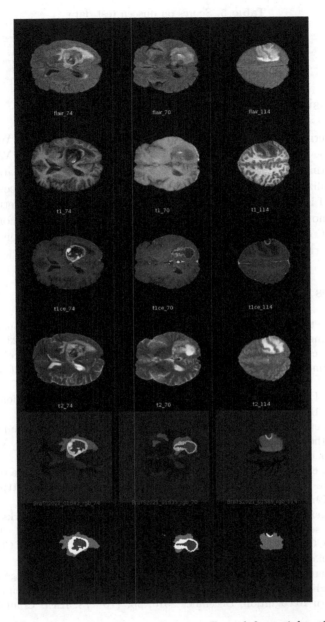

Fig. 3. Examples of predictions on test data set. From left to right, these are axial plane slices 74, 70, and 114 of BraTS2021 01642, 01633, and 01589 IDs respectively. The Dice scores for 01642 are 0.83,0.90,0.89 for labels 1, 2, and 4 respectively. The Dice scores for 01633 are 0.92,0.69,0.86 for labels 1, 2, and 4 respectively. The Dice scores for 01589 are 0.39,0.93,0.90 for labels 1, 2, and 4 respectively. From top to bottom - FLAIR, T1, T1ce, T2, segmentation overlayed on the pseudo RGB image, and predicted segmentation image. For predicted segmentation image, the label colors are: 0-black, 1-dark grey, 2-light grey, 4-white

Table 5. Scores on unseen test data

Label	Dice_ET	Dice_WT	Dice_TC	Sensitivity_ET	Sensitivity_WT	Sensitivity_TC	Specificity_ET	Specificity_WT	Specificity_TC	Hausdorff95_ET	Hausdorff95_WT	Hausdorff95_TC
Mean	0.8116	0.8966	0.8373	0.8256	0.9059	0.8408	0.9997	0.9991	0.9997	20.9267	9.9305	18.4267
StdDev	0.2404	0.0973	0.2571	0.2508	0.1005	0.2548	0.0003	0.0009	0.0007	77.7105	16.2809	66.9952
Median	0.8938	0.9279	0.9392	0.9256	0.9431	0.9432	0.9998	0.9993	0.9998	1.4142	3.7416	2.2361
25quantile	0.8131	0.8815	0.8648	0.8318	0.8718	0.8612	0.9996	0.9989	0.9997	1.0	2.0	1.4142
75quantile	0.9423	0.9539	0.9665	0.9597	0.9708	0.9735	0.9999	0.9997	0.9999	2.8284	8.2915	5.4772

4   Discussion

We have experimented with different encoders, and loss functions. We found the dice loss to be superior to focal loss or cross categorical entropy. We intend to spend more time with variations on Dice loss – slower learning rate as well as GDL (generalized dice loss) which offers ability to add class specific weights. Future line of investigation includes using a 3D CNN that may better preserve contextual information across the slices. A quicker approach to incorporate volume information could be thought of by providing layer information from above and below at the final decoding step.

References

1. Baid, U., et al.: The RSNA-ASNR-MICCAI BraTS 2021 benchmark on brain tumor segmentation and Radiogenomic classification. arXiv 2107.02314, July 2021
2. Bakas, G., et al.: Advancing the cancer genome atlas glioma MRI collections with expert segmentation labels and radiomic features. Nat. Sci. Data **4**(170117), 1–13 (2017)
3. Menze, B.H., et al.: The multimodal brain tumor image segmentation benchmark (BRATS). IEEE Trans. Med. Imaging **34**(10), 1993–2024 (2015)
4. Bakas, S., et al.: Segmentation labels and radiomic features for the pre-operative scans of the TCGA-GBM collection [Dataset]. Cancer Imaging Arch. (2017). https://doi.org/10.7937/K9/TCIA.2017.KLXWJJ1Q
5. Bakas, G., et al.: Segmentation labels and radiomic features for the pre-operative scans of the TCGA-LGG collection. Cancer Imaging Arch. (2017). https://doi.org/10.7937/K9/TCIA.2017.GJQ7R0EF
6. Ronneberger, O., Fischer, P., Brox, T.: U-Net: convolutional networks for biomedical image segmentation. In: Navab, N., Hornegger, J., Wells, W.M., Frangi, A.F. (eds.) MICCAI 2015. LNCS, vol. 9351, pp. 234–241. Springer, Cham (2015). https://doi.org/10.1007/978-3-319-24574-4_28
7. He, K., Zhang, X., Ren, S., Sun, J.: Deep residual learning for image recognition. In: Proceedings of the IEEE Computer Society Conference on Computer Vision and Pattern Recognition, December 2016, pp. 770–778. IEEE Computer Society (2015)
8. Implementation of Segnet, FCN, UNet, PSPNet and other models in Keras. https://github.com/divamgupta/image-segmentation-keras
9. Sudre, C.H., Li, W., Vercauteren, T., Ourselin, S., Jorge Cardoso, M.: Generalised dice overlap as a deep learning loss function for highly unbalanced segmentations. In: Cardoso, M.J., et al. (eds.) DLMIA/ML-CDS -2017. LNCS, vol. 10553, pp. 240–248. Springer, Cham (2017). https://doi.org/10.1007/978-3-319-67558-9_28
10. Sudre, C.H., Li, W., Vercauteren, T., Ourselin, S., Jorge Cardoso, M.: Generalised dice overlap as a deep learning loss function for highly unbalanced segmentations.

In: Cardoso, M.J., et al. (eds.) DLMIA/ML-CDS -2017. LNCS, vol. 10553, pp. 240–248. Springer, Cham (2017). https://doi.org/10.1007/978-3-319-67558-9_28

11. Simonyan, K., Zisserman, A.: Very deep convolutional networks for large-scale image recognition. In: 3rd International Conference on Learning Representations, ICLR 2015 - Conference Track Proceedings, 2014-September. International Conference on Learning Representations, ICLR (2014)

12. Hanif, F., et al.: Glioblastoma multiforme: a review of its epidemiology and pathogenesis through clinical presentation and treatment. Asian Pac. J. Cancer Prev. **18**(1), 3–9 (2017)

13. Mrugala, M.M.: Advances and challenges in the treatment of glioblastoma: a clinician's perspective. Discov Med. **15**(83), 221–30 (2013)

14. Çiçek, Ö., Abdulkadir, A., Lienkamp, S., Brox, T., Ronneberger, O.: 3D U-Net: learning dense volumetric segmentation from sparse annotation (2016)

15. Chen, W., Liu, B., Peng, S., Sun, J., Qiao, X.: S3D-UNet: separable 3D U-Net for brain tumor segmentation. In: Crimi, A., Bakas, S., Kuijf, H., Keyvan, F., Reyes, M., van Walsum, T. (eds.) BrainLes 2018. LNCS, vol. 11384, pp. 358–368. Springer, Cham (2019). https://doi.org/10.1007/978-3-030-11726-9_32

Brain Tumor Segmentation (BraTS) Challenge Short Paper: Improving Three-Dimensional Brain Tumor Segmentation Using SegResnet and Hybrid Boundary-Dice Loss

Cheyu Hsu[1], Chunhao Chang[2], Tom Weiwu Chen[1], Hsinhan Tsai[3], Shihchieh Ma[2], and Weichung Wang[2(✉)]

[1] Division of Medical Oncology, Department of Oncology, National Taiwan University Hospital, Taipei, Taiwan
[2] MeDA Lab and Institute of Applied Mathematical Sciences, National Taiwan University, Taipei, Taiwan
wwangntu@gmail.com
[3] Department of Computer Science and Information Engineering, National Taiwan University, Taipei, Taiwan

Abstract. The advancements in biotechnology and healthcare have led to the increasing use of artificial intelligence in medical imaging analysis. Recently, image recognition technology such as deep learning has become an important tool used for the detection and diagnosis of tumors. As labeling and annotation of tumors are time-consuming, it is necessary to design an approach that can automatically and accurately label tumors. Training a convolutional neural network (CNN) is possible to automatically interpret medical images more accurately, thereby assisting physicians in their diagnosis. In this paper, we describe an automated segmentation model by combining SegResnet and different loss functions to segment brain tumors in multimodal magnetic resonance imaging (MRI) scans and accelerate the tumor annotation process. By adding refinements to our training process, including region-based training, postprocessing, we were able to achieve Dice scores of 0.8159, 0.8734, and 0.9193, and Hausdorff Distance (95th percentile) of 20.02, 7.99, and 4.12 for the enhancing tumor (ET), whole tumor (WT), and tumor core (TC) respectively on the validation dataset.

Keywords: Brain tumor · MRI scans segmentation · SegResnet · Dice loss · Boundary loss

1 Introduction

Malignant brain tumor accounts for 1.7% of all cancer types, and was noticed with poor survival [1]. Studies have shown that high grade brain tumors, such as high-grade glioma, results in poor survival rate than low grade glioma [2]. Different MRI sequence help localized the boundary of brain tumors. Accurate segmentation of brain tumors may help

A. Crimi and S. Bakas (Eds.): BrainLes 2021, LNCS 12963, pp. 334–344, 2022.
https://doi.org/10.1007/978-3-031-09002-8_30

subsequent treatment such as surgery or radiotherapy. Though, manual segmentation of brain tumors is laborious and time-consuming for physicians.

Therefore, recent advances have been focusing on incorporating deep learning to replace basic manual imaging assessments with imaging techniques that can automatically analyze tumor scans, which can help accelerate and improve the diagnosis. As a result, deep learning is being increasingly employed in medical imaging. The main problem arises within the field of three-dimensional (3D) medical image segmentation research: the applicability results from the inability to effectively implement the deep learning models into medical facilities and related research. Most existing models have failed during the deployment stage due to memory constraints and limited resource availability.

In recent years, convolutional neural network (CNN)-based models, such as U-Net, SegNet, and ResNet, have frequently been employed to address the issues of brain tumor segmentation. However, it is difficult to determine and build the most effective architectures for all targeted problems. Hence, our team employed SegResnet, which employs residual blocks and convolution blocks in an encoder-decoder architecture, as a more efficient model for MRI scans segmentation tasks.

Furthermore, we incorporate dice loss to calculate the difference between our predicted results and the ground truth, by this way, our model can gradually be trained to overlap the predicted results and ground truth. Boundary loss is also employed in our model to measure the boundary edge similarity between the ground truth and the prediction mask. For the tumor-based evaluation, our main goal is to calculate the loss value of all tumors detected by our model to check the learning condition as well as the overall performance of the model. Above all, our approach has potential in future deployment and contributions that are listed as follows:

1. An approach is introduced that integrates SegResnet with hybrid loss for accurate segmentation in brain tumors.
2. A robust technique that has acceptable generalizability in the BraTS 2021 dataset is introduced.

2   Method

Our experimental results were carried out with SegResnet as the basis of our network architecture. We employed a train-validation-test split of 8:1:1. Further, we incorporated dice loss as the loss function. The overall workflow of our automatic segmentation process is presented in Fig. 1, the input MRI Scans are pre-processed and trained before eventually being evaluated and segmented.

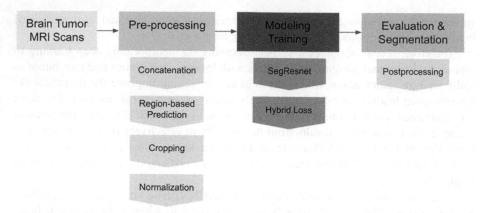

Fig. 1. The workflow of the automatic segmentation process

2.1 Datasets

This retrospective study was approved by RSNA-ASNR-MICCAI BraTS. The dataset was taken from BraTS2021 datasets, consisting of 1,251 training samples and 219 validation samples of multi-institutional routine clinically acquired multi-parametric MRI (mpMRI) scans of glioma with brain tumors. All scans have the same size of 240 x 240 x 155.

Each patient folder includes four 3D MRI scans, including T1, T2, T1 with contrast agent (T1ce), and Fluid Attenuation Inversion Recover (FLAIR). The ground truth labels include Label 0, identifying the background region, Label 1, identifying the necrotic and non-enhancing tumor core, Label 2, identifying the peritumoral edema, and Label 4, identifying the gadolinium-enhanced tumor.

2.2 Preprocessing

Only minimal image preprocessing is required as the BraTS database has been properly curated, de-skulled, registered, cropped to the same size of 240 x 240 x 155, and resampled uniformly to 1 x 1 x 1 mm^3. Our pre-processing method includes four distinct steps: concatenation, region-based prediction, cropping, and normalization. Detailed information is as follows:

1. Concatenation:
   We combined the multimodal MRI scans of each patient into a single input to be trained in the same model, to allow the model to learn identifying features of tumor regions not only from within a single MRI scan but also from the difference between MRI scans produced from different settings. The T1ce, T1, T2, and FLAIR MRI scans of size 240 x 240 x 155 were merged together in the channel dimension to form a final input size of 4 x 240 x 240 x 155.
2. Region-Based Prediction
   The ground truth labels of MRI scans separated the tumor regions into the necrotic and non-enhancing tumor core, the peritumoral edema, and the gadolinium-enhanced

tumor. However, for identification purposes using MRI scans, due to similar intensities and other identifying characteristics of the tumor sub-regions, we combined Label 1 and Label 4 to form the tumor core (TC), Label 1, Label 4, and Label 2 to form the whole tumor (WT) and label as the enhancing tumor (ET), as used by Wang et al. [3]. As a result of this step, the original label of 0, 1, 2, 4 were separated into three channels of binarized labels and combined into a ground truth label of size 3 x 240 x 240 x 155.

3. Cropping:
Image cropping aims to improve the composition and the aesthetic quality of an image by removing extraneous content from it [4]. In the training phase of our experiment, we cropped the input MRI scans into a fixed size of 224 x 224 x 144. In contrast to previous years BraTS competitions, where GPU size was a constraint, and sizes of 128 x 128 x 128 or 96 x 96 x 96 were employed, we utilized a crop size that is very close to the original image of 240 x 240 x 155, that can be divisible by 8, and can allow the network to learn directly from entire brain regions.

4. Normalization:

In preprocessing of MRI images, a normalization method is a critical step. This is because unhealthy brain images are challenging to segment, as the tumor-bearing locations vary with inconsistencies in sizes and shapes. In addition, in the BraTS 2021 dataset, each patient folder includes four complimentary 3D MRI images of differing modalities. As a result, we employed z-score normalization ($z - score(x) = \frac{x-mean(X)}{std(X)}$ where $x \in$ X)$z - score(x) = \frac{x-mean(X)}{std(X)}$ where xX on the images to prevent any biases due to different modalities or inherent variability in MRI images. Channel-wise mean and standard deviation values were calculated by only including the foreground voxels.

2.3 Data Augmentation

We added data augmentation to allow the model to learn from a larger and more diverse set of images, to add to model robustness and increase model generalizability. We applied a 50% chance random flipping of images in all three channels, a 100% chance random scaling of voxel intensity in the range of 0.9 to 1.1 and another 100% chance random shifting of voxel intensity between the values of −0.1 and 0.1.

2.4 Network Architecture: C2FNAS

NVIDIA developed C2FNAS, a method that combines NAS with 3D medical image segmentation as shown in Fig. 1. The search procedure is divided into two stages: coarse and fine stages. The coarse stage searches the network topology, while the fine stage finds the most suitable operation configuration on each node for the current topology [5].

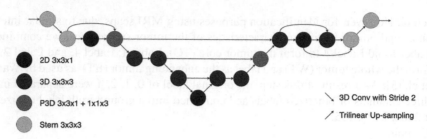

Fig. 2. Architecture of C2FNAS

2.5 Network Architecture: SegResNet

SegResNet is the model architecture name, based on the winning model employed by Myronenko [6] in his 2018 paper, which was the winner of the BraTS 2018 competition. The architecture is built upon the encoder-decoder framework, with a proportionally larger encoder, responsible for extracting data features, and a corresponding decoder structure to construct the segmentation masks. Myronenko [6] also included a variational autoencoder (VAE) branch to regularize the encoder using the output of the encoder as its input. This branch is not included in the architecture used in this paper, as the data size of the BraTS 2021 competition includes 1,251 patients, each with four MRI modalities, which is many times the data set size available for the BraTS 2018 competition, which included only 285 cases.

For the encoder portion of the architecture, ResNet blocks are used, which includes a skip connection and two convolution blocks and ReLu activation layer. Group normalization is utilized to avoid performance penalties associated with Batch normalization with small batch sizes. The downsampling convolution utilizes strided convolution, which progressively increases feature size by two, using 3x3x3 stride two kernels, PReLu activation, with an initial number of filters chosen to be 16. The encoder part of the architecture is four layers deep, with respectively one, two, two and four ResNet blocks per layer.

As shown in Fig. 2, The decoder portion of the architecture utilizes a similar block as the encoder portion. The three layers of the decoder architecture each have one ResNet block component, which is preceded by an upsampling step, using a 1x1x1 conclusion block to reduce the number of features a factor of two, and increasing the spatial dimension by a scaling factor of two using linear interpolation. The end of the decoder includes a normalization step, an in-place ReLu activation, and a 1x1x1 convolution block to output three channel masks of equal size to the four channel input images. Overall, our model proved to be an efficient architecture for the segmentation of brain MRI scans (Fig. 3).

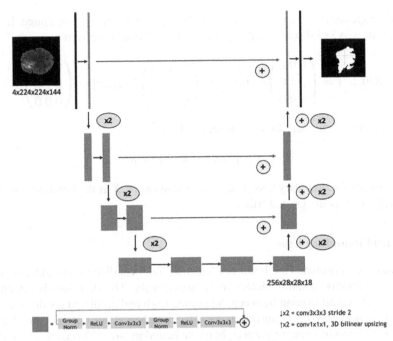

4x224x224x144

256x28x28x18

↓x2 = conv3x3x3 stride 2
↑x2 = conv1x1x1, 3D bilinear upsizing

= Group Norm → ReLU → Conv3x3x3 → Group Norm → ReLU → Conv3x3x3 → ⊕

Fig. 3. Architecture of SegResNet

2.6 Dice Loss

In classification tasks, binary cross-entropy is often used to determine the loss. However, one notable property of this loss is the ease to classify a loss with nontrivial magnitude. When the labels of the dataset are imbalanced, anomalies are considered less or, in other words, anomalies are more difficult for the model to recognize. Consequently, the label imbalance problem is common in anomaly detection or segmentation tasks as the region of interest (ROI) is always a small region. dice loss, also called the overlap index, is a region-based loss function that is widely used in medical image segmentation tasks. In edge detection tasks, the predicted edge pixels and ground truth can be regarded as two sets. By applying dice loss, the two sets can be trained to overlap gradually. For three-dimensional binary segmentation, dice loss can be written as follows:

$$Dice(\theta) = \frac{2|X| \cap |Y|}{|X| + |Y|} \tag{1}$$

where X, $Y \in \{0, 1\}^{M \times N \times L}$ is the ground true mask for any 3D space M, N, and L, and the prediction mask, respectively, while the operation |.| represents the volume of the mask.

2.7 Boundary Loss

Boundary loss is incorporated to measure the boundary edge similarity between the ground truth and the prediction mask. Laplacian filter, which is a common convolution kernel in image analysis, was used to detect the edge of the pixel-wise image. If we let K (kernel) be a 3x3x3 discrete Laplacian filter, then K can be derived as:

$$K[0, :, :] = \begin{pmatrix} 0 & 0 & 0 \\ 0 & 1 & 0 \\ 0 & 0 & 0 \end{pmatrix} K[1, :, :] = \begin{pmatrix} 0 & 1 & 0 \\ 1 & -6 & 1 \\ 0 & 1 & 0 \end{pmatrix} K[2, :, :] = \begin{pmatrix} 0 & 0 & 0 \\ 0 & 1 & 0 \\ 0 & 0 & 0 \end{pmatrix} \quad (2)$$

Consequently, boundary loss can be derived as:

$$L_B(\theta) = [F(X) \times K - Y \times K]^2 \quad (3)$$

where L_B stands for boundary loss, F is the neural network, X is the input data, K stands for Kernel, and Y is the ground truth.

2.8 Hybrid Boundary Loss

In our model, we combined the boundary loss with the focal dice loss to address various imbalance problems in tumor detection simultaneously. The dice loss is effective at increasing the overall overlap between the ground truth and predicted results. However, segmentation accuracy for boundary areas is lacking, hence, we combine the dice loss with boundary loss to increase the weight of the boundary area. This hybrid loss can be used to enhance the segmentation accuracy by applying 3D information of MRI scans to a two-dimensional (2D) SegResnet network. We achieved a better result by implementing dice loss and boundary loss separately.

$$DICE(\theta) + L_B(\theta) \quad (4)$$

2.9 Postprocessing

Not all glioma patients present with an enhancing tumor. In submitting the validation prediction labels to the Synapse server, a Dice score of one and a Hausdorff value of zero are awarded when both model output and ground truth segmentation masks do not include enhancing tumors. However, only a single voxel in model output is enhancing tumor when ground truth segmentation mask has no enhancing tumor will result in a Dice score of zero and a Hausdorff value of 373.128664. This has a significant impact on the performance of the model in regards to enhancing tumors in the validation phase. As a result, we applied a postprocessing step that checked when the model output enhancing tumor voxel count is lower than a certain threshold, these voxel values are readjusted to indicate necrotic and non-enhancing tumor core. This threshold value is determined through a grid value, applying the same postprocessing step to the training phase model output, and comparing the processed model output with the training phase ground-truth label, then using the threshold with the best Dice score, and applying the same threshold value to the validation phase model output [7].

3   Results

Using BraTS 2021 training dataset (1,251 cases) without any additional in-house data. Our model was encoded in Pytorch (https://pytorch.org/) and MONAI (https://monai.io/), implemented in Clara Train version 4.0, trained on GPU- Nvidia Quadro RTX 8000. During training, we used random crops of size 224x224x144 which ensures that most image content remains within the crop area. These datasets were provided with unknown glioma grades and unknown segmentation. We concatenated four 3D MRI scans into 4-channel input images. The output of the model is 3-channel region-based predictions, using sigmoid. Figure 4 shows the FLAIR image, ground truth label, and the predicted results.

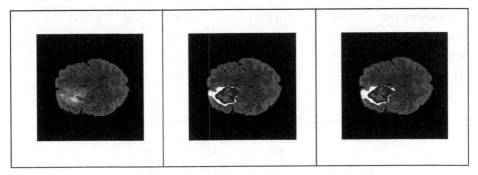

Fig. 4. From the left to right are, respectively, the FLAIR image, the ground truth label, and the prediction, showing good model prediction for ET, TC, WT. (In this figure, ET is labeled green, TC is the union of green and red, and WT includes all visible labels.) (Color figure online)

By comparing training results between C2FNAS and SegResnet, SegResnet provided better results as shown in Fig. 5. Hence, SegResnet is an appropriate method in this study.

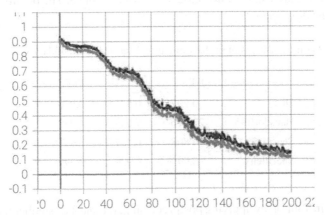

Fig. 5. Comparison of training loss between C2FNAS and SegResnet. (The orange line represents the result of SegResnet while the blue line represents that of C2FNAS.) (Color figure online)

First of all, we evaluated the performance of our model on the training set of 1,251 images, with the results shown in Table 1. From the result, it is clear that the prediction of the model improved by incorporating boundary loss. We then uploaded our model predictions of the validation dataset to the BraTS 2021 server for evaluation, against the validation dataset of 219 cases. The results of per class dice, Hausdorff distance, sensitivity, and specificity are listed in Table 2.

Table 1. The result of the training dataset (SegResnet with & without (w/o) boundary loss, using filter size 32, and crop to 128 x 128 x 128)

	Validation mean dice	Validation mean dice ET	Validation mean dice TC	Validation mean dice WT
W/o boundary loss	0.907	0.882	0.911	0.928
With boundary loss	0.909	0.888	0.911	0.931
Initial filter 32	0.900	0.879	0.894	0.929
128 x 128 x 128	0.894	0.876	0.900	0.908

Table 2. The result of the validation dataset

	ET	TC	WT
Dice	0.798	0.873	0.919
Hausdorff95	23.534	7.996	4.123
Sensitivity	0.808	0.875	0.934
Specificity	0.999	0.999	0.999

By adding boundary loss, the result should have improved. However, the Dice score of the validation dataset slightly decrease as shown in Table 3. The possible reasons are discussed in the next section.

Table 3. The result of the validation dataset (with boundary loss)

	ET	TC	WT
Dice	0.797	0.871	0.920
Hausdorff95	28.116	7.604	4.232
Sensitivity	0.808	0.867	0.931
Specificity	0.999	0.999	0.999

As shown in Table 4, by applying postprocessing, ET and TC (smaller tumor regions) increase. Hence, postprocessing can improve the model performance especially for smaller regions of the tumors.

Table 4. The result of the validation dataset (after postprocessing)

	ET	TC	WT
Dice	0.815	0.873	0.919
Hausdorff95	20.020	7.996	4.123
Sensitivity	0.826	0.875	0.934
Specificity	0.999	0.999	0.999

4 Discussion

In this paper, we proposed a method for the automatic segmentation of brain tumors on MRI scans, which shows potential in the generalizability and applicability across local hospitals.

4.1 Model Performance Evaluation

The performances of the training and validation sets in our experiment are similar, with roughly identical results for WT, a bigger drop for TC, and then an about 0.1 Dice score gap for ET. This difference in dice score is inversely proportional to the difference in the size of the target region, with WT being the largest and ET the smallest. As our model uses a multi-channel training framework, whether the segmentation mask of WT, TC, and ET are produced simultaneously through a single iteration of the model, the loss value is also computed through an effective aggregation of all three channels without weighing for the amount of contribution each channel has to the final loss value, the channel with the largest contribution would then result in higher performance compared to other channels. While experimenting with the training dataset, we have adjusted the initial filter count, the crop size, crop sample count, and network architecture. These changes either resulted in a worse or similar performance in regards to validation Dice score.

Performance result was expected to improve with the inclusion of boundary loss, as an integral over the interface between regions instead of an unbalanced integral over the regions should mitigate difficulties associated with unbalanced datasets. In addition, adding boundary loss should contribute to Hausdorff distance performance. There was indeed a small increase in training set result, with the largest improvement evident in the WT Dice score. However, the validation result showed that the model with boundary loss had a slightly worse performance in ET and TC Dice score and a slight improvement in WT Dice score, although the difference was small, in the range of 0.001, 0.002. A possible reason for this unexpected result is that the BraTS dataset doesn't really include small tumors and the difference in the performance of the two models could be noise. Another possibility stems from the way our boundary loss was calculated and the weight assigned to the loss. Currently, the losses from the three channels are simply summed. Adjusting for relative importance with appropriate weights might result in better model Performance.

Acknowledgments. Data used in this publication were obtained as part of the RSNA-ASNR-MICCAI Brain Tumor Segmentation (BraTS) Challenge project through Synapse ID (syn25829067).

References

1. Hawkes, N.: Cancer survival data emphasise importance of early. BMJ (Clinical research ed.) **364**(l408), (2019)
2. Grover, V.P., Tognarelli, J.M., Crossey, M.M., Cox, I.J., Taylor-Robinson, S.D., McPhail, M.J.: Magnetic resonance imaging: principles and techniques: Lessons for clinicians. J. Clin. Exp. Hepatol. **5**(3), 246–255 (2015)
3. Wang, G., Li, W., Ourselin, S., Vercauteren, T.: Automatic brain tumor segmentation using cascaded anisotropic convolutional neural networks. In: Crimi, A., Bakas, S., Kuijf, H., Menze, B., Reyes, M. (eds.) Brainlesion: Glioma, Multiple Sclerosis, Stroke and Traumatic Brain Injuries 2017, LNCS, vol. 10670, pp. 178–190. Springer, Cham (2018)
4. Zeng, H., Li, L., Cao, Z., Zhang, L.: Reliable and efficient image cropping: a grid anchor-based approach (2019). https://arxiv.org/abs/1904.04441v1
5. Yu, Q., et al.: C2FNAS: Coarse-to-Fine Neural Architecture Search for 3D Medical Image Segmentation (2019). https://arxiv.org/abs/1912.09628
6. Myronenko, A.: 3D MRI brain tumor segmentation using autoencoder regularization (2018). https://arxiv.org/pdf/1810.11654.pdf
7. Isensee, F., Kickingereder, P., Wick, W., Bendszus, M., Maier-Hein, K.: No New-Net (2018). https://arxiv.org/abs/1809.10483
8. Baid, U., et al.: The RSNA-ASNR-MICCAI BraTS 2021 Benchmark on Brain Tumor Segmentation and Radiogenomic Classification (2021). arXiv:2107.02314
9. Bakas, S., et al.: Advancing the cancer genome atlas glioma MRI collections with expert segmentation labels and radiomic features. Nature Scientific Data **4**(170117), (2017)
10. Bakas, S., et al.: Segmentation labels and radiomic features for the pre-operative scans of the TCGA-GBM collection. The Cancer Imaging Archive (2017)
11. Bakas, S., et al.: Segmentation labels and radiomic features for the pre-operative scans of the TCGA-LGG collection. The Cancer Imaging Archive (2017)
12. Menze, B.H., et al.: The multimodal brain tumor image segmentation benchmark (BRATS. IEEE Trans. Med. Imaging **34**(10), 1993–2024 (2015)

A Deep Learning Approach to Glioblastoma Radiogenomic Classification Using Brain MRI

Aleksandr Emchinov[✉]

Moscow Institute of Physics and Technology, Moscow, Russia
aleksandr.emchinov@phystech.edu
https://mipt.ru/english/

Abstract. A malignant brain tumor known as a glioblastoma is an extremely life-threatening condition. It has been proven that the existence of a specific genetic sequence in the tumor known as MGMT promoter methylation is a favourable prognostic factor and a sign of how well a patient will respond to chemotherapy. Currently, the only way to identify the presence of the MGMT promoter is to perform a genetic analysis that requires surgical intervention. The development of an accurate method for determining the presence of the MGMT promoter using only MRI would help to reduce the number of surgeries. In this work, we developed a method for glioblastoma classification using just MRI by choosing an appropriate loss function, neural network architecture and ensembling trained models. This problem was successfully solved as part of the "RSNA-MICCAI Brain Tumor Radiogenomic Classification" competition, and the proposed algorithm was included in the top 5% of best solutions.

Keywords: Deep learning · Medical imaging · Brain tumor classification · Glioblastoma classification · MGMT promoter detection

1 Introduction

With the advent of artificial intelligence, the field of medicine is rapidly evolving. Based on human data collected with the help of various devices, it is possible to make diagnoses and even create new methods of treatment. It is also possible to prevent the progression of certain diseases.

The Radiological Society of North America (RSNA) has teamed up with the Medical Image Computing and Computer Assisted Intervention Society (the MICCAI Society) to improve diagnosis and treatment planning for patients with glioblastoma. The decreasing number of surgeries required for glioblastoma classification is one of the most important priorities in modern medicine. Therefore, developing technologies that allow medical analysis to be performed without surgical intervention is a vital technological and scientific task. Creating tools based

Supported by the RSNA and the MICCAI Society.

on machine learning may help to meet this challenge. RSNA and MICCAI have organized an international competition designed to solve this problem. The main goal of the competition is to develop computer vision algorithms to determine the presence of the MGMT promoter using only MRI scans of patients with glioblastoma.

Consequently, the purpose of this paper is to develop an algorithm which predicts the presence of the MGMT promoter using just MRI. Several approaches have been developed over the past five years to tackle this problem [1–4] and we now have many approaches to classify, detect and segment brain tumors on MRI scans in general [5–8].

In this paper, we present a solution for glioblastoma classification using just MRI, presented in the "RSNA-MICCAI Brain Tumor Radiogenomic Classification" [9] competition on the Kaggle platform.

Our approach is based on 3D convolutional neural networks [10–12]. It is one of the most prominent methods for various classification tasks in different areas of medicine. Our proposed algorithm classifies MGMT status with a high area under the receiver operating characteristic. It was chosen over more than 1500 other solutions to be awarded a silver medal.

The remainder of this work is organized as follows. Sections 2 and 3 discuss data and evaluation method provided by the competition organizers. Section 4 is a step-by step description of our algorithm to classify MGMT status by input images. Our results are presented in Sect. 5. Section 6 summarizes our approach and is followed by the acknowledgements in Sect. 7.

2   Data

The labeled dataset of the MRI scans was provided by the RSNA and MICCAI [13–17]. The challenge data was divided into three cohorts:

1. Training data
2. Validation data (Public Test)
3. Testing data (Private Test)

All these cohorts are structured as follows: each patient has their own folder. These folders contain four sub-folders, each of which corresponds to its own type of MRI scan. The following types of scans were available in the data:

1. Fluid Attenuated Inversion Recovery (FLAIR)
2. T1-weighted pre-contrast (T1w)
3. T1-weighted post-contrast (T1wCE)
4. T2-weighted (T2)

Figure 1 shows an example of these types of MRI scans of data given by the competition organizers.

The database used in the competition included MRI of approximately 1000 patients. Annotations of the presence of MGMT existed for all samples. Training data included 585 directories with MRI(training data), validation data included

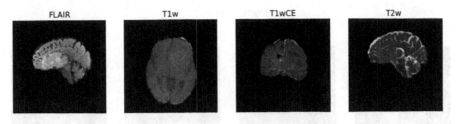

Fig. 1. An MRI example

87 directories(public test data), and testing data included approximately 400 directories(private test data).

However, we faced problems with three directories($[00109, 00123, 00709]$) and excluded them from the training set. The listed patients lack one or more MRI sequences. Therefore, we used 582 directories for training.

All images in the sub-folders were given in dcm-file format. Each of these images has a resolution of 256×256. The training set included annotations with labels to show the presence of the MGMT promoter. The training data is class-balanced. Figure 2 shows class distribution.

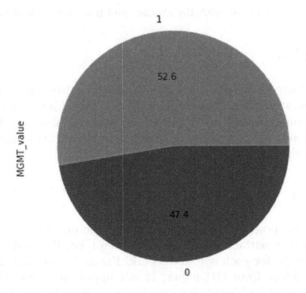

Fig. 2. Class distribution

Figure 3 shows an example of the presence and absence of the MGMT promoter. An MGMT_value which is equal to 1 highlights the presence of the MGMT promoter. Correspondingly, an MGMT_value which is equal to 0 highlights the absence of the MGMT promoter.

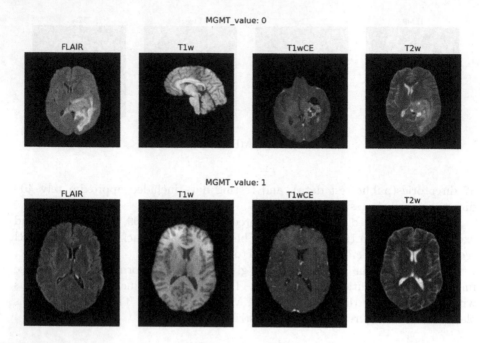

Fig. 3. MRI scans of patients with the absence and presence of the MGMT promoter

3   Evaluation

In order to evaluate the models' performance, the organizers chose the area under the receiver operating characteristic(AUC-ROC) [18]. This metric is widely used in machine learning to estimate the quality of binary classification. ROC analysis is used particularly often in medicine to estimate the quality of new methods of medical diagnosis.

4   Methods

In this paper, we propose a solution based on the ensembling of four neural networks, with one neural network for each scan type. We used 3D ResNet-34 architecture [19,20] for each neural network. Figure 4 shows 3D ResNet neural network architecture from [21] paper. In our approach we use 3D ResNet-34 architecture adapted for binary classification by adding the final fully connected layer for two classes. We also employed a special loss function to train the networks. Afterwards, it was necessary to choose a strategy for how to perform cross-validation. Moreover, ensembling the results of all weights of neural networks was used to achieve a higher value of AUC-ROC and make our model more stable. In this section, we describe each of the above processes one by one.

layer name	output size	18-layer	34-layer	50-layer	101-layer	152-layer
conv1	112×112	7×7, 64, stride 2				
conv2_x	56×56	3×3 max pool, stride 2				
		$\begin{bmatrix} 3\times3,\,64 \\ 3\times3,\,64 \end{bmatrix}\times2$	$\begin{bmatrix} 3\times3,\,64 \\ 3\times3,\,64 \end{bmatrix}\times3$	$\begin{bmatrix} 1\times1,\,64 \\ 3\times3,\,64 \\ 1\times1,\,256 \end{bmatrix}\times3$	$\begin{bmatrix} 1\times1,\,64 \\ 3\times3,\,64 \\ 1\times1,\,256 \end{bmatrix}\times3$	$\begin{bmatrix} 1\times1,\,64 \\ 3\times3,\,64 \\ 1\times1,\,256 \end{bmatrix}\times3$
conv3_x	28×28	$\begin{bmatrix} 3\times3,\,128 \\ 3\times3,\,128 \end{bmatrix}\times2$	$\begin{bmatrix} 3\times3,\,128 \\ 3\times3,\,128 \end{bmatrix}\times4$	$\begin{bmatrix} 1\times1,\,128 \\ 3\times3,\,128 \\ 1\times1,\,512 \end{bmatrix}\times4$	$\begin{bmatrix} 1\times1,\,128 \\ 3\times3,\,128 \\ 1\times1,\,512 \end{bmatrix}\times4$	$\begin{bmatrix} 1\times1,\,128 \\ 3\times3,\,128 \\ 1\times1,\,512 \end{bmatrix}\times8$
conv4_x	14×14	$\begin{bmatrix} 3\times3,\,256 \\ 3\times3,\,256 \end{bmatrix}\times2$	$\begin{bmatrix} 3\times3,\,256 \\ 3\times3,\,256 \end{bmatrix}\times6$	$\begin{bmatrix} 1\times1,\,256 \\ 3\times3,\,256 \\ 1\times1,\,1024 \end{bmatrix}\times6$	$\begin{bmatrix} 1\times1,\,256 \\ 3\times3,\,256 \\ 1\times1,\,1024 \end{bmatrix}\times23$	$\begin{bmatrix} 1\times1,\,256 \\ 3\times3,\,256 \\ 1\times1,\,1024 \end{bmatrix}\times36$
conv5_x	7×7	$\begin{bmatrix} 3\times3,\,512 \\ 3\times3,\,512 \end{bmatrix}\times2$	$\begin{bmatrix} 3\times3,\,512 \\ 3\times3,\,512 \end{bmatrix}\times3$	$\begin{bmatrix} 1\times1,\,512 \\ 3\times3,\,512 \\ 1\times1,\,2048 \end{bmatrix}\times3$	$\begin{bmatrix} 1\times1,\,512 \\ 3\times3,\,512 \\ 1\times1,\,2048 \end{bmatrix}\times3$	$\begin{bmatrix} 1\times1,\,512 \\ 3\times3,\,512 \\ 1\times1,\,2048 \end{bmatrix}\times3$
	1×1	average pool, 1000-d fc, softmax				
FLOPs		1.8×10^9	3.6×10^9	3.8×10^9	7.6×10^9	11.3×10^9

Fig. 4. 3D ResNet architectures for ImageNet. Building blocks are shown in brackets.

4.1 Loss Function

We used a distribution-based loss as a loss function. This strategy allowed us to achieve a higher AUC-ROC value and is one of the key features of the proposed solution. The loss is binary cross-entropy, which is given by the following formula:

$$L_{\mathrm{BCE}}(y, \hat{p}) = -\big[y \log \hat{p} + (1 - y) \log(1 - \hat{p})\big], \tag{1}$$

where y and $\hat{p}$ are the true label and the predicted probability respectively. As an experiment, we tried some other losses such as AUC Loss [22]. However, it showed no better convergence in comparison to the chosen binary cross-entropy loss. As a result, we decided on the latter and minimized it during the training process.

4.2 Cross-validation

We came up with one strategy to perform cross-validation. It involved dividing training directories across folds and stratifying them by according to whether or not the MGMT promoter was present. As a result of this data partitioning strategy, each fold is class-balanced. This strategy gave good results on our validation as well as on the public test data.

As we mentioned above, there are 582 directories in the training set. We divided them across five folds in a straightforward manner. Table 1 shows the number of patients in each fold.

Table 1. Fold-patient relationships

Number of folds	0	1	2	3	4
Number of patients with the MGMT promoter	62	61	61	61	61
Number of patients without the MGMT promoter	55	56	55	55	55
Total number of patients	117	117	116	116	116

4.3   Model Training

In order to solve the glioblastoma classification problem, we trained the 3D convolutional neural network for each MRI scan type. As mentioned in the previous subsection, the training process was performed using cross-validation on five folds for every scan type. As a result, we trained five sets of weights for the FLAIR scan type, five sets for the T1w, five sets for the T1wCE and five sets for the T2, bringing us to twenty trained neural networks in total.

To analyze each type of MRI scan, we used 3D ResNet-34 neural network architecture. We trained all of the neural networks in the same way with the similar hyper parameters.

The 3D neural network inputs are three dimensional tensors. We have formed each input tensor in such a way that it consists of 64 MRI scan' slices. Therefore, the dimensions of the inputs are $256 \times 256 \times 64$.

The number of epochs was limited to twenty, binary cross-entropy loss was used as the loss function, and Adam [23] was used as the optimizer.

We used an exponential scheduler [24] to change the learning rate during the training process for better convergence.

We used the value of the area under the ROC curve to control models' performance. We used it for stopping the training in the case of the AUC-ROC not improving on the validation data. This means that if the metric value on the validation data does not improve over a certain number of epochs, we stop the training process.

As the final weights of neural networks used for inference, we chose the weights from the epochs corresponding to the minimum validation loss value for each fold.

The training parameter values are shown in Table 2. If some parameters are missing, it is assumed that they are equal to the default values in PyTorch version 1.7.0.

Table 2. Training parameters of models

Parameter	Value
Neural network architecture	3D ResNet-34
Maximum number of epochs	20
Number of epochs for stopping early	5
Image size	256×256
Number of images in tensor	64
Batch size	6
Loss function	Binary cross entropy loss
Optimizer	Adam
Initial learning rate	1e–4
Weight decay	0
Learning rate scheduler	ExponentialLR
Gamma	0.9

In the Sect. 4.4 we present the training results for each scan type.

4.4 Training Results

Firstly, we take a look at the results of training on the FLAIR scan type. The results are shown in Table 3. The `Best epoch` column corresponds to the number of epochs with the minimum value of validation loss during the training. The average value of AUC-ROC validation is equal to 0.5958.

Table 3. Training results for FLAIR

Fold	Best epoch	Train loss	Valid loss	Train AUC-ROC	Valid AUC-ROC
0	8	0.676546	0.671917	0.598528	0.653666
1	3	0.686666	0.692509	0.571688	0.537471
2	0	0.775976	0.685472	0.527897	0.608048
3	1	0.728562	0.689620	0.537806	0.569001
4	3	0.695735	0.676547	0.556580	0.611028

The results of training on the T1w scan type are presented in Table 4. The average value of AUC-ROC validation is equal to 0.5994.

Table 4. Training results for T1w

Fold	Best epoch	Train loss	Valid loss	Train AUC-ROC	Valid AUC-ROC
0	9	0.661846	0.673121	0.648144	0.611730
1	8	0.667267	0.686279	0.628896	0.637881
2	5	0.686730	0.672385	0.577440	0.615201
3	1	0.712726	0.688672	0.505365	0.559762
4	2	0.690482	0.683943	0.559775	0.572578

Now we consider the results of training on the T1wCE scan type. The results are shown in Table 5. The average value of AUC-ROC validation is equal to 0.5652. This value is a little less than the average AUC-ROC as seen in the FLAIR and T1w scan types.

Table 5. Training results for T1wCE

Fold	Best epoch	Train loss	Valid loss	Train AUC-ROC	Valid AUC-ROC
0	9	0.678149	0.686935	0.598592	0.597067
1	4	0.692633	0.696199	0.564675	0.517564
2	0	0.774426	0.686005	0.490756	0.576751
3	5	0.687899	0.687936	0.556072	0.566617
4	3	0.691288	0.698215	0.556764	0.568107

Finally, we take a look at the results of training on the T2 scan type. The results are shown in Table 6. The average value of AUC-ROC validation is equal to 0.5758. As we can this value is a little less than the average AUC-ROC as seen in the FLAIR and T1w scan types and at the same time is a little more than that of T1wCE.

Table 6. Training results for T2

Fold	Best epoch	Train loss	Valid loss	Train AUC-ROC	Valid AUC-ROC
0	5	0.699441	0.671432	0.532416	0.629326
1	5	0.678554	0.688316	0.610037	0.551815
2	2	0.684151	0.698637	0.581974	0.522206
3	3	0.694851	0.688126	0.554871	0.555291
4	4	0.683007	0.670093	0.589768	0.620566

4.5   Training Summary

As we can see, each trained neural network listed above gives good AUC-ROC values on validation data. The quality of neural networks trained on the FLAIR and T1w scan types is slightly better than that of the models trained on T1wCE and T2. However, the quality of all our trained classifiers is better than random classifier quality. We therefore have twenty trained and validated models to predict the presence of MGMT promoter using just MRI.

4.6   Model Ensembling

We noticed that using models trained on just one MRI scan type gives worse results than using all twenty models. Consequently, we combined models to ensemble in order to increase the score and stability of our solution. That is, we averaged the output of twenty neural networks (five are 3D ResNet-34 trained on the FLAIR scan type, five are 3D ResNet-34 trained on the T1w scan type, yet another five are 3D ResNet-34 trained on the T1wCE scan type and the last five are 3D ResNet-34 trained on the T2w scan type).

5   Results

Figure 5 summarizes each step described in the previous sections. It reflects how an input is processed by the ensemble to arrive at our results.

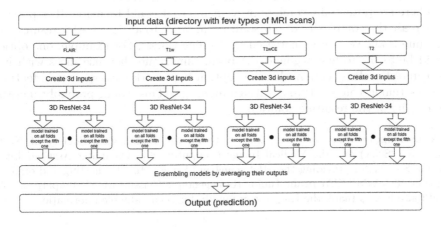

Fig. 5. Algorithm scheme

Our solution takes about one hour to predict the entire amount of private data, while the time limit was nine hours.

This ensemble won a silver medal in the "RSNA-MICCAI Brain Tumor Radiogenomic Classification" competition, finishing among the top 5% of all solutions. Table 7 shows the results of the proposed solution on the public and private datasets. Moreover, the AUC-ROC calculated based on our cross-validation are close to both scores. This means that we chose the right strategy for cross-validation and avoided overfitting.

Table 7. AUC-ROC on public and private datasets

Test	Area under ROC
Public	0.65010
Private	0.58295

Our code is freely available as a public notebook on Kaggle[1].

6 Discussions

In this paper, we presented an efficient and appropriate algorithm for glioblastoma classification. The core of the proposed solution to this problem is an ensemble consisting of a combination of 3D ResNet-34 neural networks trained on four MRI scan types. To achieve better convergence during training and improve the performance of the algorithm, the binary cross-entropy loss was chosen as the loss function. We averaged the outputs of twenty neural networks to increase the score and stability of the resulting method.

There are potentially some improvements that could be made. It is possible to increase the complexity of our solution in order to achieve better results (the run-time is allowed to be increased up to nine times). For example, one option would be to try to first segment the brain tumor and then use slices with just the tumor for classification. Another option is to work with geometric features such as tumor volume, tumor surface area, etc. This would probably increase the quality of the resulting solution.

Acknowledgements. We would like to thank the Radiological Society of North America (RSNA) and the Medical Image Computing and Computer Assisted Intervention Society for providing the MRI scans and Kaggle, Inc. for hosting and organizing the "RSNA-MICCAI Brain Tumor Radiogenomic Classification" competition. We would also like to thank the Kaggle community for their valuable information.

References

1. Yogananda, C.G.B., et al.: MRI-based deep-learning method for determining glioma MGMT promoter methylation status. Am. J. Neuroradiol. **42**(5), 845–852 (2021). https://doi.org/10.3174/ajnr.A7029

---

[1] https://www.kaggle.com/greylord1996/resnet50-all-mri?scriptVersionId=76647838.

2. Chen, X., et al.: Automatic prediction of MGMT status in glioblastoma via deep learning-based MR image analysis.; automatic prediction of MGMT status in glioblastoma via deep learning-based MR image analysis. BioMed. Res. Int. (2020). 10.1155/2020/9258649

3. Korfiatis, P., Kline, T., Lachance, D., Parney, I., Buckner, J., Erickson, B.: Residual deep convolutional neural network predicts MGMT methylation status. J. Digital Imaging. **30**, 622–628 (2017). https://doi.org/10.1007/s10278-017-0009-z

4. Han, L., Kamdar, M.: MRI to MGMT: predicting methylation status in glioblastoma patients using convolutional recurrent neural networks. Pac. Symp. Biocomput. **23**, 331–342 (2018)

5. Sadad, T., Rehman, A., Munir, A., Saba, T., Abbasi, R.: Brain tumor detection and multi-classification using advanced deep learning techniques. Microsc. Res. Techn. **84**, 1296–1308 (2021). https://doi.org/10.1002/jemt.23688

6. Magadza, T., Viriri, S.: Deep learning for brain tumor segmentation: a survey of state-of-the-art. J. Imaging. **7**, 19 (2021). https://doi.org/10.3390/jimaging7020019

7. Grampurohit, S., Shalavadi, V., Dhotargavi, V., Kudari, M., Jolad, S.: Brain tumor detection using deep learning models, pp. 129–134 (2020). https://doi.org/10.1109/INDISCON50162.2020.00037

8. Jayanthi, P., Muralikrishna, I., Esther, E.: Deep learning in oncology- a case study on brain tumor. Int. Cancer Res. Ther. **3**, 1–5 (2019)

9. Research code competition: RSNA-MICCAI Brain Tumor Radiogenomic Classification.https://www.kaggle.com/c/rsna-miccai-brain-tumor-radiogenomic-classification

10. Ji, S., Xu, W., Yang, M., Yu, K.: 3D convolutional neural networks for human action recognition. IEEE Trans. Pattern Anal. Mach. Intell. **35**, 495–502 (2010). https://doi.org/10.1109/TPAMI.2012.59

11. Fritscher, K., Raudaschl, P., Zaffino, P., Spadea, M.F., Sharp, G.C., Schubert, R.: Deep neural networks for fast segmentation of 3D medical images. In: Ourselin, S., Joskowicz, L., Sabuncu, M.R., Unal, G., Wells, W. (eds.) MICCAI 2016. LNCS, vol. 9901, pp. 158–165. Springer, Cham (2016). https://doi.org/10.1007/978-3-319-46723-8_19

12. Casamitjana, A., Aduriz, S., Vilaplana, V.: 3D Convolutional neural networks for brain tumor segmentation: a comparison of multi-resolution architectures, pp. 150–161 (2016). https://doi.org/10.1007/978-3-319-55524-9_15

13. Baid, U., et al.: The RSNA-ASNR-MICCAI BraTS 2021 Benchmark on Brain Tumor Segmentation and Radiogenomic Classification (2021). arXiv:2107.02314

14. Menze, B.H., Jakab, A., Bauer, S., Kalpathy-Cramer, J., Farahani, K., Kirby, J., et al.: The multimodal brain tumor image segmentation benchmark (BRATS). IEEE Trans. Med. Imaging **34**(10), 1993–2024 (2015). https://doi.org/10.1109/TMI.2014.2377694

15. Bakas, S., et al.: Advancing the cancer genome atlas glioma MRI collections with expert segmentation labels and radiomic features. Nat. Sci. Data **4**, 170117 (2017). https://doi.org/10.1038/sdata.2017.117

16. Bakas, S., et al.: Segmentation labels and radiomic features for the pre-operative scans of the TCGA-GBM collection. Cancer Imaging Arch. (2017). https://doi.org/10.7937/K9/TCIA.2017.KLXWJJ1Q

17. Bakas, S., et al.: Segmentation labels and radiomic features for the pre-operative scans of the TCGA-LGG collection. Cancer Imaging Arch. (2017). https://doi.org/10.7937/K9/TCIA.2017.GJQ7R0EF

18. Yang, S., Berdine, G.: The receiver operating characteristic (ROC) curve. Southwest Resp. Critical Care Chron. **5**, 34–36 (2017). https://doi.org/10.12746/swrccc. v5i19.391

19. He, K., Zhang, X., Ren, S., Sun, J.: Deep residual learning for image recognition. 7 (2015)

20. Hara, K., Kataoka, H., Satoh, Y.: Learning spatio-temporal features with 3d residual networks for action recognition, pp. 3154–3160 (2017). https://doi.org/10. 1109/ICCVW.2017.373

21. He, K., Zhang, X., Ren, S., Sun, J.: Deep residual learning for image recognition, pp. 770–778 (2016). https://doi.org/10.1109/CVPR.2016.90

22. Yuan, Z., Yan, Y., Sonka, M., Yang, T.: Large-scale robust deep AUC maximization: a new surrogate loss and empirical studies on medical image classification. In: Proceedings of the IEEE/CVF International Conference on Computer Vision (ICCV), pp. 3040–3049 (2021)

23. Kingma, D., Ba, J.: Adam: a method for stochastic optimization. In: International Conference on Learning Representations (2014)

24. Li, Z., Arora, S.: An Exponential Learning Rate Schedule for Deep Learning (2019)

Radiogenomic Prediction of MGMT Using Deep Learning with Bayesian Optimized Hyperparameters

Walia Farzana, Ahmed G. Temtam, Zeina A. Shboul, M. Monibor Rahman,
M. Shibly Sadique, and Khan M. Iftekharuddin[✉]

Vision Lab, Electrical and Computer Engineering, Old Dominion University Norfolk,
Norfolk, VA 23529, USA
{wfarz001,atemt001,zshbo001,mrahm006,msadi002,kiftekha}@odu.edu

Abstract. Glioblastoma (GBM) is the most aggressive primary brain tumor. The standard radiotherapeutic treatment for newly diagnosed GBM patients is Temozolomide (TMZ). O6-methylguanine-DNA-methyltransferase (MGMT) gene methylation status is a genetic biomarker for patient response to the treatment and is associated with a longer survival time. The standard method of assessing genetic alternation is surgical resection which is invasive and time-consuming. Recently, imaging genomics has shown the potential to associate imaging phenotype with genetic alternation. Imaging genomics provides an opportunity for noninvasive assessment of treatment response. Accordingly, we propose a convolutional neural network (CNN) framework with Bayesian optimized hyperparameters for the prediction of MGMT status from multimodal magnetic resonance imaging (mMRI). The goal of the proposed method is to predict the MGMT status noninvasively. Using the RSNA-MICCAI dataset, the proposed framework achieves an area under the curve (AUC) of 0.718 and 0.477 for validation and testing phase, respectively.

Keywords: Glioblastoma · Convolutional Neural Network (CNN) ·
Radio-genomics · MGMT · Bayesian optimization · Classification

1 Introduction

The most prevalent malignant primary brain tumor in adults is glioblastoma (GBM) which accounts for 48.3% of all malicious brain tumors [1]. The first line radiotherapeutic treatment for GBM patients is Temozolomide (TMZ). The methylation state of the O6-methylguanine-DNA-methyltransferase (MGMT) gene promoter has been a significant biomarker for tumor response to TMZ treatment [2]. MGMT methylation status is associated with prolonged survival time in GBM patients [3]. The standardized method for evaluation of MGMT status is surgical resection which is invasive and time-consuming. Recently, different studies [4,5] have found that genetic alternations are linked to phenotypic changes and can be detected using magnetic resonance imaging (MRI) features.

A. Crimi and S. Bakas (Eds.): BrainLes 2021, LNCS 12963, pp. 357–366, 2022.
https://doi.org/10.1007/978-3-031-09002-8_32

Predicting MGMT status using MRI features can be broadly categorized into two categories: application of machine learning (ML) or deep learning (DL) models. Several studies focused on quantitative and qualitative feature extraction from pre-operative MRI, and then predicting MGMT status utilizing the extracted features in different ML models. V. G. Kanas et al. [6] apply quantitative and qualitative features extracted from segmented tumors, and then apply several dimensionality reduction methods for multivariate analysis of MGMT status. Another study by T. Sasaki et al. [7], the authors apply supervised principal component analysis to predict MGMT status utilizing shape and texture features. On the other hand, Authors in [8] apply different architectures of residual CNN to predict MGMT status. P. Chang et al. [9] focus on 2D CNN filters to extract features, and then apply principal component analysis (PCA) for dimensionality reduction of features that is used in the classification of genetic mutations. The study by E. Calabrese et al. [10] has cascaded deep learned based tumor segmentation with MGMT classification. After 3D tumor segmentation on multiparametric MRI sequence, pyradiomics is utilized for extraction of image features followed by random forest method to analyze the likelihood of MGMT status in patients. Most of the studies require extensive image pre-processing, feature extraction, and tumor segmentation before classifying MGMT methylation status.

In this work, we propose a deep learning-based approach with CNN that does not require tumor segmentation and feature extraction. In addition, to find the optimal hyperparameters in CNN we utilize Bayesian Optimization method.

2   Method

2.1   Description of Dataset

The dataset [11–15] is divided into three cohorts as follows: training, validation and testing. The training dataset consists of 585 patients. Each patient has four modalities of MRI scans in DICOM (Fig. 1): Fluid Attenuated Inversion Recovery (FLAIR), T1-weighted pre-contrast (T1w), T1-weighted post-contrast (T1wCE), and T2-weighted (T2). The MGMT status distribution of the training cohort is as follows: 307 patients are methylated, and 278 patients are unmethylated. The validation cohort consists of 87 patients. Note that the ground truth of validation data and testing data are kept private by the challenge organizers.

2.2   Radiogenomic Classification Model

A convolution neural network is a stacking of convolutional layers. The layers can be categorized into different stages where each stage has a same type of convolutional layer. Each convolution filter is made up of image pixel values that are modified throughout training. The model's parameters are adjusted variables that can be approximated or learned from the data and incorporated within the learning process [16]. The model parameters are not selected manually

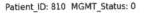
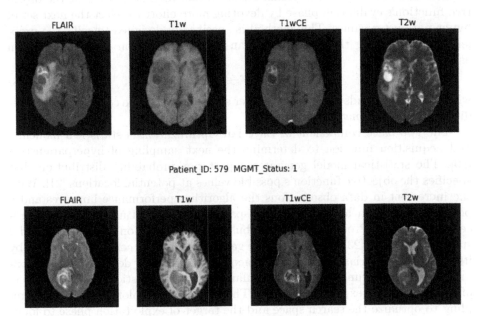

Fig. 1. Representation of MRI modalities with MGMT Status. MGMT status (0) and (1) indicates unmethylated and methylated status.

such as weights in neural network. Hyperparameters are factors that impact the model's training or behavior. Hyperparameters are non-model parameters that cannot be anticipated from the data set but can be customized by subject matter experts or via trial and error until an acceptable accuracy is attained [17].

To obtain high accuracy in classification tasks, users must properly handle the hyperparameter setting procedure, which varies depending on the algorithm and data collection. This procedure can be carried out by using the algorithm's default values or manually configuring them. Another alternative is to use data-dependent hyperparameter-tuning approaches, which aim to reduce the algorithm's estimated generalization error over a hyperparameter search space [17]. There are different methods such as random search, grid search, and Bayesian optimization to automatically configure the hyperparameters. Grid Search evaluates the learning algorithm using all possible hyper-parameter combinations [18]. Every parameter has the same chance of influencing the process. In Grid Search's there are a lot of hyper-parameters to set, and the algorithm's evaluation phase is highly expensive. Random searches utilize the same search space as Grid search using a random process. This method does not produce as accurate results as Grid Search, but it takes less time to compute. The first two approaches are computationally expensive because random combination of hyperparameters are considered. Bayesian Optimization use sequential method for global optimization of objective function [19].

The main idea behind Bayesian Optimization method is to limit the objective function's evaluation phase by devoting more effort to select the next set of hyper-parameter values. This method is specifically designed to solve the problem of determining the maximum of an objective function $f: X \to \mathbb{R}$, given as,

$$argmax_{x \in X} f(x) \tag{1}$$

where, X corresponds to hyperparameter space which can be considered as three-dimensional hypermeter space [19].

The two basic component of Bayesian Optimization is statistical modeling and acquisition function to determine the next sampling of hyperparameters [20]. The statistical model generates a posterior probability distribution that specifies the objective function's possible values at potential locations [21]. With the increment in data observations the algorithm performance improves and a potential region on hyperparameters space is determined using Gaussian Process. A Gaussian Process (GP) is a robust prior distribution on functions and a stochastic process [23]. A multi-variate gaussian process is completely defined by its mean and covariance matrix. The acquisition function determines the maximum of objective function at a particular point. The aquistion function consists of exploration and exploitation phase. The objective of exploration phase is sampling to optimize the search space and the target of exploitation phase to focus on reduced search space to select optimum samples [24].

The Bayesian optimization method employs a surrogate model that is fitted to the real model's observations [25]. In this case, the real model is the Convolutional Neural Network (CNN) with hyperparameters selected for an iteration. In each iteration, it quantifies the uncertainty in the surrogate model using Gaussian process [26]. Then for next iteration, hyperparameter set is chosen using an acquisition function that balances the need to explore the whole search space versus focusing on high-performing sections of the search space.

The proposed pipeline in the Fig. 3 shows data augmentation steps in input data. After the input is provided in the CNN model (Fig. 2), hyperparameter optimization is performed utilizing the Bayesian Optimization method which provides the tunned model with optimized hyperparameters [27]. The tunned model is utilized for a classification model of the methylation status.

2.3 Training Stage

In the training phase, we randomly split the data into 80% training and 20% validation on the basis on methylation and unmethylation status. In training phase, we consider only the T1-weighted post-contrast (T1wCE) modality of MRI. The pre-processing steps consist of selecting fixed number of slices for each patient. At first, we sort out the middle slice number from the list of slices

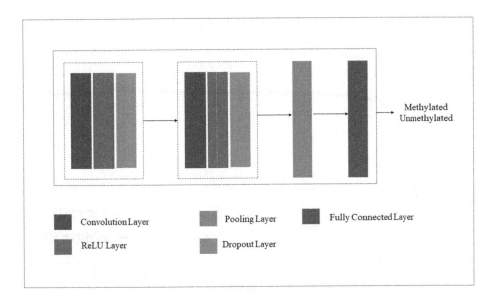

Fig. 2. Architecture of Convolutional Neural Network (CNN) model in pipeline.

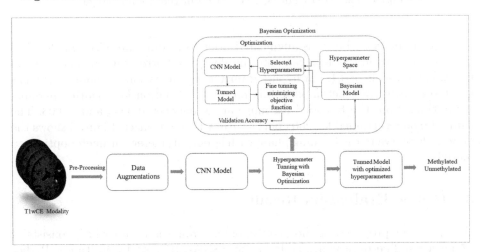

Fig. 3. Overview of the proposed radiogenomic classification pipeline.

for each patient. Afterwards, the slices that are in the range of 25% above the middle slice and 75% below the middle slice is selected with a fixed interval. The interval is three but if a patient data contains less than 10 slices then the interval is changed to one. The selected slices are resized into 32×32-pixel value and normalized between 0 and 255.

W. Farzana et al.

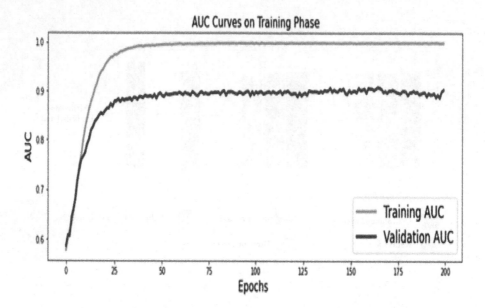

Fig. 4. The Area Under Curve (AUC) in the training stage.

The pre-processed data is augmented prior to feeding into CNN model. The data augmentation includes random flip along the horizontal axis and random rotation with scale of 0.1. For hyperparameters optimization the number of trials is 20 and objective function is to minimize the validation loss. During parameter optimization, the bounded learning rate is between 0.0003 and 0. 003. The tunned model is trained for 200 epochs with Adam optimizer. Figure 4 shows the area under curve in the training phase with hyperparameter parameter optimized model.

3 Online Evaluation Results

We apply our proposed method to the online validation data which consists of 87 patients. The data is available in the RSNA-MICCAI Brain Tumor Radiogenomic classification competition under the Kaggle Platform [15]. We apply the pre-processing steps that are discussed in the previous section. The area under curve (AUC) value in the validation phase is 0.718. In addition, the proposed method is utilized on testing data which is kept private by the challenge organizers. The area under (AUC) value in the testing phase is 0.477. The performance of classification model is shown in the Table 1.

Table 1. Performance of classification model using online evaluation

Phase	Area Under Curve (AUC)
Validation	0.718
Testing	0.477

4 Discussion

In this study, we have applied CNN with Bayesian hyperparameters optimization for classification of MGMT status in Glioblastoma (GBM) patients from MRI. As it can be seen the model performance on testing data drops compared to validation data which might be caused by the lack of generalization of model in the testing data. Moreover, the predictive feature (MGMT) is not directly visible in imaging data which is rather a genomic biomarker identified by molecular analysis in tissue specimens. However, several studies [28–30] have shown that genetic alterations express themselves as phenotypic changes that can be identified by MRI features extracted from the segmented tumor. In our proposed framework, we do not consider tumor segmentation to extract features from the segmented tumor. We utilize the pre-processed DICOM directly to evaluate the methylation status in GBM patient. The goal of the proposed method is to simulate the real-world clinical scenario and asses how well the model generalizes the data obtained from different sources.

The selected slices contain the middle slice and slices selected at a regular interval for each patient. The CNN with Bayesian optimized hyperparameters assist the model to obtain better classification accuracy as depicted in Fig. 4 and in the validation phase of the challenge as shown in Table 1. The training phase contains a simple architecture of CNN and tunned with hyperparameters that is obtained by reducing an objective function in Bayesian process. Therefore, the tunning of the hyperparameters improve the performance when the data distribution is similar in training and validation phase. The dataset consists of multiple image samples from 18 institutions [31]. The source of data and distribution of test data is completely different [31] and hence the classification model is unable to generalize the new data distribution and the selected hyperparameters are not the optimized ones in testing data.

Bayesian Optimization is included in the pipeline to obtain hyperparameters that assist in better classification performance by optimizing the search space. The objective of the Bayesian approach is to reduce the validation loss in each trial and shrink the hyperparameter space after each trail. After completion of pre-defined trials on training data, best hyperparameters are included in the final training of the classification model. However, such hyperparameter optimization may not be able to generalize to data from different source.

5   Conclusion

In this paper, we propose a CNN model with Bayesian Optimized hyperparameters to classify MGMT methylation status in glioblastoma patients. Bayes Optimization is applied to obtain the hyperparameters for the CNN model. The goal of this work is to predict the MGMT status using non-invasive MRI features. The proposed approach does not require extensive tumor segmentation, image pre-processing, and feature extraction steps to predict MGMT status. The proposed method is evaluated on validation and testing dataset provided by RSNA-MICCAI. The validation and testing area under curve (AUC) were 0.718 and 0.477 respectively.

Acknowledgements. We acknowledge partial support from National Institutes of Health grant # R01 EB020683.

References

1. Ostrom, Q.T., et al.: CBTRUS statistical report: primary brain and other central nervous system tumors diagnosed in the United States in 2012–2016. Neuro. Oncol. **21**(Suppl 5), 1–100 (2019)
2. Liu, D., et al.: Imaging-genomics in glioblastoma: combining molecular and imaging signatures. Front. Oncol. **11**, 2666 (2021)
3. Nam, J.Y., De Groot, J.F.: Treatment of glioblastoma. J. Oncol. Pract. **13**(10), 629–638 (2017)
4. Korfiatis, P., et al.: MRI texture features as biomarkers to predict MGMT methylation status in glioblastomas. Med. Phys. **43**(6), 2835–2844 (2016)
5. Hajianfar, G., et al.: Noninvasive O6 Methylguanine-DNA methyltransferase status prediction in glioblastoma multiforme cancer using magnetic resonance imaging radiomics features: univariate and multivariate radiogenomics analysis. World Neurosurg. **132**, 140–161 (2019)
6. Kanas, V.G., et al.: Learning MRI-based classification models for MGMT methylation status prediction in glioblastoma. Comput. Methods Programs Biomed. **140**, 249–257 (2017)
7. Sasaki, T., et al.: Radiomics and MGMT promoter methylation for prognostication of newly diagnosed glioblastoma. Sci. Rep. **9**(1), 1–9 (2019)
8. Korfiatis, P., Kline, T.L., Lachance, D.H., Parney, I.F., Buckner, J.C., Erickson, B.J.: Residual deep convolutional neural network predicts MGMT methylation status. J. Digital Imaging **30**(5), 622–628 (2017). https://doi.org/10.1007/s10278-017-0009-z
9. Chang, P., et al.:Deep-learning convolutional neural networks accurately classify genetic mutations in gliomas. Am. J. Neuroradiol. **39**(7), 1201–1207 (2018)
10. Calabrese, E., et al.: A fully automated artificial intelligence method for non-invasive, imaging-based identification of genetic alterations in glioblastomas. Sci. Rep. **10**(1), 1–11 (2020)
11. Baid, U., et al.: The RSNA-ASNR-MICCAI BraTS 2021 Benchmark on Brain Tumor Segmentation and Radiogenomic Classification. https://arxiv.org/abs/2107.02314. Accessed 09 Aug 2021

12. Menze, B.H., et al.: The multimodal brain tumor image segmentation benchmark (BRATS). IEEE Trans. Med. Imaging. **34**(10), 1993–2024 (2015). https://doi.org/10.1109/TMI.2014.2377694

13. Bakas, S., et al.: Advancing The Cancer Genome Atlas glioma MRI collections with expert segmentation labels and radiomic features. Nat. Sci. Data. **4**, 170–171 (2017). https://doi.org/10.1038/sdata.2017.117

14. Bakas, S., et al.: Segmentation labels and radiomic features for the pre-operative scans of the TCGA-GBM collection. In: The Cancer Imaging Archive (2017). https://doi.org/10.7937/K9/TCIA.2017.KLXWJJ1Q

15. Bakas, S., et al.: Segmentation labels and radiomic features for the pre-operative scans of the TCGA-LGG collection. In: The Cancer Imaging Archive (2017). https://doi.org/10.7937/K9/TCIA.2017.GJQ7R0EF

16. Luo, G.: A review of automatic selection methods for machine learning algorithms and hyper-parameter values. Netw. Model Anal. Health Inform. Bioinform. **5**, 1–6 (2016)

17. Bergstra, J., Bengio, Y.: Random search for hyper-parameter optimization. J. Mach. Learn. Res. **13**, 281–305 (2012)

18. Mersmann, O., Trautmann, H., Weihs, C.: Resampling methods for metamodel validation with recommendations for evolutionary computation. Evol. Comput. **20**, 249–275 (2012)

19. Alibrahim, H., Ludwig, S.A.: Hyperparameter optimization: comparing genetic algorithm against grid search and Bayesian optimization. In: 2021 IEEE Congress on Evolutionary Computation (CEC), Kraków, Poland (2021). https://doi.org/10.1109/CEC45853.2021.9504761

20. Dewancker, I., McCourt, M.J., Clark, S.C.: Bayesian Optimization for Machine Learning : A Practical Guidebook. arXiv:abs/1612.04858 (2016)

21. Bergstra, J., Bardenet, R., Bengio, Y., Kégl, B.: Algorithms for hyper-parameter optimization. In: 24th International Conference on Neural Information Processing Systems (NIPS 2011), Red Hook, NY, USA (2011)

22. Frazier, P.: A Tutorial on Bayesian Optimization. arXiv:abs/1807.02811 (2018)

23. Rasmussen, C.E.: Gaussian processes in machine learning. In: Bousquet, O., von Luxburg, U., Rätsch, G. (eds.) ML -2003. LNCS (LNAI), vol. 3176, pp. 63–71. Springer, Heidelberg (2004). https://doi.org/10.1007/978-3-540-28650-9_4

24. Borgli, R.J., Kvale Stensland, H., Riegler, M.A., Halvorsen, P.: Automatic hyper-parameter optimization for transfer learning on medical image datasets using Bayesian optimization. In: 13th International Symposium on Medical Information and Communication Technology (ISMICT), Oslo, Norway (2019)

25. Fraccaroli, M., Lamma, E., Riguzzi, F.: Automatic setting of DNN hyper-parameters by mixing Bayesian optimization and tuning rules. In: Nicosia, G., et al. (eds.) LOD 2020. LNCS, vol. 12565, pp. 477–488. Springer, Cham (2020). https://doi.org/10.1007/978-3-030-64583-0_43

26. Guillemot, M., Heusèle, C., Korichi, R., Schnebert, S.: Maxime petit and liming Chen: tuning neural network hyperparameters through Bayesian optimization and Application to cosmetic formulation data (2019)

27. Snoek, J., Larochelle, H., Adams, R.P.: Practical Bayesian optimization of machine learning algorithms. Adv. Neural Inf. Process. Syst. **2012**, 2951–2959 (2012)

28. Liu, D., et al.: Imaging-genomics in glioblastoma: combining molecular and imaging signatures. Front. Oncol. **11**, 2666–2021 (2021). https://www.frontiersin.org/article/10.3389/fonc.2021.699265

29. Hajianfar, G., et al.: Noninvasive O6 Methylguanine-DNA methyltransferase status prediction in glioblastoma multiforme cancer using magnetic resonance imaging radiomics features: univariate and multivariate radiogenomics analysis. World Neurosurg. **132**, 140–161 (2019). https://doi.org/10.1016/j.wneu.2019.08.232
30. Korfiatis, P., et al.: MRI texture features as biomarkers to predict MGMT methylation status in glioblastomas. Med. Phys. **43**(6), 2835–2844 (2016). https://doi.org/10.1118/1.4948668
31. RSNA-MICCAI Brain Tumor Radiogenomic Classification-Kaggle. https://www.kaggle.com/c/rsna-miccai-brain-tumor-radiogenomic-classification. Accessed 09 Aug 2021

Comparison of MR Preprocessing Strategies and Sequences for Radiomics-Based MGMT Prediction

Daniel Abler[1]([✉]) [iD], Vincent Andrearczyk[1] [iD], Valentin Oreiller[1] [iD],
Javier Barranco Garcia[2] [iD], Diem Vuong[2] [iD], Stephanie Tanadini-Lang[2] [iD],
Matthias Guckenberger[2] [iD], Mauricio Reyes[3] [iD], and Adrien Depeursinge[1] [iD]

[1] Institute of Information Systems, University of Applied Sciences Western
Switzerland (HES-SO), Sierre, Switzerland
{Daniel.Abler,Vincent.Andrearczyk,Valentin.Oreiller,
Adrien.Depeursinge}@hevs.ch
[2] Department of Radiation Oncology, University Hospital Zurich, Zurich, Switzerland
{Javier.Barranco,Diem.Vuong,Stephanie.Tanadini-Lang,
Matthias.Guckenberger}@usz.ch
[3] ARTORG Center for Biomedical Research, University of Bern, Bern, Switzerland
Mauricio.Reyes@artorg.unibe.ch

Abstract. Hypermethylation of the O6-methylguanine-DNA-methyl-transferase (MGMT) promoter in glioblastoma (GBM) is a predictive biomarker associated with improved treatment outcome. In clinical practice, MGMT methylation status is determined by biopsy or after surgical removal of the tumor. This study aims to investigate the feasibility of non-invasive medical imaging based "radio-genomic" surrogate markers of MGMT methylation status.

The imaging dataset of the RSNA-ASNR-MICCAI Brain Tumor Segmentation (BraTS) challenge allows exploring radiomics strategies for MGMT prediction in a large and very heterogeneous dataset that represents a variety of real-world imaging conditions including different imaging protocols and devices. To characterize and optimize MGMT prediction strategies under these conditions, we examined different image preprocessing approaches and their effect on the average prediction performance of simple radiomics models.

We found features derived from FLAIR images to be most informative for MGMT prediction, particularly if aggregated over the entire (enhancing and non-enhancing) tumor with or without inclusion of the edema. Our results also indicate that the imaging characteristics of the tumor region can distort MR-bias-field correction in a way that negatively affects the prediction performance of the derived models.

Keywords: GBM-MGMT · Radiomics · MR-standardization

This work was supported by the Swiss National Science Foundation (SNSF, grant 205320_179069) and the Swiss Personalized Health Network (SPHN) via the IMAGINE project.

1   Introduction

Brain tumors are a rare condition with about 330 000 yearly incidents (227 000 deaths) worldwide [14]. Despite their comparably low incidence rate, brain cancers cause the highest average number of years of life lost among all cancers [3]. Gliomas represent 75% of primary malignant brain tumors in adults [9]. Glioblastoma (GBM) is the most frequent and most malignant sub-type of glioma, and accounts for about 50% of primary malignant brain cancer. Surgical resection to the maximal safe extent is the primary treatment for newly diagnosed GBM, followed by radiation and chemotherapy. However, due to the tumor's infiltrative growth, resection, even if macroscopically complete, leaves behind tumor cells and the tumor typically recurs at the margins of the resection cavity. Following surgery, addition of Temozolomide (TMZ) chemotherapy to radiotherapy treatment has been the standard of care since 2005. Despite active multi-institutional and international research efforts, GBM patients continue to have a poor prognosis with a 5-year survival rate of about 5.5% [9].

The quest for more personalized oncologic treatment allocation has driven research into genetic and molecular biomarkers. A few of these have been reported to have prognostic and/or predictive implications for GBM tumors. Among those, hypermethylation of the O6-methylguanine-DNA-methyltransferase (MGMT) gene has been shown to be associated with improved outcome in (GBM) and is now considered a favorable prognostic factor and a predictor of chemotherapy response for GBM patients [16]. MGMT encodes for an important DNA repair protein; it's expression may be suppressed by methylation of the promoter region, which results in decreased DNA repair capability and thus increased susceptibility to the damaging effects of DNA-targeting treatments, such as alkylating agents like TMZ and also radiation therapy.

Genetic and molecular profiling is an invasive process that involves tissue extraction from the tumor via stereotactic/needle biopsies; it is inherently prone to sampling bias and therefore may not capture the tumor's spatial heterogeneity, a particular hallmark of GBM. Detection of a tumor's MGMT status from routine clinical imaging, on the other hand, could provide a non-invasive detection approach that would not suffer from the sampling restrictions inherent to surgical biopsies. Recent research into such "radio-genomic" imaging-markers has been fueled by the premise that biomedical images may contain information about the underlying pathophysiology which, even if hidden from the human eye, can be captured via quantitative image analysis [5].

Evidence for imaging markers of MGMT promoter methylation in GBM, however, remains mixed. A systematic review and meta-analysis [17] of 22 studies (published before March 2018) that investigated MR-imaging features linked to MGMT promoter methylation identified reduced edema, elevated apparent diffusion coefficient (ADC) and low perfusion as likely imaging characteristics of promoter methylated MGMT. The review found increased performance for studies using ADC or perfusion measures and recommends including the corresponding MR sequences in imaging protocols.

More recent studies indicate AUCs between 0.74 to 0.87 [6–8,10,19] and accuracies of 0.76 to 0.83 [4,12] for a variety of "classical radiomics" and deep learning models.

These studies were performed on single-institution datasets [7,12], public data collections [4,6], or a combination of both [8,10] and were all limited to fewer than 300 patients across training and test sets. The most heterogeneous dataset appears to have been investigated in [10] which employed a cohort of 133 patients (from the public TCIA GBM collection and from Guangzhou General Hospital) for training and another cohort of 60 patients (from two further hospitals) for independent validation.

This study presented in this manuscript was performed on the imaging dataset of the 2021 RSNA-ASNR-MICCAI Brain Tumor Segmentation (BraTS) challenge which aggregates imaging information from five public repositories and an undisclosed number of institutional data collections. Images were acquired "under standard clinical conditions, but with different equipment and imaging protocols, resulting in a vastly heterogeneous image quality reflecting diverse clinical practice across different institutions" [1].

This diversity allows exploring the performance of radiomic strategies for MGMT prediction in the presence of significant heterogeneity (protocols, device-manufacturers and generations) that must be expected in real-world applications. To this end, we first examined different data preprocessing approaches and their effect on average prediction performance of simple radiomics models. Using the most promising preprocessing strategy and most informative MR-sequence, we then investigated which tumor compartments and groups of radiomic features drive MGMT prediction.

2   Materials and Methods

2.1   Data

This study used the public dataset of the RSNA-ASNR-MICCAI Brain Tumor Segmentation (BraTS) Challenge 2021 [1,2,13]. The private test set of the RSNA-ASNR-MICCAI challenge was not considered in the analysis because our image processing workflow relied on tumor segmentation tools that could not be automatized fully for deployment as Jupyter notebook as required for submission via the Kaggle portal, see Sect. 2.2 for further details.

Data for the MGMT prediction task of the BraTs challenge (task 2) consisted in pre-operative MR-imaging for 585 patients with GBM; brain tumor, as well as information about the tumor's MGMT promoter methylation. MR imaging comprised four MR sequences per patient: T1-weighted (T1), T1 contrast (T1c) after administration of Gadolinium contrast agent, T2-weighted MRI (T2) and FLAIR (FLAIR). All images were provided in DICOM format, after application of a skull-stripping technique that preserved space and resolution of the original images [1]. The tumors' MGMT status was provided as a binary variable that indicates either absence or presence of promoter methylation of the MGMT gene.

The imaging of three of the 585 patients was incomplete with missing information in at least a subset of the four MR-sequences. These patients (IDs 109, 123, 709) were excluded from further processing.

The imaging dataset was highly heterogeneous, comprising MRIs collected from multiple public and institutional resources. Consequently, imaging protocols and quality varied greatly across the dataset. For example, MR slice spacing (thickness) varied between 0.22 to 11.00 mm (0.43 to 6.00 mm) with different acquisition planes across MR sequences and patients.

2.2   Image Pre-processing

All images were processed according to the workflow depicted in Fig. 1: First, complete patient imaging datasets containing all four MRI sequences (T1, T1c, T2, FLAIR) were selected and DICOM images converted to the NIfTI format. Brain masks were created by removing the zero-background from the skull-stripped images. Independently, the tumors present in each patient's imaging dataset were segmented, as described in this section. Exploiting the availability of brain masks and tumor regions of interest (ROIs), the original images were subjected to further pre-processing followed by feature extraction.

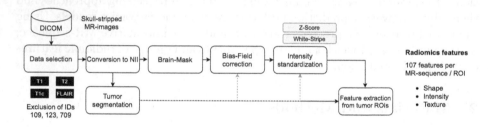

Fig. 1. Image processing workflow.

Tumor Segmentation. Each patient's tumor was segmented using the automatic GBM segmentation software DeepBraTumIA[1]. DeepBraTumIA requires T1, T1c, T2 and FLAIR sequences as input to identify the enhancing tumor (ET), non-enhancing tumor (NET) and edema subregions. Masks for each of these ROIs are output in a co-registered reference frame, as well as in the original frame of the respective MR original sequence. At the time of writing, the tool required user interaction via a GUI to initiate the automatic segmentation process. As this process could not be fully automatized, submission through the challenge portal via Python Jupyter notebook was not possible. Instead, validation was performed on subsets of the public data as described in Sect. 2.3.

---

[1] https://www.nitrc.org/projects/deepbratumia/, as of November 2021.

Table 1. Investigated MR-image preprocessing approaches.

Config ID	Bias-field correction	Standardization	Mask
A	Yes	white-stripe	Brain
B	Yes	z-score	Brain
C	No	z-score	Brain
D	No	z-score	Brain w/o tumor
E	Yes	z-score	Brain w/o tumor

Intensity Standardization. Non-quantitative MR imaging lacks a physical/anatomical reference-scale that would allow direct quantitative comparison of image intensity across vendors and imaging protocols. To enable comparability in the absence of such a reference, statistical standardization techniques are employed that aim at aligning the intensity distributions found in anatomical reference structures across individual image acquisitions. Frequently used reference-regions in the context of brain-MRI are the brain's white-matter component (white-stripe standardization) or the entire brain anatomy (z-score standardization over brain mask). Both approaches operate on the assumption that each constituent of the brain anatomy results in imaging voxels of a characteristic MR intensity and that the relative proportion of those constituents remains relatively stable across individuals. The latter assumption is clearly violated in the case of GBM patients whose tumor lesion may replace a substantial portion of healthy brain tissue and represents a source of strong inter-individual variability in the imaging appearance.

Given the strong heterogeneity of the RSNA-ASNR-MICCAI dataset, we considered effective standardization to be critical to extracting a robust MGMT-related signal from the imaging data. For this reason, we investigated a range of preprocessing strategies that included different combinations of (a) application of bias-field correction, (b) standardization method and (c) the brain regions to which those two steps were applied.

Table 1 summarizes the tested strategies. Bias-field correction and z-score standardization were performed using the respective SimpleITK [11] functions. For white-stripe standardization we relied on a modified version of the implementation in [15][2]. Processing with "brain" mask included all non-zero voxels of the skull-stripped images. For processing with "brain w/o tumor" mask, all tumor subregions detected by the automatic segmentation approach were removed from the "brain" mask.

Radiomics Feature Extraction. In addition to the tumor subregions provided by the automatic segmentation approach, further masks were created corresponding to different combinations of those subregions. We only included combinations of ROIs that typically result in a contiguous volume, and therefore

---

[2] https://github.com/jcreinhold/intensity-normalization, as of November 2021.

did not consider the combination of non-enhancing tumor and edema. Table 2 summarizes all relevant ROIs.

Table 2. Tumor sub-regions used for feature extraction

ROI name	Tumor subregion(s)
ROI_1	Edema
ROI_2	Enhancing tumor (ET)
ROI_3	Non-enhancing tumor (NET)
ROI_1-2	Edema & ET
ROI_2-3	ET & NET
ROI_1-2-3	ET & NET & edema

We used pyradiomics [18] to extract shape-based, intensity and texture features (n=107) from each ROI (Table 2) and MR-sequence resulting from the different pre-processing configurations (Table 1). The preprocessed images were resampled to a spatial resolution of 1.00 mm × 1.00 mm × 1.00 mm prior to feature extraction. Image intensity values were shifted to positive values and the "bin_width" parameter for gray value discretization was chosen in such a way that the full range of intensity values after standardization could be well captured by approximately 64 bins.

2.3   Modeling Experiments

This study aimed at identifying (a) the most suitable pre-processing approach for the provided imaging dataset and (b) sets of radiomics features, ROI and MR-modality combinations that carry predictive information of MGMT-status. To address these goals, we performed two sets of modeling experiments that will be reported here.

In a first experiment, we investigated the change of global performance trends with the preprocessing approach. The second experiment, focused on identifying the specific features and ROIs that provide most relevant information for the globally best performing pre-processing combination.

As indicated in Sect. 2.1, all experiments performed in this study relied exclusively on the public data set of the challenge which was divided into subsets (stratified by MGMT status) for model development (training-set: 80%) and testing of the final prediction model on unseen data (test-set: 20%), respectively. Initial experiments showed the final test performance to be highly sensitive to those splits, probably due to the high degree of heterogeneity of the imaging data. To obtain representative performance results despite this variability, we repeated model development and final evaluation steps multiple times using different train/test splits of the dataset, as illustrated in Fig. 2. The specific feature and model selection strategies employed for each of the experiments are further detailed in the following subsections.

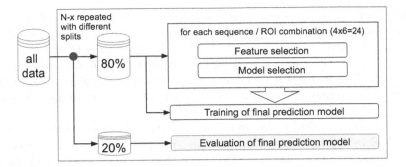

Fig. 2. Model development and final evaluation was performed multiple times using different training/test splits of the full dataset ($N = 50$ for experiment-1, $N = 15$ for experiment-2).

Experiment-1: Performance Trends in Function of Preprocessing Strategy. The first experiment aimed at uncovering global performance trends in function of the chosen preprocessing strategy.

For each combination of MR sequence and ROI (24 combinations), a set of features was selected by choosing the 20 (individually) most predictive features, identified by univariate F-score ranking, and discarding strongly correlated features (Pearson correlation coefficient exceeding 0.7) from this group. The selected features were standardized and the hyperparameters of a family of linear classifiers (including support-vector classifiers with linear kernel, logistic regression, with L2, L1 and combined penalties) were optimized to maximize AUC in 5-fold cross-validation, resulting in a single "best model" per MR-sequence and ROI. Finally, the combination of MR-sequence and ROI that yielded the highest-performing "best model" in cross-validation was selected as final prediction model, and evaluated on the unseen split of the dataset.

This process was repeated for 50 different train/test splits by varying the random seed of the the stratified split procedure, resulting in 50 independently selected combinations of prediction model, MR-sequence and ROI.

The entire feature selection, training and evaluation process was repeated with features derived from the five different pre-processing configurations in Table 1.

Experiment-2: Identification of Predictive Features and ROIs for Optimal Preprocessing Strategy and Most Informative MR-sequence. The second experiment aimed at identifying the specific set of radiomic features that carry predictive information of MGMT status for the different ROIs of the best-performing preprocessing approach and MR sequence resulting from the first experiment.

The feature selection approach in this experiment relied on repeated hyper-parameter optimization of Elastic-Net classifiers in 5-fold cross-validation. Each such optimization resulted in a set of models with varying cross-validation performance and varying number of selected features. From this set of models, we chose the best-performing model with no more than 20 features and extracted its features. For a given training set, this feature selection process was repeated 15 times by varying the random seed for cross-validation splitting, resulting in 15 feature sets. The features from those sets were then aggregated and ordered by their selection frequency, resulting in a ranking of the most-frequently selected features across the 15 selection repetitions.

From the top-ranked (most frequently selected) features, we built a prediction model by 5-fold cross-validation and grid search over the space of linear classifiers and hyper-parameters. The most promising of these models (highest cross-validation performance) was selected as final prediction model. This prediction model was evaluated on the test-split which had not been used in the feature selection and training process.

To obtain robust estimates of test-performance, we repeated the above process (feature selection, model training, model evaluation) for 15 different train/test splits by varying the random seed of the stratified splitting procedure. This resulted in 15 independently selected feature sets, prediction models and their corresponding test performances for each ROI and MR-sequence combination.

2.4 Statistical Analysis

Average AUC performance on the test-sets was compared across the different preprocessing approaches in experiment-1, and across tumor ROIs in experiment-2. To test the null hypothesis that two sets of performance measurements originate from the same distribution, an independent 2-sample t-test was performed when both sets of measurements were normally distributed and of equal variance. Welch's t-test was performed in case of normal distribution and un-equal variance, and Mann-Whitney U test in case of non-normal distribution. P-values < 0.05 were interpreted as "significant" rejection of the null hypothesis, and are reported in the manuscript.

3   Results

3.1   Experiment-1: Identification of Favorable Preprocessing Strategies and Most Informative MR-sequence

Figure 3 summarizes the test performance of the single-sequence, single-ROI prediction models evaluated in experiment-1, Sect. 2.3, in function of pre-processing configuration.

Models based on features derived from preprocessing configurations {C, D, E} performed significantly better ($p < 0.05$) compared to models based on preprocessing configurations {A and B}, Fig. 3(a), with mean AUC of 0.54 ± 0.05 to 0.55 ± 0.05 vs. 0.52 ± 0.04, Table 3. Within these sets, no statistically significant performance differences were observed. Both configuration sets differ in their approach towards bias-field correction: For preprocessing configurations {A, B}, the bias field was estimated over the entire brain volume; configurations {C, D, E} either did not attempt to correct for the bias-field, or excluded the tumor from bias-field estimation. The individually highest performing models from configurations {C, D, E} were based on the MR-FLAIR sequence, Fig. 3(b).

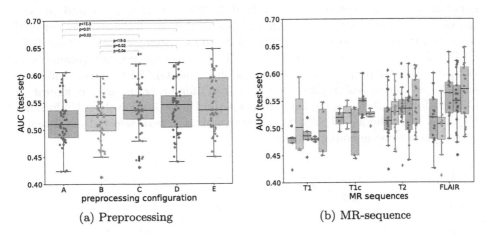

(a) Preprocessing (b) MR-sequence

Fig. 3. Distribution of test-AUC of 50 best performing classifiers resulting from experiment-1, Sect. 2.3. Models based on features derived from preprocessing configurations {C, D, E} perform significantly better ($p < 0.05$) than those based on features derived from configurations {A, B}, Fig. 3(a). Within these groups, no significant differences in overall performance were observed. Highest performing models from configurations {C, D, E} were based on MR-FLAIR Fig. 3(b)

Table 3. Average cross-validation and test performance (AUC) of 50 best performing classifiers resulting from experiment-1 in function of preprocessing approach.

Config ID	A	B	C	D	E
Validation AUC	0.60±0.02	0.61±0.01	0.61±0.01	0.61±0.02	0.62±0.01
Test AUC	0.52±0.04	0.52±0.04	0.54±0.05	0.54±0.05	0.55±0.05

3.2 Experiment-2: Identification of Predictive Feature Groups and ROIs

Figure 4 summarizes the prediction performance of experiment-2 using features derived from MR-FLAIR sequences preprocessed according to approach C, Fig. 4(a), and approach D, Fig. 4(b), respectively.

Highest test performance was achieved by models derived from ROI_2-3 and ROI_1-2-3, reaching AUCs of 0.56±0.04 to 0.56±0.05 (preprocessing configuration C) and 0.55±0.05 to 0.56±0.04 (preprocessing configuration D), respectively, Table 4. In both preprocessing configurations, the performance of models from these ROIs was significantly higher than performance of models from ROI_2 alone. For configuration C, the performance of models from these ROIs was also significantly higher than performance of models from ROI_3, but not from ROI_1. The opposite was found for configuration D.

Figure 5 shows the 15 features that were most frequently included in the 15 independently developed ROI-specific prediction models resulting from experiment-2. Features selected for ROI_3, ROI_2-3, ROI_1-2-3 and preprocessing configurations C and D are displayed. Multiple features were selected consistently across both best-performing ROIs (ROI_2-3 and ROI_1-2-3): GLDM-DependenceNonUniformityNormalized and shape (SurfaceVolumeRatio vs Sphericity) for preprocessing configuraton C, and GLCM-ClusterProminence and shape (SurfaceVolumeRatio vs Sphericity) for preprocessing configuration D. Also for ROI_3, the same three features (GLRLM-GrayLevelNonUniformity, GLCM-ClusterShade, GLSZM-SmallAreaEmphasis) were selected consistently across preprocessing configurations.

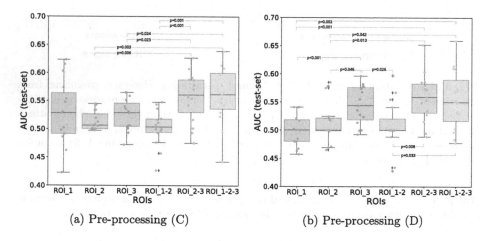

(a) Pre-processing (C)   (b) Pre-processing (D)

Fig. 4. Distribution of test-AUC for ROI-specific models resulting from the model selection and evaluation approach proposed in experiment-2. Features were derived from MR-FLAIR images preprocessed according to configuration C, Fig. 4(a), and D, Fig. 4(b), respectively. Models based on features derived from ROI_2-3 and ROI_1-2-3 performed significantly best across the tested preprocessing configurations.

Table 4. Average cross-validation and test performance (AUC) of 15 repetition of experiment-2 Sect. 2.3 based on MR-FLAIR images preprocessed according to configuration C and D.

AUC	ROI_1	ROI_2	ROI_3	ROI_1-2	ROI_2-3	ROI_1-2-3
(C) Validation	0.58±0.02	0.57±0.02	0.59±0.03	0.57±0.02	0.59±0.03	0.60±0.02
(C) Test	0.53±0.06	0.51±0.02	0.52±0.03	0.50±0.03	0.56±0.04	0.56±0.05
(D) Validation	0.56±0.03	0.57±0.04	0.59±0.03	0.55±0.02	0.60±0.03	0.60±0.02
(D) Test	0.50±0.03	0.51±0.04	0.54±0.03	0.51±0.04	0.56±0.04	0.55±0.05

4   Discussion

This study investigated the effect of different preprocessing strategies on MGMT prediction performance. The observed significant performance difference between preprocessing configurations {A, B} vs {C, D, E} indicates that inclusion of the tumor region in the bias-field estimation process deteriorates the resulting models' ability to predict MGMT status. This negative effect on modeling outweighed any other potential gains that bias-field correction may have conferred to the

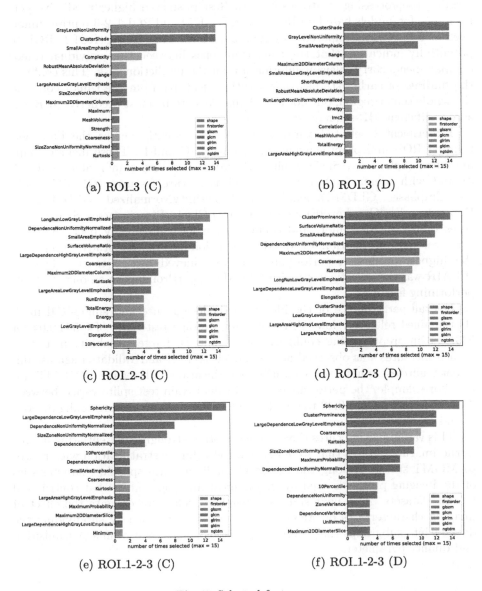

(a) ROI_3 (C)

(b) ROI_3 (D)

(c) ROI_2-3 (C)

(d) ROI_2-3 (D)

(e) ROI_1-2-3 (C)

(f) ROI_1-2-3 (D)

Fig. 5. Selected features

prediction task. Our experiments did not provide clear indications for the relative superiority of different standardization techniques on overall performance (white-stripe vs z-score based on intensity statistics of the entire brain with or without tumor regions). However, when disaggregated by MR-sequence, predictors based on preprocessing approaches {C, D, E} applied to FLAIR sequences appeared to outperform all other approaches.

Focusing on FLAIR sequences, we then investigated predictive performance and relevant features separately for each ROI and for two of the three well performing preprocessing strategies (C, D). Results showed higher predictive performance for models based on ROI_2-3 (ET, NET) and ROI_1-2-3 (entire tumor: edema, ET, NET) compared to individual tumor sub-regions (ROI_1, ROI_2), potentially indicating that the transition zones between the individual tumor compartments carry relevant information for the prediction task. This confirms the findings of earlier studies that identified features from the tumor core and the whole tumor region, but not the edema alone, to be most predictive [6,10,12] across different MR-sequences.

Experiment-2 selected various features consistently across the best performing ROIs and preprocessing configurations C and D. These include shape measures (Sphericity, SurfaceVolumeRatio) of the core tumor alone (ROI_2-3) and with edema (ROI_1-2-3), as well as texture features (GLSZM-SmallAreaEmphasis, GLDM-DependenceNonUniformityNormalized, GLDM-LargeDependenceLowGrayLevelEmphasis, GLCM-ClusterProminence). Shape measures of the active tumor, and edema region have previously been shown to carry relevant information for MGMT prediction [6]. Another study [8] reported the highest prediction performance to be achieved by T2 texture features (FLAIR was not investigated) with GLCM-ClusterProminence among the best-performing features.

Overall performance of the identified single-sequence and single-ROI models remained relatively low with maximum average test-AUC of 0.56 ± 0.04 for ROI_2-3 in preprocessing configurations C and D. Large variability in performance measures was observed across models trained and validated against different train/test splits despite ensuring stratification with regard to MGMT status. For example, the performance of individual train test splits varied between AUC 0.47 to 0.63 and 0.48 to 0.65 for ROI_2-3 and preprocessing configurations C and D, respectively.

This variability indicates the presence of other strongly differentiating factors in the imaging dataset that were not controlled for by stratification with regard to MGMT status. Among the potential candidates are specific characteristics of the imaging protocols used by the different imaging centers that contributed to this datasets. As a next step, we therefore seek to investigate the effect of imaging characteristics on MGMT prediction performance by subdividing the dataset into subgroups that share a more homogeneous set of image acquisition and quality parameters.

References

1. Baid, U., et al.: The RSNA-ASNR-MICCAI BraTS 2021 Benchmark on Brain Tumor Segmentation and Radiogenomic Classification. arXiv:2107.02314, September 2021
2. Bakas, S., et al.: Advancing the cancer genome atlas glioma MRI collections with expert segmentation labels and radiomic features. Sci. Data **4**(1), 1–3 (2017). https://doi.org/10.1038/sdata.2017.117
3. Burnet, N.G., Jefferies, S.J., Benson, R.J., Hunt, D.P., Treasure, F.P.: Years of life lost (YLL) from cancer is an important measure of population burden–and should be considered when allocating research funds. Br. J. Cancer (2005). https://doi.org/10.1038/sj.bjc.6602321
4. Chang, P., et al.: Deep-learning convolutional neural networks accurately classify genetic mutations in gliomas. Am. J. Neuroradiol. **39**(7), 1201–1207 (2018). https://doi.org/10.3174/ajnr.A5667
5. Gillies, R.J., Kinahan, P.E., Hricak, H.: Radiomics: images are more than pictures. Data. Radiol. **278**(2), 563–577 (2016). https://doi.org/10.1148/radiol.2015151169
6. Hajianfar, G., et al.: Noninvasive O6 methylguanine-DNA methyltransferase status prediction in glioblastoma multiforme cancer using magnetic resonance imaging radiomics features: univariate and multivariate radiogenomics analysis. World Neurosurg. **132**, e140–e161 (2019). https://doi.org/10.1016/j.wneu.2019.08.232
7. Kihira, S., et al.: Multiparametric MRI texture analysis in prediction of glioma biomarker status: added value of MR diffusion. Neuro-Oncol. Adv. 3(1), vdab051 (2021). https://doi.org/10.1093/noajnl/vdab051
8. Korfiatis, P., et al.: MRI texture features as biomarkers to predict MGMT methylation status in glioblastomas: MRI texture features to predict MGMT methylation status. Med. Phys. **43**(6Part1), 2835–2844 (2016). https://doi.org/10.1118/1.4948668
9. Lapointe, S., Perry, A., Butowski, N.A.: Primary brain tumours in adults. The Lancet **392**(10145), 432–446 (2018). https://doi.org/10.1016/S0140-6736(18)30990-5
10. Li, Z.-C., et al.: Multiregional radiomics features from multiparametric MRI for prediction of MGMT methylation status in glioblastoma multiforme: a multicentre study. Eur. Radiol. **28**(9), 3640–3650 (2018). https://doi.org/10.1007/s00330-017-5302-1
11. Lowekamp, B.C., Chen, D.T., Ibáñez, L., Blezek, D.: The design of SimpleITK. Front. Neuroinform. **7**, 1–8 (2013). https://doi.org/10.3389/fninf.2013.00045
12. Lu, Y., et al.: Machine learning-based radiomic, clinical and semantic feature analysis for predicting overall survival and MGMT promoter methylation status in patients with glioblastoma. Magn. Reson. Imaging **74**, 161–170 (2020). https://doi.org/10.1016/j.mri.2020.09.017
13. Menze, B.H., et al.: The multimodal brain tumor image segmentation benchmark (BRATS). IEEE Trans. Med. Imaging **34**(10), 1993–2024 (2015). https://doi.org/10.1109/TMI.2014.2377694
14. Patel, A.P., et al.: Global, regional, and national burden of brain and other CNS cancer, 1990–2016: a systematic analysis for the global burden of disease study 2016. The Lancet Neurol. **18**(4), 376–393 (2019). https://doi.org/10.1016/S1474-4422(18)30468-X

15. Reinhold, J.C., Dewey, B.E., Carass, A., Prince, J.L.: Evaluating the impact of intensity normalization on MR image synthesis. In: Angelini, E.D., Landman, B.A. (eds.) Medical Imaging 2019: Image Processing. p. 126. SPIE, San Diego, United States, March 2019. https://doi.org/10.1117/12.2513089

16. Rivera, A.L., et al.: MGMT promoter methylation is predictive of response to radiotherapy and prognostic in the absence of adjuvant alkylating chemotherapy for glioblastoma. Neuro-Oncol. **12**(2), 116–121 (2010). https://doi.org/10.1093/neuonc/nop020

17. Suh, C., Kim, H., Jung, S., Choi, C., Kim, S.: Clinically relevant imaging features for MGMT promoter methylation in multiple glioblastoma studies: a systematic review and meta-analysis. Am. J. Neuroradiol. **39**, 1439–1445 (2018). https://doi.org/10.3174/ajnr.A5711

18. van Griethuysen, J.J., et al.: Computational radiomics system to decode the radiographic phenotype. Cancer Res. **77**(21), e104–e107 (2017). https://doi.org/10.1158/0008-5472.CAN-17-0339

19. Xi, Y.b., et al.: Radiomics signature: a potential biomarker for the prediction of MGMT promoter methylation in glioblastoma: GBM radiomics features reflect MGMT. J. Magn. Reson. Imaging **47**(5), 1380–1387 (2018). https://doi.org/10.1002/jmri.25860

FeTS

FedCostWAvg: A New Averaging for Better Federated Learning

Leon Mächler[6(✉)], Ivan Ezhov[1,3], Florian Kofler[1,2,3], Suprosanna Shit[1,3], Johannes C. Paetzold[1,3,5], Timo Loehr[1,3], Claus Zimmer[2], Benedikt Wiestler[2], and Bjoern H. Menze[1,3,4]

[1] Department of Informatics, Technical University Munich, Munich, Germany
[2] Department of Diagnostic and Interventional Neuroradiology, School of Medicine, Klinikum rechts der Isar, Technical University of Munich, Munich, Germany
[3] TranslaTUM - Central Institute for Translational Cancer Research, Technical University of Munich, Munich, Germany
[4] Department of Quantitative Biomedicine, University of Zurich, Zürich, Switzerland
[5] ITERM Institute Helmholtz Zentrum Muenchen, Neuherberg, Germany
[6] Ecole Normale Supérieure, Paris, France
leon-philipp.machler@ens.fr

Abstract. We propose a simple new aggregation strategy for federated learning that won the MICCAI Federated Tumor Segmentation Challenge 2021 (FETS), the first ever challenge on Federated Learning in the Machine Learning community. Our method addresses the problem of how to aggregate multiple models that were trained on different data sets. Conceptually, we propose a new way to choose the weights when averaging the different models, thereby extending the current state of the art (FedAvg). Empirical validation demonstrates that our approach reaches a notable improvement in segmentation performance compared to FedAvg.

Keywords: Federated learning · Brain tumor segmentation · Multi-modal medical imaging · MRI · MICCAI challenges · Machine learning

1 Introduction

1.1 Motivation

Preserving data privacy is of paramount importance for confidentiality-critical fields such as the medical domain. Today it is not uncommon that large volumes of private medical records are illegally released to the *dark web* [1]. To prevent such incidents, often large amounts of resources are allocated but cannot guarantee full security. Among many precautions, reducing human (including IT specialists) exposure to the data is highly desirable to reduce the chance of compromising data protection by human failure.

© The Author(s), under exclusive license to Springer Nature Switzerland AG 2022
A. Crimi and S. Bakas (Eds.): BrainLes 2021, LNCS 12963, pp. 383–391, 2022.
https://doi.org/10.1007/978-3-031-09002-8_34

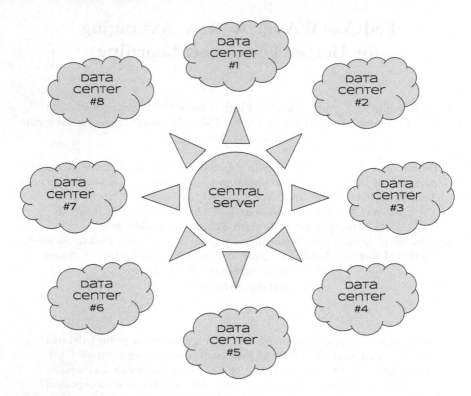

Fig. 1. Schematic illustration of the federated learning concept. Within multiple data centers, a model is trained for our task. Next, parameters are sent to the central server, where aggregation of the parameters takes place. An aggregated global configuration of the parameters is broadcasted back to the centers. The procedure repeats until convergence or some other limit is reached.

1.2   The Typical Training Scenario

In machine learning, a common scenario today looks like this: One or more institutions (companies, research institutes, governments, etc.) gather data, share it with data scientists who, in turn, train some sort of a model using the data. For example, a group of hospitals share MRI scans of tumors with the medical community to help with the development of an automatic tumor segmentation model. One problem with this approach is that the data, once it is shared, might get leaked, misused, or stolen from the developers. Other hurdles include legal reasons that might make it impossible for the hospitals to share and pool the data in the first place.

1.3   Federated Learning

Conventional machine learning requires exposing training data to a learning algorithm and its developers. When several data sources are involved, the pooling together of the data to create a single data set is also required. New approaches like *Federated learning* (FL) [2] allow to separate model training from developer access while also not requiring any pooling of data. FL was introduced in a series of seminal works starting from 2015 [3–5]. FL is a protocol consisting of two alternating steps: a) independent training of models on local entities with their respective unique corpus of data, and b) broadcasting back of only the weights of the trained models to a central entity where the weights are aggregated and a new model is redistributed. The choice of which type of model or network to perform step (a) is dictated by the task (e.g., classification, segmentation, etc.) and can be made based on the state-of-the-art in the respective task. The new FL scenario looks like this: A developer sends his or her model to all the institutions that own training data, the institutions locally train the model for the developer and send the newly trained models back. In this way, the developer can train their model while never getting any access to the data. In this setting however a new problem arises.

1.4   The Aggregation Problem

How to aggregate the different models that come back? A naive approach to solve the problem would be:

1. Send an initial model to the first data center
2. Get back a newly trained model and send it to the second data center
3. Repeat until all data centers have trained the model once

Approaches like this are called sequential learning and fail due to a phenomenon called "catastrophic forgetting" [6]. Effectively what would happen is that the final model would only be trained on the data of the last center and would not have generalized to the entire corpus of data. It would simply forget what was learned in the previous center as soon as it gets trained by the next. The state-of-the-art approach tries to avoid this phenomenon by including feedback from every center in each update.

1.5   State of the Art

The seminal work of learning deep networks from decentralized data [5] proposed as a solution a plain coordinate-wise mean averaging (FedAvg) of the model weights coming separately from multiple centers. Recently [7] proposed a valuable extension to FedAvg, which takes invariance of network weights to permutations into account. In [8] (FedProx), the authors adjust the training loss of a local model to enforce closeness of local and global model updates. Despite methodological advances, there is neither theoretical nor practical evidence for the right recipe when choosing an aggregation strategy. In this paper, we propose a new idea on how to do aggregation. Similar to other initiatives [9–12], the FETS challenge[1] [13] is organized to benchmark different weight aggregation

---

[1] https://fets-ai.github.io/Challenge/.

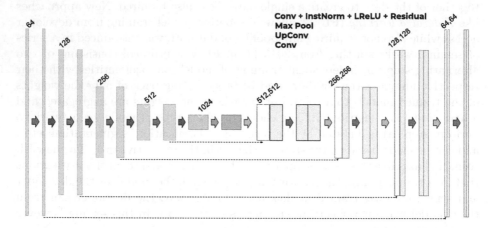

Fig. 2. 3D U-net architecture as provided by the FETS challenge.

strategies on the clinically important glioma segmentation problem [13–17]. We contribute to the initiative by proposing an effective extension to the FedAvg strategy. When compared with the other submissions, our model significantly outperformed all of them and won the challenge. On top of that we tested the model locally on a smaller corpus of data to compare it to FedAvg. It notably improves performance compared with FedAvg at no additional compute time.

2 Methodology

2.1 Segmentation Network

The segmentation network is a 3D-Unet. It was provided by the challenge organizers and remained unchanged during all experiments. The architecture is composed of an encoder with residual branches followed by a decoder. We use the *LeakyReLu* activation function [18] along with instance normalization [19] - for mitigating the covariate shift. Dice serves as loss function. Figure 2 illustrates the schematic of the network.

2.2 Federated Cost Weighted Averaging (FedCostWAvg)

The gold standard federated averaging (FedAvg) approach updates the global model as an average of all local models weighted by the respective sizes of the training data set. The new model M_{i+1} is calculated as follows:

$$M_{i+1} = \frac{1}{S} \sum_{j=1}^{n} s_j M_i^j \tag{1}$$

where s_j is the number of samples that model M^j was trained on in round i and $S = \sum_j s_j$. We propose a new weighting strategy that includes the amount by which the cost function decreased during the last step. Using FedCostWAvg, the new model M_{i+1} is calculated as following:

$$M_{i+1} = \sum_{j=1}^{n}(\alpha\frac{s_j}{S} + (1 - \alpha)\frac{k_j}{K})M_i^j \tag{2}$$

with:

$$k_j = \frac{c(M_{i-1}^j)}{c(M_i^j)}, K = \sum_j k_j \tag{3}$$

where $c(M_i^j)$ is the cost of the model j at timestep i that is simply calculated from the cost function that is being used to train the models locally. α is a parameter ranging between 0 and 1 that can be chosen to determine the balance between data size and cost improvement. In our experiments, a value of $\alpha = 0.5$ performed best. Intuitively, this weighting strategy adjusts not only for the training data set size but also for the size of the local improvements that were made during the last training round. Local updates which only marginally improved the local cost will influence the global update to a lesser extent than those which had a bigger impact.

3   Results

The method won the challenge and significantly outperformed all other submitted methods; Tables 1 and 2 summarize the performance upon convergence.

In addition we used the provided data (which is a smaller subset of the challenge data) to test the performance of FedCostWAvg against FedAvg in order to visualize the convergence behaviour. We trained and validated the model on 369 samples which were unevenly distributed over 17 data centers. The training-validation split was 80/20, the learning rate was $1e-4$ and we did 10 epochs per federated round. Please note that computational resources were limited so no exhaustive grid search to find optimal hyperparameters was feasible, also training could not run long enough to achieve maximal performance. Figures 3, 4 and 5 depict the performances over communication rounds. Also note that of course the most informative comparison between methods was done in the challenge itself with more data and many different initialisations. This comparison serves only as a visualization of how different convergence behaviours look like for one initialisation. We observe an improvement for almost all classes and metrics, when using our proposed method. The exemption is the DICE Enhanced Tumor Metric. Note though that the difference is not significant and the methods have not yet converged.

Table 1. Final performance of FedCostWAvg in the FETS challenge, DICE and sensitivity

Label	DICE WT	DICE ET	DICE TC	Sens. WT	Sens. ET	Sens. TC
Mean	0,8248	0,7476	0,7932	0,8957	0,8246	0,8269
StdDev	0,1849	0,2444	0,2643	0,1738	0,2598	0,2721
Median	0,8936	0,8259	0,9014	0,948	0,9258	0,9422
25th quantile	0,8116	0,7086	0,8046	0,9027	0,7975	0,8258
75th quantile	0,9222	0,8909	0,942	0,9787	0,9772	0,9785

Table 2. Final performance of FedCostWAvg in the FETS challenge, specificity, Hausdorff95 distance and communication cost

Label	Spec WT	Spec ET	Spec TC	H95 WT	H95 ET	H95 TC	Comm. Cost
Mean	0,9981	0,9994	0,9994	11,618	27,2745	28,4825	0,723
StdDev	0,0024	0,0011	0,0014	31,758	88,566	88,2921	0,723
Median	0,9986	0,9996	0,9998	5	2,2361	3,0811	0,723
25th quantile	0,9977	0,9993	0,9995	2,8284	1,4142	1,7856	0,723
75th quantile	0,9994	0,9999	0,9999	8,6023	3,5628	7,0533	0,723

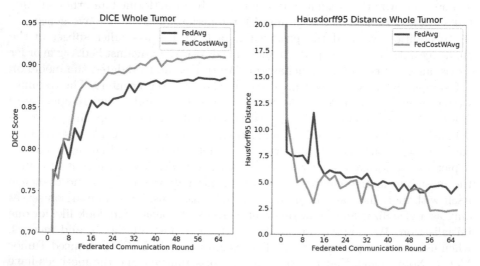

Fig. 3. Comparison of the DICE whole tumor metric per federated round for FedCost-WAvg vs. FedAvg. Note of course that the bigger the DICE score, the better and the smaller the Hausdorff95 distance, the better.

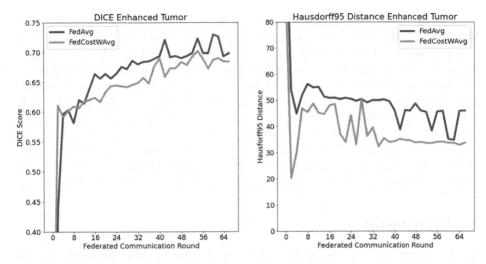

Fig. 4. Comparison of the DICE enhanced tumor metric per federated round for Fed-CostWAvg vs. FedAvg. Note of course that the bigger the DICE score, the better and the smaller the Hausdorff95 distance, the better.

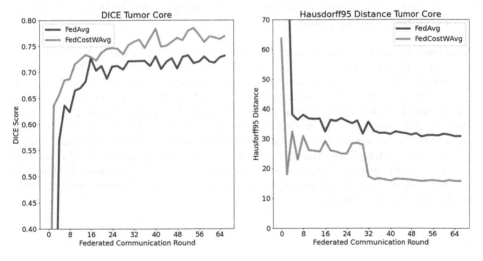

Fig. 5. Comparison of the DICE tumor core metric per federated round for FedCost-WAvg vs. FedAvg. Note of course that the bigger the DICE score, the better and the smaller the Hausdorff95 distance, the better.

3.1   Discussion

While these results already show a clear improvement over FedAvg, it is unclear whether other hyperparameters would have achieved an even better result. Due to limitations in training resources a proper grid search was not feasible.

The simple and straightforward interpretation of the mechanism of FedCost-WAvg is amplification of more informative updates against less informing ones. It could be seen as a diminishing returns acknowledging method. A deeper insight might be the interpretation as resembling a PID controller[2] [20]. When one reframes the federated learning problem as a control problem, then the central server that does the averaging is equivalent to a control unit that is included in a feedback loop. When one would then extend this logic to the averaging approach, it might be intelligent to view FedCostWAvg as an approximation of a PID controller, where the newly added term corresponding to the drop in cost is effectively functioning as the derivative part and the data size term as the proportional one. Future research could try to include the integral term as well.

4   Conclusion

In this paper, we describe a method for model aggregation developed for the MICCAI Federated Tumor Segmentation Challenge (FETS). The novelty of the method lays in including local cost improvements when calculating the weights for averaging models which are trained at different centers. The approach is validated on a brain tumor segmentation task and achieves the best performance among all participating teams.

Acknowledgement. Bjoern Menze, Benedikt Wiestler, and Florian Kofler are supported through the SFB 824, subproject B12. Supported by Deutsche Forschungsgemeinschaft (DFG) through TUM International Graduate School of Science and Engineering (IGSSE), GSC 81. Suprosanna Shit and Ivan Ezhov are supported by the Translational Brain Imaging Training Network (TRABIT) under the European Union's 'Horizon 2020' research & innovation program (Grant agreement ID: 765148). With the support of the Technical University of Munich - Institute for Advanced Study, funded by the German Excellence Initiative. Ivan Ezhov is also supported by the International Graduate School of Science and Engineering (IGSSE). Johannes C. Paetzold and Suprosanna Shit are supported by the Graduate School of Bioengineering, Technical University of Munich.

References

1. Healthcareitnews.com: Tens of thousands of patient records posted to dark web. https://www.healthcareitnews.com/news/tens-thousands-patient-records-posted-dark-web. Accessed 16 July 2021
2. Rieke, N., et al.: The future of digital health with federated learning. NPJ Digital Med. **3**(1), 1–7 (2020)
3. Konečný, J., McMahan, H.B., Yu, F.X., Richtárik, P., Suresh, A.T., Bacon, D.: Federated learning: strategies for improving communication efficiency. CoRR abs/1610.05492 (2016)
4. Konečný, J., McMahan, B., Ramage, D.: Federated optimization: distributed optimization beyond the datacenter. CoRR abs/1511.03575 (2015)

---

[2] The credit for this observation goes to David Naccache.

5. McMahan, B., Moore, E., Ramage, D., Hampson, S., y Arcas, B.A.: Communication-efficient learning of deep networks from decentralized data. In: Artificial intelligence and statistics, pp. 1273–1282. PMLR (2017)
6. McCloskey, M., Cohen, N.J.: Catastrophic interference in connectionist networks: The sequential learning problem. In Bower, G.H., (ed.) Psychology of Learning and Motivation, vol. 24, pp. 109–165. Academic Press (1989)
7. Yurochkin, M., Agarwal, M., Ghosh, S., Greenewald, K., Hoang, N., Khazaeni, Y.: Bayesian nonparametric federated learning of neural networks. In: International Conference on Machine Learning, pp. 7252–7261. PMLR (2019)
8. Sahu, A.K., Li, T., Sanjabi, M., Zaheer, M., Talwalkar, A., Smith, V.: On the convergence of federated optimization in heterogeneous networks. arXiv preprint arXiv:1812.06127 (2018)
9. Sekuboyina, A., et al.: Verse: a vertebrae labelling and segmentation benchmark. arXiv preprint arXiv:2001.09193 (2020)
10. Payette, K., et al.: A comparison of automatic multi-tissue segmentation methods of the human fetal brain using the feta dataset. arXiv e-prints (2020)
11. Paetzold, J.C., et al.: Whole brain vessel graphs: a dataset and benchmark for graph learning and neuroscience (vesselgraph). arXiv preprint arXiv:2108.13233 (2021)
12. Bilic, P., et al.: The liver tumor segmentation benchmark (LITS). arXiv preprint arXiv:1901.04056 (2019)
13. Pati, S., et al.: The federated tumor segmentation (FETS) challenge. arXiv preprint arXiv:2105.05874 (2021)
14. Bakas, S., et al.: Advancing the cancer genome atlas glioma MRI collections with expert segmentation labels and radiomic features. Sci. Data 4(1), 1–13 (2017)
15. Reina, G.A., et al.: OpenFL: an open-source framework for federated learning. arXiv preprint arXiv:2105.06413 (2021)
16. Sheller, M.J., et al.: Federated learning in medicine: facilitating multi-institutional collaborations without sharing patient data. Sci. Rep. 10(1), 1–12 (2020)
17. Kofler, F., et al.: Brats toolkit: translating brats brain tumor segmentation algorithms into clinical and scientific practice. Front. Neurosci. 14, 125 (2020)
18. Maas, A.L., et al.: Rectifier nonlinearities improve neural network acoustic models. In: Proceedings of ICML, Vol. 30, Citeseer (2013)
19. Ulyanov, D., Vedaldi, A., Lempitsky, V.: Instance normalization: the missing ingredient for fast stylization. arXiv preprint arXiv:1607.08022 (2016)
20. Bellman, R.E.: Adaptive Control Processes. Princeton University Press, Princeton (2015)

Federated Learning Using Variable Local Training for Brain Tumor Segmentation

Anup Tuladhar[1,2](✉) (iD), Lakshay Tyagi[3] (iD), Raissa Souza[1,2,4] (iD),
and Nils D. Forkert[1,2,5,6] (iD)

[1] Department of Radiology, Cumming School of Medicine,
University of Calgary, Calgary, AB, Canada
anup.tuladhar@ucalgary.ca
[2] Hotchkiss Brain Institute, University of Calgary, Calgary, AB, Canada
[3] Department of Chemical Engineering, Indian Institute of Technology Kanpur, Kanpur,
Uttar Pradesh, India
[4] Biomedical Engineering Program, University of Calgary, Calgary, AB, Canada
[5] Department of Clinical Neurosciences, Cumming School of Medicine, University of Calgary,
Calgary, AB, Canada
[6] Alberta Children's Hospital Research Institute, University of Calgary, Calgary, AB, Canada

Abstract. The potential for deep learning to improve medical image analysis is
often stymied by the difficulty in acquiring and collecting sufficient data to train
models. One major barrier to data acquisition is the private and sensitive nature of
the data in question, as concerns about patient privacy, among others, make data
sharing between institutions difficult. Distributed learning avoids the need to share
data centrally by training models locally. One approach to distributed learning is
federated learning, where models are trained in parallel at local institutions and
aggregated together into a global model. The 2021 Federated Tumor Segmentation (FeTS) challenge focuses on federated learning for brain tumor segmentation
using magnetic resonance imaging scans collected from a real-world federation of
collaborating institutions. We developed a federated training algorithm that uses
a combination of variable local epochs in each federated round, a decaying learning rate, and an ensemble weight aggregation function. When testing on unseen
validation data our model trained with federated learning achieves very similar
performance (average DSC score of 0.674) to a central model trained on pooled
data (average DSC score 0.685). When our federated learning algorithm was evaluated on unseen training and testing data, it achieved similar performances on the
FeTS challenge leaderboards 1 and 2 (average DSC scores of 0.623 and 0.608,
respectively). This federated learning algorithm offers an approach to training deep
learning learning models without the need to share private and sensitive patient
data.

Keywords: Distributed learning · Federated learning · Convolutional neural
network · Medical image analysis · Brain · Tumor segmentation · MICCAI ·
FeTS · BraTS

1 Introduction

Deep neural networks, and convolutional neural networks (CNNs) in particular, have shown promising results for various classification and segmentation tasks in medical imaging [1]. To achieve these high accuracies, deep learning models often need to be trained on a large quantity and variety of training data, *i.e.*, patient data in the case of medical imaging. The standard approach for training deep learning models is centralized learning, where models are trained on a single repository of collected data. However, this centralized training approach is difficult to implement in healthcare, as there is a lack of large clinical databases for model training and optimization. Although large amounts of imaging data are collected daily, concerns about patient privacy, data security, and legal and administrative hurdles make data collection into a single repository both difficult and unfavorable [2–4]. Thus, alternatives to centralized training of deep learning models are needed to create accurate and robust models for healthcare and medical imaging applications, especially in case of rare diseases.

Distributed learning is an alternative to centralized learning that circumvents the need for data sharing and a centralized repository. In distributed learning, model training occurs locally at each site, *e.g.* healthcare center. After local training, the models from each collaborating healthcare institution are sent back to a central server that combines these local models into a single global model. This global model is effectively trained on a larger amount and variety of patient data to ideally achieve accuracies greater than any locally trained model and similar performance compared to a model trained with central learning. Meanwhile, the patient data never leaves the local institution, which retains control over how the data is used. Thus, distributed learning is a promising approach to train deep learning models on sensitive and private patient data.

Federated learning is one approach to the distributed learning problem that aggregates model parameters, most often the gradient updates or model weights, from parallelly trained local models into a global model [6–8]. This global model then makes an inference on new data. This approach is in contrast to distributed learning by ensembling [5], which has local models make independent inferences on data and aggregates their predictions, and distributed learning using a traveling model [9, 10], which trains a single model at one site at a time.

The inaugural Federated Tumor Segmentation (FeTS) [11] challenge at the 2021 International Conference on Medical Image Computing & Computer Assisted Intervention (MICCAI) is the first challenge for federated learning in medical imaging [12]. The overall aim of the challenge is the construction and evaluation of CNN models for brain tumor segmentation using multi-institutional clinical datasets whilst, importantly, avoiding data sharing and data pooling. The 2021 FeTS challenge is composed of two tasks:

1. Task 1, Federated Training, is focused on methods for federated weight aggregation from locally-trained models using a pre-defined segmentation algorithm.
2. Task 2, Federated Evaluation, is focused on developing segmentation algorithms that generalize to unseen samples and collaborating institutions not involved in training.

In this paper, we focus on Task 1, Federated Training. We implemented federated learning using variable local training, where the number of epochs per federated training round and learning rate vary over the course of federated training. Additionally, we investigated multiple weight aggregation functions and implemented an ensemble aggregation function. We compared our federated learning model to a model trained using central learning, where all the data is pooled together and trained at a single location.

2   Methods

2.1   Challenge Dataset

The 2021 FeTS challenge uses clinically acquired multi-institutional, multi-parametric magnetic resonance imaging (MRI) images from the 2020 RSNA-MICCAI Brain Tumor Segmentation (BraTS) challenge [13–16]. The challenge dataset is comprised of 341 pre-processed patient brain imaging samples and accompanying manual segmentations from 17 contributing institutions. Each patient sample consisted of four MRI modalities: native T1-weighted, post-contrast T1-weighted, T2-weighted, and T2 Fluid Attenuated Inversion Recovery (FLAIR) volumes. The scans were acquired across multiple sites with different protocols and scanners, and were provided preprocessed for this challenge. Manual segmentations of the tumor tissue were performed by four annotators using a standardized annotation protocol and were verified by expert neuro-radiologists [15, 16]. Three tissue class segmentations were available for each sample: contrast enhanced tumor (ET), tumor core (TC), and whole tumor (WT).

The challenge dataset was partitioned for federated learning based on their source institution. As institutions vary significantly on their size and patient population, the data partitioning is heterogenous and reflective of a real-world situation. Two partitions of the data were specified by the organizers:

1. Partition 1 is the real data distribution from the 17 participating institutions, with a median institution size of 8 samples, minimum size of 3 samples and maximum size of 129 samples (Fig. 1A).
2. Partition 2 is an artificial data distribution based on partition 1 that splits the five largest institutions based on median whole tumor size across all institutions. The median institution size of Partition 2 is 11 samples, the minimum institution size is 3 samples and the maximum institution size is 65 samples (Fig. 1B).

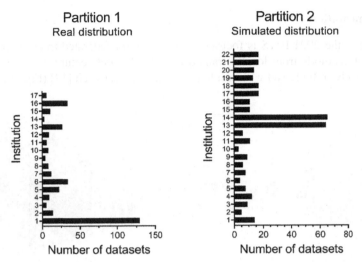

Fig. 1. Challenge data distribution for data partition 1, the real institution distribution, and partition 2, the simulated institution distribution.

For model training and validation, the 341 challenge samples were randomly separated into a training set (80%) and validation set (20%) at an institutional level. In other words, at each institution, 80% of the data was assigned to the training set and 20% of the data was assigned to the validation set.

2.2 Testing on Unseen Data

The 2021 FeTS challenge had two types of testing datasets. The first is the "Challenge Validation Set", which we will refer to as the visible test set, which provides imaging data but not the ground truth segmentations. The inferences made on the visible test set are evaluated by the organizers through the online evaluation platform, which compares the submitted model segmentations to the withheld ground truth segmentations. As per the challenge guidelines, participants must train the model on partition 2 before making inferences on the visible test set in order to obtain valid results.

The second is the "Challenge Test Set", which we will refer to as the hidden test set in the following. Both, the imaging data and segmentations on a set of unseen data, are withheld from participants. Submitted training algorithms for Task 1 will be trained on a hidden training partition, also withheld from participants, and the resultant model will be evaluated on the hidden test set. Both, training and testing for the "Challenge Test Set", were done by challenge organizers, who then provided results to participants.

Due to a complication in the 2021 FeTS challenge, two evaluations were done on the "Challenge Test Set", referred to as "Leaderboards". The first evaluation, "Leaderboard 1", used challenge code before the initial submission deadline. The second evaluation, "Leaderboard 2", used an updated version of challenge code after an error was found in the "Leaderboard 1" challenge code. Our submission described in this paper was developed for "Leaderboard 1" and used "as-is" for "Leaderboard 2".

2.3 Segmentation CNN

As Task 1 of the 2021 FeTS is focused on methods for federated training and weight aggregation methods from locally trained models, the architecture was pre-specified. More precisely, a 3D U-Net with residual connections was used [12] (Fig. 2).

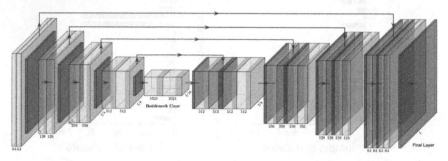

Fig. 2. The segmentation U-Net architecture specified for Task 1. Figure taken from [12].

2.4 Federated Training

The challenge uses the central parameter server approach to federated training, as opposed to decentralized federated learning. In the central parameter server approach, a centralized aggregation server controls federated training rounds and performs local model aggregation. Briefly stated, at the beginning of each federated round, the server distributes the current model weights to all participating institutions for local training. After local training, contributing institutions send the updated model to the server, which combines the model weights together to produce an updated model, completing one federated round.

In each federated training, we trained local models in parallel at all institutions. We investigated modifications to the learning rate, epochs in a federated round, and methods for aggregating the weights from local models.

2.5 Evaluation

The trained models are evaluated on their segmentation performance using the Dice similarity coefficient (DSC) and 95th percentile Hausdorff distance (95%HD). The DSC measures the overlap between segmentations, *e.g.* model segmentations and human annotations, where 0 indicates no overlap and 1 indicates perfect overlap. The Hausdorff distance measures the distance between two point sets, *i.e.* edges of the model segmentation and edges of human annotation edges; the 95%HD uses the 95th percentile of Hausdorff distances, reducing the impact of segmentations with noisy edges. The DSC and 95%HD are calculated for each type of segmentation (ET, TC, and WT). Additionally, the metrics are also reported for the average of the three segmentations, *e.g.* $DSC_{AVG} = 1/3(DSC_{WT} + DSC_{TC} + DSC_{ET})$.

We report results primarily on split 2, the artificial data distribution, as this was the data partition designated by the challenge to be used for evaluation on the visible testing set ("Challenge Validation").

We also report results from "Challenge Test Set" provided to us by challenge organizers. These are results from our final algorithm trained on a hidden training data partition and tested on a hidden test set. We report results for both "Leaderboard 1" and "Leaderboard 2".

3   Results and Discussion

We first established baseline federated training performance using a constant learning rate (5e-3) over 10 federated rounds, 1 epoch of local training per federated round, and federated averaging using the mean of weights of locally trained weights (Fig. 3). This was compared against central learning, where all training samples were pooled into one institution. The central model was trained with the same learning rate (5e-3) for 5 epochs (Fig. 3). Overall, our baseline federated model performed worse than the central model, with a lower DSC ($DSC_{AVG} = 0.607$ for federated baseline vs. $DSC_{AVG} = 0.726$ for central training) and higher 95%HD ($95\%HD_{AVG} = 25.17$ for federated baseline vs. $95\%HD_{AVG} = 15.95$ for central training). Furthermore, federated learning required more cumulative epochs than central training, as the initial rounds of federated training showed poor performance due to the low amounts of data at local institutions.

We investigated changes in learning rate, epochs per round, and weight functions aggregation independently, varying the respective values for one hyper-parameter (*e.g.* learning rate) while keeping the others (*e.g.* epochs per round and weight aggregation) at baseline values.

3.1   Learning Rate

First, we investigated learning rate decay using three types of functions: linear decay, exponential decay, and polynomial decay (Fig. 4A). For all three functions, the initial learning rate was 5e-3 and the final learning rate at the end of federated training was 1e-6. Local models were trained for 1 epoch per round for 10 rounds, and the mean weight aggregation function was used.

All models trained with decaying learning rates performed better than the constant learning rate used in the federated baseline (5e-3). Models trained with federate learning performed poorly when learning rates were higher in the initial training rounds (i.e. in the linear and polynomial decay functions) (Fig. 4). While linear and polynomial decay had similar 95%HD scores, linear decay resulted in overall better DSC. Thus, our final model used a linear decay function.

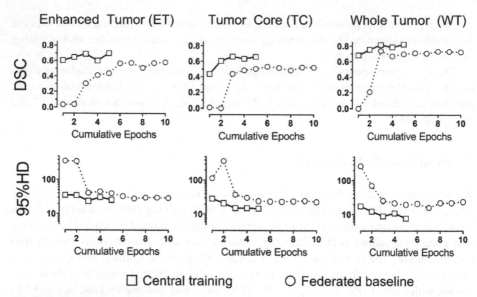

Fig. 3. Baseline federated learning model showed overall poorer performance on the validation data against a central learning model trained on all available at a single site.

3.2 Epochs Per Round

Next, we investigated both constant and variable epochs per round (EpR) throughout the course of federated training. For constant EpR, we used 0.5, 1, and 2 as parameter values. To control for the total number of cumulative epochs across all federated training, we fixed the total epochs to 10 and varied the number of rounds (*i.e.* 20 rounds for 0.5 EpR, 10 rounds for 1 EpR, and 5 rounds for 2 EpR). The learning rate was set to 5e-3 and the mean weight aggregation function was used.

Overall, the 1 EpR parameter used in the baseline model had the best performance on the validation data ($DSC_{AVG} = 0.607$; $95\%HD_{AVG} = 25.17$). Although 0.5 EpR and 2 EpR had better 95%HD scores ($95\%HD_{AVG} = 18.23$ for 0.5 EpR; $95\%HD_{AVG} = 23.97$), the DSC was noticeably worse ($DSC_{AVG} = 0.578$ for 0.5 EpR; $DSC_{AVG} = 0.523$ for 2 EpR).

For variable EpR, we fixed the total number of rounds to 10, and varied the number of epochs in each round. We investigated increasing the number of EpR and increasing and decreasing the number of EpR in a pyramid-like shape (low numbers of EpR at the initial and finial rounds, and high numbers of EpR in the middle rounds) (Fig. 5A). Increasing the number of EpR over the course of federated training resulted in substantial degraded performance, with lower DSC and higher 95%HD scores (Fig. 5B). This is likely due to overfitting to local model data at the latter stages of training due to the high number of epochs on small local datasets.

The pyramid-like changes in EpR, with high amounts of local rounds in the middle of federated training and low amounts of local rounds in the beginning and end of federated training (Fig. 5A) resulted in improved DSC scores compared to the federated baseline model. This was more noticeable in the "big pyramid", which had a maximum number

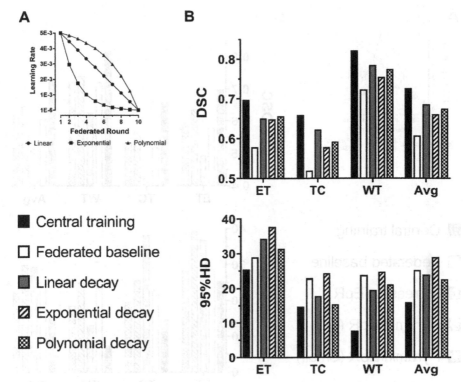

Fig. 4. Federated learning using decaying learning rates. (A) Three types of learning rate decay functions were investigated. (B) DSC and 95%HD scores for validation data on federated learning with decaying learning rates were compared against the central training and federated baseline models.

of local epochs of 5, compared to the "small pyramid", which had a maximum number of local epochs of 2. The 95%HD was best with the "small pyramid" variable EpR. However, given the substantial improvement in DSC score, our final model used the "large pyramid" variable EpR scheme.

3.3 Weight Aggregation Function

Finally, we investigated different functions for aggregating weights. The general approach used to aggregate weights was federated averaging, where matching weights from locally trained models with identical architectures are averaged together across collaborating institutions. The baseline weight averaging function used was an arithmetic mean. We investigated three additional averaging functions: weighted arithmetic mean, median, and geometric median. The weighted arithmetic mean used the number of training examples at a given institution as a weighting factor when calculating the arithmetic mean of weights. Additionally, we investigated ensembling the three weight averaging methods, so that the federated averaged weight is a combination of the weight estimate from the weighted arithmetic mean (50%), median (10%), and geometric median (40%); the

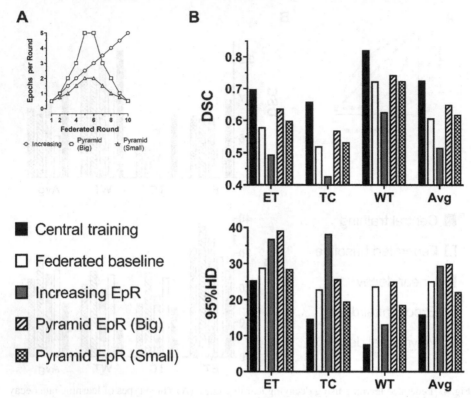

Fig. 5. Variable Epochs per Round (EpR) over the course of federated training. (A) Three types of variable EpR round were investigated. (B) DSC and 95%HD scores on validation data for federated learning with variable EpR were compared against the central training and federated baseline models.

ensemble weights were determined experimentally. Models were trained for 10 rounds at 1 epoch per round and the learning rate was set at 5e-3.

Of the individual weight aggregation functions, the weighted mean consistently performed the best across the regions of interest (ET, TC, WT) and metrics (DSC, 95%HD) (Fig. 6). The median and geometric median were comparable to each other, but generally worse than the baseline federated model that used the unweighted mean.

Compared to the federated baseline, the ensemble also significantly improved performance. On average, the ensemble was comparable to the weighted mean function, and improved DSC scores for WT segmentation. Given this, our final model used the ensemble weight aggregation function.

3.4   Final Model Results on "Challenge Validation Set"

Our final model was trained using 10 federated rounds with a variable number of epochs per round ("Big Pyramid", Fig. 5A), using a linearly decaying learning rate (from 5e-3 to 1e-6, Fig. 4A), and used an ensemble of weighted arithmetic mean, median and

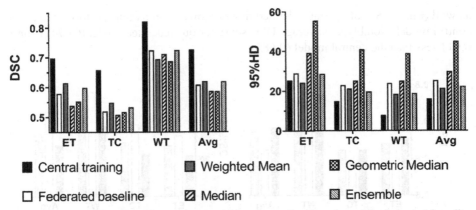

Fig. 6. Federated learning using alternate weight aggregation functions. The federated baseline used an unweighted mean to average model weights. The weighted mean used the number of local training examples at a given institution as a weighting factor when calculating the mean. DSC and 95%HD scores are reported on the validation data.

geometric median (50%, 10% and 40%, respectively) (Fig. 6). Overall, the model performed significantly better than the federated baseline model (Fig. 7). In some cases, such as DSC_{ET}, DSC_{WT}, $95\%HD_{ET}$, our final federated model matched central model performance.

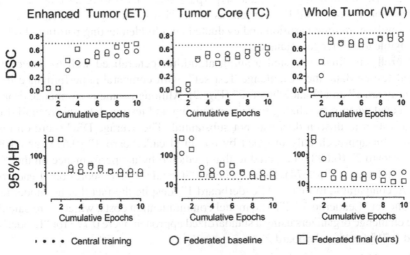

Fig. 7. Our finalized federated learning model using a "pyramid-shaped" variable number of epochs per round, a linearly decaying learning rate, and an ensemble of weight aggregation functions. DSC and 95%HD scores are reported on the validation data.

Finally, we evaluated our finalized federated training algorithm on unseen data using the visible testing set, also known as the "Challenge Validation" set. Our final federated model showed marked improvements compared to the federated baseline on this dataset as well (Fig. 8). Similarly, our federated model showed comparable performance to the central model. Notably, the average DSC score for our federated model (0.674) is only 0.011 less than the central model (0.685).

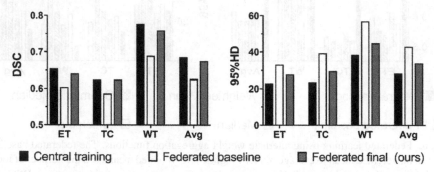

Fig. 8. Our finalized federated model performance (DSC and 95%HD scores) on the visible testing set, also known as the "Challenge Validation set".

3.5 Final Model Results on "Challenge Test Set"

Our final model was evaluated by challenge organizers on "Leaderboard 1" and "Leaderboard 2". The training algorithm and hyperparameters used were developed using the codebase for "Leaderboard 1" and used "as-is" for "Leaderboard 2". Models were trained using a hidden training partition and evaluated on a hidden testing partition; both were only visible to challenge organizers.

Overall, our final federated training algorithm generalized well to unseen training and testing data, the "Challenge Test set", with comparable performance in both "Leaderboard 1" and "Leaderboard 2" (Fig. 9). Although some performance drop is to be expected when generalizing to unseen training and testing data, this overall drop in generalization to unseen data was not substantial. The average DSC score on unseen data for our approach only dropped by 8% in "Leaderboard 1" (0.623) and 10% in "Leaderboard 2" (0.608) compared to that predicted by the performance on the "Challenge Validation set" (0.674). Notably, both DSC and 95%HD scores on "Leaderboard 2" were comparable to that on "Leaderboard 1", despite the fact that no model tuning was done for "Leaderboard 2". The model communication costs, which were calculated by the challenge organizers using a standardized approach, were 0.773 for "Leaderboard 1" and 0.715 for "Leaderboard 2".

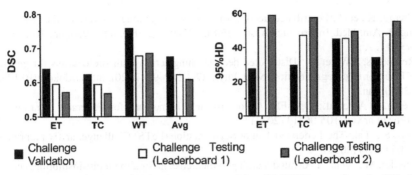

Fig. 9. Our finalized federated model performance (DSC and 95%HD scores) on the "Challenge Validation" and "Challenge Testing" sets (Leaderboard 1 and Leaderboard 2).

Acknowledgements. This work was supported by the Natural Sciences and Engineering Research Council of Canada Postdoctoral Fellowship (AT) and Discovery Grant (NDF), MITACS Globalink Research Internship (LT), University of Calgary BME Research Scholarship (RS), Canada Research Chairs program (NDF), the River Fund at Calgary Foundation (NDF), and the Canadian Institutes of Health Research (CIHR).

Conflicts of Interest. The authors declare that the research was conducted in the absence of any commercial or financial relationships that could be construed as a potential conflict of interest.

References

1. Lo Vercio, L., et al.: Supervised machine learning tools: a tutorial for clinicians. Journal of Neural Engineering **17**(6), 062001 (Oct 9 2020). https://doi.org/10.1088/1741-2552/abbff2
2. Hinton, G.: Deep learning-a technology with the potential to transform health care. JAMA - Journal of the American Medical Association, **320**(11), pp. 1101–1102. American Med-ical Association (Sep 18 2018). https://doi.org/10.1001/jama.2018.11100
3. Kaissis, G.A., Makowski, M.R., Rückert, D., Braren, R.F.: Secure, privacypreserving and federated machine learning in medical imaging. Nat. Mach. Intell. **2**(6), 305–311 (Jun 2020). https://doi.org/10.1038/s42256-020-0186-1
4. MacEachern, S.J., Forkert, N.D.: Machine learning for precision medicine. Genome **64**(4), 416–425 (2021). https://doi.org/10.1139/gen-2020-0131. Epub 2020 Oct 22 PMID: 33091314 Apr
5. Tuladhar, A., Gill, S., Ismail, Z., Forkert, N.D.: Building machine learning models without sharing patient data: A simulation-based analysis of distributed learning by en-sembling. J. Biomed. Inform. **106**, 103424 (2020). https://doi.org/10.1016/j.jbi.2020.103424. Jun.
6. McMahan, H.B., Moore, E., Ramage, D., Hampson, S., Arcas, B.A.: Communication-Efficient Learning of Deep Networks from Decentralized Data. Arxiv (2016)
7. Yang, Q., Liu, Y., Chen, T., Tong, Y.: Federated machine learning: Concept and applications. ACM Trans. Intell. Syst. Technol. **10**(2), 1–19 (2019). https://doi.org/10.1145/3298981. Jan.
8. Kaissis, G.A., Makowski, M.R., Rückert, D., Braren, R.F.: Secure, privacy-preserving and federated machine learning in medical imaging. Nature Machine Intelligence **2**(6), 305–311 (2020). https://doi.org/10.1038/s42256-020-0186-1

9. Chang, K., et al.: Distributed deep learning networks among institutions for medical imaging. J. Am. Med. Informatics Assoc. **25**(8), 945–954 (2018). https://doi.org/10.1093/jamia/ocy017. Aug.

10. Remedios, S.W., et al.: Distributed deep learning across multisite datasets for generalized CT hemorrhage segmentation. Med. Phys. **47**(1), 89–98 (2020). https://doi.org/10.1002/mp.13880. Jan.

11. Reina, G.A., et al.: OpenFL: An open-source framework for Federated Learning. arXiv preprint arXiv:2105.06413 (2021)

12. Pati, S., et al.: The Federated Tumor Segmentation (FeTS) Challenge. arXiv preprint arXiv:2105.05874 (2021)

13. Sheller, M.J., et al.: Federated learning in medicine: facilitating multi-institutional collaborations without sharing patient data. Nat. Sci. Rep. **10**, 12598 (2020). https://doi.org/10.1038/s41598-020-69250-1

14. Bakas, S., et al.: Advancing the cancer genome atlas glioma MRI collections with expert segmentation labels and radiomic features. Nature Scientific Data **4**, 170117 (2017). https://doi.org/10.1038/SDATA.2017.117

15. Bakas, S., et al.: Segmentation labels and radiomic features for the pre-operative scans of the TCGA-GBM collection. The Cancer Imaging Archive (2017). https://doi.org/10.7937/K9/TCIA.2017.KLXWJJ1Q

16. Bakas, S., et al.: Segmentation labels and radiomic features for the pre-operative scans of the TCGA-LGG collection. The Cancer Imaging Archive (2017). https://doi.org/10.7937/K9/TCIA.2017.GJQ7R0EF

Evaluation and Analysis of Different Aggregation and Hyperparameter Selection Methods for Federated Brain Tumor Segmentation

Ece Isik-Polat[1]([⊠])[ID], Gorkem Polat[1][ID], Altan Kocyigit[1][ID],
and Alptekin Temizel[1,2][ID]

[1] Graduate School of Informatics, Middle East Technical University, Ankara, Turkey
{eceisik,gorkem.polat,kocyigit,atemizel}@metu.edu.tr
[2] Neuroscience and Neurotechnology Center of Excellence, Ankara, Turkey

Abstract. Availability of large, diverse, and multi-national datasets is crucial for the development of effective and clinically applicable AI systems in the medical imaging domain. However, forming a global model by bringing these datasets together at a central location, comes along with various data privacy and ownership problems. To alleviate these problems, several recent studies focus on the federated learning paradigm, a distributed learning approach for decentralized data. Federated learning leverages all the available data without any need for sharing collaborators' data with each other or collecting them on a central server. Studies show that federated learning can provide competitive performance with conventional central training, while having a good generalization capability. In this work, we have investigated several federated learning approaches on the brain tumor segmentation problem. We explore different strategies for faster convergence and better performance which can also work on strong Non-IID cases.

Keywords: Federated learning · Collaborative learning · Brain tumor segmentation · Medical imaging

1 Introduction

Computer-aided approaches utilizing deep learning models have become prominent in the domain of medical image processing [18]. The amount and diversity of training data used to develop these models are important for model success and generalizability [25–27]. Currently, the inadequacy of medical data sources and labeled data have become a bottleneck and led to poor performance of the deep learning based solutions [30]. In order to overcome these issues, there are several initiatives to form diverse datasets to train reliable and robust models that have good generalization ability and clinical usability. EndoCV Challenges incorporates diverse endoscopy video frames from several institutions worldwide, including different modalities and organs to utilize deep learning methods to detect artifacts and diseases [1,2,21,22]. BraTS Challenges brings multi-institutional multi-parametric magnetic resonance imaging (mpMRI) scans for the analysis of brain tumors and the dataset has been continuously growing [6]. Although these initiatives are very important for reliable and clinical-ready models, they are not feasible to scale because it requires a tremendous work. First of all, it is difficult to represent whole distribution (e.g., minority and under-represented groups) as it requires healthy collaborations with many institutions and immense annotations. Secondly, data properties such as image modalities and resolutions are in a constant change that leads to distribution shift over time; therefore, collecting and processing all the data for once does not work either. Moreover, due to the data privacy regulations, collecting sensitive patient data from different institutions and hospitals is not always applicable. The federated learning (FL) concept offers a solution in such situations where data privacy and ownership are a problem by enabling collaborators train a common global model without disclosing their local data [15,19]. Several studies employing FL approaches in the medical domain have reported successful results [8,25,26]. These studies have drawn the attention of researchers into FL for medical imaging and made it a popular research field recently.

In this study, we propose various FL approaches for the Federated Tumor Segmentation (FeTS) Challenge [20]. For the Task-1 of the challenge, the participants are provided with an FL environment setup that is based on the OpenFL [24] framework and they are requested to develop strategies for the development of the methods in order to extract much of the knowledge from the collaborators. In this task, the participants are allowed to modify four functions: 1) custom performance metrics, 2) collaborator selection, 3) hyperparameter selection, and 4) custom aggregator. Our proposed methods took the 3rd place in the competition.

2   Related Work

Recently, the use of FL has been increasing in the medical field. In [11], Huang et al. proposed Loss-based Adaptive Boosting Federated Averaging (LoAdaBoost FedAvg) on critical care database data called as MIMIC-III [13]. In this method, the collaborators with higher losses than the previous round median loss are retrained before sending to the server for model aggregation. In [16], Li et al. have proposed a federated learning system for brain tumor segmentation on BraTS 2018 dataset [6] and have shown the trade-off between privacy protection costs and model performance. Similarly, in [26], Sheller et al. have compared federated learning and other data private collaborative learning approaches such as institutional incremental learning and cyclic institutional incremental learning on brain tumor segmentation task. This study has shown that FL can overcome institutional biases and form a global model that has better generalization where data amount and data diversity are inadequate. In [8], Dou et al. have used FL architecture to detect chest CT abnormalities in COVID-19 patients and showed that federated global model outperforms in terms of generalizability on external datasets better than individual models and their ensemble.

3   Data

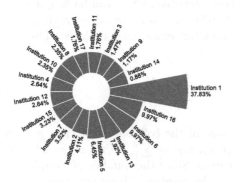 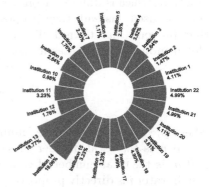

(a) Natural split, *partitioning_1*.

(b) Artificial split, *partitioning_2*: 5 largest institutions are splitted further according to the tumor sizes.

Fig. 1. The data distribution in the training dataset splits.

The Federated Tumor Segmentation (FeTS) challenge 2021 is the first challenge in the federated medical imaging area. The challenge data set is composed of multi-institutional magnetic resonance images from the International Brain Tumor Segmentation (BraTS) challenge and other independent institutions in the FeTS initiative [3–5,20,24]. The training set contains 341 images, institution-based split of which is given in Fig. 1. The validation and the tests sets contain 111 and 166 images, respectively. The segmentation annotations of the challenge dataset were performed by annotators whose experience levels vary with respect to their clinical and academic backgrounds. Then, these annotations were approved by two experienced board-certified neuroradiologists with more than 12 years of experience [20].

4   Methods

4.1   Aggregator

In a real-life FL setting, the data distribution of collaborators is non independent identically distributed (non-IID) because collaborators may have different data distribution and the number of observations. The difference in device capabilities, user demographic information, or geographic location can be major reasons for the non-IIDness [14,19].

When collaborators have access to differing amounts of data and when they use the same number of epochs E in their local training, they would perform different numbers of local updates τ. If a collaborator has n_i samples, number of local gradient descent (GD) iterations is $\tau_i = En_i/B$, where B is the mini-batch size. In [29], Wang et al. have shown that the heterogeneity in collaborators' local progresses causes convergence to a stationary point of mismatched objective function, which is different from the true objective, when vanilla weighted averaging is used. Instead, they propose FedNova, a normalized averaging method that prevents bias toward clients performing more local updates. The shared global model is updated as in Eq. 1.

$$x^{t+1} = x^t - \tau_{\text{eff}} \sum_{i=1}^{m} p_i \frac{\Delta_i^t}{\tau_i^t} \tag{1}$$

where p_i denotes the relative sample size of the collaborator i (i.e., $p_i = n_i/n$ where n is the total number of samples), $\tau_{\text{eff}} = \sum_{i=1}^{m} p_i \tau_i$, $\Delta_i^t = x^t - x_i^{t+1}$, and m is the total number of collaborators. Since the number of samples n_i for collaborator i is directly proportional to the number of local iteration τ_i and the relative sample size p_i, this formula can be rewritten as in Eq. 2.

$$\tau_i = \frac{p_i nE}{B}$$

$$\tau_{\text{eff}} = \sum_{i=1}^{m} \frac{p_i^2 nE}{B}$$

$$x^{t+1} = x^t - \frac{nE}{B}(p_1^2 + p_2^2 + \cdots + p_m^2) \sum_{i=1}^{m} \frac{B}{nE} \Delta_i^t$$

$$x^{t+1} = x^t - \underbrace{(p_1^2 + p_2^2 + \cdots + p_m^2)}_{constant} \sum_{i=1}^{m} \Delta_i^t$$

$$x^{t+1} = x^t - \gamma \sum_{i=1}^{m} \Delta_i^t \tag{2}$$

where γ refers to the aggregator learning rate, which can be increased or decreased according to FL training needs. As given in Eq. 2, FedNova corresponds to a uniform averaging with adjustable step size (or learning rate) on the aggregator. FedNova aims to prevent exacerbation of client drifts caused by relative sample sizes p_i. When there is a significant difference between the number of samples in the collaborators, as in the FeTS Challenge dataset, FedAvg creates a bias toward the collaborators having more samples (Fig. 2). Although validation set (named Val-1 in Sect. 5) results reported during the training may seem good as its data distribution directly comes from the training set, out-of-distribution performance results may not be satisfactory. Wang et al. [29] have shown that FedNova generally achieves 6–9% higher accuracy than FedAvg on a non-IID version of CIFAR-10 dataset.

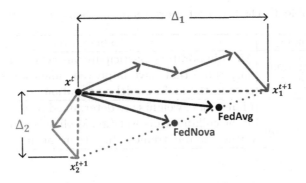

Fig. 2. Naive weighted averaging (FedAvg) creates bias toward collaborators having higher number of samples, which may adversely affect the out-of-distribution performance. On the other hand, FedNova gives equal weights to all collaborators acting as a regularizer.

Another approach to deal with convergence issues when collaborators' data distribution is non-IID is Federated Averaging with server momentum (FedAvgM). The momentum on top of the Stochastic Gradient Descent (SGD) has proven to provide a significant success in accelerating the training and dampening the oscillations [9]. In [10], Hsu et al. have shown that as the level of non-IIDness increases, the performance of the FedAvgM stays relatively constant while federated averaging falls rapidly. Moreover, [23] has shown the improved effect of adaptive optimizers such as Adam and RMSProp, which are based on momentum, on top of the federated averaging.

In FedAvgM, the average of the gradients are added to the accumulated gradient which is multiplied by a β parameter to adjust effect of the momentum as shown in Eq. 3. Then this weighted accumulated gradient is used to update weights of the current communication round as in Eq. 4. Here, an aggregator learning rate γ can be used to adjust the step size on the server (in our experiments β is chosen as 0.9 and γ is chosen as 1).

$$\Delta w^{t+1} = \sum_{i=1}^{m} p_i \Delta w_i^{t+1}$$

$$v^{t+1} = \beta v^t + \Delta w^{t+1} \tag{3}$$

$$w^{t+1} = w^t - \gamma v^{t+1} \tag{4}$$

where p_i denotes the relative sample size of the collaborator i (i.e., $p_i = n_i/n$ where n is the total number of samples), and m is the total number of collaborators.

Along with FedNova and FedAvgM, other aggregator functions (Table 1) have been implemented and experimented in the FeTS Challenge. However, in this article, only the results for FedNova and FedAvgM are presented. Please visit https://github.com/eceisik/FeTS_Challenge_METU_FL_Team to see all implemented methods by the METU FL Team.

Table 1. The list of other aggregator methods implemented.

Function name	Explanation
Make aggregation with improved nodes	All collaborators participate in each round of FL, but only those that have improved validation scores participate in the main model aggregation
Coordinate-wise median aggregation	Main model weights are determined by taking the median of the collaborators weights. Median is more robust to the outliers and extreme values than mean

4.2 Collaborator Selection

How to choose collaborators that will take part in each round is another important dimension of the FeTS Challenge. We used "all_collaborators_train" as a collaborator choice function and all collaborators participated in each FL round.

We implemented two alternative collaborator choice functions given in Table 2. If the focus is on the convergence time metric, the method called as "choose random nodes with faster ones" could be more preferable. This method does not introduce any extra communication delays, because once a random collaborator is selected, only those that are faster than the selected one participate in the training for the FL round (i.e., selected collaborator creates an upper bound for the other selected collaborators in terms of time). Although the number of collaborators participate in each round varies, the working mechanism tends to favor the fastest collaborators. Being fast, in this case, depends on two factors namely the amount of available computation/communication resources and the number of samples in a collaborator. On the other hand, the institutions having fewer patient images may be over represented, which is a disadvantage of this method.

4.3 Hyperparameter Selection

For the hyperparameter selection, an adaption of AdaComm [28] with a learning rate scheduling scheme is used. AdaComm [28] is an adaptive communication strategy that saves communication delay and enables fast convergence by federated averaging less frequently in early training rounds and later increasing communication frequency. In [28], experimental converge analysis was examined on wall-clock time instead of communication round. It is shown that using more local updates in the early rounds of training resulted in a faster decrease in loss but also a higher error. For this reason, it starts with a large number of updates per round and gradually decreases as the model starts to converge.

In the original version of AdaComm, the method is based on the number of local updates in an IID setting. However, in the challenge, the data distribution is extremely uneven. While Institute-1 has 37.83% of the data, Institute-14 has 0.88% of the whole training data (Fig. 1). Using the same number of local updates for each collaborator could potentially cause over-representation of some

Table 2. The list of other collaborator choice methods implemented.

Function name	Explanation
Choose random nodes with faster ones	For the first round, all collaborators participate in the training and round time statistics are recorded. After the first round, a random collaborator is selected and participates in the current FL round with other collaborators that are faster than itself
Random collaborators train	A random subset of collaborators are selected for each FL round

small data provider institutions. By considering the non-IID nature of the data distribution, our aggregation method mechanism, and the fact that the number of local updates is directly proportional to the number of epochs, we adapted this method based on the decaying number of epoch (AdaptiveEpoch). Basically, the number of epochs per round at each FL round decays according to the relative difference between the initial loss and current round loss as stated in Eq. 5.

$$E_t = \left\lceil \sqrt{\frac{F(x_{T=t})}{F(x_{T=0})}} E_0 \right\rceil \tag{5}$$

where T denotes the number of FL rounds, t denotes the round number, E_t denotes the number of epochs at a given round t, and $F(x)$ is the objective function with respect to model parameters denoted by x.

Learning rate scheduling is a commonly used technique to train deep neural networks in a centralized manner [9]. Studies show that learning rate scheduling is also necessary for FedAvg to converge to an optimum point of loss function [17]. However, there are many strategies for scheduling and there is no benchmark for their performances. In this study, we have adopted *decay learning rate on plateau* approach. This strategy brings two new parameters namely *patience* and *decay factor*. In our implementation, learning rate scheduling tracks the target performance metric, which is the mean Dice score for ET, TC and WT labels, and if there is no improvement on the target performance metric for a *patience* number of round, the learning rate is updated by scaling with the *decay factor*. Experiments show that learning rate scheduling provides faster convergence, more relaxed learning rate selection, higher convergence score, and reduced oscillations when training converges [9]. The list of hyperparameter selection methods are given in Table 3. For AdaptiveEpoch initial epoch E_0 is set to 8; for the LR scheduling, the initial LR is set to 0.0002 and patience is set as 15. For the constant hyperparameters, default values were used (LR = 0.00005, epoch per round = 1).

Table 3. The list of other hyperparameter selection methods.

Function name	Explanation
Constant hyperparameters	Use fixed hyperparameters for each FL round
LRScheduling hyperparameters	Learning rate decays according to the value of average Dice score with given patience scheme
AdaptiveEpoch	The number of epochs per round decays according to the decrease in the initial loss

5   Experimental Results and Discussion

Before the FL training, the training dataset is split into train and validation sets as 80% and 20%, respectively. The performance results of the aggregated and individual models on validation sets are logged at each FL round (it is integrated with the FeTS Challenge source code). Unless otherwise stated, all reported performance metrics and loss graphs belong to this validation set of *partitioning_2.csv*. The mean Dice score refers to the average of Dice scores of ET, TC, and WT labels.

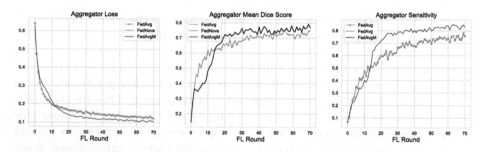

Fig. 3. The performance comparison of FedAvg, FedNova, and FedAvgM.

Figure 3 shows the performances of FedAvg, FedNova, and FedAvgM on aggregator mean dice score, aggregator loss, and aggregator sensitivity metrics. Since medical datasets may contain institutional biases [26] and FedAvg have an undesirable effect of favoring these biases, FedNova is expected to have better performance on the non-training sets. However, since samples of institutions' distributions of training and validation sets are similar to each other, we observe nearly identical performance for both FedAvg and FedNova. Yet, models built with FedNova are expected to have better inferences on the out-of-distribution dataset [29], and as such, they are expected to be more suitable for real-life use-case scenarios. On the other hand, FedAvgM outperforms both FedAvg and FedNova on all metrics. Therefore, we have preferred FedAvgM as the aggregator method in the FeTS challenge.

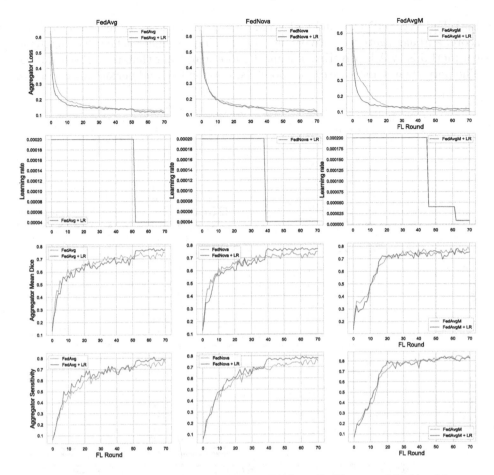

Fig. 4. The impacts of LR scheduling on FedAvg, FedNova, and FedAvgM.

Figure 4 shows the effect of the LR scheduling approach on each aggregation method. For both FedAvg and FedNova, it can be observed on both loss function and performance metrics that LR scheduling has an evident effect on their performances. In particular, a sharp increase on performance metrics occurs when the LR is decayed. On the other hand, LR scheduling has no improvement on FedAvgM. One possible reason might be since FedAvgM converges much faster than the FedAvg and FedNova, it may have directly reached the optimum region where it does not need any scheduling. However, it should be noted that we have used fixed values for starting learning rate, decay rate, and patience parameters; therefore, more experiments with different set of values should be performed to make a comment on effect of LR scheduling on FedAvgM.

AdaptiveEpoch helps training converge in fewer rounds with higher performance due to having more local epochs than using the constant hyperparameters as seen in Fig. 5. The AdaptiveEpoch method improves the performance of both FedAvg, FedNova, and FedAvgM on aggregator loss, aggregator mean dice score, and aggregator sensitivity metrics. The improvement achieved on aggregator methods by AdaptiveEpoch is much more significant than the LR scheduling. The performance increase can be observed both on loss and performance metrics.

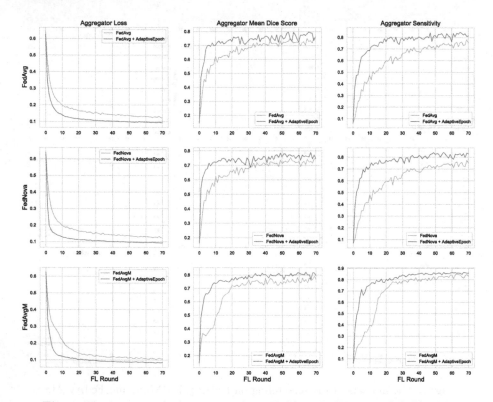

Fig. 5. The impacts of adaptive epoch on FedAvg, FedNova, and FedAvgM.

Figure 6 shows the performance comparison of different hyperparameter strategies on FedAvgM. Accordingly, LR scheduling, AdaptiveEpoch, and AdaptiveEpoch+LR scheduling improves the baseline model performance. AdaptiveEpoch and AdaptiveEpoch+LR scheduling provides faster convergence than LR scheduling. However, there is no significant difference between AdaptiveEpoch and AdaptiveEpoch+LR scheduling. Due to the time and resource constraints, the number of FL round was set to 70 for all experiments, which in turn limited the effect of LR scheduling and AdaptiveEpoch+LR scheduling due to incomplete decaying of LR.

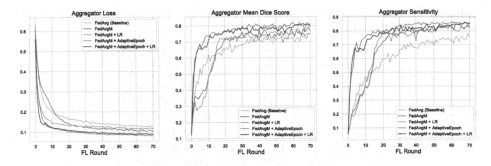

Fig. 6. The impacts of hyperparameter setting strategies on FedAvgM

Table 4 shows the mean dice score and convergence score obtained on the validation set. These experiments are performed by using *partitioning-2* as data split. The convergence score is computed as the area under the validation learning curve where the horizontal axis is the runtime, and the vertical axis is the performance. Most of the time, FedAvgM outperforms others and achieves the best mean Dice score and the convergence score for all hyperparameter choice strategies except for LR scheduling. It is expected and in line with the results that are presented in Fig. 4. Nevertheless, the convergence score is based on the validation set reported during the FL training; therefore, the comparison of convergence scores on an out-of-distribution set is still an open question.

Table 4. The mean Dice score and convergence scores on the validation set.

	Validation mean dice			Convergence score		
	FedAvg	FedNova	FedAvgM	FedAvg	FedNova	FedAvgM
Constant Hyperparameters	0.753	0.753	**0.793**	0.770	0.770	**0.788**
LR Scheduling	**0.782**	0.776	0.781	**0.761**	0.759	0.744
AdaptiveEpoch	0.796	0.790	**0.821**	0.797	0.797	**0.804**
AdaptiveEpoch+LR Scheduling	0.783	0.787	**0.814**	0.781	0.785	**0.795**

Table 5 presents the results of the our challenge submission on the challenge test set with convergence score of 0.770. The results are provided by the FeTS initiative.

Table 5. The scores were obtained on Leader Board 2 of Task 1 that our team (METU FL) won the 3rd rank in the FeTS Challenge.

	μ	σ	Q_1	Q_2	Q_3
Dice_ET	0.719	0.268	0.676	0.811	0.887
Dice_WT	0.794	0.228	0.807	0.882	0.917
Dice_TC	0.741	0.286	0.674	0.870	0.931
Sensitivity_ET	0.817	0.277	0.812	0.930	0.974
Sensitivity_WT	0.860	0.236	0.869	0.942	0.977
Sensitivity_TC	0.832	0.278	0.861	0.945	0.981
Specificity_ET	0.999	0.002	0.999	0.999	0.999
Specificity_WT	0.998	0.004	0.998	0.998	0.999
Specificity_TC	0.999	0.003	0.999	0.999	0.999
Hausdorff95_ET	34.430	96.022	1.414	2.449	9.027
Hausdorff95_WT	19.199	57.799	3.162	5.431	10.355
Hausdorff95_TC	35.288	91.651	2.236	6.240	17.051

6   Conclusion

In this study, we perform comprehensive experiments to compare different hyper-parameter selection strategies and aggregation methods. The experiments reveal that FedAvgM has better performance than FedAvg and FedNova. Moreover, it is shown that the AdaptiveEpoch approach provides performance increase and faster convergence. However, LR scheduling is not effective with FedAvgM or AdaptiveEpoch. Therefore, it can be said that methods that work well individually may not work well together when combined, or one can reduce the effectiveness of the other. For instance, while AdaptiveEpoch results in better validation mean dice scores and convergence scores than using constant hyper-parameter strategy, when it is combined with LR scheduling, all mean dice and convergence scores get worse for all aggregation methods (see Table 4).

During the experiments, all collaborators have participated in the local training process for all rounds. Instead, collaborator choosing methods such as clustering collaborators based on the update similarity or increasing the likelihood of being chosen collaborators that improved the performance for the random collaborator choice can be utilized to improve performance.

Moreover, in the medical image domain, there is generally high interobserver variability in annotations, which can be considered label noise. For example, if an institution's label quality is low, the model coming from that institution will adversely affect the global model; therefore, weights coming from that institution should be handled carefully. There are defense mechanisms such as KRUM [7], BARFED [12], or trimmed mean [31] that can overcome the attacks in federated learning to some extent. These defense strategies may be used to overcome the label noise.

7 GPU Training Times

Computation time and cost, as well as energy consumption, are important factors determining the direction of future research and adoption of the technology in real life. Table 6 shows the detailed GPU training times of the experiments that are run on single NVIDIA A100-80GB GPU. LR scheduling has no significant effect on the training times. On the other hand, although AdaptiveEpoch strategy brings an increase in performance metrics, its usage nearly doubles the total training time due to longer round times.

Table 6. The detailed GPU training times (hour).

	FedAvg	FedNova	FedAvgM	Total
Constant Hyperparameters	36.7	36.4	34.8	**107.9**
LR Scheduling	35.1	36.7	36.8	**108.6**
AdaptiveEpoch	67.2	69.0	68.9	**205.1**
AdaptiveEpoch+LR Scheduling	65.5	65.8	66.4	**197.7**
Total	**204.5**	**207.9**	**206.9**	**619.3**

Acknowledgment. This work has been supported by Middle East Technical University Scientific Research Projects Coordination Unit under grant number GAP-704-2020-10071. The numerical calculations reported in this paper were performed using TUBITAK ULAKBIM, High Performance and Grid Computing Center (TRUBA resources).

References

1. Ali, S., et al.: Deep learning for detection and segmentation of artefact and disease instances in gastrointestinal endoscopy. Med. Image Anal. **70**, 102002 (2021)
2. Ali, S., et al.: An objective comparison of detection and segmentation algorithms for artefacts in clinical endoscopy. Sci. Rep. **10**(1), 1–15 (2020)
3. Bakas, S., et al.: Segmentation labels and radiomic features for the pre-operative scans of the TCGA-GBM collection. The cancer imaging archive. Nat. Sci. Data **4**, 170117 (2017)
4. Bakas, S., et al.: Segmentation labels and radiomic features for the pre-operative scans of the TCGA-LGG collection. Cancer Imaging Archive **286** (2017)
5. Bakas, S., et al.: Advancing the cancer genome atlas glioma MRI collections with expert segmentation labels and radiomic features. Sci. Data **4**(1), 1–13 (2017)
6. Bakas, S., et al.: Identifying the best machine learning algorithms for brain tumor segmentation, progression assessment, and overall survival prediction in the brats challenge. arXiv preprint arXiv:1811.02629 (2018)
7. Blanchard, P., El Mhamdi, E.M., Guerraoui, R., Stainer, J.: Machine learning with adversaries: byzantine tolerant gradient descent. In: Proceedings of the 31st International Conference on Neural Information Processing Systems, pp. 118–128 (2017)

8. Dou, Q., et al.: Federated deep learning for detecting COVID-19 lung abnormalities in CT: a privacy-preserving multinational validation study. NPJ Digital Med. **4**(1), 1–11 (2021)

9. Goodfellow, I., Bengio, Y., Courville, A.: Deep Learning. MIT Press, Cambridge (2016). http://www.deeplearningbook.org

10. Hsu, T.M.H., Qi, H., Brown, M.: Measuring the effects of non-identical data distribution for federated visual classification. arXiv preprint arXiv:1909.06335 (2019)

11. Huang, L., Yin, Y., Fu, Z., Zhang, S., Deng, H., Liu, D.: LoAdaBoost: loss-based AdaBoost federated machine learning with reduced computational complexity on IID and non-IID intensive care data. PLoS ONE **15**(4), e0230706 (2020)

12. Isik-Polat, E., Polat, G., Kocyigit, A.: BARFED: byzantine attack-resistant federated averaging based on outlier elimination. arXiv preprint arXiv:2111.04550 (2021)

13. Johnson, A.E., et al.: MIMIC-III, a freely accessible critical care database. Sci. Data **3**(1), 1–9 (2016)

14. Kairouz, P., et al.: Advances and open problems in federated learning. arXiv preprint arXiv:1912.04977 (2019)

15. Li, T., Sahu, A.K., Talwalkar, A., Smith, V.: Federated learning: challenges, methods, and future directions. IEEE Signal Process. Mag. **37**(3), 50–60 (2020)

16. Li, W., et al.: Privacy-preserving federated brain tumour segmentation. In: Suk, H.-I., Liu, M., Yan, P., Lian, C. (eds.) MLMI 2019. LNCS, vol. 11861, pp. 133–141. Springer, Cham (2019). https://doi.org/10.1007/978-3-030-32692-0_16

17. Li, X., Huang, K., Yang, W., Wang, S., Zhang, Z.: On the convergence of FedAvg on non-IID data. arXiv preprint arXiv:1907.02189 (2019)

18. Litjens, G., et al.: A survey on deep learning in medical image analysis. Med. Image Anal. **42**, 60–88 (2017)

19. McMahan, B., Moore, E., Ramage, D., Hampson, S., Arcas, B.A.: Communication-efficient learning of deep networks from decentralized data. In: Artificial Intelligence and Statistics, pp. 1273–1282. PMLR (2017)

20. Pati, S., et al.: The federated tumor segmentation (FeTS) challenge (2021)

21. Polat, G., Isik Polat, E., Kayabay, K., Temizel, A.: Polyp detection in colonoscopy images using deep learning and bootstrap aggregation. In: Proceedings of the 3rd International Workshop and Challenge on Computer Vision in Endoscopy (EndoCV 2021) @ ISBI, vol. 2886, pp. 90–100 (2021)

22. Polat, G., Sen, D., Inci, A., Temizel, A.: Endoscopic artefact detection with ensemble of deep neural networks and false positive elimination. In: EndoCV@ ISBI, pp. 8–12 (2020)

23. Reddi, S.J., et al.: Adaptive federated optimization. In: International Conference on Learning Representations (2021). https://openreview.net/forum?id=LkFG3lB13U5

24. Reina, G.A., et al.: OpenFL: an open-source framework for federated learning. arXiv preprint arXiv:2105.06413 (2021)

25. Rieke, N., et al.: The future of digital health with federated learning. NPJ Digital Med. **3**(1), 1–7 (2020)

26. Sheller, M.J., et al.: Federated learning in medicine: facilitating multi-institutional collaborations without sharing patient data. Sci. Rep. **10**(1), 1–12 (2020)

27. Sun, C., Shrivastava, A., Singh, S., Gupta, A.: Revisiting unreasonable effectiveness of data in deep learning era. In: Proceedings of the IEEE International Conference on Computer Vision (ICCV), October 2017

28. Wang, J., Joshi, G.: Adaptive communication strategies to achieve the best error-runtime trade-off in local-update sgd. In: Talwalkar, A., Smith, V., Zaharia, M. (eds.) Proceedings of Machine Learning and Systems, vol. 1, pp. 212–229 (2019). https://proceedings.mlsys.org/paper/2019/file/c8ffe9a587b126 f152ed3d89a146b445-Paper.pdf

29. Wang, J., Liu, Q., Liang, H., Joshi, G., Poor, H.V.: Tackling the objective inconsistency problem in heterogeneous federated optimization. In: Advances in Neural Information Processing Systems 33 (2020)

30. Yang, Q., Liu, Y., Chen, T., Tong, Y.: Federated machine learning: concept and applications. ACM Trans. Intell. Syst. Technol. (TIST) 10(2), 1–19 (2019)

31. Yin, D., Chen, Y., Kannan, R., Bartlett, P.: Byzantine-robust distributed learning: towards optimal statistical rates. In: International Conference on Machine Learning, pp. 5650–5659. PMLR (2018)

Multi-institutional Travelling Model for Tumor Segmentation in MRI Datasets

Raissa Souza[1,2,3]([✉]) [iD], Anup Tuladhar[1,2,3] [iD], Pauline Mouches[1,2,3] [iD],
Matthias Wilms[1,2] [iD], Lakshay Tyagi[4] [iD], and Nils D. Forkert[1,2,5,6] [iD]

[1] Department of Radiology, Cumming School of Medicine, University of Calgary,
Calgary, AB T2N 4N1, Canada
raissa.souzadeandrad@ucalgary.ca
[2] Hotchkiss Brain Institute, University of Calgary, Calgary, AB T2N 4N1, Canada
[3] Biomedical Engineering Graduate Program, University of Calgary,
Calgary, AB T2N 4N1, Canada
[4] Department of Chemical Engineering, Indian Institute of Technology Kanpur,
Kanpur, Uttar Pradesh, India
[5] Department of Clinical Neurosciences, Cumming School of Medicine,
University of Calgary, Calgary, AB T2N 4N1, Canada
[6] Alberta Children's Hospital Research Institute, University of Calgary,
Calgary, AB T2N 4N1, Canada

Abstract. Administrative, ethical, and legal reasons are often preventing the central collection of data and subsequent development of machine learning models for computer-aided diagnosis tools using medical images. The main idea of distributed learning is to train machine learning models locally at each site rather than using centrally collected data, thereby avoiding sharing data between health care centers and model developers. Thus, distributed learning is an alternative that solves many legal and ethical issues and overcomes the need to directly share data. Most previous studies simulated data distribution or used datasets that are acquired in a controlled way, potentially misrepresenting real clinical cases. The 2021 Federated Tumor Segmentation (FeTS) challenge provides clinically acquired multi-institutional magnetic resonance imaging (MRI) scans from patients with brain cancer and aims to compare federated learning models. In this work, we propose a travelling model that visits each collaborator site up to five times with three distinct travelling orders (ascending, descending, and random) between collaborators as a solution to distributed learning. Our results demonstrate that performing more training cycles is effective independent of the order that the models are transferred among the collaborators. Moreover, we show that our model does not suffer from catastrophic forgetting and successfully achieves a similar performance (average Dice score 0.676) compared to standard machine learning implementations (Dice score 0.667) trained using the data from all collaborators hosted at a central location.

Keywords: Distributed learning · Travelling model · FeTS · BraTS

ⓒ The Author(s), under exclusive license to Springer Nature Switzerland AG 2022
A. Crimi and S. Bakas (Eds.): BrainLes 2021, LNCS 12963, pp. 420–432, 2022.
https://doi.org/10.1007/978-3-031-09002-8_37

1 Introduction

In recent years, novel machine learning methods have achieved human-like performance for many problems in the computer vision and medical image analysis domains [1]. However, a major reason that prevents a broad application of these novel artificial intelligence methods for computer-aided diagnosis using medical images is the limited access to datasets due to strict legal, technical, and ethical regulations that aim to protect patient data [2–4]. For instance, regulations such as the United States Health Insurance Portability and Accountability Act (HIPAA) [5] and European General Data Protection Regulation (GDPR) [6] determine how personally identifiable data should be stored, exchanged, and manipulated, limiting healthcare facilities to share information with each other.

To overcome data access problems, a recent approach called distributed learning has emerged, which aims to locally train machine learning models at each data contributor site, thereby avoiding the need to share data at a central location. This approach is especially relevant for applications where a single collaborator does not have enough data for training accurate and generalizable models, which is especially the case for rare diseases for which only few patients are seen at a single health care center [7].

Today, distributed learning is mostly implemented using federated learning of artificial neural networks (ANN). In federated learning, independent machine learning models are trained at each collaborator site in parallel and then combined into a global model. Contrary, in this work, we develop and evaluate a so-called travelling model for distributed learning, also known as single weight transfer and cyclical weight transfer. It consists of training a single model sequentially, at one collaborator site per time, travelling from one collaborator to the next one during training [8–12]. It is hypothesized that the final model trained using a traveling approach is able to leverage knowledge from the diversity of all samples with a similar performance than corresponding models trained using a centralized database.

The 2021 Federated Tumor Segmentation (FeTS) challenge aims at comparing state-of-the-art distributed learning methods that effectively aggregate weights and leverage data from multiple collaborators, given a pre-defined segmentation algorithm. Most previous studies investigating distributed learning described in literature simulated data distribution or used datasets that are acquired in a controlled way, likely misrepresenting real clinical cases [7,9]. The FeTS challenge intends to address these issues by providing clinically acquired multi-institutional magnetic resonance imaging (MRI) scans from previous Brain Tumor Segmentation (BraTS) challenges [13–15], and data from independent collaborators that are part of FeTS initiative [16,18] to provide a common ground to compare different distributed learning approaches.

For this work, we implemented a travelling machine learning framework to solve the proposed challenge. We compared the proposed distributed learning model to a standard central learning implementation and investigated the influence of the order by which the model travels among the collaborators and the number of visits on its performance.

2   Material and Methods

2.1   Dataset

FeTS provided 341 pre-processed brain imaging datasets from patients with brain tumours including four MRI modalities: T1-weighted (T1), post-contrast T1-weighted (T1Gd), T2-weighted (T2), and T2-weighted Fluid Attenuated Inversion Recovery (T2-FLAIR) volumes, resulting in a total of 1364 scans for the 341 patients. The scans were acquired across multiple sites with different protocols and scanners.

For each patient, a corresponding brain tumor segmentation is available with separate labels for the enhancing tumor (ET) tissue, core tumor (CT) tissue, and whole tumor (WT) tissue. The manual segmentation was performed by up to four raters using the same annotation protocol, described in [12], that was later approved by expert neuro-radiologists.

Two csv files describing the distribution of the datasets among 17 (partitioning one) and 22 (partitioning two) collaborators were also provided by the FeTS challenge. It is important to note that the data is not equally distributed, with some collaborators providing data for up to 50 patients while other centers provide data for less than ten patients.

Furthermore, the FeTS challenge released datasets from 111 patients containing the same MRI modalities but without ground truths labels for a validation of the distributed models on unseen data.

2.2   Method Training Aggregator

The pre-defined algorithm provided for the challenge is a U-Net segmentation architecture with residual connections. The U-Net is an encoder-decoder structure, which consists of convolutional layers and downsampling layers in the encoder and upsampling layers in the decoder. In order to improve context and feature re-usability, the defined architecture includes skip connections that concatenate feature maps paired across the encoder and the decoder layer. It also includes residual connections that take advantage of information from previous layers to boost its performance [16].

The general idea of the proposed travelling model is to train a single U-Net segmentation model at one collaborator at time. Briefly, we define the order that we want to visit the collaborators and then initiate the model training at the first collaborator of the sequence. When the training is completed at a collaborator, the model with the learned parameters is sent to the next collaborator. This process is repeated until the model reaches the end of the sequence. The whole traveling process can also be repeated for multiple cycles, which may improve the model performance and avoid catastrophic forgetting [17], which means that the model forgets patterns learned at previous collaborators. The final model is always defined as the last model generated after the last visit to all collaborators.

For model development and evaluation using the publicly available training data, the datasets were shuffled and for each collaborator 80% of the datasets

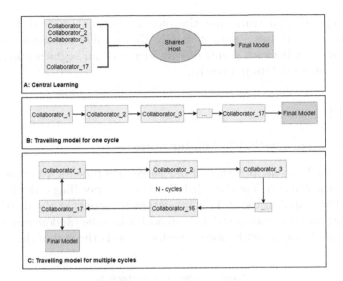

Fig. 1. Model training aggregators investigated (A) central learning, (B) single weight transfer and (C) cyclical weight transfer.

were used for training the model and 20% for internal validation of the trained model. In this work, we tested different aggregation methods and compared their performance. First, we trained the segmentation model provided by the FeTS challenge with a standard central learning approach, pooling the data to a central database (Fig. 1A). Second, we trained a travelling model for one cycle. With this method, the model visits each collaborator only one time as illustrated in Fig. 1B. Finally, as shown in Fig. 1C, we performed multiple cycle visits. This setup only differs from the previous approach by sending the model to each collaborator more than once. We investigated the model performance for 2, 3, 4, and 5 cycles in this work.

We also investigated how the order by which the model is transferred between collaborators affects its ability to learn and generalize. Therefore, we investigated three distinct transfer schemes: ascending and descending orders according to the number of samples available at each collaborator, and a random order.

We used one epoch per cycle for all experiments, which means that we used all available data at least once at each collaborator. An optimizer rate of 0.05 was used during training.

2.3 Validation

After training our models for the given dataset partitioning, we inferred the labels for the provided unseen validation dataset. Then, generated segmentation labels were uploaded to the challenge system to obtain the evaluation results.

The FeTS evaluation system provides the Dice score and the Hausdorff95 metrics for each image. Briefly, the Dice score measures the overlap of two segmentations (ground truth and the model's output). It is defined between 0 and 1 where 1 indicates a perfect match. Hausdorff95 measures the 95th percentile of distances between points on one edge set (our segmentation) to points on the other edge set (ground truth).

3   Results

3.1   Experiments with 17 Collaborators

First, we verified the performance of our three experiments using the data consisting of 17 institutions. The data distribution and travelling order for all experiments are illustrated in Fig. 2. It is important to note that the distribution for the ascending and descending orders is smooth while the random order randomly placed the collaborators with more samples towards the end of the sequence.

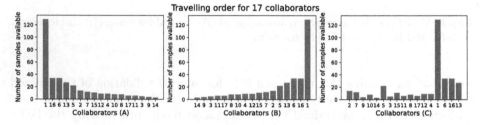

Fig. 2. Data distribution and travelling order for 17 collaborators: (A) descending order, (B) ascending order, and (C) random order.

The internal validation results for the above distributions are shown in Figs. 3 and 4. We evaluated travelling models for 1–5 cycles and compared the results to our baseline model (central learning) represented as a green line in the graphs.

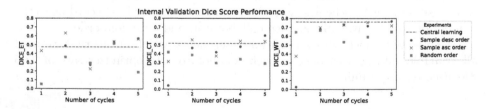

Fig. 3. Dice score performance evaluation results for travelling models with 1–5 cycles for 1 epoch per round travelling in different orders for partitioning one (17 collaborators).

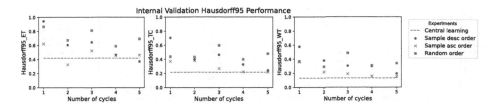

Fig. 4. Hausdorff95 performance evaluation results (values are divided by one hundred) for travelling models with 1–5 cycles for 1 epoch per round travelling in different orders for partitioning one (17 collaborators).

Analyzing the Dice scores for the whole tumor segmentation and one training cycle in Fig. 3, it becomes obvious that the random order led to the best results (0.647) followed by the ascending (0.375) and descending (0.025) order, but they performed worse compared to the baseline model (0.759). This might indicate that the network is mainly learning from the last collaborators of the sequence, forgetting the data seen at the first collaborators. However, investigating the models with more cycles, it becomes evident that this scenario changes. For two cycles, the order does not seem important in any experiment resulting in indistinguishable scores (0.667, 0.678, 0.696). For three, four, and five cycles, the ascending and descending orders led to similar results, which were also comparable to the baseline model. On the other hand, the random order performance improved as the number of cycles increased.

The Hausdorff95 metric demonstrated that the ascending order led to results that are more similar to the baseline model for all segmentations and cycles. It also indicates that as the number of cycles increases, the travelling order does not matter and all experiments tend to converge to similar results.

The results of the validation of the developed models using the unseen data is shown in Figs. 5 and 6. The metrics clearly show that the number of cycles is the major determinant for the generalizability of the network. It also reinforces the observation that with more cycles, the order of data contributors is less important, catastrophic forgetting does not happen, and all experiments (average Dice score for five cycles 0.672) achieve results comparable to the baseline score (0.667).

Thus, the results show that our distributed learning model does not forget patterns learned from previous collaborators. Travelling models with more than one cycle demonstrated to be more effective, and all orders converge to central learning results with an increasing number of cycles.

3.2 Experiments with 22 Collaborators

Finally, we evaluated the performance of the proposed distributed learning models based on the training data from 22 collaborators as illustrated in Fig. 7. It is important to highlight that this distribution is not as smooth as the previous one.

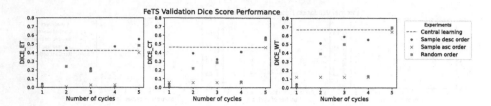

Fig. 5. Validation Dice scores for experiments with 1 epoch per round for partitioning one (17 collaborators).

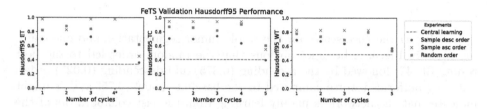

Fig. 6. Validation Hausdorff95 scores, values are divided by one hundred, for experiments with 1 epoch per round for partitioning one (17 collaborators). *Notice that random order with 4 cycles results in an outlier for the enhancing tumour segmentation measuring 3.7.

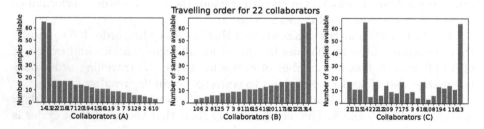

Fig. 7. Data distribution and travelling order for 22 collaborators: (A) descending order, (B) ascending order, and (C) random order.

As can be seen in Fig. 7(C), the database for 22 collaborators is more evenly distributed for the random order compared to the random distribution for the 17 collaborator database. Therefore, the collaborators that provide the majority of data are not concentrated towards the end of the sequence in this case.

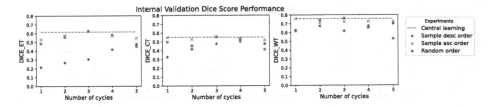

Fig. 8. Dice score performance evaluation results for travelling models with 1–5 cycles for 1 epoch per round travelling in different orders for partitioning two (22 collaborators).

In contrast to the previous results, the model trained with one cycle led to a performance comparable to the baseline model. While the ascending order achieved the same result as central learning (0.758), the descending and random orders achieved similar results (0.629, 0.619), which resulted in Dice scores only 0.14 worse than central learning. This difference might be due to the data distribution that does not have the majority of samples available at a single collaborator (Fig. 8).

Furthermore, travelling models with more than two cycles demonstrated the same trends as seen before. For two cycles, all order schemes resulted in Dice score differences of up to 0.1 (0.675, 0.711, 0.740). In addition to that, the ascending order achieved scores similar to the baseline model for all cycles numbers. Moreover, for five cycles, the descending order achieved a similar score compared to the ascending order, demonstrating once again that increasing the number of cycles improves performance and indicating that the order is not important as no catastrophic forgetting was observed.

Even though the Hausdorff metric performance was not as good for enhancing tumor and core tumor segmentations, with some outliers, it showed acceptable results for the whole tumor segmentation with all experiments leading to similar results compared to the baseline model (Fig. 9).

Validation metrics demonstrated similar trends compared to the training metrics. The ascending order performance was better for all cycles except for two cycles, resulting in scores similar to the descending and random orders (average Dice score 0.521). However, comparing these metrics to the validation metrics for 17 collaborators, the 22 collaborators results were worse and showed more variations when compared to the training results (Figs. 10 and 11).

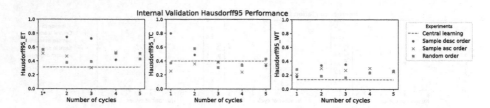

Fig. 9. Hausdorff95 performance evaluation results, values are divided by one hundred, for travelling models with 1–5 cycles for 1 epoch per round travelling in different orders for partitioning two (22 collaborators). *Notice that for tumor core segmentation, the central learning model results in an outlier measuring 3.7 and ascending order for 1 cycle is an outlier for the enhancing tumour segmentation measuring 1.2.

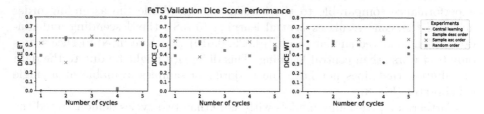

Fig. 10. Dice Score validation of experiments with 1 epoch per round for partitioning two (22 collaborators).

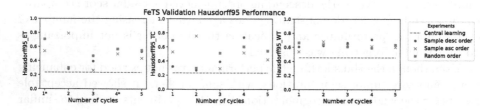

Fig. 11. Hausdorff95 validation results, values are divided by one hundred, with 1 epoch per round for partitioning two (22 collaborators). *Notice that for ascending order for 1 and 4 cycles are outliers for the enhancing tumour segmentation measuring 3.5.

3.3 Leaderboard Validation

For the final validation of our work, we needed to select one of our models to be evaluated by the challenge leaderboard on a hidden test set. In order to verify our assumption that as number of cycles increases the order loses importance, we submitted our random order travelling model to be evaluated for five cycles, using the same learning rate (0.05) used for our validations. A comparison of our evaluation and leaderboards' evaluation can be seen in Figs. 12 and 13.

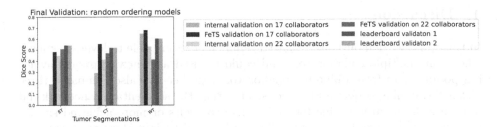

Fig. 12. Dice score comparison for random order models for 5 cycles. Light blue represents our internal validation for 17 collaborators, dark blue represents FeTS validation for 17 collaborators, light pink represents our internal validation for 22 collaborators, dark pink represents FeTS validation for 22 collaborators, and red and orange represent the results provided by FeTS challenge for leaderboard 1 and 2.

Figure 13 compares Dice scores for our internal and external validations for 17 and 22 institutions, and leaderboards validation as provided by the FeTS challenge on a hidden test set. The leaderboard evaluation achieved results (WT: 0.602) comparable to evaluations done for 17 institutions (WT internal: 0.647, WT external: 0.679), which suggests that our assumption that the number of cycles is more important for travelling models than travelling order is indeed correct.

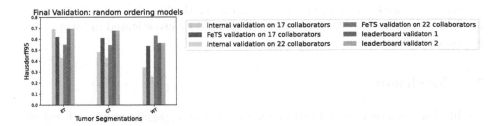

Fig. 13. Hausdorff95 comparison for random ordering models for 5 cycles. Light blue represents our internal validation for 17 collaborators, dark blue represents FeTS validation for 17 collaborators, light pink represents our internal validation for 22 collaborators, dark pink represents FeTS validation for 22 collaborators, and red and orange represent the results provided by FeTS challenge for leaderboard 1 and 2.

Furthermore, Fig. 13 shows Hausdorff95 results for the same models. The results are consistent with the results found for the Dice score results whereas the leaderboard evaluation and our evaluations for 17 institutions led to similar results. This demonstrates that our approach is robust and generalizable enough to be applied in different scenarios.

4   Discussion

In this work, we demonstrated that travelling models are able to leverage knowledge from multiple collaborators and could be used as a new approach avoiding pooling data from different collaborators together. We also compared three distinct travelling orders and demonstrated that the segmentation network did not suffer from catastrophic forgetting, as two cycles or more achieved similar results for the three different travelling orders and their performance converge with increasing number of cycles.

Moreover, we observed that when the data is more evenly distributed among the collaborators and there is not a single collaborator holding the majority of the data, the ascending travelling order achieved results comparable to the baseline model for the different number of cycles, while the descending and random travelling orders achieved improved results when the number of cycles is increasing. On the other hand, when the data distribution is smooth and there is a single institution providing most of the data, all experiments showed that performance improves as number of cycles increases. However, the one cycle models did not perform as well as the baseline model.

Overall, the validation performance for 17 collaborators indicated that fewer collaborators and a smoother data distribution is better when compared to the 22 collaborators results with a more uneven distribution.

Furthermore, we believe that as the number of cycles increases, the network performance will improve and, when reaching a certain number of cycles, all experiments should converge to results similar to the baseline model's accuracy level. However, the use of additional cycles should be investigated in future work to confirm this assumption.

5   Conclusion

We implemented distributed learning methods that aggregate weights effectively within a traveling model, leveraging knowledge from data of multiple collaborators with real world distribution, thereby avoiding the need to share data centrally.

The simplicity of the methodology and ability to learn remotely are important benefits of this method, which might convince health care centers to collaborate and take advantage of it in the future eliminating data sharing bureaucracy.

Acknowledgement. This work was supported by University of Calgary BME Research Scholarship (RS), the Natural Sciences and Engineering Research Council of Canada Postdoctoral Fellowship (AT) and Discovery Grant (NDF), MITACS Globalink Research Internship (LT), Canada Research Chairs program (NDF), the River Fund at Calgary Foundation (NDF), and Canadian Institutes of Health Research (NDF).

Disclosures. The authors declare that there is no conflict of interest.

References

1. Lo Vercio, L., et al.: Supervised machine learning tools: a tutorial for clinicians. J. Neural Eng. **17**(6), 062001 (2020). https://doi.org/10.1088/1741-2552/abbff2
2. Hinton, G.: Deep learning-a technology with the potential to transform health care. JAMA **320**(11), 1101–1102 (2018). https://doi.org/10.1001/jama.2018.11100
3. Kaissis, G.A., Makowski, M.R., Rückert, D., Braren, R.F.: Secure, privacy-preserving and federated machine learning in medical imaging. Nat. Mach. Intell. **2**(6), 305–311 (2020). https://doi.org/10.1038/s42256-020-0186-1
4. MacEachern, S.J., Forkert, N.D.: Machine learning for precision medicine. Genome **64**(4), 416–425 (2021). https://doi.org/10.1139/gen-2020-0131
5. HIPAA. US Department of Health and Human Services (2020). https://www.hhs.gov/hipaa/index.html
6. GDPR. Intersoft Consulting (2016). https://gdpr-info.eu
7. Tuladhar, A., Gill, S., Ismail, Z., Forkert, N.D.: Building machine learning models without sharing patient data: a simulation-based analysis of distributed learning by ensembling. J. Biomed. Inform. **106**, 103424 (2020). https://doi.org/10.1016/j.jbi.2020.103424
8. Yang, Q., Liu, Y., Chen, T., Tong, Y.: Federated machine learning: concept and applications. ACM Trans. Intell. Syst. Technol. **10**(2), 1–19 (2019). https://doi.org/10.1145/3298981
9. Chang, K., et al.: Distributed deep learning networks among institutions for medical imaging. J. Am. Med. Inform. Assoc. **25**(8), 945–954 (2018). https://doi.org/10.1093/jamia/ocy017
10. Remedios, S.W., et al.: Distributed deep learning across multisite datasets for generalized CT hemorrhage segmentation. Med. Phys. **47**(1), 89–98 (2020). https://doi.org/10.1002/mp.13880
11. Reina, G.A., Gruzdev, A., Foley, P., Perepelkina, O., Sharma, M., Davidyuk, I., et al.: OpenFL: an open-source framework for Federated Learning. arXiv preprint arXiv:2105.06413 (2021)
12. Sheller, M.J., Edwards, B., Reina, G.A., Martin, J., Pati, S., Kotrotsou, A., et al.: Federated learning in medicine: facilitating multi-institutional collaborations without sharing patient data. Nat. Sci. Rep. **10**, 12598 (2020). https://doi.org/10.1038/s41598-020-69250-1
13. Bakas, S., Akbari, H., Sotiras, A., Bilello, M., Rozycki, M., Kirby, J.S., et al.: Advancing the cancer genome atlas glioma MRI collections with expert segmentation labels and radiomic features. Nat. Sci. Data **4**, 170117 (2017). https://doi.org/10.1038/SDATA.2017.117
14. Bakas, S., Akbari, H., Sotiras, A., Bilello, M., Rozycki, M., Kirby, J., et al.: Segmentation labels and radiomic features for the pre-operative scans of the TCGA-GBM collection. Cancer Imaging Archive (2017). https://doi.org/10.7937/K9/TCIA.2017.KLXWJJ1Q
15. Bakas, S., Akbari, H., Sotiras, A., Bilello, M., Rozycki, M., Kirby, J., et al.: Segmentation labels and radiomic features for the pre-operative scans of the TCGA-LGG collection. Cancer Imaging Archive (2017). https://doi.org/10.7937/K9/TCIA.2017.GJQ7R0EF

16. Pati, S., Baid, U., Zenk, M., Edwards, B., Sheller, M.J., Reina, G.A., et al.: The Federated Tumor Segmentation (FeTS) Challenge, arXiv preprint arXiv:2105.05874 (2021)
17. Kirkpatrick, J., et al.: Overcoming catastrophic forgetting in neural networks. Proc. Natl. Acad. Sci. **114**, 3521–3526 (2017)
18. The Federated Tumor Segmentation (FeTS) Challenge https://www.fets.ai/. Accessed 22 July 2021

Efficient Federated Tumor Segmentation via Normalized Tensor Aggregation and Client Pruning

Youtan Yin[2], Hongzheng Yang[3], Quande Liu[1(✉)], Meirui Jiang[1],
Cheng Chen[1], Qi Dou[1], and Pheng-Ann Heng[1,4]

[1] Department of Computer Science and Engineering,
The Chinese University of Hong Kong, Hong Kong SAR, China
{qdliu,qdou}@cse.cuhk.edu.hk
[2] Department of Computer Science and Technology, Zhejiang University,
Hangzhou, China
[3] Department of Computer Science and Engineering, Beihang University,
Beijing, China
[4] Guangdong-Hong Kong-Macao Joint Laboratory of Human-Machine
Intelligence-Synergy Systems, Shenzhen Institute of Advanced Technology,
Chinese Academy of Sciences, Shenzhen, China

Abstract. Federated learning, which trains a generic model for different
institutions without sharing their data, is a new trend to avoid training
with centralized data, which is often impossible due to privacy issues. The
Federated Tumor Segmentation (FeTS) Challenge 2021 has two tasks for
participants. Task 1 aims at effective weight aggregation methods given a
pre-defined segmentation algorithm for clients training. While task 2 looks
for robust segmentation algorithms evaluated on unseen data from remote
independent institutions. In federated learning, heterogeneity in the local
clients' datasets and training speeds results in non-negligible variations
between clients in each aggregation round. The naive weighted average
aggregation of such models causes objective inconsistency. As for task 1,
we devise a tensor normalization approach to solve the objective inconsistency. Furthermore, we propose a client pruning strategy to alleviate
the negative impact on the convergence time caused by the uneven training time among local clients. Our method achieves a projected convergence score of 74.32% during the training phase. For task 2, we dynamically adapt model weights at test time by minimizing the entropy loss
to address the domain shifting problem for unseen data evaluation. Our
method finally achieves dice scores of 90.67%, 86.23%, and 78.90% for the
whole tumor, tumor core, and enhancing tumor, respectively, on the task's
validation data. Overall, the proposed solution ranked first for task 2 and
third for task 1 in the FeTS Challenge 2021.

Keywords: Federated learning · Brain tumor segmentation ·
nnU-Net · Test-time adaptation

The first two authors contributed equally. The work was done when they did summer
internship at CUHK.

1   Introduction

It is widely accepted that segmentation for magnetic resonance imaging of the brain is beneficial for clinical treatment [1]. Although the Brain Tumor Segmentation (BraTS) challenges' [2–4] state-of-the-art average Dice has reached an uplifting score as high as around 85 [5,6] on the test set, applying these algorithms in the real world remains challenging due to regulatory and privacy hurdles [7]. Clinical institutions usually do not allow access to each other's data, in which scenario models cannot be trained with centralized data. Federated learning (FL) [8–19] trains local models using each institution's data and aggregates local models' weights to the global model. This server-clients framework solves the above issue well. In this trend, the Federated Tumor Segmentation (FeTS) Challenge [20] is the first Challenge proposed for FL. The Challenge is structured in two explicit tasks, and we participate in both of the tasks.

Task1 requires customizing core functions of a baseline federated learning system implementation, aiming to improve the baseline consensus models. There are four functions we can adjust: (i) **Aggregation Function:** In which way the clients will aggregate their wights to the global model. (ii) **Collaborator Training Selection:** Which set of collaborators will be selected to train in each aggregation round. (iii) **Hyperparameters for training:** Hyperparameters for training: Hyperparameters for collaborators' training stage. We can only custom two aspects according to the official API. One is the learning rate for each local model, and the other one is batches or epochs per round. Notice that we can only set either batch or epoch, and all collaborators share the same hyperparameters for each communication round. (iv) **Validation Function:** Validation metrics used for local clients and the global model. Except for the above four functions, all other details in the federated learning pipeline have been prepared by the organizers and are the same for all participants. Participants will be ranked considering both the performance and convergence speed in task 1.

For this task, noting that our task provides a heavy, uneven partition of data, we should design methods to address this issue. Meanwhile, this task asks for a general algorithm that can be applied without involving local training settings [21,22] like adjusting gradient descent. Putting all these factors together, we find Fed-Nova [23], which eliminates objective inconsistency while preserving fast error convergence, is the most appropriate aggregation function for this task. In addition, as the convergence speed is also an important metric, we propose a client pruning strategy to "prune" the clients if their local training time is larger than a threshold in the first ten aggregation rounds. This method is proven to be effective in speeding up the convergence process a lot with a cost of slight performance drop in early rounds, thus guaranteeing an increase of the projected convergence score.

Task2 expects robust segmentation algorithms evaluated on unseen data during the testing phase without any limitations to participants. Specifically, participants will submit a trained model with their inference code, and models will be evaluated on data from various remote independent institutions, which is not released to participants.

For this task, we need to design algorithms to enhance the generalization ability of our model to perform better on unseen data. Models work well if the training datasets can represent the distribution of the test datasets. However, there is often a mismatch between training and test cases regarding their acquisition details in medical image segmentation, especially in this Challenge, the test data coming from different institutions. According to [5,24,25], they observe a depressing performance drop when shifting from the training dataset to the test dataset, which confirms the fact that there is a deviation between the training dataset and the test dataset in the FeTS Challenge. We propose to dynamically adapt model's parameters by optimizing the entropy loss calculated on its test dataset predictions. Entropy is an unsupervised objective as it only requires model predictions and not annotations. According to previous research [26], a noticeable performance improvement can be achieved for one iteration on each test set's case without altering training and violating the inferencing time limitation of 180s per case.

2   Solution for Task 1

Task 1 aims to develop effective weight aggregation and clients sampling strategy for real-world medical federated optimization. The local network architecture and training algorithm for tumor segmentation are pre-defined by organizers. Given the data partition across multiple individual institutions, our job is to design task-specific aggregation function for global model updates, clients chosen for each federated round and the training hyper-parameters like learning rate and local epoches.

2.1   Efficient Federated Aggregation with Tensor Normalization

In each communication round, the clients participating in federated optimization are highly heterogeneous in the number of local stochastic gradient descent iterations. To alleviate this problem, we propose to re-normaliaze aggregated tensors at each round. Assuming there are totally m clients, the update rule of federated learning can be written as:

$$x^{t+1} - x^t = \sum_{i=1}^{m} p_i \delta_i^t \tag{1}$$

where p_i is the relative sample size at client i, x^t denotes the model parameters at round t and δ_i^t is the local parameters change at client i.

To alleviate the objective inconsistency problem [23] caused by heterogeneous number of local iterations, we re-weight the aggregated local tensors for fair federated aggregation and rewrite the update rule as:

$$x^{t+1} - x^t = -(\sum_{i=1}^{m} p_i \tau_i) \sum_{i=1}^{m} p_i \frac{\delta_i^t}{\|a_i^t\|_1} \tag{2}$$

where τ_i is the number of local updates at client i which varies widely across all clients and $\|a_i^t\|_1$ is a normalizing scalar defined by how stochastic gradients are locally accumulated, i.e. local optimizers. This update rule is taken from FedNova [23].

For SGD with momentum [27] used in this challenge, a_i can be set as $a_i = [1 - \rho^{\tau_i}, 1 - \rho^{\tau_i-1}, ..., 1 - \rho]/(1 - \rho)$ where ρ is the momentum factor.

Comparing to previous algorithms such as FedAvg, local parameters change in our method is re-scaled based on different number of local iterations for each client. Thus the inconsistency optimization can be eliminated and faster convergence is achieved in real clinical scenarios.

2.2 Pruning of Slower Local Clients for Fast Federated Training

In realistic scenarios, federated collaborators are also heterogeneous in different computation, download and upload speeds. Within the same communication round, slower clients will consistently need more wall-clock cpu time to finish the download, upload and training tasks. This speed gap across participating clients will harm the parallel performance of federated learning thus incurring a slower convergence rate.

To address this issue, we design a client pruning mechanism to adaptively filter out some slower clients. Specifically, we collect the simulated time of last round for each client as the pruning basis:

$$Times = [s_1^{t-1}, s_2^{t-1}, ..., s_m^{t-1}] \tag{3}$$

where s_m^t denotes the simulated time for client m at round $t - 1$

Then we calculate a threshold μ according to mean value of $Times$ as following:

$$\mu = (\frac{1}{m} \sum_{i=1}^{m} s_i^{t-1}) * \alpha \tag{4}$$

where α is a hyper-parameter to control the filter range. We empirically set it as 0.8. All clients with simulated time above threshold μ will be filtered and do not participate in the federated optimization. This pruning mechanism will be performed only for the first c rounds to save the overall computation time as well as preserve the global model performance. In practice, to collect the simulated time, all clients will participate the federated training at odd rounds and we perform the pruning strategy at even rounds.

2.3 Learning Rate and Local Iterations/epochs

We carried out experiments on static and dynamic learning rate schedules to find out the most appropriate hyper-parameters. Supposing η stands for learning rate, η_0 represents the initial learning rate, t represents aggregation round. Then for static learning rate schedule, learning rate for each round is simply:

$$\eta = \eta_0 \tag{5}$$

For dynamic learning rate schedule, we proposed the polynomial decay in the form:

$$\eta = \eta_0 * (1 - \frac{t}{t_{max}})^\epsilon \tag{6}$$

where t_{max} refers to the max training round number and ϵ is the polynomial factor.

As for the iterations/epochs, we conduct experiments under $\eta = 1e - 3$ with static schedule. In general, local epochs between every aggregation round are set to 1 in federated learning because this guarantees the balance between convergence performance and speed. Though we still test other settings and observe that increasing epoch indeed improves performance lightly but with a cost of an increase in training time to convergence while decreasing batches speeds up convergence significantly. However, its final segmentation performance drops sharply, respectively.

3   Solution for Task 2

We base our algorithms on the rank one team of the BraTS 2020 Challenge. We refer to [5] for a detailed description and a thorough baseline.

3.1   Backbone Architecture

We integrate the best BraTS-specific modifications discussed in [5] to complete our backbone. According to the source code (GitHub), these optimizations are further improved after the BraTS 2020 Challenge. We follow the latest ones.

Specifically, this pipeline adopts a pure nnU-Net as network architecture. The input patch is cropped from randomly selected training cases to the size of $128 \times 128 \times 128$, then the encoder generates a $4 \times 4 \times 4$ feature map with five downsampling steps. The number of the encoder's first layer's convolutional kernels is set to 32 and doubled with each layer up to a maximum of 320. The decoder architecture mirrors the encoder, which upsamples the feature map back to the original input size. Leaky ReLUs and BN are used as nonlinearities and normalizations in the network. Furthermore, brain tumor-specific operations involve improved data augmentation, region-based dice loss optimization, and a threshold to filter predictions.

3.2   Dynamic Adaptation of Parameters at Test Time

As mentioned in [26], lower entropy indicates reasonable performance. At the same time, higher entropy reflects notable domain shift. Based on this observation, we implement a test time dynamic parameter adaptation by updating the model's weights to minimize the entropy loss calculated from the prediction on the test set for one iteration. This little trick has been proven to work well and not increase much time in domain shift tasks [28,29].

Specifically, our test-time objective is to minimize the entropy loss L_e (in [26]) of model predictions $\hat{y} = M_\theta(x^t)$, supposing M represents the model itself and θ represents the model's weights. x^t means model input at test time. The entropy loss is given as follows:

$$L_e = -\Sigma_c(\hat{y}_c * \log(\hat{y}_c + \epsilon)) \tag{7}$$

where c represents each class, in this task 3 classes respectively, and ϵ represents an add-on hyperparameter, which avoids the logarithm of zero. As region-based training uses sigmoid activations at the end of the model layers, resulting in three binary classifications, we calculate the mean entropy loss of each region's output.

4   Experiments

4.1   Dataset

Based on the previous BraTS Challenge, the FeTS Challenge provides the MRI dataset with their source information indicating the relationship between each case and their original institutions. Task 1 and task 2 share the same training data with 341 cases [4,20,30–33]. The Challenge also provides information on how to partition the training data into non-IID institutional subsets. There are two partitions. Partition one is the originating institution split, and partition two is derived from partition one by further splitting the "larger" institutions according to whether a record's tumor size fell above or below the mean size for that institution. As a supplement, participants are given un-labeled data, which can be evaluated on the online platform, to assess their algorithms before the testing stage.

We employ pre-processed training and validation data from FeTS 2021 Challenge and mainly use the provided partition-2 for data split across different institutions. In the FeTS 2021 Challenge dataset, three kinds of regions have been manually segmented as annotations, including the whole tumor (consisting of all three original classes), the tumor core (the original non-enhancing and necrosis + enhancing tumor), and the enhancing tumor (the original enhancing tumor). All images have been pre-processed and further partitioned into 22 clients according to their original institutions and tumor sizes. MRI scans can be highly heterogeneous among participating clients in this Challenge as various scanners and image protocols were employed.

4.2   Implementation Details

As for task 1, we implement FedNorm (federated aggregation with tensor normalization) and the client pruning mechanism based on the open-fl framework. The momentum factor in FedNorm was set as 0.6 based on the experimental results in this challenge. For client pruning, we choose to filter out slower clients for the first 10 rounds. We adopt the polynomial decaying learning rate with an initial value of 5e-4, polynomial factor of 0.9, and max training epoch of 1000. We perform one epoch for local client training at each communication round. All experiments were conducted under a fixed train validation split and random seed to make our results convincing and deterministic.

As for task 2, the backbone's details are described as follow: **(i) Training settings:** The loss function is the sum of dice and cross-entropy loss with an SGD optimizer with the initialize learning rate of 1e-2 and a Nesterov momentum of 0.99, training 200 epochs with 250 iterations. An polynomial learning rate decay schedule which is the same of task 1 is used. The batch size is 2. **(ii) Data augmentation:** We use the following combination in [5]:

- increase the probability of applying rotation and scaling from 0.2 to 0.3.
- increase the scale range from (0.85, 1.25) to (0.65, 1.6)
- select a scaling factor for each axis individually.
- use elastic deformation with a probability of 0.2 and scale range (0, 0.25).
- use additive brightness augmentation with a probability of 0.3.
- Increase the aggressiveness of the gamma augmentation to range (0.5, 1.6).

(iii) Postprocessing threshold: We follow the example of the official implementation directly to filter the prediction values for enhancing tumor regions if there are less than 200 positive predictions. **(iv) Test-time Dynamic adaptation:** The add-on hyperparameter value ϵ is 1e-6 and we update all of the model's weights with a case of test data at each step for one iteration.

4.3   Results

Abbreviations. We will represent our methods using the following abbreviations. **(i) FedAvg:** refers to the weighted average aggregation. **(ii) FedNorm:** refers to the Fed-Nova aggregation described in Sect. 2.1. **(iii) WT:** refers to the whole tumor region. **(iv) TC:** refers to the tumor core region. **(v) ET:** refers to the enhancing tumor region.

Evaluation Metrics. As for task 1, both the performance of our algorithm and convergence speed will be taken into consideration. Specifically, besides the Dice coefficient (Dice) and Hausdorff distance-95% (HD95), a projected convergence score, calculated by multiplying the Dice with the programs' total running time, is used to assess convergence speed. Moreover, during the training process, Sensitivity (TP/P) and Specificity (TN/N) are also provided by the organizers.

For task 2, there is no exact ranking algorithm before we submit our algorithm. So we adopt the commonly used Dice as criteria.

Ablation Study for Task 1. As shown in Table 1, it is observed that FedNorm consistently outperforms FedAvg under dice performance and convergence score metric, demonstrating the effectiveness of our method for fair federated aggregation. Furthermore, we fine-tune the FedNorm scheme by adjusting the (i)learning

Table 1. Ablation study for task 1

Method			Rounds	Dice [%]				Convergence score
Aggre. Func.	Filt. Clien.	Learn. Rate		ET	TC	WT	Mean	
FedAvg	✗	5e-4	40	0.7563	0.6201	0.7655	0.7140	0.7114
FedNorm	✗		40	0.7560	0.6376	0.7698	0.7211	0.7190
FedNorm	first 5	5e-4	50	0.7421	0.6304	0.7633	0.7119	0.7103
	first 10		50	0.7573	**0.6431**	0.7724	**0.7243**	**0.7432**
	first 20		50	0.7543	0.6358	0.7602	0.7168	0.7122
FedNorm	✗	1e-3	40	**0.7897**	0.5930	0.6707	0.6845	0.7167
	✗	5e-4	40	0.7560	0.6376	0.7698	0.7211	0.7190
	✗	dynamic 1e-3	40	0.7597	0.6074	0.7426	0.7033	0.7227
	✗	dynamic 5e-4	40	0.7535	0.6090	**0.7981**	0.7202	0.7261

Table 2. Test results for task 1

Task	LeaderBoard 1				LeaderBoard 2				LeaderBoard 1				LeaderBoard 2			
Label	ET	WT	TC	Avg.	ET	WT	TC	Avg	ET	WT	TC	Avg	ET	WT	TC	Avg
	Dice Coefficient (Dice) ↑								Hausdorff Distance (HD) ↓							
Mean	0.5200	0.7027	0.5878	0.6035	0.6689	0.7771	0.6528	0.6996	57.17	43.46	51.71	50.78	42.47	19.85	40.76	34.36
Std	0.2590	0.2348	0.2926	0.2621	0.2791	0.1861	0.2776	0.2476	94.14	28.86	79.59	67.53	95.82	23.80	79.30	66.31

Table 3. Ablation study for task 2

Model	ET	WT	TC	Average
80% clients	0.7696	0.8933	0.8445	0.8358
All training data	0.7782	0.9073	0.8473	0.8443
test time + all training data	**0.7890**	**0.9067**	**0.8622**	**0.8526**

rate from set {1e-3,5e-4} with (ii)constant/polynomial decay/cosine cycle (T = 10/20) and (iii)more epochs (2)/partially batches (50% or 25%) strategies and achieve the highest performance with epoch one and polynomial learning rate decaying setting beginning at 5e-4. We add the client pruning strategy that filters out time-consuming clients in the first c rounds for faster convergence with the above basis. The value of c is chosen from set 5,10,20. Notably, the convergence score of 74.32 is achieved when we perform client pruning for the first ten rounds, indicating that rejecting time-consuming clients to participate in federated optimization can further improve the convergence speed on top of the FedNorm scheme. And the results are sensitive to the hyper-parameter c. After extensive experiments, we set it as 10.

In the end, we obtained the performance of our method on the test dataset from the organizers as Table 2 shows. The results show that the mean dice score has dropped from 72.43 to 60.35.

Ablation Study for Task 2. We train two models for task 2. One uses the fixed train and validation split in task 1, and another one drops the last 20% of

Table 4. Test results for task 2

Unseen data	Dice ↑		HD95 ↓		Sensitivity ↑		Specificity ↑	
	mean	std	mean	std	mean	std	mean	std
ET	0.7602	0.2736	56.666	110.22	0.7758	0.2806	0.9996	0.0006
WT	0.8715	0.1311	11.198	21.208	0.8814	0.1229	0.9993	0.0007
TC	0.7731	0.2393	15.693	28.515	0.8669	0.1637	0.9992	0.0008
Average	0.8016	0.2147	27.852	53.316	0.8414	0.1891	0.9994	0.0007

clients as unseen test data to simulate the domain shift problem, with the first 80% of clients' data then randomly divided into train and validation set in a ratio of 8:2. The two models are both trained using the backbone discussed in Sect. 3.1. As we can see from Table 3, the model trained with complete training data still performs better than the 80% one on the validation platform with about one percent dice scores improvement. So we finally choose the model in the second row as our submission. Finally, we add test time adaptation to the submission model and observe an approximate one-point increase for enhancing tumor and tumor core while slightly dropping for the whole tumor (Fig. 1).

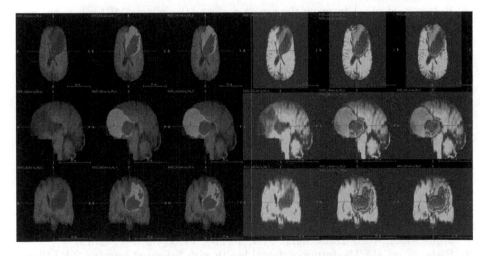

Fig. 1. Visualisation for task 2: We visualise case 100 in validation set. From left to right, the pictures are the original image, the segmentation result before adaptation and after adaptation, following by their corresponding entropy map. From top to bottom, in turn are the slices observed along z, y, and x axes.

Also, we obtained the performance on the test dataset as Table 4 shows. Compared to the sharp performance drop from training set to test set in task 1, the results show that our test time adaptation may mitigate the impact of the domain shifting problem to some degree.

Since we only had the training set and validation set without ground truth, we visualized the case in which the overall segmentation results were good-corresponding Dice is high. As we can see from the figure, the entropy map after adapting is smoother than the one without adapting. However, the effect is not significant because there is no severe domain shifting between the training set and the validation set recognized by the Challenge's organizer.

Acknowledgement. This work was supported by Key-Area Research and Development Program of Guangdong Province, China (2020B010165004), Hong Kong RGC TRS Project No. T42-409/18-R, National Natural Science Foundation of China with Project No. U1813204 and Shenzhen-HK Collaborative Development Zone.

References

1. Pati, S., et al.: Reproducibility analysis of multi-institutional paired expert annotations and radiomic features of the Ivy glioblastoma atlas project (Ivy GAP) dataset. Med. Phys. **12**, 6039–6052 (2020)
2. Menze, B.H., et al.: The multimodal brain tumor image segmentation benchmark (BRATS). IEEE Trans. Med. Imaging **34**(10), 1993–2024 (2015)
3. Bakas, S., et al.: Identifying the best machine learning algorithms for brain tumor segmentation, progression assessment, and overall survival prediction in the brats challenge (2019)
4. Bakas, S., et al.: Advancing the cancer genome atlas glioma MRI collections with expert segmentation labels and radiomic features. Sci. Data **4**, 170117 (2017)
5. Isensee, F., Jäger, P.F., Full, P.M., Vollmuth, P., Maier-Hein, K.H.: nnU-Net for brain tumor segmentation. In: Crimi, A., Bakas, S. (eds.) BrainLes 2020. LNCS, vol. 12659, pp. 118–132. Springer, Cham (2021). https://doi.org/10.1007/978-3-030-72087-2_11
6. Isensee, F., Jaeger, P.F., Kohl, S.A.A., Petersen, J., Maier-Hein, K.H.: nnU-Net: a self-configuring method for deep learning-based biomedical image segmentation. Nat. Methods **18**(2), 203–211 (2021)
7. Annas, G.J.: HIPAA regulations - a new era of medical-record privacy? N. Engl. J. Med. **348**(15), 1486–1490 (2003)
8. McMahan, H.B., Moore, E., Ramage, D., Hampson, S., y Arcas, B.A.: Communication-efficient learning of deep networks from decentralized data (2017)
9. Yang, T., et al.: Applied federated learning: improving google keyboard query suggestions (2018)
10. Yang, Q., Liu, Y., Chen, T., Tong, Y.: Federated machine learning: concept and applications. ACM Trans. Intell. Syst. Technol. (TIST) **2**, 1–19 (2019)
11. Rieke, N., et al.: The future of digital health with federated learning. NPJ Digital Med. **1**, 1–7 (2020)
12. Sheller, M.J., et al.: Federated learning in medicine: facilitating multi-institutional pruning without sharing patient data. Sci. Rep. **1**, 1–12 (2020)
13. Dou, Q., et al.: Federated deep learning for detecting COVID-19 lung abnormalities in CT: a privacy-preserving multinational validation study. NPJ Digital Med. **4**(1), 1–11 (2021)
14. Roth, H.R., et al.: Federated learning for breast density classification: a real-world implementation. In: Albarqouni, S., et al. (eds.) DART/DCL -2020. LNCS, vol. 12444, pp. 181–191. Springer, Cham (2020). https://doi.org/10.1007/978-3-030-60548-3_18

15. Li, W., et al.: Privacy-preserving federated brain tumour segmentation. In: Suk, H.-I., Liu, M., Yan, P., Lian, C. (eds.) MLMI 2019. LNCS, vol. 11861, pp. 133–141. Springer, Cham (2019). https://doi.org/10.1007/978-3-030-32692-0_16
16. Kaissis, G.A., Makowski, M.R., Rückert, D., Braren, R.F.: Secure, privacy-preserving and federated machine learning in medical imaging. Nat. Mach. Intell. **2**(6), 305–311 (2020)
17. Li, D., Kar, A., Ravikumar, N., Frangi, A.F., Fidler, S.: Federated simulation for medical imaging. In: Martel, A.L., et al. (eds.) MICCAI 2020. LNCS, vol. 12261, pp. 159–168. Springer, Cham (2020). https://doi.org/10.1007/978-3-030-59710-8_16
18. Sheller, M.J., Reina, G.A., Edwards, B., Martin, J., Bakas, S.: Multi-institutional deep learning modeling without sharing patient data: a feasibility study on brain tumor segmentation. In: Crimi, A., Bakas, S., Kuijf, H., Keyvan, F., Reyes, M., van Walsum, T. (eds.) BrainLes 2018. LNCS, vol. 11383, pp. 92–104. Springer, Cham (2019). https://doi.org/10.1007/978-3-030-11723-8_9
19. Silva, S., Gutman, B.A., Romero, E., Thompson, P.M., Altmann, A., Lorenzi, M.: Federated learning in distributed medical databases: meta-analysis of large-scale subcortical brain data. In: ISBI, pp. 270–274. IEEE (2019)
20. Pati, S., et al.: The federated tumor segmentation (FeTS) challenge (2021)
21. Guo, P., Wang, P., Zhou, J., Jiang, S., Patel, V.M.: Multi-institutional collaborations for improving deep learning-based magnetic resonance image reconstruction using federated learning (2021)
22. Mohri, M., Sivek, G., Suresh, A.T.: Agnostic federated learning (2019)
23. Wang, J., Liu, Q., Liang, H., Joshi, G., Poor, H.V.: Tackling the objective inconsistency problem in heterogeneous federated optimization (2020)
24. Liu, Q., Chen, C., Qin, J., Dou, Q., Heng, P.-A.: FedDG: federated domain generalization on medical image segmentation via episodic learning in continuous frequency space. In: CVPR (2021)
25. Chen, C., Liu, Q., Jin, Y., Dou, Q., Heng, P.-A.: Source-free domain adaptive fundus image segmentation with denoised pseudo-labeling. In: de Bruijne, M., et al. (eds.) MICCAI 2021. LNCS, vol. 12905, pp. 225–235. Springer, Cham (2021). https://doi.org/10.1007/978-3-030-87240-3_22
26. Wang, D., Shelhamer, E., Liu, S., Olshausen, B., Darrell, T.: Tent: fully test-time adaptation by entropy minimization (2021)
27. Liu, C., Belkin, M.: Accelerating SGD with momentum for over-parameterized learning. arXiv preprint arXiv:1810.13395 (2018)
28. Karani, N., Erdil, E., Chaitanya, K., Konukoglu, E.: Test-time adaptable neural networks for robust medical image segmentation. Med. Image Anal. **68**, 101907 (2021)
29. Sun, Y., Wang, X., Liu, Z., Miller, J., Efros, A., Hardt, M.: Test-time training with self-supervision for generalization under distribution shifts (2020)
30. Reina, G.A., et al.: OpenFL: an open-source framework for federated learning (2021)
31. Bakas, S., Akbari, H., Sotiras, A., Bilello, M., Rozycki, M., Kirby, J.: Segmentation labels and radiomic features for the pre-operative scans of the TCGA-GBM collection (brats-TCGA-GBM). Cancer Imaging Archive (2017)
32. Bakas, S., Akbari, H., Sotiras, A., Bilello, M., Rozycki, M., Kirby, J.: Segmentation labels and radiomic features for the pre-operative scans of the TCGA-LGG collection (brats-TCGA-LGG). Cancer Imaging Archive (2017)
33. Liu, Q., Yang, H., Dou, Q., Heng, P.-A.: Federated semi-supervised medical image classification via inter-client relation matching. arXiv preprint arXiv:2106.08600 (2021)

Federated Learning for Brain Tumor Segmentation Using MRI and Transformers

Sahil Nalawade[1]($\boxtimes$), Chandan Ganesh[1], Ben Wagner[1], Divya Reddy[1], Yudhajit Das[1], Fang F. Yu[1], Baowei Fei[3], Ananth J. Madhuranthakam[1,2], and Joseph A. Maldjian[1,2]

[1] Department of Radiology, University of Texas Southwestern Medical Center, Dallas, TX, USA
{Sahil.Nalawade,
ChandanGanesh.BangaloreYogananda}@UTSouthwestern.edu
[2] Advanced Imaging Research Center, University of Texas Southwestern Medical Center, Dallas, TX, USA
[3] Department of Bioengineering, University of Texas at Dallas, Richardson, TX, USA

Abstract. This work focuses on training a deep learning network in a federated learning framework. The Federated Tumor Segmentation Challenge has 2 separate tasks. Task-1 was to design an aggregation logic for a given network, which is trained in a federated learning framework. Task-2 of the challenge was to train a network that is robust and generalizable in a federated testing environment. 341 subjects were used for training both tasks of the challenge. This data was distributed across 17 collaborators, which were then used to train an individual network for each collaborator. A new weight aggregation logic was developed. The network weights in this logic were determined based on the average validation dice scores of each collaborator. A concise model was obtained using the developed weighted aggregation logic. The Dice scores for task-1 on the validation dataset for whole tumor, tumor core, and enhancing tumor were 0.767, 0.612, and 0.628 respectively. The Dice scores for task-2 on the validation dataset for whole tumor, tumor core, and enhancing tumor were 0.874, 0.773, and 0.721 respectively.

Keywords: Federated learning · Brain tumor · Segmentation · Transformers · Deep learning · Convolutional neural network

1 Introduction

Gliomas are one of the most aggressive and heterogeneous types of brain tumors and can be further classified into high-grade gliomas (HGG) and low-grade gliomas (LGG). Despite the development of new therapeutic strategies, average patient survival has only improved by 15 months [1] and only 10% of the glioblastoma patients survive over 5 years [1, 2]. Magnetic resonance imaging (MRI) remains the modality of choice for guiding diagnosis and treatment planning. A crucial step in glioma research involves segmenting the tumor into its sub-components. Brain tumor segmentation of MRI images remains a challenging task as the intensity difference of image voxels within the tumor are difficult to segregate. This is made further challenging due to broad variations in tumor shape,

A. Crimi and S. Bakas (Eds.): BrainLes 2021, LNCS 12963, pp. 444–454, 2022.
https://doi.org/10.1007/978-3-031-09002-8_39

size, and location. To address the problem of high variability in patient data, an automated deep learning network can be used for segmenting the tumor sub-components. However, a robust, generalizable deep learning network needs to be trained using data collected from multiple different institutions. Such an approach to data collection unfortunately faces privacy, regulatory, and administrative challenges.

Federated learning (FL) is a distributed machine learning approach for training large-scale decentralized datasets where the data remains on individual devices or institutions. Specifically, FL is an approach of "bringing the code to the data instead of data to the code" [3]. This addresses some of the challenges posed by data privacy, regulatory issues, ownership, and location of the data. The Federated tumor segmentation (FeTS) challenge [2] was introduced to avoid the above problems of data privacy and regulatory issues by using FL [4–8]. The FeTS challenge uses the data from different platforms, including the BraTS 2020 challenge [9] as well as several independent institutions, providing a platform for sharing a unique brain tumor dataset with known ground truth segmentations. The segmentation regions-of-interest (ROIs) were either performed manually from scratch or were fine-tuned by experts [2].

The primary purpose of the challenge was two-fold. First, to generate a consensus segmentation model that will be able to learn from the data held at multiple institutions. Second, to evaluate a trained segmentation model in a federated configuration. The primary goals were evaluated by 2 different tasks:

1. Task-1: This task utilized a network provided by the organizers and was trained in a federated configuration. The primary goal of this task was to develop an optimal weight aggregation approach towards creating a consensus model that has gained knowledge from federated learning across multiple distinct institutions.
2. Task-2: This task utilized federated testing across different sites of the FeTS initiative that were not part of the training dataset to evaluate network performance across institutions, MRI scanners, image acquisition techniques, and patient populations. The primary goal of this task was to evaluate the generalizability of networks trained using the federated approach.

In this study, we propose an aggregation logic for task-1 based on the validation scores. Dice scores were used as one of the metrics for evaluating the performance. The functions for hyper-parameter selection and model aggregation were fine-tuned based on the average dice score. We also propose a Medical Segmentation Transformer (MST), which is a transformer-based network architecture used for task-2 of the FeTS challenge. Deep learning-based brain tumor segmentation has achieved benchmark results in the previous BraTS challenges [10, 11]. Recent advancements in the transformer-based models in the field of natural language processing, vision, and segmentation tasks have shown even more promising results [12–14]. MST has an encoder and decoder block which are composed of convolutional layers. This network uses a local and global branch for training, which helps to learn not only the information present in the full resolution image but also from patches extracted from the image. MST has advantages to learn from smaller datasets which can be leveraged for training the network in a federated learning environment [15].

2   Materials and Methods

The FeTS challenge data was provided by the BraTS Challenge 2020 as well as independent institutions [9, 16–19]. The data partitions from the organizers were partition-1 and partition-2, which consisted of 17 and 22 collaborators (institutions), respectively. We selected partition-1 for the FeTS challenge, which corresponded to a total of 341 subjects [2]. Each subject's data consisted of native T1-weighted (T1w) images, contrast-enhanced T1-weighted (T1ce) images, T2-weighted (T2w) images, and T2-weighted Fluid Attention Inversion Recovery (FLAIR) images. The segmentation ROI was also provided by the organizers, which was composed of 4 labels. The segmentation labels had values of 1 for necrotic tumor, 2 for edema, 4 for enhancing tumor, and 0 for everything else. The data in partition-1 was further divided into groups of unequal numbers ranging from 3 to 129 subjects. This data was used for training and in-training validation for each institution.

2.1   Data and Preprocessing

The data provided for the FeTS challenge were pre-processed using the Cancer Imaging Phenomics Toolkit (CaPTk) [20–22]. All MRI images (T1w, T2w, T1ce, and FLAIR) were co-registered to the same anatomical template (SR-124) [23] using the Greedy registration algorithm [24]. This assured a fixed spatial resolution of 1 mm^3 for all MRI sequences. The next step of skull stripping was performed on the co-registered MRI sequences using a deep learning-based algorithm specifically designed for the glioma images. These skull-stripped images were then used to perform the annotations for the FETS challenge. The annotators used either a completely manual method for segmentation or a hybrid approach, where an initial automated algorithm was used to segment the tumor that was subsequently refined by manual segmentations. The annotations are described in detail by Pati et al. [2].

2.2   Network Architecture

2.2.1   Task-1

The network architecture used for training task-1 of the federated training was provided by the challenge organizers. It was based on the U-Net architecture [25] with residual connections. In the domain of medical imaging, U-Net and residual connections have yielded robust results [10, 26–30]. The encoder-decoder network was selected for the federated learning as it captures the information from multiple resolutions. The encoder part is comprised of convolutional and down-sampling layers, whereas the decoder part is comprised of the up-sampling layers and the skip connections. The details of the network architecture are described by Pati et al. [2].

2.2.2 Task-2

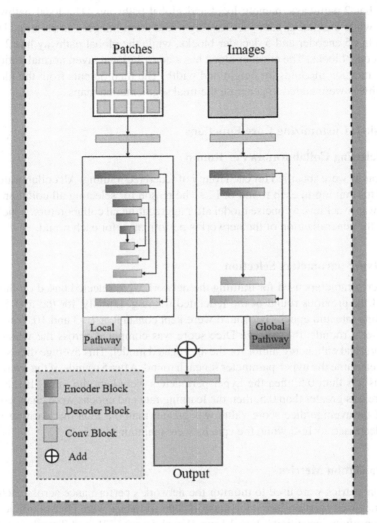

Fig. 1. Network architecture for Medical Segmentation Transformer (MST) for Task-2.

The network architecture for MST was based on the transformer encoder-decoder architectures, which takes advantage of the self-attention structure (Fig. 1). This network structure helps in learning the long-range dependencies and also representations that are highly expressive [31]. MST has a gated axial-attention module which was included as an additional control for the self-attention modules. The axial attention module comprised two different self-attention modules. The first self-attention module computes the feature maps along the height axis and the other computes along the width axis. Relative positional encodings are added to the self-attention module while computing affinities. This encoding helps in making the affinities more sensitive to positional information.

Wang et al. [14] proposed an attention-based model which uses the combination of axial attention modules and positional encodings for the image segmentation task. This network has 2 pathways, namely local and global pathways. The local pathway uses patches, while the global pathway uses high-resolution images for training. The local pathway has 5 encoder and 5 decoder blocks, while the global pathway has 2 encoder and 2 decoder blocks. The encoder block has a convolutional layer, normalization layer, and self-attention modules for height and width. The final outputs from the global and local pathway were added to generate the final segmentation maps.

2.3   Task-1: Customizing Core Functions

2.3.1   Selecting Collaborators Per Round

Collaborators were specified for each round of federated training. All collaborators were selected for training in each round of FL. The reason for selecting all collaborators for training was to achieve a concise model after aggregating all collaborators, which would enhance the generalization of the network's performance for each round.

2.3.2   Hyper-parameters Selection

The hyper-parameters used for training the network were selected based on the performance of the previous round of the federated training. Initially, for the first 5 rounds, the learning rate and epochs per round were kept constant at 1e-3 and 10, respectively. Later, after 5 rounds, the average Dice score was computed across the whole tumor, tumor core, and enhancing tumor for the aggregated model. This average dice score was used to determine the hyper-parameter for each round. After 5 rounds, if the average Dice score was less than 0.5, then the hyper-parameters were kept the same. If the average dice score was greater than 0.5, then the learning rate and epochs were changed to 1e-4 and 5. If the average dice score value was greater than 0.8 then the learning rate was further decreased to 1e-5 while the epochs were maintained at 5.

2.3.3   Validation Metrics

Validation metrics were used to monitor the network's performance across each round. The metrics used for monitoring the network's performance were Dice coefficient (Dice score), sensitivity, specificity, Focal Loss (Focal score) [32], and Tversky score [33]. The equations for dice coefficient, Focal score, and Tversky score are shown below:

$$Dice\ coefficient = \frac{2 * |GT \cap PR|}{|GT| + |PR|} \tag{1}$$

GT: Ground Truth
PR: Predicted tumor mask

$$Focal\ score(p_t) = \alpha(1 - p_t)^\gamma \log(p_t) \tag{2}$$

α: 1.0
γ: 2.0

p_t: models' estimated probability

$$Tversky\ score = \frac{TP}{TP + \alpha * FP + \beta * FN} \qquad (3)$$

TP: True Positive
FP: False Positive
FN: False Negative
α: 0.7
β: 1.0

2.3.4 Model Aggregation

The network parameters from all collaborators were compiled for each round of federated training. The average dice score was computed across the whole tumor, tumor core, and enhancing tumor for each collaborator. An importance factor/weight was assigned for each collaborator based on the average dice score. The higher the validation dice score of a collaborator, the greater was the importance factor/weight assigned to the corresponding network. The aggregation of all networks was done based on the logic of the weighted average, where all networks were given a particular weight proportional to their average validation dice score.

2.4 Task-2: Model Generalization

2.4.1 Training

The transformer network was used for training across all the collaborators and was evaluated using the validation dataset provided by the organizer. The network was trained in a slice-wise manner, i.e., the axial slices from each subject were used for training the network. To avoid the problem of data leakage, slices from training and in-training validation were kept separate. This was carried out by performing a subject-wise split between training and in-training validation. The network was trained by distributing the data for each collaborator into 80% for training and 20% for in-training validation. The in-training validation set aids in improving network performance during training. The individual segmentation networks for the whole tumor, tumor core, and enhancing tumor were set to train for 50 epochs, with a learning rate of 0.001, and the cost function used for training was negative log-likelihood. Three separate networks were implemented to circumvent the problems of overfitting and misclassification. The performance of the networks was monitored on both training and in-training validation data. Hyperparameter tuning and model checkpoint was implemented based on the performance of the networks on in-training validation data as mentioned in the Sect. 2.3.2 (Hyper-parameters selection).

2.4.2 Testing

The outputs from individual networks of the whole tumor, tumor core, and enhancing tumor were used to fuse the final tumor segmentation maps. The segmentation label for edema was obtained by subtracting the tumor core from the whole tumor. The segmentation label for necrosis was obtained by subtracting the enhancing tumor from the tumor core. All tumor sub-components were assigned a unique value similar to the values in the ground truth.

The networks trained for segmenting the tumor sub-components were used to test the validation dataset. All the algorithms were to put together as a package and dockerized to test the testing dataset.

3 Results

The results for both tasks were tested on both the validation and testing dataset. The results for the validation dataset were computed using the validation portal for the challenge, and the testing results were provided by the organizers. The metrics used for evaluation were dice score and Hausdorff distance [34].

3.1 Task-1

Table 1. Quantitative results of task-1.

Task 1	Dice scores			Hausdorff distance		
Weighted aggregation network	WT	TC	ET	WT	TC	ET
	0.767	0.612	0.628	31.075	30.089	29.482

The testing pipeline for task-1 of the challenge was provided by the organizers. Table 1 shows the quantitative results for task-1 of the challenge. The Dice score and Hausdorff distance on the validation dataset were 0.767 and 31.08 for the whole tumor, 0.61 and 30.09 for tumor core, and 0.63 and 29.48 for enhancing tumor respectively.

Table 2. Quantitative results of task-1 on Leaderboard 1and leaderboard 2.

Task 1	Dice scores			Hausdorff distance		
Test data LB 1	WT	TC	ET	WT	TC	ET
	0.682	0.551	0.599	37.821	50.359	54.511
Test data LB 2	0.731	0.603	0.640	36.117	40.956	43.867

Table 2 shows the quantitative results for task-1 of the challenge on Leaderboard 1 and leaderboard 2 respectively.

3.2 Task-2

Table 3 shows the quantitative results for task-2 of the challenge on both Validation and test dataset.

Table 3. Quantitative results of task-2 on Validation and Test dataset.

Task 2	Dice scores			Hausdorff distance		
Validation dataset	WT	TC	ET	WT	TC	ET
	0.874	0.773	0.721	22.218	36.955	22.083
Testing dataset	0.773	0.637	0.677	34.536	52.701	66.550

4 Discussion

The primary purpose of task-1 of the FeTS challenge was to improve the baseline consensus model. The metrics of Dice score, Focal score, and Tversky score were monitored throughout the training process. Hyper-parameter selection was set with a dynamic learning rate. This helped in decreasing the training time of the network. Initially, for the first 5 rounds, the learning rates and epochs were assigned relatively high values since the initial learning would require more time to learn the important tumor features from the images. This helped us to improve the initial Dice score for all collaborators across training and in-training validation. After round 5, the learning rate and epochs were reduced to have a better network convergence, as learning the feature maps would be more specific to the collaborators and would require less time. Average Dice score across tumor sub-components was monitored for selecting the best training hyper-parameters. The model aggregation function also utilized the average Dice score for aggregating the networks across collaborators. Since the weight for each collaborator was based on the Dice score performance, the networks were ranked from worst to the best and the network with the top Dice score was assigned the highest weight. This approach was followed for each round, which helped in improving the performance of the consensus model. A single network architecture was used to segment all three tumor sub-components and monitoring the average Dice score helped the network to learn the feature maps with equal importance for all sub-components. Lastly, the aggregation function in combination with the hyper-parameter selection was able to learn quickly, converge faster, and achieve improved results for each round.

The MST network used for training and evaluation of task-2 of the challenge was able to generate robust segmentation outputs. The segmentation outputs for the whole tumor, tumor core, and enhancing tumor showed high Dice scores on the validation dataset. Transformer network encodes long-range dependencies, and hence, it can learn and segment not only the larger components but also the smaller tumor regions. The global and local pathways in the network help in learning not only the long-range dependencies from the full resolution image but also finer imaging details from the image patches. The network was trained for segmenting individual labels, which made the network less complex and more efficient by greatly reducing both misclassifications and overfitting.

5 Conclusion

A fully automated tumor segmentation pipeline was developed for segmenting gliomas into their sub-components using federated learning. Federated learning enables learning features from datasets located at the institutional level. This approach can be used for datasets located in different geographical locations, overcoming issues of privacy, regulatory, and locality of data. The federated evaluation across multiple institutions can help to improve research as well as clinical workflows for reliable tumor segmentation to guide diagnosis and treatment planning.

References

1. Ostrum, Q., et al.: CBTRUS statistical report: primary brain and central nervous system tumors diagnosed in the United States in 2008–2012. Neuro Oncol. **17**, v1–v62 (2015)
2. Pati, S., et al.: The Federated Tumor Segmentation (FeTS) Challenge. arXiv:2105.05874 (2021)
3. Bonawitz, K., et al.: Towards Federated Learning at Scale: System Design. arXiv:1902.01046 (2019)
4. McMahan, B., Moore, E., Ramage, D., Hampson, S., y Arcas, B.A.: Communication-efficient learning of deep networks from decentralized data. In: Artificial Intelligence and Statistics, pp. 1273–1282. PMLR (2017)
5. Yang, T., et al.: Applied Federated Learning: Improving Google Keyboard Query Suggestions. arXiv:1812.02903 (2018)
6. Yang, Q., Liu, Y., Chen, T., Tong, Y.: Federated machine learning: concept and applications. ACM Trans. Intell. Syst. Technol. **10**, 1–19 (2019)
7. Rieke, N., et al.: The future of digital health with federated learning. NPJ Digit. Med. **3**, 1–7 (2020)
8. Sheller, M.J., et al.: Federated learning in medicine: facilitating multi-institutional collaborations without sharing patient data. Sci. Rep. **10**, 1–12 (2020)
9. Menze, B.H., et al.: The multimodal brain tumor image segmentation benchmark (BRATS). vol. 34, pp. 1993–2024 (2014)
10. Isensee, F., et al.: Abstract: nnU-Net: self-adapting framework for u-net-based medical image segmentation. In: Handels, H., Deserno, T.M., Maier, A., Maier-Hein, K.H., Palm, C., Tolxdorff, T. (eds.) Bildverarbeitung für die Medizin 2019: Algorithmen – Systeme – Anwendungen. Proceedings des Workshops vom 17. bis 19. März 2019 in Lübeck, pp. 22–22. Springer Fachmedien Wiesbaden, Wiesbaden (2019). https://doi.org/10.1007/978-3-658-25326-4_7
11. Kamnitsas, K., et al.: Efficient multi-scale 3D CNN with fully connected CRF for accurate brain lesion segmentation. Med. Image Anal. **36**, 61–78 (2017)
12. Devlin, J., Chang, M.-W., Lee, K., Toutanova, K.: Bert: Pre-training of Deep Bidirectional Transformers for Language Understanding. arXiv:1810.04805 (2018)
13. Dosovitskiy, A., et al.: An Image is Worth 16 × 16 Words: Transformers for Image Recognition at Scale. arXiv:2010.11929 (2020)
14. Wang, H., Zhu, Y., Green, B., Adam, H., Yuille, A., Chen, L.-C.: Axial-deeplab: stand-alone axial-attention for panoptic segmentation. In: Vedaldi, A., Bischof, H., Brox, T., Frahm, J.-M. (eds.) Computer Vision – ECCV 2020: 16th European Conference, Glasgow, UK, August 23–28, 2020, Proceedings, Part IV, pp. 108–126. Springer International Publishing, Cham (2020). https://doi.org/10.1007/978-3-030-58548-8_7
15. Reina, G.A., et al.: OpenFL: An Open-source Framework for Federated Learning. arXiv: 2105.06413 (2021)

16. Bakas, S., et al.: Identifying the best machine learning algorithms for brain tumor segmentation, progression assessment, and overall survival prediction in the BRATS challenge (2018)
17. Bakas, S., et al.: Advancing the cancer genome atlas glioma MRI collections with expert segmentation labels and radiomic features. Sci. Data **4**, 170117 (2017)
18. Bakas, S., et al.: Segmentation labels and radiomic features for the pre-operative scans of the TCGA-LGG collection. The Cancer Imaging Archive 286 (2017)
19. Bakas, S., Akbari, H., Sotiras, A.: Segmentation labels for the pre-operative scans of the TCGA-GBM collection. The Cancer Imaging Archive. (2017)
20. Davatzikos, C., et al.: Cancer imaging phenomics toolkit: quantitative imaging analytics for precision diagnostics and predictive modeling of clinical outcome. J. Med. Imaging **5**, 011018 (2018)
21. Pati, S., et al.: The cancer imaging phenomics toolkit (captk): technical overview. In: Crimi, A., Bakas, S. (eds.) Brainlesion: Glioma, Multiple Sclerosis, Stroke and Traumatic Brain Injuries: 5th International Workshop, BrainLes 2019, Held in Conjunction with MICCAI 2019, Shenzhen, China, October 17, 2019, Revised Selected Papers, Part II, pp. 380–394. Springer International Publishing, Cham (2020). https://doi.org/10.1007/978-3-030-46643-5_38
22. Rathore, S., et al.: Brain cancer imaging phenomics toolkit (brain-CaPTk): an interactive platform for quantitative analysis of glioblastoma. In: Crimi, A., Bakas, S., Kuijf, H., Menze, B., Reyes, M. (eds.) Brainlesion: Glioma, Multiple Sclerosis, Stroke and Traumatic Brain Injuries, pp. 133–145. Springer International Publishing, Cham (2018). https://doi.org/10.1007/978-3-319-75238-9_12
23. Rohlfing, T., Zahr, N.M., Sullivan, E.V., Pfefferbaum, A.: The SRI24 multichannel atlas of normal adult human brain structure. Hum. Brain Mapp. **31**, 798–819 (2010)
24. Yushkevich, P.A., Pluta, J., Wang, H., Wisse, L.E., Das, S., Wolk, D.: Fast automatic segmentation of hippocampal subfields and medial temporal lobe subregions in 3 Tesla and 7 Tesla T2-weighted MRI. Alzheimers Dement. **7**, P126–P127 (2016)
25. Ronneberger, O., Fischer, P., Brox, T.: U-net: convolutional networks for biomedical image segmentation. In: Navab, N., Hornegger, J., Wells, W.M., Frangi, A.F. (eds.) Medical Image Computing and Computer-Assisted Intervention – MICCAI 2015: 18th International Conference, Munich, Germany, October 5-9, 2015, Proceedings, Part III, pp. 234–241. Springer International Publishing, Cham (2015). https://doi.org/10.1007/978-3-319-24574-4_28
26. Thakur, S., et al.: Brain extraction on MRI scans in presence of diffuse glioma: multi-institutional performance evaluation of deep learning methods and robust modality-agnostic training. Neuroimage **220**, 117081 (2020)
27. Bangalore Yogananda, C.G., et al.: A novel fully automated MRI-based deep-learning method for classification of IDH mutation status in brain gliomas. Neuro Oncol. **22**, 402–411 (2020)
28. Murugesan, G.K., et al.: Multidimensional and multiresolution ensemble networks for brain tumor segmentation. In: Crimi, A., Bakas, S. (eds.) Brainlesion: Glioma, Multiple Sclerosis, Stroke and Traumatic Brain Injuries: 5th International Workshop, BrainLes 2019, Held in Conjunction with MICCAI 2019, Shenzhen, China, October 17, 2019, Revised Selected Papers, Part II, pp. 148–157. Springer International Publishing, Cham (2020). https://doi.org/10.1007/978-3-030-46643-5_14
29. Nalawade, S.S., et al.: Brain Tumor IDH, 1p/19q, and MGMT Molecular Classification Using MRI-based Deep Learning: Effect of Motion and Motion Correction. bioRxiv (2020)
30. Nalawade, S., et al.: Classification of brain tumor isocitrate dehydrogenase status using MRI and deep learning. J. Med. Imaging **6**(1–13), 13 (2019)

31. Valanarasu, J.M.J., Oza, P., Hacihaliloglu, I., Patel, V.M.: Medical transformer: gated axial-attention for medical image segmentation. In: de Bruijne, M., Cattin, P.C., Cotin, S., Padoy, N., Speidel, S., Zheng, Y., Essert, C. (eds.) MICCAI 2021. LNCS, vol. 12901, pp. 36–46. Springer, Cham (2021). https://doi.org/10.1007/978-3-030-87193-2_4
32. Lin, T.-Y., Goyal, P., Girshick, R., He, K., Dollár, P.: Focal loss for dense object detection. In: Proceedings of the IEEE International Conference on Computer Vision, pp. 2980–2988 (2017)
33. Salehi, S.S.M., Erdogmus, D., Gholipour, A.: Tversky loss function for image segmentation using 3D fully convolutional deep networks. In: Wang, Q., Shi, Y., Suk, Heung-Il., Suzuki, K. (eds.) machine Learning in Medical Imaging, pp. 379–387. Springer International Publishing, Cham (2017). https://doi.org/10.1007/978-3-319-67389-9_44
34. Huttenlocher, D.P., Klanderman, G.A., Rucklidge, W.J.: Comparing images using the Hausdorff distance. IEEE Trans. Pattern Anal. Mach. Intell. 15, 850–863 (1993)

Adaptive Weight Aggregation in Federated Learning for Brain Tumor Segmentation

Muhammad Irfan Khan[1]([✉]), Mojtaba Jafaritadi[1,2], Esa Alhoniemi[1],
Elina Kontio[1], and Suleiman A. Khan[3]

[1] Turku University of Applied Sciences, 20520 Turku, Finland
{irfan.khan,mojtaba.jafaritadi,esa.alhoniemi,elina.kontio}@turkuamk.fi
[2] Stanford University, Stanford, CA 94305, USA
[3] University of Helsinki, 00100 Helsinki, Finland
suleimkh@amazon.com

Abstract. We introduce similarity weighted aggregation, a principled and efficient method for regularized weight aggregation in federated learning. Our method is adapted to non-IID collaborators and is simultaneously cost-efficient. This is the first method to propose a sliding-window to select the collaborators, to the best of our knowledge. We demonstrate our method on the federate training task of the FeTS 2021 challenge. We proposed two variations coined Similarity Weighted Aggregation (SimAgg) and Regularized Aggregation (RegAgg). SimAgg results on internal validation data demonstrate that the proposed method outperforms the baseline FedAvg. The method SimAgg by our team HT-TUAS won 2nd position on both leaderboards in FeTS2021 challenge. SimAgg is the only method to be among the top performing methods on both the leaderboards, making it robust and reliable to data variations. Our solution is open sourced at: https://github.com/dskhanirfan/FeTS2021

Keywords: Brain tumors · Cancer · Collaborative learning ·
Federated learning · FeTS challenge · Lesion segmentation · Weight
aggregation

1 Introduction

Federated Learning (FL) can facilitate healthcare organizations to collaborate and share information without compromising patients privacy. This is in contrast to many medical imaging studies that use data stored in a centralized database, where the curation of image data, prepossessing, and model development are done with full access to the sensitive and delicate patient information. Moreover, by using secure FL infrastructures we can potentially eliminate tedious and time-consuming ethical permission process for using medical images.

A. Crimi and S. Bakas (Eds.): BrainLes 2021, LNCS 12963, pp. 455–469, 2022.
https://doi.org/10.1007/978-3-031-09002-8_40

Federated learning is a computational paradigm for distributed or decentralized machine learning where training data is shared via multiple collaborators and a central server learns a consensus model by aggregating locally-computed updates [14]. In other words, FL allows distributed adaption of AI development in a privacy-preserving fashion such that private data never leaves the local data storage (e.g. a medical device, academic research center, clinical trial site, and medical data repository). With the advent of strict regulations like GDPR (EU) and HIPAA (US) the usability spectrum of Federated Learning is diverse [1,20]. In FL, multiple collaborators – also referred to as devices or clients – contribute to a learning task. This approach allows clients to collaboratively train a shared inference model while holding all the training data on the local storage privately, decoupling the ability to do machine learning from the need to keep the data in one centralized location [18]. Hence, only certain model updates may leave the client's secure computational environment, enabling the aggregation of the learned parameters into a single generalized (global) model without disclosing the raw data to the third parties. The communication between the clients usually involves a central orchestrator that receives and aggregates client's updates [12].

Decentralized training of an inference model in a federated fashion is an iterative process, in which a subset of clients are selected to receive the current global model in each iteration. Each client runs several epochs, for example in a stochastic gradient descent optimization problem where a neural network is trained with certain mini-batches, and communicates its model update back to the server. The differences between the local models and the received global model are considered as model updates, for which the server aggregates them from the contributing clients to obtain an improved global model. This process continues to the next iteration until a desired performance is obtained [11]. Figure 1 shows a high-level schema of the federated learning framework for healthcare institutions.

In general, algorithms for FL face three main challenges: 1) statistical heterogeneity in weight aggregation, 2) communication efficiency, and 3) privacy with security [12,22]. An efficient aggregation strategy, i.e. combining the models of all clients, is essential for the successful implementation of FL in real-life applications. Numerous aggregation strategies have been studied, of which Federated Averaging (FedAvg) [14] is one of the most well-known FL methods. This approach considers the normalized number of non-Independent Identical Distribution (non-IID) data in each client to aggregate the models in the server. However, FedAvg does not address the weight divergence challenge due to the strongly skewed data distributions. FedProx [13] handles statistical heterogeneity in the network by constraining the local solvers so that they do not deviate significantly from the global model. This is achieved using a proximal weight term, however, FedProx works on the client side. Existing research on dealing with the statistical challenge of federated learning focuses on the ideas of inverse distance aggregation [23], temporal weighting [6], knowledge transfer [9], knowledge distillation and augmentation [10], multi-task learning [7], and meta-learning [5].

Communication efficiency in many FL settings is the primary bottleneck, which requires adequate cost management strategies such as decreasing the

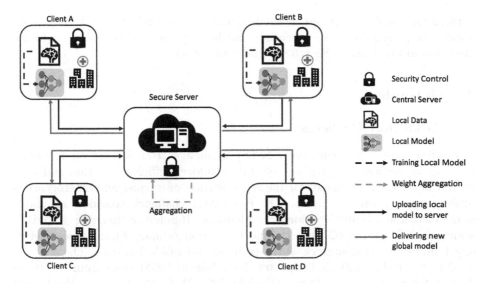

Fig. 1. General workflow of an FL-trained model and the key components in a federated learning setting [22]. Private clients A–D (e.g. healthcare institutions) communicate the local weight updates with a central secure server at regularly occurring intervals to learn a global model; the server aggregates the updates and sends back the parameters of the updated global model to the clients.

number of clients, reducing the update size, and reducing the number of updates. Hence, the existing research on communication-efficient FL is divided into four major categories: model compression, client selection, update reducing, and peer-to-peer learning [12,22].

From privacy-preserving point of view, it is also important to securely aggregate the model parameters or weights to avoid possibilities of leakage of information and vulnerability to adversarial inference and inversion [8,11,15]. Even well-generalized deep models can potentially leak a considerable amount of information about the input training data [15]. Even worse, certain neural networks trained on sensitive data (e.g., medical image data) can memorize the training data [8]. Secure aggregation protocols such as secure multiparty computation (SMC) and differential privacy (DP) have been proposed to alleviate the risk of adversarial attacks and further enhance privacy guarantees in FL [19,21]. We leave dealing with the privacy-preserving and security challenges for the future works.

Our main contributions in this paper are 1) the establishment of an efficient adaptive regularized weight aggregation approach on the FeTS 2021 multi-modal brain MRI data; 2) the implementation of a practical algorithm that can be applied to this setting; and 3) an extensive evaluation of the proposed weight aggregation approach. This paper is organized as follows: in Sect. 2, we describe the methodologies including our two FL weight aggregation strategies by our experiment setting. In Sect. 3, we describe FL experiments and evaluate the performance of the proposed methods quantitatively and in Sect. 4, we discuss about the presented work, potentials and limitations, and describe our future direction in FL. Finally, Sect. 5 concludes this work.

2   Methods

2.1   FeTS 2021 Challenge

Federated Tumor Segmentation (FeTS) Challenge 2021 focuses on federated learning in medical imaging, and intends to address efficient creation and evaluation of a consensus model for the segmentation of intrinsically heterogeneous brain tumors, namely gliomas. The FeTS 2021 challenge considers an ample multi-institutional multi-parametric Magnetic Resonance Imaging (mpMRI) scans of glioblastoma (GBM), the most common primary brain tumor, before any kind of resection surgery as the training and validation data. The datasets used in the FeTS 2021 challenge are the subset of GBM cases from the Brain Tumor Segmentation Challenge (BraTS) 2020 [2–4]. BraTS offers the largest fully annotated and publicly available database for AI model development for the objective of brain tumor segmentation methods.

The FeTS 2021 data release consists of a training set and two partitions each providing information for how to split the training data into non-IID institutional subsets[1]. The training dataset includes 341 subjects with High-Grade Gliomas (HGG) and Low-Grade Gliomas (LGG). All FeTS mpMRI scans, provided as NIfTI files (`.nii.gz`), had four $240 \times 240 \times 155$ structural MRI images including native (T1), post-contrast T1-weighted (T1Gd), T2-weighted (T2), and T2 FLuid Attenuated Inversion Recovery (FLAIR) volumes. A sample image is shown in Fig. 2. Annotations comprise the pathologically confirmed segmentation labels with similar volume size of $240 \times 240 \times 155$ including the GD-enhancing tumor (ET - label 4), the peritumoral edematous/invaded tissue (ED - label 2), and the necrotic tumor core (NCR - label 1). All these provided MRI scans were collected from multiple institutions and certain pre-processing steps such as rigid registration, brain extraction, alignment, $1 \times 1 \times 1$ mm resolution resampling, and skull stripping were applied as described in [2–4].

We deployed Intel Federated Learning (OpenFL) [17] framework for training brain tumor segmentation model—an encoder-decoder U-shape type of convolutional neural network provided by FeTS2021 challenge—using the data-private collaborative learning paradigm of FL. OpenFL considers two main components: 1) the collaborator which uses a local dataset to train the global model and 2) the aggregator which receives model updates from each collaborator and fuses them to form the global model. Our experiments were performed on a cluster workstation with running NVIDIA TITAN V100 GPU and 350 GB memory.

---

[1] https://github.com/FETS-AI/Challenge/tree/main/Task_1.

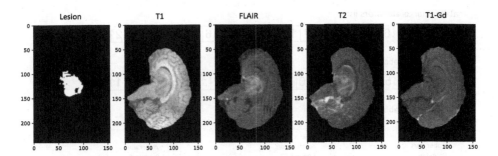

Fig. 2. Sample images from all MRI modalities with the corresponding GBM lesion.

2.2 Method 1: Similarity Weighted Aggregation (SimAgg)

We developed an adaptive machine-learning approach coined similarity weighted aggregation for efficient aggregation of model parameters at the server. Our approach is suitable for both IID as well as non-IID data. Specifically, our strategy is focused on collaborator selection and parameter aggregation policy.

Collaborator Selection. For the collaborator selection, we use a subset of the available collaborators (for example, 20%) in each round. To allow for systems heterogeneity where collaborators can contribute in a non-deterministic fashion, we simulate random selection of collaborators in each round. However, to ensure that the model sees all collaborators the same number of times at regular intervals, we implement a sliding window over the randomized collaborator index as shown in Fig. 3. In this setup, once all collaborators have participated in updates, a new randomized order is computed for better learning. We use a sliding window instead of random collaborator selection to ensure participation of all collaborators. We used a sliding-window size equal to 20% of the collaborators in each partition. In partition 1, the sliding-window size was set to three as the total number of collaborators was 17. In partition 2, the sliding-window size was set to four as the total number of collaborators was 22.

Weight Aggregation. A fundamental issue with non-IID data is that model parameters coming from the collaborators can diverge. To overcome such a scenario we use weighted aggregation of the collaborators at the server. The collaborators are weighted based on how similar they are to their non-weighted average. This simple yet effective mechanism can help in learning a master model that is representative of most of the collaborators at each round, see Algorithm 1.

Specifically, at round r, the parameters p_{C^r} of the participating collaborators C^r are collected at the server. The average of these parameters is calculated as:

$$\hat{p} = \frac{1}{|C^r|} \Sigma_{i \in C^r} p_i. \tag{1}$$

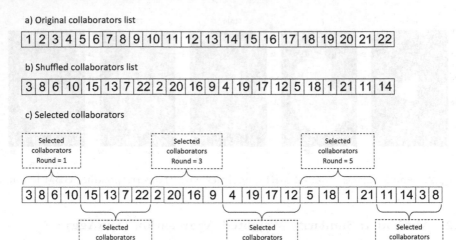

Fig. 3. Collaborator selection strategy. In a) the model receives a list of initial collaborators, in b) collaborator order is randomized to help better learning, and in c) collaborators are selected for each round using a sliding window. Once the collaborator list is entirely used, it is shuffled again and the process starts again from step b).

We subsequently calculate the similarity of each collaborator $c \in C^r$ with the average parameter values from all collaborators as

$$sim_c = \frac{\Sigma_{i \in C^r} |p_i - \hat{p}|}{|p_c - \hat{p}| + \epsilon}, \tag{2}$$

where $\epsilon = 1e - 5$ (small positive constant), and normalize to obtain similarity weights as follows:

$$u_c = \frac{sim_c}{\Sigma_{i \in C^r} sim_i}. \tag{3}$$

The collaborators closer to the average receive a higher similarity score while those further away obtain a lower value. In the extreme case this approach can expel the diverging collaborator.

In order to adjust for the effect of varying number of samples in each collaborator $c \in C^r$, we use a second weighting factor that favors collaborators with larger sample sizes:

$$v_c = \frac{N_c}{\Sigma_{i \in C^r} N_i}, \tag{4}$$

where N_c is the number of examples in collaborator c.

Using the weights obtained using Eqs. 3 and 4, the similarity weighted parameter values (p^m) are computed as:

$$w_c = \frac{u_c + v_c}{\Sigma_{i \in C^r}(u_i + v_i)}. \qquad (5)$$

Finally, the parameters are aggregated as follows:

$$p^m = \frac{1}{|C^r|} \cdot \Sigma_{i \in C^r}(w_i \cdot p_i). \qquad (6)$$

The normalized aggregated parameters p^m are then dispatched to the next set of collaborators in the successive federation rounds.

Algorithm 1. SimAgg aggregation algorithm

1: **procedure** SIMILARITY WEIGHTED AGGREGATION(C^r, p_{C^r})
2:    $\epsilon \leftarrow 1e-5$ ▷ C^r = set of collaborators (at round r)
3:    $\hat{p}$ = average(p_{C^r}) using **Eq. 1** ▷ p_{C^r} = parameters of the collaborators in C^r
4:    **for** c in C^r **do**
5:        Compute similarity weights u_c using **Eqs. 2** and **3**
6:        Compute sample weights v_c using **Eq. 4**
7:    **for** c in C^r **do**
8:        Compute aggregation weights w_c using **Eq. 5**
9:    Compute master model parameters p^m using **Eq. 6**
10:   **return** p^m

2.3   Method 2: Regularized Aggregation (RegAgg)

We also developed a regularizing version of our aggregation approach. The method performs stronger penalization of diverging collaborators.

Collaborator Selection. The collaboration selection for regularized aggregation is the same as in Sect. 2.2.

Weight Aggregation. The weight aggregation methodology is adapted from Sect. 2.2 to compute the similarity and sample weights using Eqs. 3 and 4. We then compute the regularizing weights of each of the collaborator as:

$$w_c = \frac{u_c \cdot v_c}{\Sigma_{i \in C^r}(u_i \cdot v_i)}. \qquad (7)$$

Finally, the master models parameters are computed using Eq. 6. The entire process is summarized in Algorithm 2.

Algorithm 2. RegAgg aggregation algorithm

1: **procedure** REGULARIZED AGGREGATION(C^r, p_{C^r})
2:     $\epsilon \leftarrow 1e-5$ ▷ C^r = set of collaborators (at round r)
3:     $\hat{p}$ = average(p_{C^r}) using **Eq. 1** ▷ p_{C^r} = parameters of the collaborators in C^r
4:     **for** c in C^r **do**
5:         Compute similarity weights u_c using **Eqs. 2** and **3**
6:         Compute sample weights v_c using **Eq. 4**
7:     **for** c in C^r **do**
8:         Compute aggregation weights w_c using **Eq. 7**
9:     Compute master model parameters p^m using **Eq. 6**
10:     **return** p^m

---

3 Experiments

3.1 Setup

The goal of task 1 is to improve the federation process by focusing on efficient aggregation, client selection, training-per-round, compression, and communication efficiency. We have developed an efficient method that aggregates the model updates trained on individual collaborators. A data set with total of 341 multi-institutional patients was available. Supplementary information indicates the division of patients in different partitions. Partition 1 and partition 2 have 17 collaborators and 22 collaborators, respectively. Partition 1 means institutional split, while partition 2 is further divided based on the tumor size. The experimental setup uses Intel's OpenFL platform for federation learning and a predefined 3D U-shape neural network for the semantic segmentation of whole tumor, tumor core, and enhancing tumor. The metrics computed in the aggregation rounds are binary DICE similarity (whole tumor, enhancing tumor, tumor core) and Hausdorff (95%) distance (whole tumor, enhancing tumor, tumor core) as described in [16].

The hyperparameters used are shown in Table 1. Collaborator selection for SimAgg and RegAgg are shown in Fig. 3.

Table 1. Hyperparameters used in aggregation algorithms.

Leaderboard	Hyperparameter	SimAgg	RegAgg	FedAvg
1	Learning rate	5e−5	5e−5	5e−5
1	Epochs per round	5.0	1.0	1.0
2	Learning rate	5e−5	5e−5	5e−5
2	Epochs per round	5.0	5.0	1.0

3.2   Results

In this section, results are summarized for leaderboards 1 and 2 (with partitions 1 & 2). The comparison of baseline FedAvg with default setting and our aggregation methods – namely regularized aggregation and similarity weighted aggregation – shows that both of our methods rapidly converge and are stable as the learning progresses across all the measured metrics. Moreover, our methods show significant improvement in the performance.

Model Training and Performance Using Internal Validation Data. Figure 4 shows the performance comparison of model training on internal validation for partition 2 for Leaderboard 1. Figure 5 contains the same comparison for both partitions 1 and 2 of Leaderboard 2.

In Leaderboard 1, SimAgg significantly outperforms RegAgg with approximately 10–15% improvement across all DICE and Hausdorff (95%) scores. In Leaderboard 2, SimAgg performs slightly better than RegAgg and FedAvg across all DICE and Hausdorff (95%) scores.

Model Performance Using External Validation Data. Prior to the official testing phase, the performance of both of our methods was assessed using unseen external validation data provided by challenge organizers, see Tables 2, 3, and 4. From the Tables 3 and 4, we can see that SimAgg resulted in higher performance across all DICE scores. Similarly, the Hausdorff (95%) distances obtained by SimAgg method were smaller than the RegAgg for the partitions 1 & 2.

Table 2. Leaderboard 1 experiments: Trained aggregation algorithms on partition 2 performance on validation data.

	SimAgg	RegAgg
Binary DICE WT	0.7774	0.6982
Binary DICE ET	0.6793	0.5856
Binary DICE TC	0.6682	0.5664
Hausdorff (95%) WT	34.2991	50.1060
Hausdorff (95%) ET	22.8250	42.5777
Hausdorff (95%) TC	29.6163	43.1602

Model Performance Using Fully Blinded Test Set. FeTS2021 challenge organizing committee permitted one algorithm per team for ranking in the official leaderboards. Therefore, we submitted SimAgg algorithm for the leaderboard ranking since SimAgg performed better on internal and external validation data in our experiments.

The SimAgg performance stats for team HT-TUAS on the fully blinded test set for Leaderboards 1 and 2 are shown in Tables 5 and 6, respectively. These

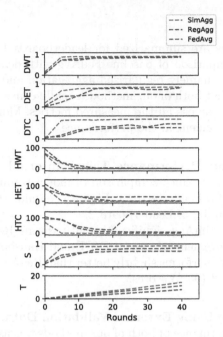

Fig. 4. Leaderboard 1 experiments: Performance metrics model training of SimAgg, RegAgg, and FedAvg for partition 2. The horizontal axis refers to the number of rounds and the vertical axis to the performance metrics. Metrics; DWT: DICE Whole Tumor, DET: DICE Enhancing Tumor, DTC: DICE Tumor Core, HWT: Hausdorff (95%) Whole Tumor, HET: Hausdorff (95%) Enhancing Tumor, HTC: Hausdorff (95%) Tumor Core, S: Projected Convergence Score, T: Simulation Time (Hours).

results ranked us as the top second team for the federated tumor segmentation challenge. In leaderboard 1, a significant discrepancy between the validation and testing datasets for the DICE and Hausdorff distance scores was visible. The discrepancy is because the wrapper function for data loader had a logical bug that the next collaborator is not selected. However, in leaderboard 2, the results on fully blind test set is better because model training is performed for 500 rounds by challenge organizers after the logical bug was removed.

Overall, SimAgg performs whole tumor segmentation better as compared to enhancing tumor segmentation and tumor core segmentation.

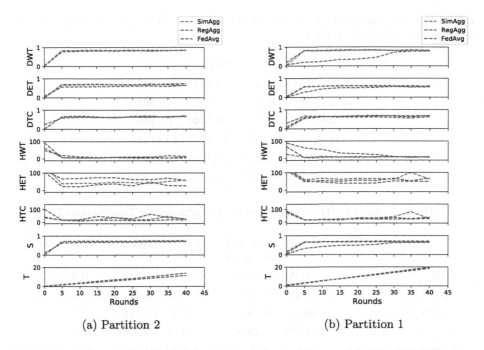

(a) Partition 2   (b) Partition 1

Fig. 5. Leaderboard 2 experiments: Performance metrics model training of SimAgg, RegAgg, and FedAvg for partition 2 (a) and partition 1 (b). The horizontal axis refers to the number of rounds and the vertical axis to the performance metrics. Metrics; DWT: DICE Whole Tumor, DET: DICE Enhancing Tumor, DTC: DICE Tumor Core, HWT: Hausdorff (95%) Whole Tumor, HET: Hausdorff (95%) Enhancing Tumor, HTC: Hausdorff (95%) Tumor Core, S: Projected Convergence Score, T: Simulation Time (Hours).

Table 3. Leaderboard 2 experiments: Trained aggregation algorithms on partition 2 performance on validation data.

	SimAgg	RegAgg
Binary DICE WT	0.8415	0.8387
Binary DICE ET	0.6993	0.6910
Binary DICE TC	0.7143	0.7110
Hausdorff (95%) WT	12.1612	12.8851
Hausdorff (95%) ET	17.2475	26.5882
Hausdorff (95%) TC	17.6554	26.3145

4 Discussion

Various methods have been proposed in the literature for federated aggregation. However, a limited set of methods work exclusively on the server side. To start with, we explored several alternatives including exponential smoothing aggre-

Table 4. Leaderboard 2 experiments: Trained aggregation algorithms on partition 1 performance on validation data.

	SimAgg	RegAgg
Binary DICE WT	0.8501	0.8265
Binary DICE ET	0.7087	0.6867
Binary DICE TC	0.7038	0.7160
Hausdorff (95%) WT	13.2122	14.1265
Hausdorff (95%) ET	15.2001	16.9239
Hausdorff (95%) TC	16.3441	18.1132

Table 5. SimAgg (HT-TUAS) test set performance on Leaderboard 1.

	Mean	Standard Deviation	Median	25quantile	75quantile
DICE WT	0.7076	0.2676	0.8259	0.5788	0.9066
DICE ET	0.6054	0.3172	0.7558	0.3633	0.8461
DICE TC	0.6502	0.3320	0.8144	0.4134	0.9082
Sensitivity ET	0.7845	0.2908	0.8967	0.7565	0.9542
Sensitivity WT	0.8471	0.1722	0.8997	0.8231	0.9410
Sensitivity TC	0.8104	0.2913	0.9328	0.8259	0.9729
Specificity WT	0.9942	0.0081	0.9985	0.9909	0.9994
Specificity ET	0.9973	0.0045	0.9993	0.9971	0.9997
Specificity TC	0.9964	0.0062	0.9993	0.9957	0.9998
Hausdorff (95%) WT	30.5343	29.3950	13.8515	4.3872	58.5597
Hausdorff (95%) ET	53.9195	98.8776	5.5649	1.4142	71.2686
Hausdorff (95%) TC	48.6906	80.4691	16.8320	3.0000	68.4579
Communication Cost	0.8562	0.8562	0.8562	0.8562	0.8562

gation and conditional threshold aggregation. However, both of these methods required user defined threshold parameters that needed tuning, hence, these approaches are not inherently generalizable to new and unseen data sets. Therefore, we designed similarity weighted aggregation and regularized aggregation that automatically adapt the weights. Unlike, our approach, FedProx [13] performs regularized weight aggregation on the client side by restricting the local solvers so that they do not deviate significantly from the global model. Our method works on the server-side by limiting the contribution of the diverging collaborators to learn the global model. Our approach has the additional advantage that it can be implemented only on the server-side so that clients with varying configurations can join the federation.

Several works have demonstrated that using a subset of random collaborators helps speed up the training of federated learning algorithms [24]. We extended

Table 6. SimAgg (HT-TUAS) test set performance on Leaderboard 2.

	Mean	Standard deviation	Median	25quantile	75quantile
DICE WT	0.8213	0.1797	0.8847	0.8055	0.9188
DICE ET	0.7438	0.2425	0.8174	0.7179	0.8868
DICE TC	0.7455	0.2662	0.859	0.6780	0.9119
Sensitivity ET	0.8423	0.2597	0.9427	0.8563	0.9820
Sensitivity WT	0.9070	0.1731	0.9619	0.9190	0.9866
Sensitivity TC	0.8510	0.2685	0.9607	0.8735	0.9881
Specificity WT	0.9979	0.0025	0.9984	0.9975	0.9991
Specificity ET	0.9993	0.0011	0.9995	0.9992	0.9998
Specificity TC	0.9988	0.0019	0.9994	0.9986	0.9998
Hausdorff (95%) WT	8.2904	10.7090	5.0990	3.0000	9.0415
Hausdorff (95%) ET	26.4082	88.3786	2.2361	1.4142	3.6056
Hausdorff (95%) TC	26.2290	74.0068	6.7082	2.4495	16.9027
Communication Cost	0.7937	0.7937	0.7937	0.7937	0.7937

the ideas here and formulated a sliding window strategy that ensures representation of all collaborators in the training process. It may be valuable to study the performance of sliding window alone without SimAgg or RegAgg aggregation in future. We used a sliding window size equal to 20% of the collaborators. The size of the sliding window is a hyper-parameter of the method and optimizing it will only further improve the model performance. A promising future work is to develop a strategy for optimizing the sliding-window size.

The FeTS 2021 data release consists of two partitions each providing information for how the training data is split into non-IID institutional and tumor size subsets. Therefore, the size and distribution of data in each collaborator can be different. Our method works well on both partitions, as the weighted aggregation approach helps learn a model that is representative of most of the collaborators at each round, with minimal impact from the outliers. While the model performs well in general when data has non-IID splits, it will be valuable to further investigate the performance on the outliers.

A limitation of this work is the small number of patients and collaborators. However, our approach has laid the groundwork for the refined development of an improved model that can be applied to newly generated data sets at scale. The aggregation algorithm can be used for generalizable ML model training for "real-world" clinical data in clinical practices and production environments on geographically distinct collaborators.

Our future research direction includes incorporation of our developed FL methods with diverse state-of-the-art privacy protection AI frameworks for data anonymization, augmentation, object detection and segmentation, and image translation. The widespread adoption of secure and private AI on medical image data still requires vigorous improvements to the generalization or personalization of the AI models. Decentralized data storage, efficient cryptographic and privacy primitives, and dedicated neural network operations are yet emerging to replace the current paradigm of data sharing and privacy preservation, enabling privacy-preserving cross-institutional research in a breadth of biomedical disciplines.

5 Conclusion

In this work, we proposed two novel weight aggregation schemes, regularized aggregation and similarity weighted aggregation, for aggregation of neural network models in a federated learning setting for brain tumor segmentation. Our extensive experiments on internal validation show that the proposed methods outperform FedAvg in terms of convergence score and communication costs. Our team HT-TUAS submitted SimAgg for ranking on official leaderboards and won 2nd position on both Leaderboards in FeTS2021 challenge. While our proposed strategies offer better aggregation benefits, providing stronger privacy guarantees, for example via differential privacy, secure multi-party computation, or a mixture of them is an interesting future research direction.

Acknowledgements. This work was supported by the Business Finland under Grant 33961/31/2020. We also acknowledge the support and computational resources facilitated by the CSC-Puhti super-computer, a non-profit state enterprise owned by the Finnish state and higher education institutions in Finland.

References

1. Annas, G.J.: HIPAA regulations-a new era of medical-record privacy? (2003)
2. Bakas, S., et al.: Segmentation labels and radiomic features for the pre-operative scans of the TCGA-GBM collection. The cancer imaging archive. Nat. Sci. Data **4**, 170117 (2017)
3. Bakas, S., et al.: Segmentation labels and radiomic features for the pre-operative scans of the TCGA-LGG collection. Cancer Imaging Archive **286** (2017)
4. Bakas, S., et al.: Advancing the cancer genome atlas glioma MRI collections with expert segmentation labels and radiomic features. Sci. Data 4(1), 1–13 (2017)
5. Beel, J.: Federated meta-learning: democratizing algorithm selection across disciplines and software libraries. Science (AICS) **210**, 219 (2018)
6. Chen, Y., Sun, X., Jin, Y.: Communication-efficient federated deep learning with layerwise asynchronous model update and temporally weighted aggregation. IEEE Trans. Neural Netw. Learn. Syst. **31**(10), 4229–4238 (2019)
7. Corinzia, L., Beuret, A., Buhmann, J.M.: Variational federated multi-task learning. arXiv preprint arXiv:1906.06268 (2019)
8. Fung, C., Yoon, C.J., Beschastnikh, I.: Mitigating sybils in federated learning poisoning. arXiv preprint arXiv:1808.04866 (2018)
9. He, C., Annavaram, M., Avestimehr, S.: Group knowledge transfer: federated learning of large CNNs at the edge. arXiv preprint arXiv:2007.14513 (2020)

10. Jeong, E., Oh, S., Kim, H., Park, J., Bennis, M., Kim, S.L.: Communication-efficient on-device machine learning: Federated distillation and augmentation under non-IID private data. arXiv preprint arXiv:1811.11479 (2018)

11. Kadhe, S., Rajaraman, N., Koyluoglu, O.O., Ramchandran, K.: FastSecAgg: scalable secure aggregation for privacy-preserving federated learning. arXiv preprint arXiv:2009.11248 (2020)

12. Kairouz, P., et al.: Advances and open problems in federated learning (2019). https://arxiv.org/abs/1912.04977

13. Li, T., Sahu, A.K., Zaheer, M., Sanjabi, M., Talwalkar, A., Smith, V.: Federated optimization in heterogeneous networks. arXiv preprint arXiv:1812.06127 (2018)

14. McMahan, B., Moore, E., Ramage, D., Hampson, S., Arcas, B.A.: Communication-efficient learning of deep networks from decentralized data. In: Artificial Intelligence and Statistics, pp. 1273–1282. PMLR (2017)

15. Nasr, M., Shokri, R., Houmansadr, A.: Comprehensive privacy analysis of deep learning: passive and active white-box inference attacks against centralized and federated learning. In: 2019 IEEE Symposium on Security and Privacy (SP), pp. 739–753. IEEE (2019)

16. Pati, S., et al.: The federated tumor segmentation (FETS) challenge. arXiv preprint arXiv:2105.05874 (2021)

17. Reina, G.A., et al.: OpenFL: an open-source framework for federated learning. arXiv preprint arXiv:2105.06413 (2021)

18. Sadilek, A., et al.: Privacy-first health research with federated learning. medRxiv (2020)

19. Truex, S., Baracaldo, N., Anwar, A., Steinke, T., Ludwig, H., Zhang, R.: A hybrid approach to privacy-preserving federated learning (2018)

20. Voigt, P., Von dem Bussche, A.: The EU General Data Protection Regulation (GDPR). A Practical Guide, 1st edn. Springer, Cham (2017). https://doi.org/10.1007/978-3-319-57959-7

21. Wei, K., et al.: Federated learning with differential privacy: algorithms and performance analysis. IEEE Trans. Inf. Forensics Secur. **15**, 3454–3469 (2020)

22. Xu, J., Glicksberg, B.S., Su, C., Walker, P., Bian, J., Wang, F.: Federated learning for healthcare informatics. J. Healthc. Inform. Res. **5**(1), 1–19 (2021)

23. Yeganeh, Y., Farshad, A., Navab, N., Albarqouni, S.: Inverse distance aggregation for federated learning with non-IID data. In: Albarqouni, S., et al. (eds.) DART/DCL -2020. LNCS, vol. 12444, pp. 150–159. Springer, Cham (2020). https://doi.org/10.1007/978-3-030-60548-3_15

24. Zhao, Y., Li, M., Lai, L., Suda, N., Civin, D., Chandra, V.: Federated learning with non-IID data. arXiv preprint arXiv:1806.00582 (2018)

A Study on Criteria for Training Collaborator Selection in Federated Learning

Vishruth Shambhat[1], Akansh Maurya[2], Shubham Subhas Danannavar[1], Rohit Kalla[1], Vikas Kumar Anand[1], and Ganapathy Krishnamurthi[1(✉)]

[1] Department of Engineering Design, IIT Madras, Chennai, India
ed17b024@smail.iitm.ac.in, gankrish@iitm.ac.in
[2] Robert Bosch Center of Data Science and AI, IIT Madras, Chennai, India

Abstract. Federated learning is an important aspect of enabling the deployment of deep learning. It addresses data privacy and security concerns by decentralizing data. In a federated learning setup, models are trained locally in the data center called collaborators, and the model weights are aggregated by a central server. We present our work towards the efficient aggregation of trained model weights from multiple institutions which is Task 1 in the federated learning challenge (FeTS 2021). We devised a scoring system for selecting appropriate collaborators every round and aggregating their weight by simple averaging. We calculate the score based on the sensitivity, dice coefficient, and Hausdorff distance of each segmentation class on validation data from every collaborator. The best collaborators are chosen serially based on the scores with higher scores indicating better performing networks. Our approach gave mean dice score of 0.58 ± 0.259 & 0.639 ± 0.176 & 0.55 ± 0.201 on Enhancing Tumor, Whole Tumor and Tumor Core respectively.

Keywords: Deep learning · Federated Learning · Brain tumor segmentation · Aggregation method · Client selection

1 Introduction

Brain tumor segmentation plays an important role in the early diagnosis of brain tumors. Deep Learning methods for segmentation speed up the process compared to the manual segmentation of the brain tumor which is a time-consuming task. The brain tumor segmentation (BraTS) challenge has contributed to making a multi-institutional dataset available to benchmark and qualitatively evaluate the performance of the segmentation algorithm.

That being said, deep Learning methods for tumor segmentation require a good amount of data. If traditional deep learning methods are to be considered then de-centralization of the data via multi-institutional collaboration is necessary. Although challenges like data privacy laws, data ownership challenges, expert knowledge for data labeling makes decentralization difficult [1,11]. To overcome this challenge, Federated Learning (FL) is being used to avoid data centralization. Federated Learning methods train models locally, weights are transferred to the central server where they are aggregated and passed on to the individual local models

2   Challenge Details

FeTS 2021 was divided into two tasks, namely task 1 and task 2. This paper focuses and presents methodology and results for task 1 only. The objective of task 1 is to find best way to aggregate the knowledge learned from segmentation model trained on individual institutions. For the task we were provided with infrastructure (software code) using federated averaging was provided to us. We were allowed to develop custom aggregation method, and perform hyper parameter tuning like client selection, training epochs, training-per-round etc. In the later section we discuss our methodology for hyper parameter tuning and aggregation method. As the task 1 concentrate on development of aggregation, the architecture of segmentation model was fixed as U-Net [10], as it has previously shown robust performance on medical imaging datasets [4,6].

3   Dataset

The data used in this paper is part of FeTS Challenge 2021. It includes multi-parametric Magnetic Resonance Imaging (mp-MRI) scans of Glioblastoma (GBM) from various institutes. According to the organizers, the dataset is a subset of GBM cases from the BraTS 2020 challenge [1,2] and the ground truth is verified by expert board-certified neuroradiologists for every subject [9]. The data can be further classified into two categories Imaging data and Non-imaging data.

3.1   Imaging Data

All the scans available in the challenge are mpMRI scans in NIfTI files (.nii.gz). There are 341 subjects in total. For each of the subjects we have five scans(.nii.gz files):

1. Native T1
2. Contrast-enhanced T1-weighted(T1-Gd)
3. T2-weighted
4. T2 Attenuated Inversion Recovery (T2-FLAIR)
5. Ground truth, segmented GBM scan.

Each scan consisting of 150 axial 2D slice images of 240×240 resolution, and skull-stripped. GBM or tumor has three sub-regions that are "Enhancing tumor" (ET), the "Tumor core" (TC), and the "Whole tumor" (WT). From the following Fig. 1 [8], one can distinguish sub regions of the brain in terms of Peritumoral

Edematous (Edema), Necrotic (NCR), and Active or ET (Enhancing Tumor). Tumor core is the union of the area of ET and NCR. While the Whole tumor is the summation of the area of the Tumor Core and Enhancing Tumor. In FeTS challenge 2021, segmentation targets have annotation values of 1 for NCR, 2 for ED, 4 for ET, and 0 for everything else.

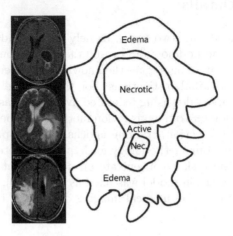

Fig. 1. Sub-regions of tumor

3.2 Non-Imaging Data

Along with all the scans, the data is accompanied by a comma-separated value (.csv) file. The CSV file covers the information on the data partitioning according to acquisition origin. Scan names and their corresponding institutional ID source are mentioned in this file. For Task 1 of the challenge [9], we are using partitioning_2.csv. This is the same as the institutions split but after further partitioning of the 5 largest institutional according to the median size of the whole tumor. The Fig. 2, shows the distribution of the number of cases over institutions. There are 22 institutions in this split. The maximum number of cases are present in institution 14 while least in institutions 10.

4   Related Work

An important problem faced in federated learning is the performance of the aggregated model on non-iid data. The paper [7] tries to understand the convergence of Federated Averaging (FedAvg) on non-iid data. They propose that the learning rate must decay for convergence to an optimal solution. They also propose a few sampling schemes:

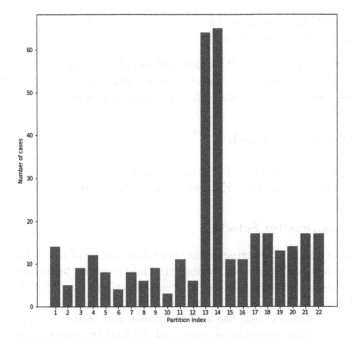

Fig. 2. Partitioning Information, X-axis represents the partitioning index, Y-axis represent counts of scans.

1. **Probabilistic Sampling** - K collaborators are sampled based on a probability p_k assigned to each collaborator, where

$$p_k = \frac{n_k}{N}$$

n_k is the number of data points with the kth collaborator and N is the total number of data points.

2. **Uniform Sampling** - Sample k collaborators with uniform probability $\frac{1}{N}$, where N is the total number of data points.

They show that choosing only K out of N collaborators has no harmful effect on the performance. This also has an added effect of reducing communication cost between the central server and the local models.

In paper [5], the authors propose one-shot federated learning, with only a single round of communication. They train local models to completion and use ensembling techniques to capture the global information from the local models. Several strategies for ensemble selection are discussed. The ones relevant to our work are the following:

1. **Cross Validation Selection** - The local models are used in the ensemble only if they achieve a baseline accuracy on the validation data. The server aggregates the k top-performing models.

2. **Data Selection** - Local models are used for ensembling only if they have a certain amount of baseline data.

Our work heavily draws from [5], where instead of ensembling the local models, we choose the top-performing models based on a combination of validation scores and then use FedAvg to aggregate the weights of the selected models.

5   Proposed Approach

We use a linear combination of dice and hausdorff Distance scores, to sort the collaborators and choose top "K" performing collaborators.

5.1   Hyperparameter Selection

To perform an efficient hyperparameter search, a subset of the data was chosen, containing 8 collaborators. This reduced the time required to conduct the experiments. The counts of each collaborator are described Fig. 3. 80% of the data was used for training, 20% for validation. A set of experiments were performed using this mini dataset. All the eight collaborators were chosen for training and weighted average aggregation was used. To find the effect of hyperparameter selection training was performed till 5 rounds and the hyperparameters like learning rate and epochs per round were varied as shown in following fashion:

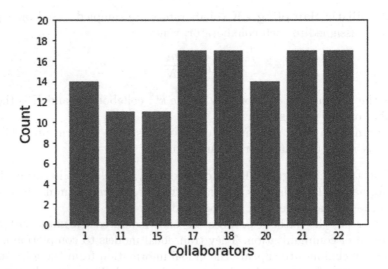

Fig. 3. Mini-collaborators distribution

1. **Constant Hyperparameters** - Learning rate of 5e-5 and 1 epochs per round
2. **Decay Learning Rate, Fixed Epochs** - Decay the learning rate by a factor of 0.9 by each round. Epochs per round = 10
3. **Decay Learning Rate and Decrease Epochs** - Decay Learning Rate and Decrease epochs as rounds increase. Epochs at every round is defined as 5 minus integer division of round number by 2. This is formulated in Eq. 1, where 'e' is epochs, and 'r' in round number. Here $\lfloor x \rfloor$, represents floor function.

$$e = 5 - \lfloor r/5 \rfloor \tag{1}$$

Table 1. Dice scores with different hyperparameter selection

Hyperparameter	WT Dice	ET Dice	TC Dice
Constant	0.488	0.875	0.047
Decay LR	0.84	0.54	0.58
Decay LR, decrease epochs	0.90	0.77	0.84

From the Table 1, we conclude that decreasing training epochs and decaying the learning rate as the rounds increased yielded better results. For running our final experiment, we have used hyperparameters selection described in Algorithm 1. Here "TR" means total number of rounds which in our case is equal to 6. Base learning rate and final learning rate were set to 3×10^{-4} and 1×10^{-5} respectively. We found these settings to work best, based on the preliminary experiments.

Algorithm 1: Hyperparameters per round

---

if round $<$(TR)/2 **then**
$\quad$| epochs_per_round (e) = TR - $\lfloor round(r)/2 \rfloor$;
else
$\quad$| epochs_per_round=2
end
if round $<$TR-1 **then**
$\quad$| learning rate = base learning rate$\times 0.9^{round}$;
else
$\quad$| learning rate = final learning rate
end
return (learning rate, epochs_per_round)

5.2   Training Collaborator Selection

Selecting the appropriate collaborators for training is crucial for the model performance. Collaborators should be selected in such a way, that they maximize the contribution to the model performance. This is a challenging task, as we do not have access to the pixel level data of each collaborator. Metrics must be defined, to assess the contribution of the collaborator data on the segmentation network. Here, we have chosen the validation scores, namely dice score and hausdorff distance.

To begin with, a simple dice thresholding was performed, wherein, after 3 rounds of training, for each round, only those collaborators whose WT dice score was greater than 0.5 were chosen for training. Figure 4(a) shows the dice score while Fig. 4(b) shows Hausdorff Distance corresponds to validation scores on the local data, after training on the local data. It is clearly observed that the model under performs on ET and TC classes. To "balance" the performance on all classes, a custom thresholding function was used.

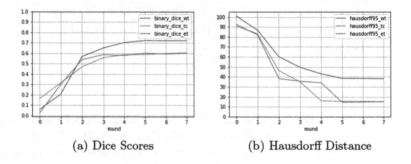

(a) Dice Scores   (b) Hausdorff Distance

Fig. 4. Validation scores after dice thresholding

Selection Algorithm: We sort the collaborators based on the validation scores obtained after local training of the model. In this approach, we define a score that is a linear combination of dice similarity coefficient and Hausdorff distance (95th percentile). For ease of notation, we will denote dice score by "D" and Hausdorff Distance by "HD". A score "S" is defined as follows, in Eq. 2:

$$[S = D + (1 - HD/100)] \tag{2}$$

Hausdorff Distance has been normalized by 100. This is purely empirical, because on average the hausdorff distance lied between 0 and 100. This number has no effect on the algorithm itself. The above score is to be maximized. This score is calculated for all 3 classes.

As an example for "WT" class, "D" and "HD" are the dice scores and Hausdorff distance for "WT" class. For each class, we calculate the score and sort the corresponding collaborators, in descending order. Doing this for the three classes WT, TC and ET, we get 3 lists of collaborators. We also sort the collaborators based on their sensitivity, in descending order. Once we have the 4 lists of sorted collaborators, one collaborator from each list is chosen, from beginning to end, until the total number of collaborators meets a certain value. After every iteration, we remove duplicates from the final list to make sure that a single collaborator appears only once in the list. This is done re-iteratively. For the first few rounds, all collaborators are trained, to let them learn the low level features of their data. Also, after every few rounds of choosing top performing collaborators, for a single round, all collaborators are chosen for training, to prevent "forgetting". In the present data distribution, collaborators 13 and 14 have around 60 data points each. We found it logical to select these collaborators every round, as they make up around 30% the overall data.

Algorithm 2 shows the working flow of our selection algorithm.

Algorithm 2: Ranked Collabs

---

if round $\leq$ 3 or (round >5 and round %4 ==1) **then**
   | return all collaborators ;
else
   | Initialize -

       – Max Accuracy = 0
       – w = [0, 0.1, 0.2, 0.3, 0.4, 0.5, 0.6, 0.7, 0.8, 0.9, 1]
       – 3 lists for Hausdorff Distance - WT_haus,TC_haus,ET_haus
       – 1 list for sensitivity - sens_score

      for record in db_iterator **do**
          wt_names.append(collaborator name);
          wt_dice.append(wt dice score);
          wt_haus.append(Hausdorff distance);
          Repeat above 3 steps for all the 3 classes ;
          sens_names.append(collaborator name);
          sens_score.append(sensitivity);
      end
      Calculate score "S" according to equation [2]. For WT,
      wt_score=[wt_dice[i] + 1-wt_haus[i]/100 for i in range(0,len(wt_dice))]
      Sort wt_names based on wt_score, in descending order for all 3 classes.
      Sort sens_name based on sens_score, in descending order
      We have 4 lists,3 lists for Hausdorff Distance for each class and sensitivity, sorted according to their respective scores
      sorted_collaborators= [ ]
      i=0
      while len(sorted_collaborators) <8 **do**
          sorted_collaborators.append(wt_names[i]+tc_names[i]+et_names[i]+sens_names[i])
          remove duplicates from sorted_collaborators, to make sure a single collaborator appears only once in the list
          i=i+1
      end
      Add collaborators 13,14 to the list if not already present
      return sorted_collaborators
end

Aggregation Algorithm: The aggregation algorithm used was weighted average aggregation. For the first few rounds, all collaborators were chosen for aggregation, but in the consecutive rounds, top performing collaborators were chosen to aggregate. The algorithm used was the same as the previous, except that the validation scores were from the same round. For example, if aggregation is to be performed for round 6, the validation scores were from round 6. Algorithm 3 shows the working flow of our Ranked Aggregation.

Algorithm 3: Ranked Aggregation

---

if round ≤ 3 **then**
  | weighted average aggregation on all collaborators ;
else
  | Sort the collaborators, as described in algorithm 2. sorted_collaborators= [ ]
  | i=0
  | **while** len(sorted_collaborators) < 7 **do**
  | | sorted_collaborators.append(wt_names[i]+tc_names[i]+et_names[i]+sens_names[i])
  | | remove duplicates from sorted_collaborators, to make sure a single collaborator
  | | appears only once in the list
  | | i=i+1
  | **end**
  | perform weighted average aggregation, using only those collaborators that are
  | present in sorted_collaborators
end

5.3 Results

Training was performed until round 7 (total of 8 rounds). The results shown in Fig. 5 were obtained on the held out validation data, which consists of approximately 20% of the training data. Taking a mean of scores among the three classes, we obtain a mean dice score of 0.81 and a hausdorff distance of 3.58.

We evaluated our model on the FeTS 2021 challenge's validation data and the scores were obtained by uploading the segmentation files to CBICA's IPP portal, shown in Table 2.

Table 2. Results on validation data (CBICA's IPP portal)

Validation scores	ET	WT	TC
Mean dice score	0.58 ± 0.259	0.639 ± 0.176	0.55 ± 0.201
Median dice score	0.659	0.6729	0.60
Mean Hausdorff95	37.47	48.92	36.69
Median Hausdorff95	27.72	51.56	23.244

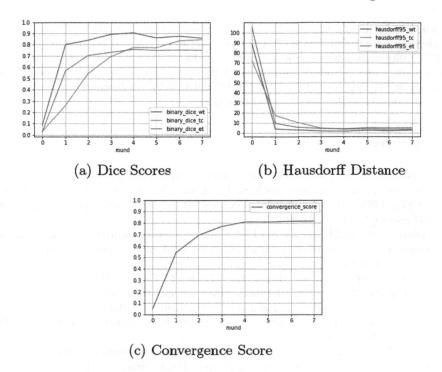

(a) Dice Scores   (b) Hausdorff Distance

(c) Convergence Score

Fig. 5. Results

5.4   Conclusion and Future Work

Our experiments suggest that there is high class imbalance in the data. Whole Tumor and Tumor Core classes are easier to detect compared to Enhanced Tumor class. Solving the class imbalance problem is difficult, as we do not have access to pixel level data [3].

Another observation is that the model overfits after training for a few rounds. This may be the due to two reasons:

1. Our learning rate of 3×10^{-4} is too high, leading to early convergence. This could also be why the model is not able to generalize well on non-IID data.
2. Due to the drawbacks of Federated Averaging. In FedAVg, coordinate-wise averaging of weights is performed and this may have a detrimental effect on the performance of the aggregated model. This is because of the permutational invariance of Neural Network parameters, wherein multiple weight combinations result in similar outputs. Federated Matched Averaging solves this problem. The paper [12] propose the Federated matched averaging (FedMA) algorithm designed for federated learning of CNNs and LSTM. This paper shows FedMA results are better for CIFAR-10 dataset even when the number of local epochs increase

Acknowledgement. We would like to acknowledge help from Shreyas N.C, Raghavendra Bhat and Pravin Chandran for providing technical help in understanding FeTS challenge 2021 framework. We would also like to thanks Robert Bosch Center for Data Science and Artificial Intelligence (RBCDSAI), Indian Institute of Technology Madras, India, Project no: CR1718CSE001RBEIBRAV for funding our project and also providing us with computational facilities.

References

1. Bakas, S., et al.: Advancing the cancer genome atlas glioma MRI collections with expert segmentation labels and radiomic features. Sci. Data **4**(1), 170117 (2017). ISSN 2052–4463. https://doi.org/10.1038/sdata.2017.117. http://www.nature.com/articles/sdata2017117
2. Bakas, S., et al.: Identifying the best machine learning algorithms for brain tumor segmentation, progression assessment, and overall survival prediction in the brats challenge (2019)
3. Chan, R., Rottmann, M., Hüger, F., Schlicht, P., Gottschalk, H.: Application of decision rules for handling class imbalance in semantic segmentation (2019)
4. Çiçek, Ö., Abdulkadir, A., Lienkamp, S.S., Brox, T., Ronneberger, O.: 3D U-Net: learning dense volumetric segmentation from sparse annotation. CoRR, abs/1606.06650 (2016)
5. Guha, N., Talwalkar, A., Smith, V.: One-shot federated learning (2019)
6. He, K., Zhang, X., Ren, S., Sun, J.: Deep residual learning for image recognition. CoRR, abs/1512.03385 (2015)
7. Li, X., Huang, K., Yang, W., Wang, S., Zhang, Z.: On the convergence of FedAvg on non-IID data (2020)
8. Liu, J., Li, M., Wang, J., Wu, F., Liu, T., Pan, Y.: A survey of MRI-based brain tumor segmentation methods. Tsinghua Sci. Technol. **19**, 578–595 (2014). https://doi.org/10.1109/TST.2014.6961028
9. Pati, S., et al.: The federated tumor segmentation (FeTS) challenge (2021)
10. Ronneberger, O., Fischer, P., Brox, T.: U-Net: convolutional networks for biomedical image segmentation. CoRR, abs/1505.04597 (2015)
11. Tresp, V., Overhage, J.M., Bundschus, M., Rabizadeh, S., Fasching, P.A., Yu, S.: Going digital: A survey on digitalization and large scale data analytics in healthcare (2016)
12. Wang, H., Yurochkin, M., Sun, Y., Papailiopoulos, D., Khazaeni, Y.: Federated learning with matched averaging (2020)

Center Dropout: A Simple Method for Speed and Fairness in Federated Learning

Akis Linardos$^{(\boxtimes)}$ ⓘ, Kaisar Kushibar ⓘ, and Karim Lekadir ⓘ

Department of Mathematics and Computer Science, University of Barcelona, 08007
Barcelona, Spain
linardos.akis@gmail.com

Abstract. This work tackles the Federated Training Task put forth by
FeTS 2021. The goal of the task is to manipulate the aggregation algorithm, including aspects like client selection and training-per-round, in
order to improve the generalizability of the segmentation algorithm as
well as the communication cost. Our work proposes Center Dropout, a
simple modification to the vanilla algorithm that does not train on the
entire consortium on every round, but selects a random assortment of
the total collaborators and proportionally increases the amount of local
learning. This way, underrepresented centers are not consistently overwhelmed by the bigger ones during aggregation steps and communication
costs are cut down. We also test another modification that smooths the
weights of the aggregation algorithm to improve fairness across centers.
We find that both techniques show benefits in terms of generalization
performance, and using several variants of the Center Dropout method,
we also achieve a significant boost in speed.

Keywords: Federated learning · Brain tumor segmentation · FETS
challenge

1 Introduction

Federated learning was introduced by Google in 2017 as a framework that allows
models to be trained locally on edge devices circumventing problems of privacy
and data traffic [12]. The aspect of privacy is particularly relevant for medical
imaging, where data is sensitive by nature, and has led to a recent surge of
studies that utilize federated learning with particular emphasis on segmentation,
including tumors of brain MRI [4,8,9,15,17], but also for the segmentation of
prostate [16] and COVID-19 affected regions [7,11,20].

The Federated Training Task, brought forth by FeTS Challenge 2021 [13]
aimed at creating a collaborative effort to improve on the technical aspect of the
aggregation algorithm, again using the case of brain tumor segmentation as test
bed. The organizers provided the infrastructure based on the Open Federated

A. Crimi and S. Bakas (Eds.): BrainLes 2021, LNCS 12963, pp. 481–493, 2022.
https://doi.org/10.1007/978-3-031-09002-8_42

Learning (OpenFL) framework [14]. A standard U-Net was pre-selected and given to the participants, but no changes to the model's structure were allowed for the scope of the challenge. The provided data was derived from 17 institutions and included T1 and T2- weighted mpMRI scans [1–3]. It was distributed after pre-processing which involved co-registration to the same anatomical template, interpolation to the same resolution, and skull stripping. Two partitioning files were made available, one including the original institution split and one splitting the largest institutions further to a total of 22 partitions. Only the natural partitioning was used for the present study.

At present, the task emphasizes on four technical aspects of federated learning: a) Weight Aggregation, b) Client Selection, c) Training-per-Round, d) Choice Validation Functions. Given those restrictions, we propose the following technical modifications for the federated training algorithm:

– Center Dropout: a technique for alleviating some of the communication cost while preserving the overall training time. By dropping centers per round, we obtain a significant boost on the validation set over the baseline while at the same time improving on the speed of the algorithm. We also find that variant of this method significantly improves upon simulated time further while still being competitive to the baseline.
– Weight Smoothing: a modification to the weights during aggregation that increase the voting power of underrepresented institutions for increased fairness. This method was also found to improve on the generalizability of the federated model.

2   Methods

In its original version, Federated Learning distributes copies of a deep learning model across *all* centers in each round. After these models are trained locally, they are sent back to the central server where aggregation takes place. This process is also referred to as the *FederatedAveraging* algorithm [12]. In more technical terms, every copy of the model takes one step on the loss space, optimizing for its respective center c with a pre-defined learning rate λ (equal across all models and centers) using the calculated gradients g_c. The equation that describes one such step is then defined as:

$$w_{t+1}^c \longleftarrow w_t - \lambda g_c, \forall k \tag{1}$$

And the aggregation step that follows is defined as:

$$W_{t+1} \longleftarrow \sum_{c=1}^{C} \frac{n_c}{n} w_{t+1}^c \tag{2}$$

with n being the total sample size and n_c the corresponding size of center c.

An important thing to note is the fact that the aggregation step weights model parameters according to the respective size of the center they were trained on. This algorithm was first developped by Google [12] bearing in mind the needs of edge devices, where it was intuitive to give a bigger vote to the better informed models–i.e. models trained on more data. In medical imaging, it's not quite as simple. Domain shift effects may occur due to cross-center variety in scanners, acquisition protocols, and even ethnicities. Coupled with the data imbalance problem, which is also prevalent in this challenge (center 1 being richer in data than the rest by a great magnitude) and we can see how weighting the models by sample size can lead to severe bias towards the more wealthy sites.

The methods we propose here seek to address this issue, in one case by varying the centers trained in each round (so that center 1 and other sizeable centers are not always present to overwhelm the vote), as well as changing the aggregation algorithm itself, smoothing the weights towards a more balanced state (Fig. 1, Fig. 2 and Fig. 3).

2.1 Center Dropout

Federated learning distributes copies of the same model across all centers which are then trained locally and sent back to the central server for aggregation. This has the inherent problem of communication cost, as sizeable deep learning models are transferred to and fro the many sites involved. Inherently, this means that the aggregation algorithm is bound to expect the slowest member before finalizing a round. To improve on this issue, we propose Center Dropout–i.e. given C total centers, we choose $P * C$ centers for training each round where P is a fixed percentage. Equation (2) then becomes:

$$W_{t+1} \longleftarrow \sum_{c=1}^{C'} \frac{n_c}{n} w_{t+1}^c, \; where \; C' = P * C \qquad (3)$$

To be comparable and fair to a baseline (i.e. a set-up without dropout), the amount of training that goes on in a single round is scaled up so that by the end of the learning process the exact same amount of training time will have passed. For our experiments we use a fixed batch size per round rather than a epochs-per-round, so as to better control the amount of data being processed. The batch size was then proportionally increased on each experiment depending on the choice of P–i.e. the center dropout percentage. If a center has less data than the indicated batch size, it loops on it until it has trained the correct amount. This way the total amount of data processed throughout the federated training is exactly the same, while communication traffic is reduced substantially as we use a fraction of the models used in the baseline per round. An additional benefit of this is that the aggregation weights naturally change in each round to reflect the relative sample sizes of participating collaborators. That way smaller centers are not consistently overwhelmed by the bigger ones, and so the final federated model is not as biased towards the wealthiest centers.

Center Dropout can also be thought of as an intermediate solution between Federated Learning and Cyclic Institutional Incremental Learning (CIIL), an

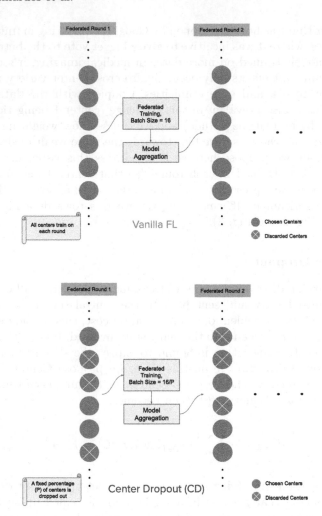

Fig. 1. In the vanilla version of federated learning, all centers train each round. To have a baseline for our experiments, we use a batch size of 16 (a center loops over its own data if it has less than that). In the case of Center Dropout (CD), we instead sample a certain amount of centers, using a batch size that is scaled up proportionally to the number of discarded centers. That way our results are comparable with the baseline, as the total training is essentially the same for a fixed amount of rounds.

alternative distributed learning technique in which a single model is transferred sequentially from center to center rather than aggregating copies of local models [6,17,18]. In essence, a Center Dropout of all centers but one would be equivalent to CIIL, as in each round there is only one model and no aggregation occurs, while a $P = 0$ (i.e., no centers dropped) is equivalent to all centers contributing in every round, which is the traditional way FL works.

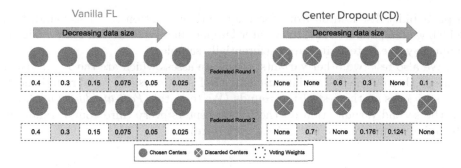

Fig. 2. Center Dropout, first intuition: Fairness. In the vanilla version of Federated Learning, the voting scheme in the aggregation step always favors the wealthiest center. This is the same in each round when all centers participate, and the weights add up to one. As we omit different centers each round, the voting scheme also changes, realigning the weights to still add up to one.

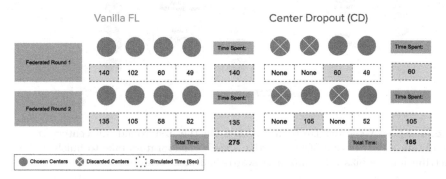

Fig. 3. Center Dropout, second intuition: Efficiency. Training moves as slow as its slowest member. By omitting centers each round, the slowest member is not always present in the pool of collaborators. This means that the total training time will tend to be much faster. In this figure, an example of two rounds in total is illustrated.

While Center Dropout takes its name and, on a high-level, its inspiration from the widely used neuron dropout [19], our method makes no changes to the network architecture during training, and is particular to federated learning. The similarity comes from the fact that Center Dropout essentially conducts dropout of collaborators per round much like the traditional technique drops out neurons per iteration during training. Furthermore, it should not be confused with Federated Dropout [5], another technique for improving communication efficiency that does not drop centers, but trains smaller versions of the global model locally instead.

Finally, using the best performing setup, we optimize this set-up for time, by running a single round with a batch size of 10, gain estimates of per-center speed and use these estimates to sample selectively based on relative speed. We use a variant that we call *Speed-Weighted* Dropout, in which case we generate a probability distribution from the relative time spent on the first round, from which we sample centers for the Center Dropout in all rounds that follow (Fig. 4). That way, the fastest sites are preferentially sampled.

We also test two other variants, where we assess which are the $P * n$ fastest centers, then on the first variant use only the fastest ones every odd round and all the slow ones on the rest of the rounds (We term this *Fast-at-odd-rounds*), and on the second variant train on the fastest centers every third round, randomly dropping centers on the rest (*Fast-every-three*).

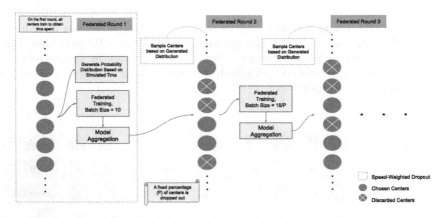

Fig. 4. Speed-Weighted Dropout (SWD): On the first round, all centers train, and we obtain a distribution of the relative speeds collaborators take to finish. Using this distribution, we bias the sampling toward the fastest centers.

2.2 Weight Smoothing

Our second approach makes no changes to the collaborators trained in each round, but manipulates the aggregation equation itself. In a recent study, one such manipulation was tested in a principled manner, replacing the original weight scheme by equal voting across all participating collaborators [10]. This was found to be competitive to the original weighting scheme that is based on the size of each institution. Here, we test equal voting as well, but also take into account a spectrum of weight values between equal weights and sample-size based weights. In particular, we test the average of the two, as well as the upper and lower quartiles of their distance (Fig. 6).

For example, given 2 centers whose initial data size would warrant a weight of (0.75,0.25) under traditional FL, the equal voting would be (0.5,0.5). We then obtain a spectrum of values between the two, corresponding to 25% (lower quartile), 50% (mean value) and 75% (upper quartile) of the distance between them. In this example, these values would be correspondingly, (0.5625, 0.4375), (0.625, 0.375), and (0.685, 0.315).

This changes equation (2) to:

$$W_{t+1} \longleftarrow \sum_{c=1}^{C} s * w_{t+1}^{c} \tag{4}$$

where s is a scalar value that can be either of the five scalars defined as:

$$s_{baseline} = \frac{n_c}{n}, \quad s_{equalVote} = \frac{1}{n}, \quad s_{avg} = \frac{\frac{n_c}{n} + \frac{1}{n}}{2} \tag{5}$$

$$s_{lowerQuartile} = \frac{\frac{n_c}{n} + s_{avg}}{2}, \quad s_{upperQuartile} = \frac{s_{avg} + \frac{1}{n}}{2} \tag{6}$$

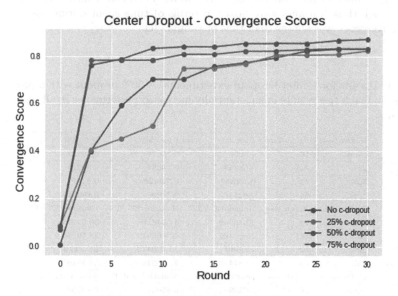

Fig. 5. The convergence scores of three CD set-ups are illustrated. A 50% c. dropout is found to converge higher than all the alternatives, while both 50% and 75% dropout converge much faster than the baseline alternative.

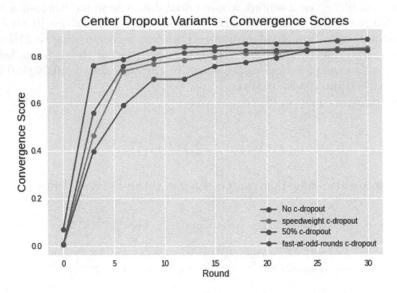

Fig. 6. The convergence scores of 50% CD and its speed-based variants are illustrated. Even though these variants were faster in terms of time spent during the 30 rounds, their convergence was slower than that of vanilla CD.

Table 1. Results for Center Dropout experiments. A 50% dropout with a proportional increase in batch size results in substantially increased performance in all segmentation metrics.

C. Dropout	Batch Size	Dice ET	Dice WT	Dice TC
None	16	0.6023	0.75637	0.60354
25%	21	0.58755	0.70387	0.60216
50%	32	**0.62857**	**0.78498**	0.6417
75%	64	0.62146	0.74899	**0.64332**
C. Dropout	Batch size	Hausdorff95 ET	Hausdorff95 WT	Hausdorff95 TC
None	16	30.40639	34.34818	30.59265
25%	21	35.62406	44.66591	38.50768
50%	32	**25.439**	**24.74043**	**25.31731**
75%	64	33.87432	38.05616	39.45167
C. Dropout	Batch size	Sensitivity ET	Sensitivity WT	Sensitivity TC
None	16	0.62994	0.85051	0.64658
25%	21	0.66112	0.87553	0.70035
50%	32	**0.69037**	0.85899	0.6968
75%	64	0.69004	**0.87832**	**0.7077**
C. Dropout	Batch size	Specificity ET	Specificity WT	Specificity TC
None	16	**0.99927**	0.99702	**0.99877**
25%	21	0.99892	0.9946	0.99798
50%	32	0.99914	**0.99737**	0.99852
75%	64	0.99902	0.99606	0.9982

Table 2. Results for variants of Center Dropout optimized for speed. The baseline refers to the traditional FL which uses no drop-out.

Center Dropout	Dice scores		
	ET	WT	TC
Baseline	0.6023	0.75637	0.60354
50%	**0.62857**	**0.78498**	0.6417
50% - Fast-every-three	0.61636	0.76677	0.60661
50% - Speed-Weighted	0.62926	0.76774	0.63153
50% - Fast-at-odd-rounds	0.61546	0.77496	0.62941
Center dropout	Hausdorff95 Scores		
	ET	WT	TC
Baseline	30.40639	34.34818	30.59265
50%	**25.439**	**24.74043**	**25.31731**
50% - Fast-every-three	29.95821	29.39877	34.822
50% - Speed-Weighted	27.97087	27.86705	29.79932
50% - Fast-at-odd-rounds	31.19735	25.66278	31.39343
Center dropout	Simulated time		
Baseline	40056.50603		
50%	36097.703293		
50% - Fast-every-three	30871.189649		
50% - Speed-Weighted	31329.380983		
50% - Fast-at-odd-rounds	**30250.973070**		

Table 3. Results for weight smoothing experiments. The lower quartile smoothing results in a significant boost in generalization performance.

Weight smoothing	Dice ET	Dice WT	Dice TC
None	0.56381	0.7629	0.6047
25%	**0.62062**	**0.79182**	**0.64865**
50%	0.54254	0.75507	0.5939
75%	0.56817	0.73514	0.5881
Equal voting	0.58637	0.77149	0.61454
Weight smoothing	Hausdorff95 ET	Hausdorff95 WT	Hausdorff95 TC
None	29.51121	33.13562	29.9334
25%	**26.23376**	**26.01608**	**27.76094**
50%	35.41347	32.53653	36.94565
75%	34.4664	33.44295	35.03869
Equal voting	30.66208	27.27246	29.08732
Weight smoothing	Sensitivity ET	Sensitivity WT	Sensitivity TC
None	0.73345	**0.86171**	**0.74909**
25%	0.65903	0.84284	0.70282
50%	**0.76691**	0.84612	0.71791
75%	0.70251	0.85442	0.70465
Equal voting	0.72821	0.83703	0.67776
Weight smoothing	Specificity ET	Specificity WT	Specificity TC
None	0.99841	0.99704	0.99793
25%	**0.99933**	**0.998**	**0.99881**
50%	0.99843	0.99625	0.99772
75%	0.99787	0.99706	0.99794
Equal voting	0.99871	0.99788	0.99868

Table 4. Final solution results in the two leaderboards.

Task-1 Leaderboard 1

	Dice_ET	Dice_WT	Dice_TC
Mean	0.55226	0.74764	0.65048
StdDev	0.27827	0.24049	0.33247
	Hausdorff95_ET	Hausdorff95_WT	Hausdorff95_TC
Mean	49.25017	25.85408	47.2764
StdDev	95.07102	28.87247	88.4407
	Sensitivity_ET	Sensitivity_WT	Sensitivity_TC
Mean	0.78496	0.88841	0.76358
StdDev	0.30752	0.15616	0.32131
	Specificity_ET	Specificity_WT	Specificity_TC
Mean	0.99677	0.99537	0.9971
StdDev	0.00467	0.00672	0.0052
	Communication Cost		
	0.798421		

Task-1 Leaderboard 2

	Dice_ET	Dice_WT	Dice_TC
Mean	0.74405	0.80927	0.7576
StdDev	0.23177	0.19344	0.26343
	Hausdorff95_ET	Hausdorff95_WT	Hausdorff95_TC
Mean	23.18087	14.84291	28.87294
StdDev	79.47217	49.55645	83.32321
	Sensitivity_ET	Sensitivity_WT	Sensitivity_TC
Mean	0.83341	0.87675	0.83323
StdDev	0.26073	0.21516	0.28683
	Specificity_ET	Specificity_WT	Specificity_TC
Mean	0.99938	0.9981	0.99913
StdDev	0.00061	0.00154	0.00124
	Communication Cost		
	0.755072		

3   Results and Discussion

We initiate our experiments by testing the Center Dropout idea, dropping out first 25% of the centers per round, then 50% and finally 75%. We use a baseline of fixed batch size 16 where no center is dropped out. The batch sizes are scaled in each Center Dropout setup, so that the (P, Batch Size) parameters correspond to (0.25, 21), (0.5, 32), (0.75, 64), thus keeping total training time equal. We run federated training for a total of 31 rounds, using a learning rate of $5 * 10^{-5}$.

The results are demonstrated in Table 1, while the gain in convergence speed is illustrated in Fig. 5. Notably, 50% dropout reaches a higher performance than the baseline and converges much faster (approximately 20 rounds earlier than the baseline).

Results are overall substantially worse for Sensitivity compared to Specificity, likely owing to the higher prevalence of healthy voxels in the brain compared to tumorous ones. Dice score is higher for WT (Whole Tumor). This is partially due to the larger volume of WT and the increased complexity of the TC and ET areas whose texture is more heterogeneous. The Hausdorff metric is boundary based, making it less sensitive to the number of voxels. In this case, performance across WT, TC and ET is more or less the same.

Building upon the best performing Center Dropout set-up that is (0.5, 32), we also test the variants that selectively sample centers based on their speed as evaluated on the first round. The results show significant gain in speed (as high as 25% reduced training time compared to the baseline) and a boost in performance over the baseline in all cases Table 2. The methods optimized for speed exhibit a benefit of approximately 14% in terms of time over the standard 50% Center Dropout, but their performance suffers, particularly on the Hausdorff95 metrics, even though they are still better than the baseline. Interestingly, although *Fast-at-odd-rounds* parses the entire data by interspersing the slowest with the fastest members it performs worse than the stochastic *Speed-Weighted* counterpart, hinting that the stochastic sampling of centers benefits performance. An important thing to note is that, although for our method we would ideally drop out centers both from the training and the validation process in each federated round, the provided infrastructure only allows dropping out collaborators from the training process. Thus some communication cost persists as models are still send to all collaborators for validation in all rounds. We could thus expect an even greater gain in speed if that part was omitted as well.

For each of our Weight Smoothing experiments, we use a total of 21 rounds down from 31 due to time limitations. We consider five set-ups: the two extremes that are the traditional FL without any smoothing, and equal voting, in which all weights have the same value, and three values in between that are the mean and the two quartiles. Our results–presented in Table 3–demonstrate that the lower quartile smoothing achieves a significant boost over the baseline in the validation set.

We finally sought to combine the two experiments, but found that naively combining our best results–i.e. lower quartile (25%) weight smoothing and a 50% center dropout–did not perform well and resulted in a loss of performance. This is unsurprising, considering that in Center Dropout the centers shift per round, and thus the weights are always shifting as well (in rounds where centers with more data are absent, underrepresented centers gain a significant vote without the need for smoothing). We believe that although Center Dropout does not combine well with the fixed Weight Smoothing method we proposed here, it would warrant further exploration with a dynamic equivalent of this technique, where the aggregation weights are smoothed each round in an adaptive way (Table 4).

Given that the CD variants did not perform as well as the simple 50% CD case, and that weight smoothing did not combine well with CD, we used the 50% CD as our final solution to the Task-1 of FeTS challenge. The method achieved first place in Leaderboard 1. The same method was used for Leaderboard 2, only the number of rounds was increased to 60. Results for both leaderboards are displayed in Fig. 4.

We believe the methods presented here show promise and warrant further exploration in real world studies in the future. There has been enough evidence of the Center Dropout's potential to improve both on speed and fairness in this simulated study. Moving forward, it would be ideal that the communication cost is measured rather than simulated, and thus the benefit of the method assessed more accurately, as well as allowing for the complete drop out of centers (validation during training also only happening on the selected centers). Selective dropout of centers and sub-partitions of centers based on other aspects (such as ethnicities, scanners, tumor sizes etc.) would also be interesting to explore. Weight Smoothing is another step towards making the aggregation more fair by being more inclusive of small sample sizes. Considering the immense inequality of data between hospitals coming from different countries, we believe these methods are a step in the right direction, and we expect more sophisticated aggregation techniques that account and optimize for fairness and better combine with Center Dropout to come into play in the future.

Acknowledgements. The authors have received funding from the European Union's Horizon 2020 research and innovation programme under grant agreement No 952103.

References

1. Bakas, S., et al.: Segmentation labels and radiomic features for the pre-operative scans of the TCGA-GBM collection. the cancer imaging archive. Nat. Sci .Data **4**, 170117 (2017)
2. Bakas, S., et al.: Segmentation labels and radiomic features for the pre-operative scans of the TCGA-LGG collection. Cancer Imaging Arch. **286** (2017)
3. Bakas, S., et al.: Advancing the cancer genome atlas glioma MRI collections with expert segmentation labels and radiomic features. Sci. Data **4**(1), 1–13 (2017)
4. Bakas, S., et al.: Identifying the best machine learning algorithms for brain tumor segmentation, progression assessment, and overall survival prediction in the brats challenge. arXiv preprint arXiv:1811.02629 (2018)
5. Caldas, S., Konečny, J., McMahan, H.B., Talwalkar, A.: Expanding the reach of federated learning by reducing client resource requirements. arXiv preprint arXiv:1812.07210 (2018)
6. Chang, K., et al.: Distributed deep learning networks among institutions for medical imaging. J. Am. Med. Inform. Assoc. **25**(8), 945–954 (2018)
7. Kumar, R., et al.: Blockchain-federated-learning and deep learning models for covid-19 detection using CT imaging. arXiv preprint arXiv:2007.06537 (2020)

8. Li, W., et al.: Privacy-preserving federated brain Tumour segmentation. In: Suk, H.-I., Liu, M., Yan, P., Lian, C. (eds.) MLMI 2019. LNCS, vol. 11861, pp. 133–141. Springer, Cham (2019). https://doi.org/10.1007/978-3-030-32692-0_16

9. Li, X., Gu, Y., Dvornek, N., Staib, L.H., Ventola, P., Duncan, J.S.: Multi-site fMRI analysis using privacy-preserving federated learning and domain adaptation: abide results. Med. Image Anal. **65**, 101765 (2020)

10. Linardos, A., Kushibar, K., Walsh, S., Gkontra, P., Lekadir, K.: Federated learning for multi-center imaging diagnostics: a study in cardiovascular disease. arXiv preprint arXiv:2107.03901 (2021)

11. Liu, B., Yan, B., Zhou, Y., Yang, Y., Zhang, Y.: Experiments of federated learning for covid-19 chest x-ray images. arXiv preprint arXiv:2007.05592 (2020)

12. McMahan, B., Moore, E., Ramage, D., Hampson, S., y Arcas, B.A.: Communication-efficient learning of deep networks from decentralized data. In: Artificial Intelligence and Statistics. pp. 1273–1282. PMLR (2017)

13. Pati, S., et al.: The federated tumor segmentation (FeTS) challenge. arXiv preprint arXiv:2105.05874 (2021)

14. Reina, G.A., et al.: Openfl: an open-source framework for federated learning. arXiv preprint arXiv:2105.06413 (2021)

15. Roy, A.G., Siddiqui, S., Pölsterl, S., Navab, N., Wachinger, C.: Braintorrent: a peer-to-peer environment for decentralized federated learning. arXiv preprint arXiv:1905.06731 (2019)

16. Sarma, K.V., et al.: Federated learning improves site performance in multicenter deep learning without data sharing. J. Am. Med. Inform. Assoc. **28**(6), 1259–1264 (2021)

17. Sheller, M.J., et al.: Federated learning in medicine: facilitating multi-institutional collaborations without sharing patient data. Sci. Rep. **10**(1), 1–12 (2020)

18. Sheller, M.J., Reina, G.A., Edwards, B., Martin, J., Bakas, S.: Multi-institutional deep learning modeling without sharing patient data: a feasibility study on brain tumor segmentation. In: Crimi, A., Bakas, S., Kuijf, H., Keyvan, F., Reyes, M., van Walsum, T. (eds.) BrainLes 2018. LNCS, vol. 11383, pp. 92–104. Springer, Cham (2019). https://doi.org/10.1007/978-3-030-11723-8_9

19. Srivastava, N., Hinton, G., Krizhevsky, A., Sutskever, I., Salakhutdinov, R.: Dropout: a simple way to prevent neural networks from overfitting. J. Mach. Learn. Res. **15**(1), 1929–1958 (2014)

20. Yang, D., et al.: Federated semi-supervised learning for Covid region segmentation in chest CT using multi-national data from China, Italy, Japan. Med. Image Anal. **70**, 101992 (2021)

Brain Tumor Segmentation Using Two-Stage Convolutional Neural Network for Federated Evaluation

Kamlesh Pawar[1,2(✉)] ⓘ, Shenjun Zhong[1,5], Zhaolin Chen[1,4] ⓘ, and Gary Egan[1,2,3] ⓘ

[1] Monash Biomedical Imaging, Monash University, Melbourne, VIC, Australia
kamlesh.pawar@monash.edu
[2] School of Psychological Sciences, Monash University, Melbourne, VIC, Australia
[3] ARC Center of Excellence for Integrative Brain Functions, Monash University, Melbourne, VIC, Australia
[4] Department of Data Science and AI, Faculty of Information Technology, Monash University, Melbourne, VIC, Australia
[5] National Imaging Facility, Melbourne, VIC, Australia

Abstract. A deep learning method is proposed for brain tumor segmentation using a two-stage encoder-decoder convolutional neural network (CNN). To improve the generalization of the proposed network for federated evaluation, we propose a two-stage encoder-decoder CNN that performs coarse segmentation at stage-I and fine segmentation at stage-II. Stage-I consists of an ensemble of three predictions on the orthogonal slices of a subject. In stage-II, the predictions of the first stage are used to crop the region of interest consisting of the tumor region and a fine grain segmentation is performed on the cropped image. A single ResUNet was used for stage-I and seven different networks were used for stage-II. Heavy data augmentation consisting of geometric transformation and random contrast was used to avoid overfitting and improve the generalization. The mean dice scores on 21 imaging sites evaluated in a federated manner achieved dice scores of 0.8659, 0.7708, and 0.7714 for the whole tumor, tumor core, and enhancing tumor respectively. The method ranked second in the federated evaluation task.

Keywords: Brain tumor segmentation · Convolutional neural network · Medical imaging

1 Introduction

Automatic brain tumor segmentation can minimize the intra-reader variability [1] in delineating tumor regions which may result in a more accurate diagnosis of the extent of disease. The brain tumor segmentation challenge (BRATS) [2–5] provides multiparametric MR image datasets to develop automated segmentation methods. Although the dataset is heterogeneous, the generalization of the methods developed using this dataset to different imaging sites is still uncertain. Training the models on large datasets from many imaging sites is needed to develop generalized models. However, the privacy

© The Author(s), under exclusive license to Springer Nature Switzerland AG 2022
A. Crimi and S. Bakas (Eds.): BrainLes 2021, LNCS 12963, pp. 494–505, 2022.
https://doi.org/10.1007/978-3-031-09002-8_43

of patient information is a constraining factor in the availability of such datasets. To address the issues of privacy and generalization, this year a separate challenge named 'Federated Brain Tumor Segmentation (FeTS)' [6, 7] was launched.

FeTS21 consists of two tasks: (i) develop federated model aggregation algorithm and train a model with the unbalanced and non-IID dataset from each imaging site; and (ii) assess the performance of a model trained on one set of data from multiple sites to another set of unseen data from different imaging sites in a federated evaluation. FeTS provides a subset of the BRATS dataset to train and validate the models in the federated environment. In this work, we focus on the second task of the challenge and develop a deep learning [8] based model to segment tumor regions using multi-parametric T1, T2, T1c, and FLAIR images. Our method uses an ensemble of 2d convolutional neural networks [9, 10] to predict the tumor region in the 3D images. Specifically, a two-stage convolutional neural network, one for coarse segmentation and another for fine-grain segmentation was used to accurately segment brain tumors. This work aimed to validate the hypothesis that an ensemble of models trained with data augmentation can achieve better accuracy and generalization.

2 Methods

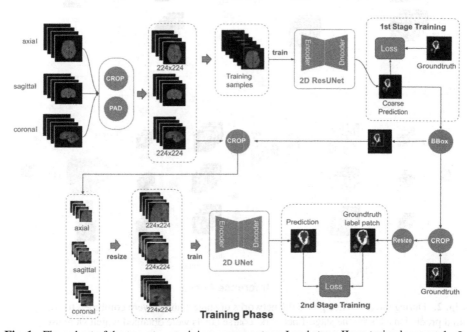

Fig. 1. Flow chart of the two-stage training process; stage-I and stage-II are trained separately. In stage-I, a Unet with Reset50 encoder was trained on 2D slices in all three orientations. In stage-II, multiple Unet's were trained using the cropped images resized to 224 × 224.

2.1 Dataset

The dataset consisted of 340 multi-parametric (T1, T2, T1c, and FLAIR) 3D images from 17 different imaging sites, with the number of images from each site varying. We used 272 images for training and 69 images were used for validating the model. The split was performed based on the number of images per site. In the validation dataset, sites with a minimum number of images were included to increase the diversity in the validation data. The validation data was composed of the images from site numbers 3, 4, 8, 9, 10, 11, 12, 14, 15, and 17.

Separately a validation dataset of 111 subjects was provided by the organizers of FeTS without ground truth labels. The segmentation labels for the validation dataset were uploaded on the compute infrastructure web link provided by the organizers to compute the results.

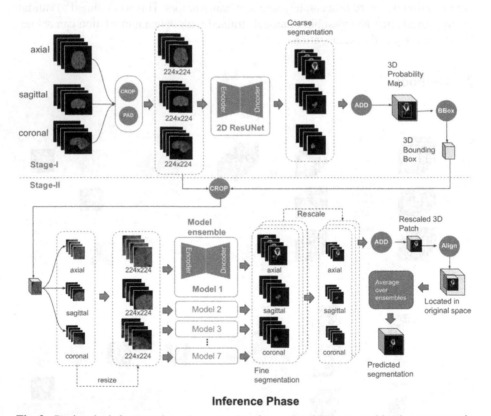

Inference Phase

Fig. 2. During the inference phase the networks of stage-I and II were combined to compute the final predictions. Using the stage-I network, coarse labels were obtained which were used to crop the input images; the cropped images were processed using the stage-II networks (seven in total). The predicted probabilities from all the predictions were added and final labels were obtained from the aggregated probability map.

2.2 Algorithm and Deep Learning Network

We proposed a two-stage deep learning based approach inspired by one of the submissions [1] of the TN-SCUI challenge to accurately segment brain tumors. Stage-I processes the whole image volume and obtains a coarse label. In stage II, only the region of interest (ROI) containing the tumor was processed thus providing better delineation of the tumor edges. Figure 1 shows the training process of the two-stage network. In stage I, a Unet with Resent50 encoder was trained to predict the labels on 2D slices of the image. The network was trained on slices in all three orientations with data augmentation, and the original slices were cropped or zero-padded to match network input dimension (i.e. 224 × 224). In the second stage-II, seven different encoder-decoder networks were trained on the cropped images and labels. The cropping was based on the bounding box generated from the coarse segmentation in the first stage. The rectangular bounding box was defined such that it covers 125% of the tumor region. The cropped regions of both the input images and labels were then resized to 224 × 244 size for training the network. We used nearest-neighbor interpolation for both image and label.

The architecture and encoders for the eight networks used in the algorithm are presented in Table 1. The architectures consisted of Unet [11, 12], Unet plus-plus [12], and feature pyramid networks (FPN) [13]; encoder consisted of resnet [14], dual path network [15], inception residual network [16], densely connected network [17] and efficientnet network [18].

Table 1. Encoder-Decoder architectures and number of parameters

Stage	Architecture	Encoder	Parameters (M)	Flops (G) per 256 × 256 image
I	Unet	Resnet-50	33.8	3.90
II	Unet	Resnet-50	33.8	3.90
II	Unet ++	Resnet-50	33.8	3.90
II	FPN	Resnet-50	26.1	4.23
II	FPN	DPN-92	37.9	0.79
II	FPN	InceptionResnetV2	56.7	4.12
II	FPN	DenseNet169	14.1	0.96
II	FPN	EfficientNet-B5	29.1	2.43

At the inference stage, an input image was fed into the stage-1 network to obtain a coarse label, then its cropped and resized part was fed into the stage-2 network to predict the fine segmentation labels (in axial, sagittal, and coronal directions) which were aggregated into the final 3D segmentation volume. Figure 2 shows the overall flow of the inference process as follows:

1. Input volume was first processed through the stage-I Unet in all three orientations, the 3D predicted probabilities were averaged, and coarse labels were obtained from the averaged probability map.
2. A bounding box was generated based on the coarse labels and was used to crop the original image and ground truth labels for feeding into the stage-II network. To calculate a bounding box we convert the predicted labels to a binary image, followed by five steps of dilation and five steps of erosion, the bounding box is then finally calculated using this binary image. The cropped input image and label were both resized to 224x224 using the nearest-neighbor interpolation.
3. Cropped and resized images from all three orientations processed through the stage-II network to predict the fine probability map in the ROI. There was a total of seven networks in stage-II.
4. The predicted probability map was resized to the original crop size using linear interpolation. The predicted probability consisted of 4 channels, i.e. one channel for each label. Each label was interpolated separately during the resizing step to make sure that the probabilities for each label are preserved.
5. The resized probability blob was stitched into the probability distribution of the whole image (4, 240, 240, 155) based on its original location.
6. Segmentation probabilities from all the predictions in stage-I and stage-II were averaged to obtain the final probability map.
7. The final segmentation labels were then obtained from the argmax of the aggregated probability map.

2.3 Preprocessing

Each slice of the images was normalized by subtracting the mean and dividing by the standard deviation of the slice. For training, data augmentation was used consisting of geometric transformations (affine, perspective, flip, rotate, crop, translation, grid distortion) and image intensity transformation (Gaussian blur, motion blur, random contrast). The probability of data augmentation was set to 0.6. Some of the data augmented images are shown in Fig. 3. Data augmentation was applied just before the inputs were fed to the network.

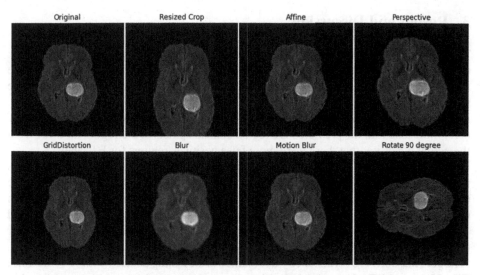

Fig. 3. Representative data augmentation examples used for training the DL network

2.4 Training

The training was performed with the Nvidia DGX V100 GPU using PyTorch deep learning library. Pytorch Segmentation library [19] was used to develop encoder-decoder Unet [11] models. The learning rate was optimized for each network based on the learning rate finder [20]. We used the Adam optimizer with logarithmic soft dice loss defined in Eq. (1). Each network was trained for 40 epochs and the model with minimum validation loss was selected as a model of choice for prediction.

$$loss = -log\left(\frac{2\sum p_p p_t}{\sqrt{\sum p_p^2 + p_t^2}}\right) \qquad (1)$$

where p_p is the predicted probability map and p_t is the true probability map and $\sum$ was over all the pixels in the sample.

2.5 Post-processing

A post-processing step was developed to minimize false-positive segmentations. The post-processing involved converting the predicted segmentation label to a binary image to determine the number of separate blobs using 8-way connectivity analysis [21]. The detected blobs were sorted by the area (number of pixels) and any blob less than 10% of the max area was considered as a false positive and removed from the predictions. A further simple post-processing step was performed which included removing all the pixels labeled as 4 if the number of such pixels was less than 500 and this threshold was found empirically using the training data. The post-processing step was applied after calculating the tumor labels using the ensembled probabilities i.e. the raw labels predicted using the ensemble network were modified using the two post-processing methods.

3 Results and Discussion

Table 2 shows the results of the online validation dataset and the test dataset used to rank the submitted algorithms. On the validation dataset which included 111 subjects, the mean dice scores were less than the median dice scores, which demonstrates that there were few cases in which the algorithms performed poorly taking the mean downwards. Hausdorff (95%) distance of 32.9 mm from ET was large compared to WT (7.2) and ET (7.1) indicating that the predicted ET region contains pixels in the region far away from the actual tumor i.e. that there were more false positives regions for ET label.

During the federated evaluation phase, the algorithm was assessed on all the datasets from 21 institutions in a federated manner. The proposed method completed all the tests, given the resources were constrained on each of the federated nodes (e.g. limits on CPU/GPU wall times and on-board memory). Mean dice scores of 86.59%, 77.08%, and 77.14% were achieved for the whole tumor (WT), tumor core(TC), and enhancing tumor (ET) sub-regions, with standard deviations of 11.3%, 23.29%, and 22.79% respectively. A larger Hausdorff (95%) distance was obtained in the testing dataset, with WT (9.1 mm), TC (23.1), and ET (51.4 mm) indicating there were more false positives predicted in the test cases. Furthermore, the method achieved high specificity scores for all the sub-regions, and also achieved sensitivity scores of 88.14% for the whole tumor, 83.96% for the tumor core, and 77.16% for the enhancing tumor.

Table 2. Dice score and Hausdorff distance for 111 subject validation datasets and online test datasets from all 21 institutions

		Whole tumor	Core tumor	Enhancing tumor	Mean
Online validation dataset	Dice score (mean)	0.8922	0.8353	0.7509	0.8261
	Dice score (median)	0.9206	0.9166	0.8653	0.9008
	95Hausdorff distance	7.2	7.1	32.9	15.7
Federated evaluation across 21 sites	Dice score (mean)	0.8659 ± 0.1130	0.7708 ± 0.2329	0.7714 ± 0.2279	0.8027 ± 0.1913
	95Hausdorff distance	9.1 ± 8.1	23.1 ± 32.1	51.4 ± 89.87	27.9 ± 43.4
	Sensitivity	0.8814 ± 0.0839	0.8396 ± 0.1421	0.7716 ± 0.2334	0.8309 ± 0.1431
	Specificity	0.9991 ± 0.0008	0.9995 ± 0.0007	0.9996 ± 0.0006	0.9994 ± 0.0007

Table 3 shows the mean dice scores per site represented across a range of percentiles (5% to 95%), calculated using the mean dice score across 21sites. At the five percentile, the mean dice scores for ET and TC were substantially lower (0.2333 and 0.3241 respectively), demonstrating that there were at least 5% of the institutions with the data substantially different from the training dataset. At the 25 percentile, the dice scores were all greater than 0.8 demonstrating that the algorithms performed well in 75% of the institutions (i.e. 15 out of 21 institutions).

Table 3. Mean dice scores per institution represented in terms of percentile calculated across 21 institutions

Metric	Region	Percentiles						
		Min	5%	25%	50%	75%	95%	Max
Dice	ET	0.0527	0.2333	0.7986	0.8601	0.8877	0.9305	0.9361
Dice	TC	0.1056	0.3241	0.8099	0.8523	0.9022	0.9521	0.9547
Dice	WT	0.5186	0.6171	0.8765	0.9023	0.9184	0.9460	0.9655
Hausdorff95	ET	1.1	1.2	2.3	20.7	32.9	285.4	327.2
Hausdorff95	TC	1.5	1.8	5.9	8.6	28.0	96.8	123.7
Hausdorff95	WT	2.4	2.4	5.7	8.2	9.9	13.8	41.7
Sensitivity	ET	0.0510	0.2329	0.7695	0.8557	0.8907	0.9440	0.9472
Sensitivity	TC	0.4129	0.4817	0.8434	0.8825	0.9048	0.9608	0.9795
Sensitivity	WT	0.5838	0.7469	0.8676	0.9014	0.9254	0.9595	0.9611
Specificity	ET	0.9971	0.9990	0.9997	0.9998	0.9999	1.0000	1.0000
Specificity	TC	0.9969	0.9986	0.9994	0.9997	0.9998	0.9999	0.9999
Specificity	WT	0.9964	0.9982	0.9990	0.9993	0.9995	0.9998	0.9998

One observation from the visual inspection was that for the images where the ground truth labels were fragmented (Fig. 4), the proposed algorithm did not perform well with lower dice scores for all three types of tumor. However, for the cases where the ground truth labels were smooth (Fig. 5), the algorithm performed well with high Dice scores.

Using 2D models might potentially have the benefits of transferring from pre-train models on large natural image datasets, e.g. ImageNet [22] and public medical imaging datasets. This is a proven technique that can improve the model performance in medical imaging tasks [23]. Compared to 3D models, there are more choices of pre-trained 2D models that can be used. 2D models require less memory compared to their 3D counterparts for both training and inference. Due to limited GPU memory, training large 3D models (deep and wide) is not feasible which can impact the overall performance of the model.

In this work we focused on two aspects of the segmentation problem, one is the accuracy and another is the generalization. The accuracy is improved by using two-stage CNN's while we rely on heavy data augmentation and large ensemble for the generalization of the model. The two-stage network was used to enable more precise segmentation of boundary regions of the tumor due to the large effective tumor size in stage-II of the network. Apart from the effective larger image size in stage-II of the net-work, the proposed methods also have a computational advantage. The stage-II network needs to perform predictions only on the tumor region which is much smaller than the whole image and hence the stage-II prediction need to be performed on a relatively small number of slices. The stage-II inference thus requires 4x-6x less computation (based on the size of the tumor) than the stage-I network. The computation saving comes from

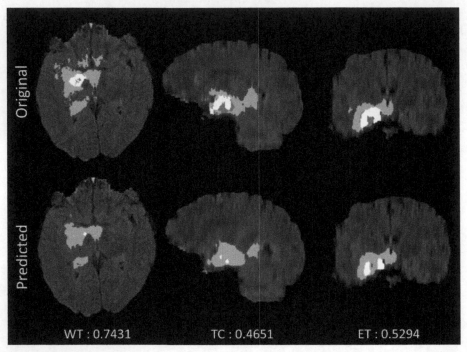

Fig. 4. Image overlay showing FLAIR image with original segmentation mask (top row) and predicted segmentation mask (bottom row). An example case where the algorithm underperformed with low Dice similarity scores; white- label 4, yellow-label 2, and orange-label 1. (Color figure online)

predicting on a few slices containing only the tumor region. This enables us to use more stage-II networks in an ensemble.

The online data set did not represent the true out of distribution scenarios and the model was trained on the similar data distribution. The mean dice scores for the three tumor regions on the online validation was 0.8261. On the other hand, the federated evaluation was performed on 21 imaging sites across the globe and represented a true data variability found in real-world scenarios. Our method achieved a mean dice score of 0.8027 which was ~2.8% degradation in the overall performance of the model. The whole tumor region degraded comparatively more (0.8922 to 0.8659) while the enhancing tumor improved (0.7509 to 7714). Although the method here is presented for the brain tumor segmentation for the federated evaluation, however, the framework of using 2D CNNs for the 3D imaging task can be translated to other MRI imaging applications such as deep learning based image reconstruction [24], motion artifact correction [25] and denoising of the images [26].

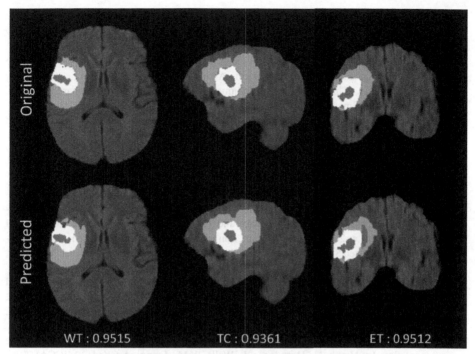

WT : 0.9515   TC : 0.9361   ET : 0.9512

Fig. 5. Image overlay showing FLAIR image with original segmentation mask (top row) and predicted segmentation mask (bottom row). An example case where the algorithm performed well with high Dice similarity scores; white- label 4, yellow-label 2, and orange-label 1. (Color figure online)

4   Conclusion

We developed an ensemble of multistage deep learning based pipelines capable of segmenting different types of tumors. A Federated evaluation on 21 imaging sites resulted in a mean dice score of 0.8027 suggesting that the proposed automated segmentation methods can segment brain tumors with an 80% match to the human reader. A little degradation in performance (~2.8%) in federated evaluation suggests that the proposed method can generalize well on the unseen out of distribution datasets.[1]

References

1. Mazzara, G.P., Velthuizen, R.P., Pearlman, J.L., Greenberg, H.M., Wagner, H.: Brain tumor target volume determination for radiation treatment planning through automated MRI segmentation. Int. J. Radiation Oncol. Biol. Phys. **59**, 300–312 (2004)
2. Bakas, S., et al.: Advancing the cancer genome atlas glioma MRI collections with expert segmentation labels and radiomic features. Scientific Data **4**, 170117 (2017)

---

[1] code repository: https://github.com/kamleshpawar17/FeTS2021

3. Bakas, S., et al.: Identifying the best machine learning algorithms for brain tumor segmentation, progression assessment, and overall survival prediction in the BRATS challenge. arXiv preprint arXiv:1811.02629 (2018)
4. Bakas, S., et al.: Segmentation labels and radiomic features for the pre-operative scans of the TCGA-LGG collection. The Cancer Imaging Archive **286** (2017)
5. Menze, B.H., et al.: The multimodal brain tumor image segmentation benchmark (BRATS). IEEE Trans. Med. Imag. **34**(10), 1993 (2015)
6. Pati, S., et al.: The federated tumor segmentation (FeTS) challenge. arXiv preprint arXiv: 2105.05874 (2021)
7. Reina, G.A., et al.: OpenFL: An open-source framework for Federated Learning. arXiv preprint arXiv:2105.06413 (2021)
8. LeCun, Y.A., Bengio, Y., Hinton, G.E.: Deep learning. Nature **521**, 436–444 (2015)
9. Pawar, K., Zhaolin Chen, N., Shah, J., Egan, G.F.: An ensemble of 2D convolutional neural network for 3D brain tumor segmentation. In: Crimi, Alessandro, Bakas, Spyridon (eds.) Brainlesion: Glioma, Multiple Sclerosis, Stroke and Traumatic Brain Injuries: 5th International Workshop, BrainLes 2019, Held in Conjunction with MICCAI 2019, Shenzhen, China, October 17, 2019, Revised Selected Papers, Part I, pp. 359–367. Springer International Publishing, Cham (2020). https://doi.org/10.1007/978-3-030-46640-4_34
10. Pawar, K., Chen, Z., Shah, N.J., Egan, G.: Residual encoder and convolutional decoder neural network for glioma segmentation. In: Crimi, A., Bakas, S., Kuijf, H., Menze, B., Reyes, M. (eds.) BrainLes 2017. LNCS, vol. 10670, pp. 263–273. Springer, Cham (2018). https://doi.org/10.1007/978-3-319-75238-9_23
11. Ronneberger, O., Fischer, P., Brox, T.: U-Net: convolutional networks for biomedical image segmentation. In: Navab, N., Hornegger, J., Wells, W.M., Frangi, A.F. (eds.) MICCAI 2015. LNCS, vol. 9351, pp. 234–241. Springer, Cham (2015). https://doi.org/10.1007/978-3-319-24574-4_28
12. Zhou, Z., Siddiquee, M.M.R., Tajbakhsh, N., Liang, J.: Unet++: a nested u-net architecture for medical image segmentation. In: Deep learning in medical image analysis and multimodal learning for clinical decision support, pp. 3–11. Springer (2018)
13. Lin, T.-Y., Dollár, P., Girshick, R., He, K., Hariharan, B., Belongie, S.: Feature pyramid networks for object detection. In: Proceedings of the IEEE conference on computer vision and pattern recognition, pp. 2117–2125 (2017)
14. He, K.M., Zhang, X.Y., Ren, S.Q., Sun, J.: Deep Residual Learning for Image Recognition. Proc Cvpr Ieee 770–778 (2016)
15. Chen, Y., Li, J., Xiao, H., Jin, X., Yan, S., Feng, J.: Dual path networks. arXiv preprint arXiv: 1707.01629 (2017)
16. Szegedy, C., Ioffe, S., Vanhoucke, V., Alemi, A.A.: Inception-v4, inception-resnet and the impact of residual connections on learning. In: Thirty-First AAAI Conference on Artificial Intelligence (2017)
17. Huang, G., Liu, Z., Van Der Maaten, L., Weinberger, K.Q.: Densely connected convolutional networks. In: Proceedings of the IEEE conference on computer vision and pattern recognition, pp. 4700–4708 (2017)
18. Tan, M., Le, Q.: Efficientnet: rethinking model scaling for convolutional neural networks. In: International Conference on Machine Learning, pp. 6105–6114. PMLR
19. Yakubovskiy, P.: Segmentation Models Pytorch. GitHub Repository (2020). https://github.com/qubvel/segmentation_models.pytorch
20. Smith, L.N.: Cyclical learning rates for training neural networks. In: 2017 IEEE winter conference on applications of computer vision (WACV), pp. 464–472. IEEE (2017)
21. Wu, K., Otoo, E., Shoshani, A.: Optimizing connected component labeling algorithms. In: Medical Imaging 2005: Image Processing, vol. 5747, pp. 1965–1976. SPIE (2005)

22. Deng, J., Dong, W., Socher, R., Li, L.-J., Li, K., Fei-Fei, L.: Imagenet: a large-scale hierarchical image database. In: 2009 IEEE conference on computer vision and pattern recognition, pp. 248–255. IEEE (2009)
23. Alzubaidi, L., Fadhel, M.A., Al-Shamma, O., Jinglan Zhang, J., Santamaría, Y.D., Oleiwi, S.R.: Towards a better understanding of transfer learning for medical imaging: a case study. Appl. Sci. **10**(13), 4523 (2020)
24. Pawar, K., Chen, Z., Shah, N.J., Egan, G.F.: A deep learning framework for transforming image reconstruction into pixel classification. IEEE Access **7**, 177690–177702 (2019)
25. Pawar, K., Zhaolin Chen, N., Shah, J., Egan, G.F.: Suppressing motion artefacts in MRI using an Inception-ResNet network with motion simulation augmentation. NMR Biomed. **35**(4), e4225 (2019). https://doi.org/10.1002/nbm.4225
26. Pawar, K., Egan, G.F., Chen, Z.: Domain knowledge augmentation of parallel MR image reconstruction using deep learning. Comput, Med. Imaging Graphics **92**, 101968 (2021). https://doi.org/10.1016/j.compmedimag.2021.101968

CrossMoDA

Using Out-of-the-Box Frameworks for Contrastive Unpaired Image Translation for Vestibular Schwannoma and Cochlea Segmentation: An Approach for the CrossMoDA Challenge

Jae Won Choi[1,2]([envelope]) [iD]

[1] College of Medicine, Seoul National University, Seoul, South Korea
[2] Department of Radiology, Armed Forces Yangju Hospital, Yangju, South Korea
jhoci@snu.ac.kr

Abstract. The purpose of this study is to apply and evaluate out-of-the-box deep learning frameworks for the crossMoDA challenge. We use the CUT model, a model for unpaired image-to-image translation based on patchwise contrastive learning and adversarial learning, for domain adaptation from contrast-enhanced T1 MR to high-resolution T2 MR. As data augmentation, we generate additional images with vestibular schwannomas with lower signal intensity. For the segmentation task, we use the nnU-Net framework. Our final submission achieved mean Dice scores of 0.8299 in the validation phase and 0.8253 in the test phase. Our method ranked 3rd in the crossMoDA challenge.

1 Introduction

Vestibular schwannomas (VS) are benign neoplasms of the nerve sheath most commonly occurring in the internal auditory canal and cerebellopontine angle. Currently, magnetic resonance (MR) imaging is the gold standard for diagnosis and surveillance of VS, and MR imaging protocols commonly include contrast-enhanced T1-weighted (ceT1) and high-resolution T2-weighted (hrT2) images [14]. In general, smaller tumors are managed with long-term preservation rather than surgical resection [6]. Therefore, volumetric measurement of VS is critical, and a research group recently demonstrated a deep learning model for automatic segmentation of VS from ceT1 and hrT2 MR images [22]. However, the necessity of the MR contrast agent in the imaging of VS has been questioned, and an abbreviated MR imaging with only hrT2 images has been proposed as a cost-effective, faster, and safe alternative to the full MR with both ceT1 and hr T2 images [2,14]. In this context, the crossMoDA (Cross-Modality Domain Adaptation for Medical Image Segmentation) challenge[1] [3] has provided unpaired annotated ceT1 and non-annotated hrT2 images, a subset of a recently released

---

[1] https://crossmoda.grand-challenge.org/.

publicly available imaging dataset [20,21]. The challenge participants were evaluated with results of segmentation of VS and the cochlea, a key anatomical structure in the treatment planning of VS, on hrT2 images.

Despite the recent rapid development of deep learning in medical imaging, few studies validate previous methods while most concentrate on novelty. The purpose of this study is to apply and evaluate out-of-the-box deep learning frameworks for the crossMoDA challenge. We use CUT^2 [17], a generic model for unpaired image-to-image translation based on patchwise contrastive learning and adversarial learning, to adapt ceT1 domain hrT2 domain. For the segmentation task in the hrT2 domain, we utilize nnU-Net^3 [10], a framework that showed state-of-the-art performance in multiple medical image segmentation challenges [12].

2   Related Work

Over the past few years, deep learning has been widely used for medical image segmentation, and many papers have shown great success in various tasks on different modalities [8,9,11]. However, most of the recent high-performing deep learning models are based on supervised learning which often requires a large amount of carefully labeled data. The collection and annotation of data is especially challenging for medical image segmentation because of the high cost of pixel-level labeling by experts and heterogeneous nature of medical data. Thus, there has been many research efforts on learning with limited supervision although they have not been as successful as fully supervised learning [19]. c Domain adaptation (DA) is a popular subcategory of transfer learning that tackles limited supervision by utilizing labeled data in source domains to execute tasks in a target domain. Unsupervised domain adaptation (UDA) refers to a domain adaptation task where only labeled data from the source domain and none from the target domain are available. Feature alignment is an approach for UDA that learns domain-invariant feature distributions across domains. One method of aligning feature spaces is through minimizing the discrepancy between the distributions based on measurements such as maximum mean discrepancy [25] and correlation alignment [23]. Also, the features spaces can be aligned via adversarial learning commonly based on domain classifier [5,24]. Another line of research in UDA is the alignment of input spaces instead of features that makes use of unsupervised image-to-image translation. The popular strategy in this field is the cycle-consistency constraint of CycleGAN [26] that inspired many networks such as UNIT [15] and U-GAT-IT [13], where bi-directional image translations are learned by two GANs. Some works address a one-sided image translation by utilizing some kind of content loss between domains. Benaim et al. [1] propose DistanceGAN that learns image translation by pairwise distances matching between images within domains. Fu et al. [4] propose GCGAN to preserve the predefined geometric transformation between the input images before and after

---

^{2} https://github.com/taesungp/contrastive-unpaired-translation.
^{3} https://github.com/MIC-DKFZ/nnUNet.

translation. Recently, Park et al. [17] propose CUT to maximize the mutual information between the translations based on patchwise contrastive learning. Few studies have assessed application of CUT in medical image analysis. In this study, we use CUT to translate from ceT1 to hrT2 images.

3 Methods

Since we focus on applications of the publicly available frameworks, there is no modification to the mathematical setting or algorithm of the original works. Also, most hyperparameters were set as in the default configurations of the frameworks. All implementations were performed with PyTorch [18] (version 1.7.1) on Nvidia RTX 3090 GPUs (single GPU training).

3.1 Data

The official training set includes ceT1 images with segmentation labels from 105 patients and hrT2 images without labels from a separate set of 105 patients. The VS (label 1) and cochlea (label 2) were manually segmented in consensus by the treating neurosurgeon and physicist using both the ceT1 and hrT2 images [21]. As stated in the official challenge rules, no additional data was included for training. The official validation set and test set include hrT2 MR images of 32 patients and 138 patients, respectively. The test phase is evaluated privately by the challenge organizers based on submissions using Docker containers during the evaluation phase of the challenge.

3.2 Preprocessing

Since the voxel spacings of the given training data are heterogeneous, we resample all cases to common voxel shaping of $0.6 \times 0.6 \times 1.0$ mm. Labels were also interpolated likewise for the ceT1 domain. For each case, the input volume is scaled to $[0.0, 1.0]$. Then, a center $z-$axis is calculated as the average of x and y coordinates of voxels with intensity higher than the 75th percentile of the whole volume. We crop the input volume with a size of 256×256 pixels in $xy-$plane around the center $z-$axis, resulting in an image shape of $256 \times 256 \times N$ voxels. Finally, we slice the volume data along the $z-$axis to acquire N images with the size of 256×256 pixels because the CUT model only supports 2D images.

3.3 Domain Adaptation

We employ two model configurations in the official PyTorch implementation of CUT, CUT and FastCUT, to train models to perform DA from ceT1 to hrT2 domain on the training set. The training parameters for CUT and FastCUT were all based on the default options except that no resizing or cropping is performed and the number of epochs with the initial learning rate and the number of epochs with decaying learning rate are both set to 25.

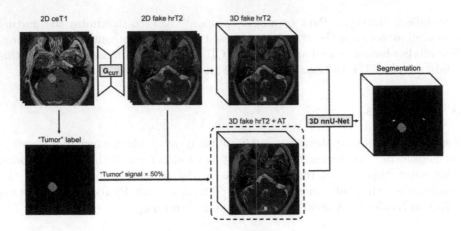

Fig. 1. Overview of our implementation of unpaired image translation with CUT and segmentation with nnU-Net. Training data is augmented by generating images with tumor signals reduced by 50% (referred to as AT).

Although DA quality is eventually evaluated in the downstream segmentation task, objective visual quality assessment is also conducted using the widely used Fréchet Inception Distance (FID) metric, which measures the distance between the distributions of sets of images [7].

3.4   Segmentation

For the segmentation task, we use the default 3D full resolution U-Net configuration of the nnU-Net framework for training and inference except that the total epochs for training was set to 250.

We apply the trained DA model on all ceT1 images in the training set to acquire fake hrT2 images. The generated fake hrT2 images are stacked along the z−axis to reconstruct a volume data for each case in the training set. The fake hrT2 volumes and labels from the corresponding ceT1 images from the training set are used for training segmentation models. We hereafter refer to the nnU-Net model trained using fake hrT2 images generated by our trained CUT model as simply CUT, and likewise for FastCUT.

On MR T2 imaging, VS is generally hyperintense but some tumors can show heterogeneous signal intensity [14]. To introduce heterogeneity of tumor signals to mimic such clinical characteristics, we generate additional training data by reducing the signal intensity of the labeled VS by 50% (hereafter referred to as AT for "augmented tumor"). Thus, with AT, 210 cases were used as training data instead of 105 cases. We evaluate segmentation results of models trained on the original training data and the data with AT.

4   Results

4.1   Domain Adaptation

The FID scores measured between real and fake hrT2 images were 32.85 for FastCUT and 11.15 for CUT. As shown in Fig. 2, while both FastCUT and CUT achieved to translate from ceT1 images to hrT2 images, fine structures including the cochlea are better depicted by CUT.

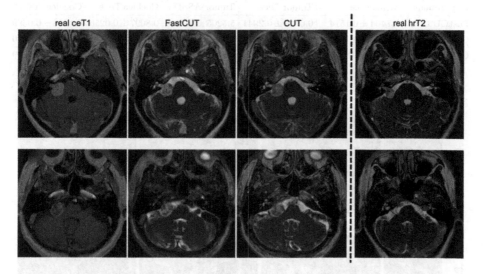

Fig. 2. Representative examples of UDA from ceT1 to hrT2. The second and third columns show fake hrT2 images generated by FastCUT and CUT from ceT1 images in the first column. For comparison, sample hrT2 images of different patients are presented in the last column.

4.2   Segmentation

All results for the segmentation task are obtained via the validation leaderboard of the crossMoDA challenge. Mean Dice scores are used to compare experiments, although other metrics including Dice scores and average symmetric surface distances (ASSD) for each label are also provided. All results are based on the ensembles of five-fold cross-validations on the training set. Ensembles are constructed by averaging softmax outputs.

Table 1 shows comparison of results on the validation set between segmentation models trained on images generated by FastCUT and CUT. Based on the higher performance of plain CUT over FastCUT, further evaluation of the effect of AT is conducted only on CUT. All metrics show better results for CUT with AT compared to plain CUT and FastCUT. Improvement of overall performance is mainly attributed to enhanced tumor segmentation as illustrated in Fig. 3. The evaluation metrics showed improvements with AT not only for VS but also for cochlea even though AT involved only altering the signal intensity of the tumors.

Table 1. Comparison of results on the validation set between segmentation models trained on images generated by FastCUT, CUT without augmented tumor, and CUT with augmented tumor.

Experiment	Mean Dice	Tumor Dice	Tumor ASSD	Cochlea Dice	Cochlea ASSD
FastCUT	0.7404 ± 0.1514	0.6711 ± 0.2941	5.5205 ± 9.0409	0.8097 ± 0.0256	0.1958 ± 0.0399
CUT w/o AT	0.7703 ± 0.1428	0.7217 ± 0.2817	1.6655 ± 1.8147	0.8188 ± 0.0219	0.1765 ± 0.0340
CUT w/ AT	$\mathbf{0.8299 \pm 0.0465}$	0.8375 ± 0.0834	1.2940 ± 1.2373	0.8223 ± 0.0235	0.1720 ± 0.0369

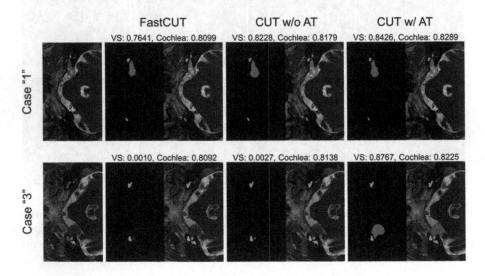

Fig. 3. Representative cases from validation set. Segmentation masks are displayed along with overlayed images and Dice scores for VS and cochlea. The first and second rows illustrate cases where tumors with cystic portions and darker signals, respectively, are better segmented by CUT with AT.

We submitted the ensemble of five-fold cross-validations of CUT with AT as the final submission for the challenge. Our method ranked 3rd in the test phase of the crossMoDA challenge with a mean Dice score of 0.8253. The mean Dice scores for tumor and cochlea were 0.8288 and 0.8217, respectively. The mean ASSD for tumor and cochlea were 1.0436 and 0.2858, respectively.

5 Discussion

In this work, we apply CUT, an unpaired image-to-image translation model, to generate fake hrT2 MR images from ceT1 MR images and nnU-Net, a framework for medical image segmentation, for segmentation of VS and cochlea on hrT2 MR images in the crossMoDA challenge. As data augmentation for the segmentation model, additional training data with lower tumor signals are generated. Our final submission achieved mean Dice scores of 0.8299 in the validation phase. In the test phase, with a mean Dice score of 0.8253, our method ranked 3rd in the crossMoDA challenge.

A significant strength of this study is that publicly available deep learning frameworks were applied on a public dataset without modifying default configurations as much as possible. Many publications on deep learning in medical image analysis focus on novel network architectures or training workflows to enhance performance. Also, they are often based on private datasets. However, specialized methods make it difficult for other researchers to reproduce the published results or apply them to different datasets or tasks. Thus, publicly available generic models may be a good choice of methods, especially in medical imaging where reproducibility and generalizability are critical to be actually used in clinical practice [16].

The current study has several limitations. First, it involves a limited number of experiments due to the circumstance of a challenge. Further experiments on different preprocessing and data augmentation may enhance performance. Also, comparison with other unsupervised image-to-image translation networks and out-of-the-box frameworks are warranted. Moreover, real hrT2 data were not used for training the segmentation model in this study. Self-training approach that retrains the segmentation model using pseudo-labels acquired from real hrT2 data would enhance segmentation results.

6   Conclusion

In conclusion, this study exploited a generic image-to-image translation network based on patchwise contrastive learning and adversarial learning to perform unsupervised domain adaptation for vestibular schwannoma and cochlea segmentation on high-resolution T2 MR images. Our results show that publicly available generic deep learning frameworks can achieve a certain degree of performance in medical imaging without a novel network or methodology.

References

1. Benaim, S., Wolf, L.: One-sided unsupervised domain mapping. arXiv preprint arXiv:1706.00826 (2017)
2. Buch, K., Juliano, A., Stankovic, K.M., Curtin, H.D., Cunnane, M.B.: Noncontrast vestibular schwannoma surveillance imaging including an mr cisternographic sequence: is there a need for postcontrast imaging? J. Neurosurg. **131**(2), 549–554 (2018)
3. Dorent, R., et al.: Crossmoda 2021 challenge: Benchmark of cross-modality domain adaptation techniques for vestibular schwnannoma and cochlea segmentation (2022)

4. Fu, H., Gong, M., Wang, C., Batmanghelich, K., Zhang, K., Tao, D.: Geometry-consistent generative adversarial networks for one-sided unsupervised domain mapping. In: Proceedings of the IEEE/CVF Conference on Computer Vision and Pattern Recognition, pp. 2427–2436 (2019)
5. Ganin, Y., Ustinova, E., Ajakan, H., Germain, P., Larochelle, H., Laviolette, F., Marchand, M., Lempitsky, V.: Domain-adversarial training of neural networks. j. Mach. Learn. Res. **17**(1), 2030–2096 (2016)
6. Goldbrunner, R., et al.: EANO guideline on the diagnosis and treatment of vestibular schwannoma. Neuro Oncol. **22**(1), 31–45 (2020)
7. Heusel, M., Ramsauer, H., Unterthiner, T., Nessler, B., Hochreiter, S.: GANs trained by a two time-scale update rule converge to a local Nash equilibrium. In: Advances in Neural Information Processing Systems, vol. 30 (2017)
8. Iantsen, A., Visvikis, D., Hatt, M.: Squeeze-and-excitation normalization for automated delineation of head and neck primary tumors in combined pet and CT images. In: Andrearczyk, V., Oreiller, V., Depeursinge, A. (eds.) HECKTOR 2020. LNCS, vol. 12603, pp. 37–43. Springer, Cham (2021). https://doi.org/10.1007/978-3-030-67194-5_4
9. Isensee, F., Jäger, P.F., Full, P.M., Vollmuth, P., Maier-Hein, K.H.: nnU-Net for brain tumor segmentation. In: Crimi, A., Bakas, S. (eds.) BrainLes 2020. LNCS, vol. 12659, pp. 118–132. Springer, Cham (2021). https://doi.org/10.1007/978-3-030-72087-2_11
10. Isensee, F., Jaeger, P.F., Kohl, S.A., Petersen, J., Maier-Hein, K.H.: nnu-net: a self-configuring method for deep learning-based biomedical image segmentation. Nat. Methods **18**(2), 203–211 (2021)
11. Isensee, F., Maier-Hein, K.H.: An attempt at beating the 3d u-net. arXiv preprint arXiv:1908.02182 (2019)
12. Isensee, F., Petersen, J., Kohl, S.A., Jäger, P.F., Maier-Hein, K.H.: nnU-Net: Breaking the spell on successful medical image segmentation. arXiv preprint arXiv:1904.08128 1, 1–8 (2019)
13. Kim, J., Kim, M., Kang, H., Lee, K.: U-GAT-IT: unsupervised generative attentional networks with adaptive layer-instance normalization for image-to-image translation (2020)
14. Lin, E., Crane, B.: The management and imaging of vestibular schwannomas. Am. J. Neuroradiol. **38**(11), 2034–2043 (2017)
15. Liu, M.Y., Breuel, T., Kautz, J.: Unsupervised image-to-image translation networks (2018)
16. Park, S.H., Han, K.: Methodologic guide for evaluating clinical performance and effect of artificial intelligence technology for medical diagnosis and prediction. Radiology **286**(3), 800–809 (2018)
17. Park, T., Efros, A.A., Zhang, R., Zhu, J.Y.: Contrastive learning for unpaired image-to-image translation (2020)
18. Paszke, A., et al.: Pytorch: an imperative style, high-performance deep learning library. In: Wallach, H., Larochelle, H., Beygelzimer, A., d' Alché-Buc, F., Fox, E., Garnett, R. (eds.) Advances in Neural Information Processing Systems 32, pp. 8024–8035. Curran Associates, Inc., Vancouver, BC (2019)
19. Peng, J., Wang, Y.: Medical image segmentation with limited supervision: A review of deep network models. IEEE Access **9**, 36827– 36851 (2021)
20. Shapey, J., et al.: Segmentation of vestibular schwannoma from magnetic resonance imaging: an open annotated dataset and baseline algorithm (2021). https://wiki.cancerimagingarchive.net/x/PZwvB

21. Shapey, J., Kujawa, A., Dorent, R., Wang, G., Dimitriadis, A., Grishchuk, D., Paddick, I., Kitchen, N., Bradford, R., Saeed, S.R., et al.: Segmentation of vestibular schwannoma from MRI, an open annotated dataset and baseline algorithm. Sci. Data **8**(1), 1–6 (2021)

22. Shapey, J., et al.: An artificial intelligence framework for automatic segmentation and volumetry of vestibular schwannomas from contrast-enhanced t1-weighted and high-resolution t2-weighted mri. J. Neurosurg. **134**(1), 171–179 (2019)

23. Sun, B., Saenko, K.: Deep CORAL: correlation alignment for deep domain adaptation. In: Hua, G., Jégou, H. (eds.) ECCV 2016. LNCS, vol. 9915, pp. 443–450. Springer, Cham (2016). https://doi.org/10.1007/978-3-319-49409-8_35

24. Tzeng, E., Hoffman, J., Saenko, K., Darrell, T.: Adversarial discriminative domain adaptation. In: Proceedings of the IEEE Conference on Computer Vision and Pattern Recognition, pp. 7167–7176 (2017)

25. Tzeng, E., Hoffman, J., Zhang, N., Saenko, K., Darrell, T.: Deep domain confusion: maximizing for domain invariance. arXiv preprint arXiv:1412.3474 (2014)

26. Zhu, J.Y., Park, T., Isola, P., Efros, A.A.: Unpaired image-to-image translation using cycle-consistent adversarial networks. In: 2017 IEEE International Conference on Computer Vision (ICCV) (2020)

Unsupervised Cross-modality Domain Adaptation for Segmenting Vestibular Schwannoma and Cochlea with Data Augmentation and Model Ensemble

Hao Li[1], Dewei Hu[1], Qibang Zhu[2], Kathleen E. Larson[3], Huahong Zhang[2], and Ipek Oguz[2(✉)]

[1] Department of Electrical and Computer Engineering, Nashville, USA
[2] Department of Computer Science, Nashville, USA
ipek.oguz@vanderbilt.edu
[3] Department of Biomedical Engineering, Vanderbilt University, Nashville, TN 37235, USA

Abstract. Magnetic resonance images (MRIs) are widely used to quantify the volume of the vestibular schwannoma (VS) and cochlea. Recently, deep learning methods have shown state-of-the-art performance for segmenting these structures. However, training segmentation models may require manual labels in target domain, which is expensive and time-consuming. To overcome this problem, unsupervised domain adaptation is an effective way to leverage information from source domain to obtain accurate segmentations without requiring manual labels in target domain. In this paper, we propose an unsupervised learning framework to segment the VS and cochlea. Our framework leverages information from contrast-enhanced T1-weighted (ceT1-weighted) MRIs and its labels, and produces segmentations for T2-weighted MRIs without any labels in the target domain. We first applied a generator to achieve image-to-image translation. Next, we combined outputs from an ensemble of different models to obtain final segmentations. To cope with MRIs from different sites/scanners, we applied various 'online' data augmentations during training to better capture the geometric variability and the variability in image appearance and quality. Our method is easy to build and produces promising segmentations, with a mean Dice score of 0.7930 and 0.7432 for VS and cochlea respectively in the validation set of the cross-MoDA challenge.

Keywords: Unsupervised domain adaptation · Segmentation · Vestibular schwannoma · Cochlea · Deep learning

1 Introduction

Vestibular schwannoma (VS) is a benign tumor of the human hearing system. For better understanding the disease progression, quantitative analysis of VS and cochlea from magnetic resonance images (MRIs) is important. Recently,

A. Crimi and S. Bakas (Eds.): BrainLes 2021, LNCS 12963, pp. 518–528, 2022.
https://doi.org/10.1007/978-3-031-09002-8_45

deep learning frameworks have been dominating the medical segmentation field [2,6,10–12,14] with state-of-the-art performances. However, supervised learning methods often require a high level of consistency between training and testing data. Consequently, such supervised methods often lack domain generalizability or ability to deal with images from various sites that have different intensity distributions, i.e., distribution shift or domain shift. Such a shift is usually caused by different image acquisition protocols or scanners; different image modalities could also be considered a domain shift problem.

Furthermore, in medical image analysis, lack of human delineations in one or multiple domains is another common issue, which is problematic for supervised learning. Unsupervised domain adaptation (UDA) is a solution for increasing generalizability of deep learning models to deal with new data from different domains.

In the cross-MoDA challenge[1], the ceT1-weighted and T2-weighted MRIs are provided, but only ceT1-weighted MRIs are labeled by experts. To obtain the segmentations on T2-weighted MRIs, we consider it as a UDA problem and propose an unsupervised cross-modality domain adaptation framework for segmenting the VS and cochlea. Our framework contains 2 parts: synthesis and segmentation. For synthesis, we apply a CycleGAN [16] to perform unpaired image translation between ceT1-weighted and T2-weighted MRIs. For segmentation, we use the generated T2-weighted MRIs as input and train an ensemble of models with various data augmentations, each of which yields candidate segmentations of VS and cochlea. We fuse those candidate segmentations to form the final segmentation.

2 Related Work

Supervised learning is an effective way for medical image segmentation when sufficient labels are available in target domain. Wang et al. [14] proposed an attention-based 2.5D convolutional neural network (CNN) to segment VS from T2-weighted MRIs with anisotropic resolution. In a following publication, Shapey et al. [12] employed this 2.5D CNN and further explored the performance of segmenting VS on both T1-weighted and T2-weighted MRIs. As we know, obtaining manual annotations is labor-intensive and time-consuming. Dorent et al. [2] introduced a novel weakly-supervised domain adaptation framework for VS segmentation on T2-weighted MRIs. In their work, only scribbles are needed as weak supervision in the target domain. They leveraged information from T1-weighted (source domain) MRIs to segment VS in the target domain based on co-segmentation and structured learning. However, in scenarios where there is no label available in target domain, UDA is a solution. Typical UDA methods try to align the image features between source domain and target domain [1,5]. Once the features are well aligned, downstream tasks, such as segmentation, are relatively easy to accomplish. CycleGAN [16] and MUNIT [4] are popular

---

[1] https://crossmoda.grand-challenge.org/.

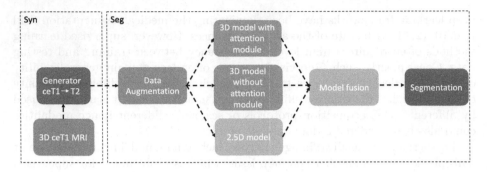

Fig. 1. Proposed overall framework. Our framework contains 2 parts: synthesis (Syn) and segmentation (Seg). We use a CycleGAN model as generator in the synthesis part. Results from the different models (and with different augmentations) are fused to obtain the final segmentation.

methods to achieve unpaired image translation. Huo et al. [5] propose an end-to-end framework for unpaired synthesis between CT and MRI images, and jointly segment the spleen on CT images without any label from CT images during training. In their framework [5], CycleGAN is used for unpaired image translation. Chen et al. [1] present a method to segment the cardiac structures from late-gadolinium enhanced (LGE) images by leveraging information from balanced steady-state free precession (bSSFP) images. Similarly, no label is used from target domain (LGE images) during training. The MUNIT is used as image translation network. While our framework is similar to the approach proposed by Huo et al. [5], we use an ensemble model with various augmentation strategies for our segmentation component to improve the robustness of our results.

3   Methods and Material

3.1   Dataset

The cross-modality domain adaptation for medical image segmentation challenge dataset (cross-MoDA[2]) contains two different MRI modalities: contrast-enhanced T1-weighted (ceT1-weighted) with an in-plane resolution of 0.4 × 0.4$mm and slice thickness between $1-1.5$ mm, and high-resolution T2-weighted with an in-plane resolution of 0.5×0.5 mm and slice thickness between 1–1.5 mm. ceT1-weighted im aging was performed with an MPRAGE sequence and T2-weighted imaging with 3D CISS or FIESTA sequence. The training set contains 105 ceT1-weighted and 105 T2-weighted MRIs, and the validation set contains 32 T2-weighted MRIs. Expert manual VS and cochlea labels are available for the 105 ceT1-weighted training MRIs. More detailed information about this dataset can be found in[3].

---

[2] https://crossmoda.grand-challenge.org/CrossMoDA/.
[3] https://wiki.cancerimagingarchive.net/pages/viewpage.action?pageId=70229053.

3.2   Overall Framework

Figure 1 displays our proposed framework. There are two parts in our framework: synthesis (Syn) and segmentation (Seg). For the Syn part, the 3D ceT1-weighted image, after undergoing pre-processing, is fed to the CycleGAN [16] pipeline to achieve image-to-image translation (ceT1-weighted to T2-weighted). Data augmentation strategies are applied on the generated T2-weighted MRIs to increase the model robustness. We send the augmented data into four different models: a 2.5D model with two different augmentation schemes, a 3D model with attention module, and a 3D model without attention module. We finally employ a union operation to fuse the outputs of each model to form the final segmentation.

3.3   Preprocessing and Postprocessing

Our preprocessing pipeline contains 5 steps: (1) non-local mean filter denoising, (2) image alignment with MNI template by rigid registration, (3) bias field correction, (4) image cropping based on region of interest (ROI), and (5) linear intensity normalization with range [0,1]. Before rigid registration, MNI template was resampled to the size of $512 \times 512 \times 128$ voxel^3, with spatial resolution $0.377 \times 0.447 \times 1.508$ mm^3. The ROIs are identified based on the labels of ceT1-weighted MRIs. We first make a common bounding box by taking the union of each bounding box over all labels. In order to cover all structures from all MRIs, the bounding box was then extended to the size $256 \times 128 \times 48$ voxel^3.

In postprocessing, we extracted the largest connected component for VS from the network output. Finally, we applied the inverse transformation from the rigid registration (step 2 of preprocessing) to move the segmentations back to their original space.

3.4   Synthesis: Image-to-Image Translation

The CycleGAN [16] framework is used for image-to-image translation in 2D. We first split the 3D cropped ROIs into 2D slices. Next, we feed those 2D slices to the CycleGAN for training; in this context, we consider the ceT1-weighted and T2-weighted MRIs to be two different domains. After the training process, we stack 2D slices back together to form a 3D MRI volume. The model convergence is determined based on the best performance by visual inspection at each epoch.

3.5   Data Augmentation

Data augmentation is widely used in medical image segmentation to help minimize the gap between datasets/domains, producing more robust segmentations. Here, we design an 'online' augmentation strategy during training and randomly apply data transformations to input images. These transformations are categorized in 3 different groups:

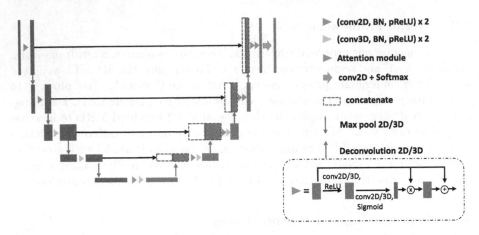

Fig. 2. Network architecture of 2.5D model from the work [12,14]. To deal with anisotropic image resolution, 2D convolutions are used in the first 2 levels, and 3D convolutions are used in levels 3–5.

- **Spatial Augmentation.** 3 types of random spatial augmentation are used: affine transformation with angle range of $[-10°, 10°]$, and scale factor from 0.9 to 1.2; elastic deformation with control points $= 7$, max displacement $= 6$; and a combination of affine and elastic deformation [9]. The same spatial augmentations and parameters are applied to both MRIs and the labels.
- **Image Appearance Augmentation.** To minimize the different image appearance between MRIs from different sites and scanners, we randomly apply multi-channel Contrast Limited Adaptive Equalization (mCLAHE) and gamma correction with γ from 0.5 to 2 to adjust image contrast.
- **Image Quality Augmentation.** In this context, image quality refers to resolution and noise level. We randomly blur the image using Gaussian kernel with σ_{blur} from 0.5 to 1.5, we add Gaussian noise with $\sigma_{noise} = 0.01$, and we sharpen the image by $I_s = I_b + (I_b - I_{bb}) \times \alpha$, where I_s is sharpened image, I_b is the image blurred with a Gaussian kernel (σ_{blur}), and I_{bb} is the image blurred twice with the same Gaussian kernel. In our case, we set $\alpha = 10, \sigma_{blur} = 1.5$.

3.6   Segmentation: 2.5D Model and Its Architecture

We leverage a 2.5D CNN [14] model to alleviate the impact of the anisotropic image resolution. Network architecture details can be found in Fig. 2. This 2.5D network uses both 2D and 3D convolutions to capture both in-slice and global information. 2D convolutions are used in the first 2 levels and 3D convolutions for the remainder. Adapted from U-Net [10], the 2.5D model contains an encoder and a decoder, and the skip connections between encoder and decoder. The max-pooling and deconvolution operations connect the features between levels. Batch normalization and parametric rectified linear unit (pReLU) are used in the network architecture. An attention module is applied to assist in segmenting

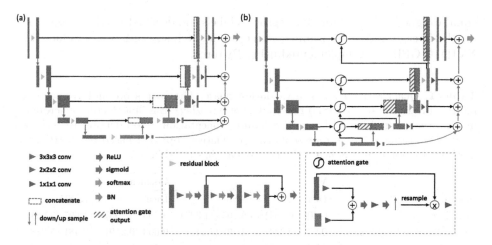

Fig. 3. The details of 3D models. Residual block and deep supervision are used in the 3D model. (a) 3D model without attention module, (b) 3D model with attention module.

the small ROI. A second 2.5D model with identical architecture was also used in the ensemble, with the only difference being in the gamma correction parameter in the augmentation stage (with $\gamma \in [0.5, 1.5]$ rather than $[0.5, 2]$).

3.7 Segmentation: 3D Model and its Architecture

We used a fully convolutional neural network for our 3D models [6]. The network architecture details can be found in Fig. 3. Similar to a 3D U-Net, it consists of an encoder and a decoder. 3D max-pooling and 3D nearest neighbor upsampling are used in both the encoder and decoder. We further reinforce the output by adding the feature maps at the end of each level. In one of our two 3D models, we employ an attention module in the skip connections to emphasize the small ROI and preserve the information from encoder to decoder. Note that the two 3D models are identical except the attention module.

3.8 Implementation Details

The Adam optimizer was used with L2 penalty of 0.00001, $\beta_1 = 0.9$, $\beta_2 = 0.999$ and an initial learning rate of 0.0002 for the CycleGAN generators [16] and 0.0001 for the segmentation models [6,12,14]. For the generators, the learning rate was left at the initial value for the first 100 epochs, and then dropped to 0 in following 100 epochs. For segmentation models, learning rate was decayed by a factor of 0.5 every 50 epochs. We evaluated our generator and segmentation models every epoch and selected the optimal model based on visual inspection of image quality for generator, and Dice score for segmentation. Based on the Dice loss [7], we defined our loss function as $1 - \text{mean}(\text{Dice})$ from multiple labels, with equal weight ($w_{FG} = 1$) for all foreground labels and decayed weight ($w_{BG} = 0.1$) for the background. The training, which has a batch size of 2, was conducted on NVIDIA GPUs and implemented using PyTorch.

Table 1. Quantitative results in validation phase. The Dice score and average symmetric surface distance (ASSD) reported as mean(stdev). Baseline denotes no cropping in pre-processing, followed by synthesis and segmentation. Crop denotes the cropped input with certain size. + represents the cumulative approach based on the previous method. Bold numbers indicate the best results in each column.

Method	VS		Cochlea	
	Dice	ASSD	Dice	ASSD
baseline	0.408 (0.284)	8.205 (11.327)	0.405 (0.195)	1.697 (3.684)
crop ($256 \times 128 \times 96\,voxel^3$)	0.637 (0.324)	2.495 (7.443)	0.603 (0.219)	2.481 (5.688)
crop ($256 \times 128 \times 48\,voxel^3$)	0.662 (0.265)	3.008 (3.916)	0.620 (0.048)	0.454 (0.158)
+ data augmentation	0.740 (0.193)	2.481 (9.592)	0.731 (0.043)	**0.288 (0.114)**
+ ensemble (proposed)	**0.794 (0.156)**	**0.634 (0.359)**	**0.741 (0.041)**	0.294 (0.060)

4   Results

4.1   Quantitative Results

Table 1 displays the quantitative results of our methods in the validation phase, reported as mean(stdev). The initial result of our method is shown as baseline in the Table 1, which uses the resampled MRIs without any cropping as input to the 3D model with attention module. Different crop sizes in the preprocessing step leads to different results, as evidenced by the results presented in Table 1. By adding various data augmentations, the performance of segmentation network is dramatically improved, 7.8% and 11.1% on Dice scores for VS and cochlea respectively. Lastly, using the model ensemble boosts the Dice score of VS to nearly 80%. We submitted the proposed method as our final result in the validation phase of the cross-MoDA challenge.

4.2   Qualitative Results

Representative qualitative results from 4 different subjects can be viewed in Fig. 4. In the first row of Fig. 4, we observe that our 2.5D method produces an accurate segmentation. Varying the augmentation parameters of the 2.5D model improves performance in some challenging cases (e.g., fourth row of Fig. 4(c)). However, in some cases, both 2.5D models under-segments the VS, which can be seen in the second and third rows of Fig. 4(b,c). In such cases, 3D models compensate for this tendency of the 2.5D models. Although the attention module has good ability to capture small ROIs, which can be observed in the second row of Fig. 4(e), it may also lead to over-fitting (first and third rows of Fig. 4(e)).

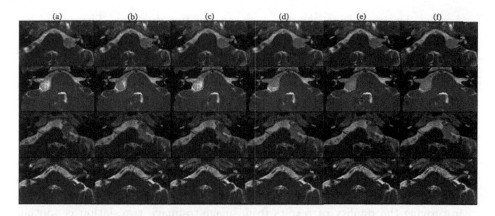

Fig. 4. Segmentation results from 4 different subjects. Red, VS, green, cochlea. (a) Input image. (b) 2.5D model with $\gamma \in [0.5, 2]$. (c) 2.5D model with $\gamma \in [0.5, 1.5]$. (d) 3D model without attention. (e) 3D model with attention. (f) Final segmentation. While each individual model has performance issues in some rows, the final model fusion step produces consistently good segmentations for all rows.

Thus, we also include a 3D model without attention module (first and third rows of Fig. 4(d)) in the model ensemble for best results. The model fusion balances the strengths of the individual models and is able to produce consistently good segmentations in a variety of images (Fig. 4(f)).

5   Discussion

There are four main design choices of our method that merit discussion: (1) cropping ROI, (2) image-to-image translation, (3) segmentation network, and (4) self-training strategy.

- **Cropping ROI.** Given the small size of the segmented objects and the overall MRI size, cropping an ROI is an essential preprocessing step. Using the cropped ROI as input not only reduces redundant computation and improves the computational efficiency by letting the network focus on the structures of interest increases accuracy. An additional benefit is the reduced GPU memory requirements. However, determining the optimal size for cropped MRIs is not straightforward. Too small ROIs might not fully contain all the structures of interest; however, too large ROIs would negatively impact the quality of the image-to-image translation and segmentation results by increasing the intensity variability in the input samples. How to balance the size of ROIs and the quality of generated MRIs from image-to-image translation remains an important problem.
- **Image-to-Image Translation.** Image-to-image translation is a critical step in our pipeline and generally in UDA problems [1,5]. Moreover, generating well-aligned pseudo T2-weighted MRIs from source domain (i.e., from ceT1-weighted MRIs) could determine the accuracy of segmentations in the target

domain, by minimizing the gap between the two domains. Thus, choosing a suitable image-to-image translation method is important. In our experiments, we employ CycleGAN [16], a popular method for unpaired image-to-image translation. However, synthesis artifacts (intensity shift between slices) appear along the depth direction of generated images in 2D CycleGAN. This is a common issue of 2D CycleGAN for translating volumetric MRIs, since slices are mapped independently from each other during training. We also found that 3D CycleGAN requires large amount of GPU memory, and the quality of images generated by using downsampled input MRIs is not satisfactory. Furthermore, patch-based 3D CycleGAN approaches could blur MRIs along the borders of the patches. However, modifying the architecture of the generator in CycleGAN pipeline could lead to satisfactory results [15]. Thus, improving the quality of results from image-to-image translation is another way to boost the performance. This argument is not only about the training manner of CycleGAN pipeline, but also more generally for methods such as CUT [8] and MUNIT [4].

- **Segmentation Network.** In our pipeline, the segmentation performance is primarily determined by the quality of the generated MRIs in the target domain. Nevertheless, given the same input MRIs, different segmentation models produce different results. In our work, we combine results from an ensemble of models to form the final segmentation, since each model could bring different advantages, even with small changes. The design choices then become the specific models and the ensembling strategy. Additional models with different hyper-parameters could thus improve the segmentation results. The good performance of the top teams in the challenge [3] suggests that the nnU-Net [13], which is a well-known framework for biomedical image segmentation, could provide a good alternative for our ensemble models. Additionally, while we currently use a simple union operation, a more sophisticated ensembling strategy could be designed to minimize the weaknesses of each model while maximizing the strengths.

- **Self-training Strategy.** Finally, the training strategy contributes to the accuracy of segmentation results. Compared to other teams [3], our training strategy is potentially the biggest limitation of our work, since we just use traditional supervised learning after generating T2-weighted MRIs. Following this training strategy, we only use the generated images instead of the real images in the segmentation task, which leads to our model lacking information in the original target domain. In an ideal situation, the features of generated T2-weighted MRIs should be very close or identical to the target domain, and the segmentation model could achieve a good accuracy by leveraging those features. However, given the limitations of image-to-image translation, not all of the generated T2-weighted MRIs are well-aligned to the target domain. Self-training could be a good approach to better handle such situations in the challenge [3]; this may involve directly segmenting real T2-weighted MRIs by a pre-trained model with generated T2-weighted MRIs as inputs, and designing an algorithm to find plausible segmentations among the results. Next, we could use these plausible segmentations as 'ground truths' to further fine-tune the pre-trained segmentation model. Iterating this process could further improve the segmentation accuracy. We believe that using such a self-training strategy would improve the final segmentation results.

6   Conclusion

In this work, we proposed an unsupervised cross-modality domain adaptation framework for VS and cochlear segmentation. There are two parts in our framework: synthesis and segmentation. We applied various 'online' data augmentations to deal with the MRIs from different sites and scanners. In addition, a model ensemble is used for increasing the performance. In the validation stage of the crossMoDA challenge, our method shows promising results.

Acknowledgments. This work was supported, in part, by NIH grant R01-NS094456.

References

1. Chen, C., et al.: Unsupervised multi-modal style transfer for cardiac MR segmentation. In: Pop, M., et al. (eds.) STACOM 2019. LNCS, vol. 12009, pp. 209–219. Springer, Cham (2020). https://doi.org/10.1007/978-3-030-39074-7_22
2. Dorent, R., et al.: Scribble-based domain adaptation via co-segmentation. In: Martel, A.L., et al. (eds.) MICCAI 2020. LNCS, vol. 12261, pp. 479–489. Springer, Cham (2020). https://doi.org/10.1007/978-3-030-59710-8_47
3. Dorent, R., et al.: Crossmoda 2021 challenge: benchmark of cross-modality domain adaptation techniques for vestibular schwnannoma and cochlea segmentation. arXiv preprint arXiv:2201.02831 (2022)
4. Huang, X., Liu, M.Y., Belongie, S., Kautz, J.: Multimodal unsupervised image-to-image translation. In: Proceedings of the European Conference on Computer Vision (ECCV), pp. 172–189 (2018)
5. Huo, Y., Xu, Z., Bao, S., Assad, A., Abramson, R.G., Landman, B.A.: Adversarial synthesis learning enables segmentation without target modality ground truth. In: 2018 IEEE 15th International Symposium on Biomedical Imaging (ISBI 2018), pp. 1217–1220. IEEE (2018)
6. Li, H., Zhang, H., Johnson, H., Long, J.D., Paulsen, J.S., Oguz, I.: MRI subcortical segmentation in neurodegeneration with cascaded 3D CNNs. In: Medical Imaging 2021: Image Processing. vol. 11596, p. 115960W. International Society for Optics and Photonics (2021)
7. Milletari, F., Navab, N., Ahmadi, S.A.: V-Net: fully convolutional neural networks for volumetric medical image segmentation. In: 2016 Fourth International Conference on 3D Vision (3DV), pp. 565–571. IEEE (2016)
8. Park, T., Efros, A.A., Zhang, R., Zhu, J.-Y.: Contrastive learning for unpaired image-to-image translation. In: Vedaldi, A., Bischof, H., Brox, T., Frahm, J.-M. (eds.) ECCV 2020. LNCS, vol. 12354, pp. 319–345. Springer, Cham (2020). https://doi.org/10.1007/978-3-030-58545-7_19
9. Pérez-García, F., Sparks, R., Ourselin, S.: Torchio: a python library for efficient loading, preprocessing, augmentation and patch-based sampling of medical images in deep learning. Comput. Methods Prog. Biomed. **208**, 106236 (2021). https://doi.org/10.1016/j.cmpb.2021.106236, https://www.sciencedirect.com/science/article/pii/S0169260721003102

10. Ronneberger, O., Fischer, P., Brox, T.: U-Net: convolutional networks for biomedical image segmentation. In: Navab, N., Hornegger, J., Wells, W.M., Frangi, A.F. (eds.) MICCAI 2015. LNCS, vol. 9351, pp. 234–241. Springer, Cham (2015). https://doi.org/10.1007/978-3-319-24574-4_28
11. Shapey, J., et al.: Segmentation of vestibular schwannoma from MRI — an open annotated dataset and baseline algorithm. Sci. Data **8**, 286 (2021). https://doi.org/10.1101/2021.08.04.21261588 medRXiv:10.1101/2021.08.04.21261588
12. Shapey, J., et al.: An artificial intelligence framework for automatic segmentation and volumetry of vestibular schwannomas from contrast-enhanced t1-weighted and high-resolution t2-weighted MRI. J. Neurosurg. **134**(1), 171–179 (2019)
13. Simpson, A.L., et al.: A large annotated medical image dataset for the development and evaluation of segmentation algorithms. arXiv preprint arXiv:1902.09063 (2019)
14. Wang, G., et al.: Automatic segmentation of vestibular schwannoma from T2-weighted MRI by deep spatial attention with hardness-weighted loss. In: Shen, D., et al. (eds.) MICCAI 2019. LNCS, vol. 11765, pp. 264–272. Springer, Cham (2019). https://doi.org/10.1007/978-3-030-32245-8_30
15. Zhang, Z., Yang, L., Zheng, Y.: Translating and segmenting multimodal medical volumes with cycle-and shape-consistency generative adversarial network. In: Proceedings of the IEEE Conference on Computer Vision and Pattern Recognition, pp. 9242–9251 (2018)
16. Zhu, J.Y., Park, T., Isola, P., Efros, A.A.: Unpaired image-to-image translation using cycle-consistent adversarial networks. In: Proceedings of the IEEE International Conference on Computer Vision, pp. 2223–2232 (2017)

Unsupervised Domain Adaptation for Vestibular Schwannoma and Cochlea Segmentation via Semi-supervised Learning and Label Fusion

Han Liu[1]([✉]), Yubo Fan[1], Can Cui[1], Dingjie Su[1], Andrew McNeil[2], and Benoit M. Dawant[2]

[1] Department of Computer Science, Vanderbilt University, Nashville, TN 37235, USA
han.liu@vanderbilt.edu
[2] Department of Electrical and Computer Engineering, Vanderbilt University, Nashville, TN 37235, USA

Abstract. Automatic methods to segment the vestibular schwannoma (VS) tumors and the cochlea from magnetic resonance imaging (MRI) are critical to VS treatment planning. Although supervised methods have achieved satisfactory performance in VS segmentation, they require full annotations by experts, which is laborious and time-consuming. In this work, we aim to tackle the VS and cochlea segmentation problem in an unsupervised domain adaptation setting. Our proposed method leverages both the image-level domain alignment to minimize the domain divergence and semi-supervised training to further boost the performance. Furthermore, we propose to fuse the labels predicted from multiple models via noisy label correction. In the MICCAI 2021 crossMoDA challenge (https://crossmoda.grand-challenge.org/), our results on the final evaluation leaderboard showed that our proposed method has achieved promising segmentation performance with mean dice score of 79.9% and 82.5% and ASSD of 1.29 mm and 0.18 mm for VS tumor and cochlea, respectively. The cochlea ASSD achieved by our method has outperformed all other competing methods as well as the supervised nnU-Net.

Keywords: Vestibular schwannoma · Cochlea · Unsupervised domain adaptation · Semi-supervised learning · Label fusion

1 Introduction

Vestibular schwannoma (VS) is a benign tumor that arises from the Schwann cells of the vestibular nerve, which connects the brain and the inner ear. To facilitate the follow-up and treatment planning of VS, automatic methods to segment the VS tumors and the cochlea from magnetic resonance imaging (MRI) have

---

H. Liu and Y. Fan—Equal contribution.

A. Crimi and S. Bakas (Eds.): BrainLes 2021, LNCS 12963, pp. 529–539, 2022.
https://doi.org/10.1007/978-3-031-09002-8_46

been proposed [1]. While the most commonly used modality for VS segmentation is contrast-enhanced T1 (ceT1), high-resolution T2 (hrT2) imaging has been demonstrated to be a possible alternative with less risk and lower cost [2].

Supervised segmentation methods have shown to be effective for VS segmentation [3], but they require to fully annotate image data which may not be an option in practice. Weakly-supervised methods require less annotation efforts, such as scribbles and bounding boxes, and sometimes they even achieve a level of performance comparable to the supervised ones [4]. In this work, we aim at segmenting the VS tumor and the cochlea in hrT2 without any hrT2 annotations during training. We consider the problem as an unsupervised domain adaptation (UDA) problem. Specifically, we are provided with a dataset consisting of ceT1 images and hrT2 images, but only the ceT1 images have the segmentation labels.

There are mainly two types of methods to tackle the UDA problem, domain alignment and techniques based on semi-supervised learning (SSL). Domain alignment focuses on reducing the distribution discrepancy by optimizing some divergence metric [5,6] or via adversarial learning [7,8]. Domain gaps can be bridged by image-level alignment [20,21], feature-level alignment [22,23], or the combination of the two [24]. On the other hand, due to the lack of labels in the target domain, techniques originating from SSL can be utilized to improve the performance. Zou et al. [9] and Zhang et al. [25] use self-training based methods which iteratively generate pseudo labels and use them to retrain the network. To alleviate the negative impact from the noisy pseudo labels, learning from noisy labels has also received increasing interest. Motivated by [15], Zhang et al. [26] use a confident learning module to characterize the label errors and correct them to achieve a more robust training. Mean teacher [28], as another SSL-based technique, can be also used in UDA to provide competitive performance [10,27]. Inspired by previous works, we focus on exploring methods that combine image-level domain alignment and SSL for UDA.

2   Methods

2.1   Problem Formulation

For an unsupervised domain adaptation problem, we have access to a source domain $D^S = \{(x_i^s, y_i^s)|i = 1, 2, \cdots, n_s\}$, and a target domain $D^T = \{x_j^t|j = 1, 2, \cdots, n_t\}$, where Y^S and Y^T share the same K classes. In our case, source and target domains correspond to ceT1 and hrT2 respectively and $K = 3$ representing background, VS and cochlea. We aim to train a segmentation network F_t that learns from the source domain and is capable to achieve robust and accurate segmentation performance on the target domain, without accessing the target domain labels Y^T.

2.2   Image-Level Domain Alignment

Image-level domain alignment is a simple but effective method to tackle UDA problem by reducing the distribution mismatch at the image-level, i.e., pseudo image synthesis. Here, we propose to train the segmentation model F_t with the pseudo target domain images $\tilde{X}^T$, which are generated by unpaired image-to-image translation. We explore both end-to-end training and two-stage training. For end-to-end training, we rely on the Contrastive Unpaired Translation (CUT) [11] as the backbone for image synthesis and add an extra segmentation module F_t on top of the synthesized images. This method is referred as **CUTSeg**. We select CUT for unpaired image-to-image translation because it can be trained faster and is less memory-intensive than the CycleGAN [12], allowing more flexibility when adding the 3D CNN-based segmentation module. During training, we first train the CUT model alone till it achieves reasonable synthesis performance. Then we train the CUTSeg end-to-end with the CUT subnetwork initialized with the pre-trained weights and the segmentation module trained from scratch. For two-stage training, we use the CycleGAN to generate pseudo hrT2 images $\tilde{X}^T$. To improve the data diversity, we train both 2D and 3D CycleGANs and collect pseudo images from different epochs. Lastly, we train a segmentation module F_t using $\tilde{X}^T$.

2.3 Semi-supervised Training

Though image-level domain alignment can minimize the domain divergence, the unlabeled target domain images X^T are not directly involved in training the segmentation model F_t. To overcome this limitation, we propose to adapt a semi-supervised learning method named Mean Teacher [13] to make better use of X^T. Specifically, a student model along with a teacher model with the same network architecture are created and both models are initialized with the best model weights obtained from Sect. 2.2. In our semi-supervised setting, the labeled images are the pseudo hrT2 images while the unlabeled images are the real hrT2 images. During training, the labeled pseudo images are fed to the student model and the segmentation loss L_{seg} is computed in a supervised manner. For unlabeled images, we first augment the same image twice with different intensity transformation parameters. The augmented images are then fed to the student model and the teacher model separately and a consistency loss L_{con} is computed. As described in Eqs. 1–4, we use Dice loss [14] and Cross-Entropy (CE) loss as L_{seg} and Mean Squared Error (MSE) loss as L_{con}, where p_{ik} is the predicted probability of the ith voxel at the kth output channel. Note that both L_{seg} and L_{con} are used to update the weights of the student model. The weights of the teacher model are updated as an exponential moving average (EMA) of the student weights, where the EMA decay coefficient is set as 0.99. As suggested in [13], the teacher prediction is more likely to be correct at the end of the training and thus the teacher model is taken as our final F_t.

$$L_{seg} = L_{Dice} + L_{CE} \tag{1}$$

$$L_{Dice} = 1 - \frac{2 \sum_k^K \sum_i^N p_{ik} y_{ik}}{\sum_k^K \sum_i^N p_{ik}^2 + \sum_k^K \sum_i^N y_{ik}^2} \tag{2}$$

$$L_{CE} = -\frac{1}{N} \sum_{k}^{K} \sum_{i}^{N} y_{ik} \log p_{ik} \tag{3}$$

$$L_{con} = \frac{1}{N} \sum_{k}^{K} \sum_{i}^{N} (p_{ik}^{Teacher} - p_{ik}^{Student})^2 \tag{4}$$

2.4   Noisy Label Correction as Label Fusion

In this challenge, we have obtained three models (as shown in Fig. 1) that were trained with different strategies and each model alone has achieved satisfactory result on the validation leaderboard. Specifically, the first model is obtained by two-stage training using the pseudo images from 2D CycleGAN, followed by a semi-supervised learning method, i.e., Mean Teacher. The second model is initialized with the teacher model and fine-tuned using the pseudo images from 3D CycleGAN. The third model is a CUTSeg model. Training details can be found in Sect. 3.1.

Empirically, ensembles tend to yield better predictive performance when there is a significant diversity among the models. Here, we propose to fuse the labels from different models by treating the label fusion task as a noisy label correction problem. We adapt a confident learning method called **CleanLab** [15] which provides exact noise estimation and label error finding. Note that we use CleanLab to directly fuse labels at the inference phase rather than update the pseudo labels iteratively during training. Specifically, we first obtain the softmax outputs of two models and convert one output to a one-hot encoded label mask. The one-hot encoded mask is considered as a 'noisy label' and corrected by the softmax outputs from the other model. Once the labels from the first two models are fused, the fused labels are treated as noisy labels and fused again with the softmax outputs from the remaining model. The labels fused from the three models are used as our final predictions.

3   Experiments and Results

3.1   Experimental Design

In this section, we describe different methods in our experiments and summarize the training details in Table 1.

Methods #1–3. First, we compare different segmentation backbones including 2D nnU-Net, 3D nnU-Net, and the 2.5D U-Net proposed in [3], which are referred to as method #1–3.

Method #4. We utilize a semi-supervised learning method named Mean Teacher to leverage the unlabeled real T2 images. Details are described in Sect. 2.3.

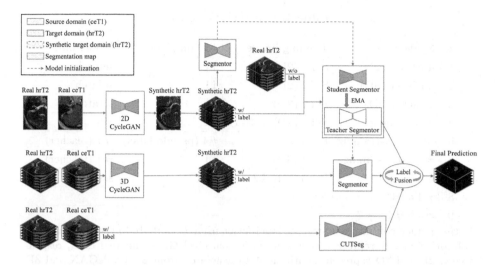

Fig. 1. The schematic diagram of our proposed method

Method #5. Here, we explore the feasibility of using self-training to improve the segmentation performance of Mean Teacher. Specifically, we use the mean teacher model to obtain the pseudo labels on the real T2 images. Then we fine-tune the teacher model obtained from method #4 with the pseudo-labeled real T2 images. The pseudo labels are iteratively updated at the end of each epoch by a confident learning method [15]. Note that methods #1–4 are trained using pseudo images generated from 2D CycleGAN.

Method #6. We incorporate more training data to further boost the performance. Specifically, we fine-tune the teacher model from method #4 on additional pseudo images generated from 3D CycleGAN.

Method #7. Here, we train an end-to-end CUTSeg model and the details can be found in Sect. 2.2.

Methods #8–9. Lastly, we fuse the predictions from different models by Clean-Lab as described in Sect. 2.4.

3.2 Data and Implementation

The dataset was released by the MICCAI challenge crossMoDA 2021 [16]. All images were obtained on a 32-channel Siemens Avanto 1.5T scanner using a Siemens single-channel head coil [17]. ceT1 images have in-plane resolution of 0.41×0.41 mm and slice thickness of 1.0 or 1.5 mm. For hrT2 images, the in-plane resolution varies from 0.47×0.47 mm to 0.55×0.55 mm and slice thickness is 1.0 or 1.5 mm. The VS and cochleae were manually segmented in consensus by

Table 1. Experimental design

#	Method	Training image	Training label	Model init.
1	nnU-Net (2D)	S-T2 (2D)	T1	scratch
2	nnU-Net (3D)	S-T2 (2D)	T1	scratch
3	U-Net (2.5D)	S-T2 (2D)	T1	scratch
4	Mean teacher	S-T2 (2D) + R-T2	T1	#3
5	#4 + self-training	R-T2	#4 (pseudo label)	#4 (teacher)
6	#4 + fine-tuning	S-T2 (3D)	T1	#4 (teacher)
7	CUTSeg	R-T1 + R-T2	T1	scratch
8	#4 ∘ #6	-	-	-
9	#4 ∘ #6 ∘ #7	-	-	-

In the method column, ∘ represents label fusion using CleanLab. In the training data column, S and R represent synthetic data from CycleGAN and real data, respectively. 2D and 3D represent synthetic data generated from 2D CycleGAN and 3D CycleGAN, respectively.

the treating neurosurgeon and physicist using both the ceT1 and hrT2 images. We randomly split the images into 185 and 25 for training and validation respectively. Since the Field of View (FoV) of the source and target domain images varies significantly, we crop each image into a cubic box, or ROI, using single-atlas registration [18]. As shown in Fig. 2, the ROI on the atlas image is manually cropped around the right side of the brain. To obtain the ROI on the left side, we flip the volume left-to-right before performing registration.

For preprocessing, in two-stage training (methods #1–6), we resample the images to the most common spacing in the target domain, i.e., (0.46875, 0.468975, 1.5) and normalize the intensity to [0, 1]. In end-to-end training (method #7), we first train a CUTSeg model for 82 epochs with an auxiliary consistency loss, which is a Mean Absolute Error (MAE) loss between the segmentation result of the real hrT2 image and the prediction from the two-stage training model. This model is used to make inferences for the testing images with in-plane resolution less than 0.5 mm. We use another CUTSeg model which is fine-tuned on the hrT2 images with in-plane resolution more than 0.5 mm to make inference for the testing images with such resolution. For all our segmentors, we use the 2.5D U-Net architecture proposed in [3]. For post-processing, we first reduce the false positive VS prediction by removing the isolated components whose center is more than 15 voxels along the z-axis from the adjacent cochlea center. Then we take the largest connected components for both VS and cochlea within each ROI.

For training, we use Adam optimizer with weight decay 10^{-4} and batch size 1. The learning rates are initialized to 5×10^{-4}, 5×10^{-5} and 2×10^{-4} for two-stage training, Mean Teacher, and CUTSeg, respectively. The hyperparameters are determined by grid-search within the range of 10^{-2} to 10^{-6}. The best hyperparameters are selected based on the segmentation performance on our

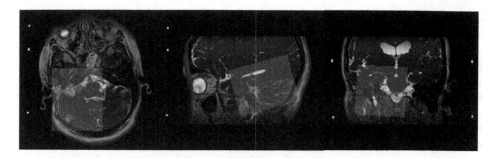

Fig. 2. An illustration of our cropped ROI on the target domain atlas image.

own validation set. The CNNs are implemented in PyTorch [19] and MONAI on a Ubuntu desktop with an NVIDIA RTX 2080 Ti GPU. For quantitative evaluation, we measure the Dice score and Average Symmetric Surface Distance (ASSD) between the segmentation results and the ground truth.

Table 2. Quantitative results on validation leaderboard

#	Method	Dice↑ (%)		ASSD↓ (mm)	
		VS	Cochlea	VS	Cochlea
1	nnU-Net (2D)	72.90 ± 22.77	68.14 ± 12.62	1.32 ± 2.83	1.27 ± 3.65
2	nnU-Net (3D)	71.77 ± 27.29	79.95 ± 4.12	2.71 ± 5.09	0.20 ± 0.07
3	U-Net (2.5D)	74.81 ± 22.14	80.39 ± 3.18	1.37 ± 2.63	0.22 ± 0.05
4	Mean teacher	80.81 ± 9.09	80.50 ± 6.36	0.63 ± 0.30	0.20 ± 0.06
5	#4 + self-training	80.73 ± 5.21	81.16 ± 4.25	0.69 ± 0.35	0.19 ± 0.04
6	#4 + fine-tuning	81.66 ± 10.5	81.24 ± 3.52	0.61 ± 0.37	0.20 ± 0.06
7	CUTSeg	81.00 ± 7.50	81.45 ± 3.53	0.66 ± 0.29	0.19 ± 0.06
8	#4 ∘ #6	82.08 ± 4.77	81.46 ± 3.51	0.58 ± 0.31	0.19 ± 0.06
9	#4 ∘ #6 ∘ #7	$\mathbf{83.02 \pm 7.72}$	$\mathbf{82.20 \pm 3.10}$	$\mathbf{0.57 \pm 0.27}$	$\mathbf{0.18 \pm 0.05}$

3.3 Experimental Results

Table 2 shows the evaluation metrics on the validation leaderboard of our developed methods. By comparing method #1–3, we notice that the 2.5D U-Net architecture inspired by [3] outperforms the 2D and 3D nnU-Nets and thus is used as the segmentation backbone in all our experiments. We also find that by incorporating the real unlabeled T2 images, our Mean Teacher model (method #4) is able to increase the VS dice score from 74.81% to 80.81%, demonstrating the effectiveness of our semi-supervised learning strategy. We observe that a smaller learning rate and appropriate model initialization, i.e., the pre-trained segmentation model weights from method #3, are critical for the effectiveness of MT. Since the Mean Teacher achieved the best performance among method #1–4 on leaderboard during validation phase, we use the best weights obtained by method #4 for model initialization for other methods, i.e., methods #5-6. By comparing method #4 and #5, we observe that self-training slightly outperforms the mean teacher model on cochlea but underperforms on VS tumor. By fine-tuning with more training data, method #6 shows slight improvements on both VS and cochlea compared to method #4. Furthermore, we find that the CUTSeg model (method #7) achieves comparable segmentation performance to method #4. Lastly, in method #8 and #9, we show that though CleanLab is unable to improve performance by iteratively updating labels during training (method #5), it is however an effective method to fuse the predictions from different models during the inference phase. In the evaluation phase, our proposed method (method #9) achieved dice scores of 79.9% and 82.5% and ASSD of 1.29 mm and 0.18 mm for VS tumor and cochlea, respectively. We note that the ASSD of cochlea achieved by our method (0.18 mm) is the lowest among all unsupervised methods and even lower than that achieved by the supervised nnU-Net (0.22 mm). The qualitative results of our method is shown in Fig. 3.

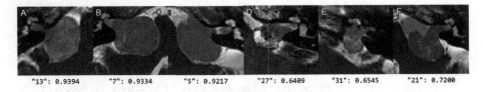

| "13": 0.9394 | "7": 0.9334 | "5": 0.9217 | "27": 0.6409 | "31": 0.6545 | "21": 0.7200 |

Fig. 3. Qualitative results on the validation set. A to C and D to F display the best and worst VS segmentation results. The image ID and the corresponding dice score are also shown. Our experiments show that VS tumors with higher inhomogeneity, e.g., D, are more difficult to segment.

4   Discussion

4.1   ROI Selection Strategy

In this challenge, we observe that the FoV of source and target domain images varies significantly. To minimize the impact of FoV difference, we manually determine a cubic box as ROI and use rigid registration to obtain the ROI from each volume as described in Sect. 3.1. Note that our ROI covers either the left or the right side region around the cochlea while most other teams use the ROIs that cover both cochleae. Arguably, our ROI selection strategy has both a positive and a negative impact on the downstream segmentation tasks. First, this strategy helps to increase the amount of training data since two ROIs can be extracted from one volume. Second, by flipping the right ROI to the left, the orientation and relative position of the cochlea within each ROI remain almost the same, which is greatly beneficial for the accuracy and robustness of cochlea segmentation. Based on the results from the validation leaderboard, all our attempted methods have achieved around 80% dice scores, which are very competitive against other teams' results. Moreover, in the evaluation leaderboard, our method has achieved an ASSD of 0.18 mm which is lower than the supervised nnU-Net of 0.22 mm, suggesting the benefits of our ROI selection strategy on cochlea segmentation. However, this strategy inevitably introduces challenges for VS segmentation. Because VS tumor can be either fully/partially included in both left and right ROIs, the merging scheme for combining the VS segmentation results from both ROIs needs to be carefully designed. In the future, it may be interesting to explore whether using ROIs with different FoVs for VS tumor and cochlea can help improve the results.

4.2 Self-training Strategy

Our experiments show that our self-training strategy cannot help to improve the segmentation performance. In contrast, both the top-two teams on the leaderboard found the self-training strategy very beneficial for their performance. Specifically, the 1st-place team updated the noisy labels by manually inspecting their qualities and filtered out the unreliable labels. On the other hand, the 2nd-place team considered the voxels with the higher probabilities as confident labels to train the next epoch. Hence, we speculate that the effectiveness of self-training may heavily depend on the filtering strategy for noisy pseudo labels. Besides, in our self-training experiments, we only used the real unlabeled data while the aforementioned teams used the combined data, i.e., pseudo T2 and real T2 images. The combined data might also be a key factor for the effectiveness of self-training. In the future, an exciting direction to improve the performance would be to develop an automatic and smart filtering strategy for self-training.

5   Conclusion

In this work, we exploited the image-level domain alignment and semi-supervised training to tackle the unsupervised domain adaptation segmentation problem. The results on the validation and evaluation leaderboard of crossMoDA challenge show that our proposed method can yield promising segmentation performance on VS tumor and cochlea on hrT2 MRI images without labels.

References

1. Vokurka, E.A., et al.: Using Bayesian tissue classification to improve the accuracy of vestibular schwannoma volume and growth measurement. Am. J. Neuroradiol. **23**(3), 459–467 (2002)
2. Coelho, D.H., et al.: MRI surveillance of vestibular schwannomas without contrast enhancement: clinical and economic evaluation. Laryngoscope **128**(1), 202–209 (2018)

3. Wang, G., et al.: Automatic segmentation of vestibular schwannoma from T2-weighted MRI by deep spatial attention with hardness-weighted loss. In: Shen, D., et al. (eds.) MICCAI 2019. LNCS, vol. 11765, pp. 264–272. Springer, Cham (2019). https://doi.org/10.1007/978-3-030-32245-8_30

4. Dorent, R., et al.: Scribble-based domain adaptation via co-segmentation. In: Martel, A.L., et al. (eds.) MICCAI 2020. LNCS, vol. 12261, pp. 479–489. Springer, Cham (2020). https://doi.org/10.1007/978-3-030-59710-8_47

5. Lee, C.-Y., et al.: Sliced wasserstein discrepancy for unsupervised domain adaptation. In: Proceedings of the IEEE/CVF Conference on Computer Vision and Pattern Recognition (2019)

6. Long, M., et al.: Learning transferable features with deep adaptation networks. In: International Conference on Machine Learning. PMLR (2015)

7. Hoffman, J., et al.: CyCADA: cycle-consistent adversarial domain adaptation. In: International Conference on Machine Learning. PMLR (2018)

8. Ganin, Y., et al.: Domain-adversarial training of neural networks. J. Mach. Learn. Res. **17**(1), 2096-2030 (2016)

9. Zou, Y., Yu, Z., Vijaya Kumar, B.V.K., Wang, J.: Unsupervised domain adaptation for semantic segmentation via class-balanced self-training. In: Ferrari, V., Hebert, M., Sminchisescu, C., Weiss, Y. (eds.) ECCV 2018. LNCS, vol. 11207, pp. 297–313. Springer, Cham (2018). https://doi.org/10.1007/978-3-030-01219-9_18

10. Perone, C.S., et al.: Unsupervised domain adaptation for medical imaging segmentation with self-ensembling. Neuroimage **194**, 1–11 (2019)

11. Park, T., Efros, A.A., Zhang, R., Zhu, J.-Y.: Contrastive learning for unpaired image-to-image translation. In: Vedaldi, A., Bischof, H., Brox, T., Frahm, J.-M. (eds.) ECCV 2020. LNCS, vol. 12354, pp. 319–345. Springer, Cham (2020). https://doi.org/10.1007/978-3-030-58545-7_19

12. Zhu, J.-Y., et al.: Unpaired image-to-image translation using cycle-consistent adversarial networks. In: Proceedings of the IEEE International Conference on Computer Vision (2017)

13. Tarvainen, A., Valpola, H.: Mean teachers are better role models: weight-averaged consistency targets improve semi-supervised deep learning results. arXiv preprint arXiv:1703.01780 (2017)

14. Milletari, F., Navab, N., Ahmadi, S.A.: V-Net: fully convolutional neural networks for volumetric medical image segmentation. In: 2016 Fourth International Conference on 3D Vision (3DV), pp. 565–571. IEEE, October 2016

15. Northcutt, C., Jiang, L., Chuang, I.: Confident learning: estimating uncertainty in dataset labels. J. Artif. Intell. Res. **70**, 1373–1411 (2021)

16. Dorent, R., et al.: CrossMoDA 2021 challenge: benchmark of cross-modality domain adaptation techniques for vestibular schwnannoma and cochlea segmentation. arXiv preprint arXiv:2201.02831 (2022)

17. Shapey, J., et al.: Segmentation of vestibular schwannoma from MRI - an open annotated dataset and baseline algorithm. Sci. Data (2021). https://doi.org/10.1101/2021.08.04.21261588

18. Avants, B.B., et al.: A reproducible evaluation of ANTs similarity metric performance in brain image registration. Neuroimage **54**(3), 2033–2044 (2011)

19. Paszke, A., et al.: PyTorch: an imperative style, high-performance deep learning library. Adv. Neural. Inf. Process. Syst. **32**, 8026–8037 (2019)

20. Zhang, Y., Miao, S., Mansi, T., Liao, R.: Task driven generative modeling for unsupervised domain adaptation: application to X-ray image segmentation. In: Frangi, A.F., Schnabel, J.A., Davatzikos, C., Alberola-López, C., Fichtinger, G. (eds.) MICCAI 2018. LNCS, vol. 11071, pp. 599–607. Springer, Cham (2018). https://doi.org/10.1007/978-3-030-00934-2_67

21. Bousmalis, K., et al.: Unsupervised pixel-level domain adaptation with generative adversarial networks. In: Proceedings of the IEEE Conference on Computer Vision and Pattern Recognition (2017)

22. Zhang, Y., et al.: Collaborative unsupervised domain adaptation for medical image diagnosis. IEEE Trans. Image Process. **29**, 7834–7844 (2020)

23. Chang, W.-L., et al.: All about structure: adapting structural information across domains for boosting semantic segmentation. In: Proceedings of the IEEE/CVF Conference on Computer Vision and Pattern Recognition (2019)

24. Chen, C., et al.: Unsupervised bidirectional cross-modality adaptation via deeply synergistic image and feature alignment for medical image segmentation. IEEE Trans. Med. Imaging **39**(7), 2494–2505 (2020)

25. Zhang, Q., et al.: Category anchor-guided unsupervised domain adaptation for semantic segmentation. Adv. Neural. Inf. Process. Syst. **32**, 435–445 (2019)

26. Zhang, M., et al.: Characterizing label errors: confident learning for noisy-labeled image segmentation. In: Martel, A.L., et al. (eds.) MICCAI 2020. LNCS, vol. 12261, pp. 721–730. Springer, Cham (2020). https://doi.org/10.1007/978-3-030-59710-8_70

27. Zhao, Z., Xu, K., Li, S., Zeng, Z., Guan, C.: MT-UDA: towards unsupervised cross-modality medical image segmentation with limited source labels. In: de Bruijne, M., et al. (eds.) MICCAI 2021. LNCS, vol. 12901, pp. 293–303. Springer, Cham (2021). https://doi.org/10.1007/978-3-030-87193-2_28

28. Tarvainen, A., Harri, V.: Mean teachers are better role models: weight-averaged consistency targets improve semi-supervised deep learning results. In: Advances in Neural Information Processing Systems, vol. 30 (2017)

nn-UNet Training on CycleGAN-Translated Images for Cross-modal Domain Adaptation in Biomedical Imaging

Smriti Joshi[1]([✉]), Richard Osuala[1], Carlos Martín-Isla[1], Victor M. Campello[1],
Carla Sendra-Balcells[1], Karim Lekadir[1], and Sergio Escalera[1,2]

[1] Artificial Intelligence in Medicine Lab, Facultat de Matemàtiques
i Informàtica, Universitat de Barcelona, Barcelona, Spain
smriti.joshi@ub.edu
[2] Computer Vision Center, Barcelona, Spain

Abstract. In recent years, deep learning models have considerably advanced the performance of segmentation tasks on Brain Magnetic Resonance Imaging (MRI). However, these models show a considerable performance drop when they are evaluated on unseen data from a different distribution. Since annotation is often a hard and costly task requiring expert supervision, it is necessary to develop ways in which existing models can be adapted to the unseen domains without any additional labelled information. In this work, we explore one such technique which extends the CycleGAN [2] architecture to generate label-preserving data in the target domain. The synthetic target domain data is used to train the nn-UNet [3] framework for the task of multi-label segmentation. The experiments are conducted and evaluated on the dataset [1] provided in the 'Cross-Modality Domain Adaptation for Medical Image Segmentation' challenge [23] for segmentation of vestibular schwannoma (VS) tumour and cochlea on contrast enhanced (ceT1) and high resolution (hrT2) MRI scans. In the proposed approach, our model obtains dice scores (DSC) 0.73 and 0.49 for tumour and cochlea respectively on the validation set of the dataset. This indicates the applicability of the proposed technique to real-world problems where data may be obtained by different acquisition protocols as in [1] where hrT2 images are more reliable, safer, and lower-cost alternative to ceT1.

Keywords: Domain adaptation · Vestibular schwannoma (VS) · Deep learning · nn-UNet · CycleGAN

1 Introduction

Deep learning techniques have achieved immense success under the assumption that the training data and test data come from the same distribution. However, this assumption frequently does not hold true in real world data due to differences

A. Crimi and S. Bakas (Eds.): BrainLes 2021, LNCS 12963, pp. 540–551, 2022.
https://doi.org/10.1007/978-3-031-09002-8_47

in acquisition conditions and techniques. In recent works, unsupervised domain adaptation has proven to be an important tool to traverse this domain gap between source data and un-annotated target data. These techniques reduce the need of expensive labelling in target domain without compromising the performance of the model. Unsupervised domain adaptation (UDA) techniques enable researchers to train models on synthetic data (for which labels can be easily generated) and adapt it to real data. In the field of medical image analysis, annotating images is not only expensive and time-consuming but it also requires tedious and labour-intensive participation of physicians, radiologists and other experts. Further, domain gaps are observed in medical data due to images obtained from different clinical centres, imaging conditions, scanner vendors [22] and the modality of the data. Since the medical field has low error tolerance, it is essential to devise techniques that can perform well even in the presence of high domain gap. In this work, we propose one such approach for segmentation of vestibular schwannoma (VS) tumour and cochlea on unannotated high-resolution T2 (hrT2) brain MRI scan given fully annotated contrast-enhanced T1 (ceT1) data.

2   Related Work

In this work, we use techniques based on unsupervised domain adaptation methods. The following section explain the variety of literature in this field.

Divergence Minimization: To align the distributions of source domain and target domain, the divergence between them is calculated by a distance metric and minimized. The most common distance metrics in the literature are maximum mean discrepancy (MMD) [5], correlation alignment (CORAL) [6], contrastive domain discrepancy (CCD) [8] and Wasserstein metric [7]. They are calculated between source and target features which are the output of a neural network.

Adversarial Learning: Generative adversarial network (GAN) [10] was proposed by Goodfellow et al. for synthetic data generation. It is based on adversarial way of learning with competing generators and discriminators. Many researchers have used the GAN architecture to propose variants specific to domain adaptation. The first of these networks called DANN [9] was proposed in 2016. In this architecture, the discriminator differentiates between source and target domains. The feature extractor is trained to fool this discriminator thereby learning domain invariant features. Another variant called WDGRL [11] modifies the GAN and replaces the classifier with a network to predict Wasserstein distance.

Domain Mapping: Divergence minimization and adversarial learning are both methods to learn domain invariant features. The alternative to this technique is to map from source domain to target domain. Here, source data can be translated pixel wise to an image that has similar distribution to target domain. This can be done via methods like CycleGAN [2] and DualGAN [24]. For larger domain gaps and complex problems like one-to-many relationships, XGAN [25] is a worthy alternative. This way of domain mapping has been used in many papers for the purpose of domain invariant learning with the aid of consistency losses [12].

Normalization: Techniques like Adaptive Batch Normalization (AdaBN) [13] and Automatic domain alignment (AutoDIAL) [14] propose normalization techniques for domain adaptation. AdaBN modulates batch norm layer statistics from source to target domain. This is a parameter free alternative to previous methods. AutoDIAL is an extension of this AdaBN which also learns the network weights by using the target data in a shared parameter space.

Pseudo-Labeling: This technique can be used in problems with relatively smaller domain gap. Saito et al. [15] proposed an asymmetric tri-training architecture with two networks trained on source domain data. If these two networks agree on the prediction for a target image, then the prediction is assumed to be its ground truth which can be used to train a third network on the target domain. Another technique [16] suses a discriminator between source and target predictions to output a confidence map indicating quality of target predictions. The predictions with high confidence are used as pseudo labels for target domain.

Domain Disentanglement: Another line of work uses the concept of domain entanglement. One of the works by Chang et al. [17] proposes three encoders: two private encoders for source and target respectively in addition to a shared encoder. The network is trained such that private encoders learn domain specific information like structure and shared encoder learns domain invariant features.

Test-Time Training: These methods used self-supervised learning to enable domain adaptation during test phase. Sun et al. [18] propose test-time parameter update using a self-supervised branch responsible for four way rotation prediction. Neerav et al. [19] propose an MRI segmentation network composed of two parts, (i) "image to normalization (I2N)" with parameter-update during training and testing and (ii) "normalization to segmentation (N2S)" which updates only during training. Similar approaches based on this principle adopt consistency training [20] and entropy minimization [21]. These methods are effective when domain gap is low between source and target data. Therefore, their applicability in our case is minimal.

In our work, we use a combination of domain mapping and pseudo-labelling techniques as discussed in the next section.

3   Method

The method adopted for domain adaptation in this work has three main steps:

1. **Pre-processing:** Selection of axial slices from MRI using maximum coordinates of bounding boxes across all available segmentation masks and resizing them to a uniform size.
2. **Mapping:** Generation of synthetic images in hrT2 domain using the 2D CycleGAN [2] architecture.

3. **Segmentation:** Training segmentation model using nnUNet [3] framework with generated images from CycleGAN.

The following sections discuss this pipeline in more detail. Figure 2 presents the main steps of the pipeline.

3.1   Dataset and Evaluation Metrics

The experiments are conducted and evaluated on the dataset [1] provided in the *Cross-Modality Domain Adaptation for Medical Image Segmentation Challenge* [23]. The dataset consists of unpaired MRI scans with ceT1 and hrT2 modalities. For the ceT1 domain, tumour and cochlea are annotated as 1 and 2 respectively while for the hrT2 domain, no label information is available. The ceT1 images have pixel dimension of 512×512 with a resolution of 0.4×0.4 mm while hrT2 images are of pixel dimensions 384×384 or 448×448 with higher resolution of 0.5×0.5 mm. Further, in hrT2 images, the number of slices along the z axis is either 20, 40 or 80. Figure 1 shows the resized axial slices of ceT1 and hrT2 images for visual demonstration of the domain gap between the two modalities. Evaluation of the experiments is conducted on the validation set of this dataset with Dice score (DSC) and Average Symmetric Surface Distance (ASSD) as performance metrics.

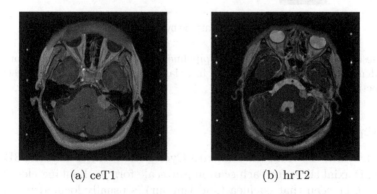

(a) ceT1   (b) hrT2

Fig. 1. Axial slices of MRI modalities present in the dataset showing VS tumour

3.2   Setup

For the development of the project, Python 3.8 was used with PyTorch 1.7.1 framework. The experiments were conducted using a Nvidia RTX 3090 GPU with 24 GB memory.

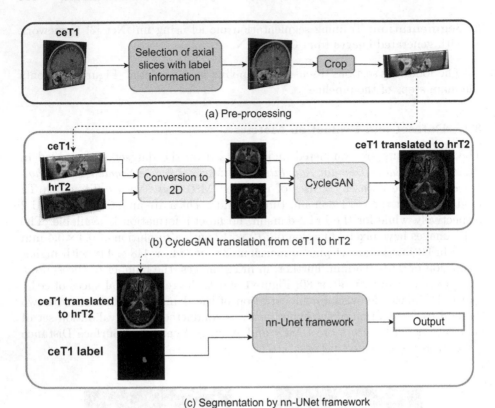

Fig. 2. Description of main steps of the pipeline. 3D images are presented from sagittal view to demonstrate the slice selection in axial direction. In 2D, slices presented are axial direction.

3.3   Preprocessing

Slice Selection: To train the standard CycleGAN architecture, the 3D data is saved as 2D axial slices for each scan in grayscale format. Looking closely at the data, it can be seen that cochlea (and tumour) is usually located in the initial axial slices of the images. Therefore, to minimize the occurrence of irrelevant data, the range of slices containing labelled information is calculated and only the slices inside this range [10, 60] are used for training. These slices are also resized to a common size of 192×224. Further, to train the segmentation model using nn-UNet, these 2D slices in the ceT1 domain are mapped to the hrT2 domain using the trained CycleGAN and concatenated to form a 3D volume of size $192 \times 224 \times 51$.

3.4 Generating Synthetic Images

The generation of synthetic images is conducted using 2D CycleGAN[1] using the axial slices of MRI scans. Figure 3 shows the translation of images from ceT1 domain to hrT2 domain. It can be observed that tumour information is preserved during the translation. All the translated slices are incorporated in the dataset without any manual selection i.e. there was no removal of slices based on visual inspection.

Configuration: Before feeding the image to the network, the images are normalized to the range $[-1, 1]$. Adam optimizer with initial learning rate of 0.00002 is used to train the generators as well as the discriminators. For augmentation, basic torchvision transforms, namely RandomHorizontalFlip (probability: 0.5) and RandomRotation (5°) are used. The remaining parameters are same as in the original configuration [2]. The model is trained for 100–150 epochs. The aforementioned hyperparameters are chosen upon visual evaluation of translated images.

To make sure that the discriminator does not overpower the generator, it is only updated when its accuracy gets too low, that is, below 0.6.

3.5 Segmentation for hrT2 Domain

Once the CycleGAN is trained, it is used to map the ceT1 data to hrT2 domain. To implement this, the individual slices are mapped and concatenated to get a volume of size $192 \times 224 \times 51$. The labels corresponding to these translated images are the corresponding slices of given ceT1 ground truth images. Further, multiple sets of images are translated using CycleGAN weights from different stages. One observation inspiring this approach was the difference in representation of tumours in generated images over the training epochs. Initial epochs of CycleGAN show brighter tumours similar to ceT1 while darker tumours are obtained in later epochs. Since both kinds of textures are present in hrT2 data, this approach was adopted to improve generalization of the network.

Our network is built upon the nn-UNet [3], a dynamic fully automatic segmentation framework for medical images leveraging the UNet, which is commonly used for segmentation tasks. For training this network, the nn-UNet configuration for 2D data is used. This is because that CycleGAN is trained on 2D images and information along the z-axis cannot be taken into consideration due to its anisotropic nature. This is also supported by the experimentation as discussed in the Sect. 4. As a part of nn-UNet pre-processing, the data is cropped (region of non-zero values only), resampled and normalised. Loss function used for training the 2D nn-UNet is a combination of dice loss and cross entropy loss. Instead of using instance normalisation as in the original configuration, batch normalization is used as the authors of [4] demonstrated that it yields better performance on brain MRI segmentation tasks.

---

[1] Code available at: https://github.com/aitorzip/PyTorch-CycleGAN.

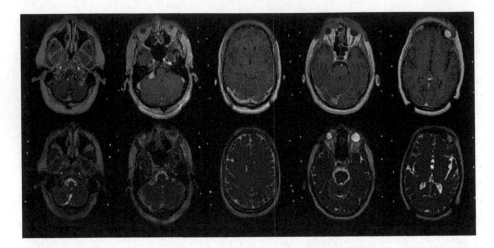

Fig. 3. The translation from ceT1 to hrT2 domain using CycleGAN for non-registered data. First row corresponds to the randomly generated axial slices corresponding to ceT1 domain while the second row shows corresponding translated synthetic images in hrT2 domain.

Augmentation: Data augmentation is an integral part of the nn-UNet framework. The following augmentations are used for training the framework in this work: Spatial transforms such as elastic deformation, rotation, scaling, random crop and intensity transformations like gaussian noise, gaussian blur, additive brightness, multiplicative brightness, contrast, simulated low resolution, gamma transform and mirroring. The file used for data augmentations can be accessed from data_augmentation_moreDA.py[2] file of nn-UNet framework.

Postprocessing in nn-UNet: For the tumour labels, all predictions but the one with the largest region in the 3D volume are removed as it indicated better performance on internal validation set generated during five-fold cross validation training by nn-UNet framework.

4   Results

On the validation data, the metrics obtained with our approach with different configurations are summarised in Table 1. 2D nn-UNet performs better than 3D nn-UNet. This is intuitive as the translated data obtained from 2D CycleGAN likely lacks some 3D coherence across domains. Pretraining the network with labelled ceT1 data makes tumour recognition better, contributing to an increase of ≈0.03 to the overall dice score. Further, adding more synthetic data from different CycleGAN weights to the training set pushes the performance even

---

[2] Code available at: https://github.com/MIC-DKFZ/nnUNet.

Table 1. Evaluation metrics on validation set. MD refers to the case where more data generated from CycleGAN weights over epochs is added to the dataset, PL refers to pseudo-labelling.

Method	Tumour				Cochlea				Total	
	Dice		ASSD		Dice		ASSD		Dice	
	Mean	Std.	Mean	Std.	Mean	Std.	Mean	Std.	Mean	Std.
3D nn-UNet	0.6072	0.2766	6.1097	8.1267	0.3212	0.0682	1.0882	2.5184	0.4642	0.1458
2D nn-UNet	0.6572	0.2131	2.3072	6.7850	0.4388	0.0980	1.0964	2.4962	0.5480	0.1224
+ pretrain	0.6999	0.1470	1.0188	0.5377	0.4460	0.0828	0.6602	0.2160	0.5730	0.0861
+ pretrain + MD	0.7120	0.1411	0.9643	0.5117	0.4779	0.0773	0.6024	0.1874	0.5950	0.0860
+ pretrain + MD + PL	**0.7291**	**0.1428**	**0.8969**	**0.4929**	**0.4944**	**0.0598**	**0.5591**	**0.1573**	**0.6117**	**0.0813**

further. Addition of real target data to the training data with pseudo-labels predicted by the former configuration also pushes the performance by overall dice value of ≈0.02.

5 Discussion

This section discusses the results in detail by analysing the predictions qualitatively and providing explanations for the observed behaviour of the network.

5.1 Improving Segmentation Quality

As seen in Table 1, there is progressive improvement in the metrics obtained by the baseline i.e. training 2D nn-UNet with fake hrT2 images and real ceT1 labels. It can be seen in Fig. 4a that the predicted segmentation does not cover the whole tumour area. Pretraining improves the results as seen in Fig. 4b and adding more generated data (Fig. 4c) expands the prediction to the complete tumour region. Finally, a smooth labelling is obtained when further trained with pseudo-labels (Fig. 4d).

Specifically, with pretraining, the network is able to localize the position of tumours and cochlea which leads to a smaller number of false positives and better recognition of existing structures. This can be observed in Fig. 5 where structures in the image are misidentified as tumour (Fig. 5a) or the actual tumour regions are not identified (Fig. 5b). After pretraining the network with ceT1 data, the tumour is identified correctly (Fig. 5c).

Further, Fig. 6 shows the advantages of pseudo-labelling based fine-tuning of the network. It helps to propagate target features in the network and better recognizes the tumour representations present in the original target data. This is important as most tumours are darker in colour in hrT2 images compared to bright tumours in ceT1. Figure 6b shows improvement over Fig. 6a as the whole region of the tumour is identified.

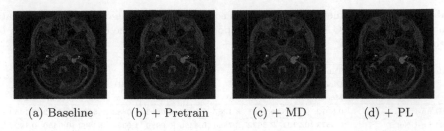

(a) Baseline   (b) + Pretrain   (c) + MD   (d) + PL

Fig. 4. Figure showing progressive improvement of label prediction. MD refers to the case where more data generated from CycleGAN weights over epochs is added to the dataset, PL refers to pseudo-labelling.

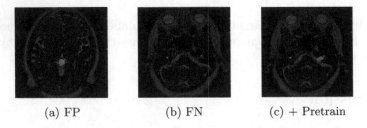

(a) FP   (b) FN   (c) + Pretrain

Fig. 5. Improvement due to pretraining with ceT1 data. Left: False positive (FP) detection for tumour label, Middle: False negative (FN) detection for tumour label, Right: Correct identification of tumour region

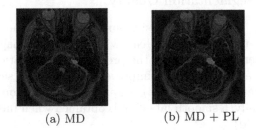

(a) MD   (b) MD + PL

Fig. 6. Improvement due to fine-tuning with pseudo-labels

5.2   Tumour Versus Cochlea

It is expected that the translation of tumour is better than cochlea during Cycle-GAN mapping as the latter is small and harder to define in ceT1 images. This can be observed in the synthetic hrT2 image shown in Fig. 7b where there is indistinct representation of cochlea at the locations indicated by Fig. 7a. However, in real hrT2 image (Fig. 7c), the cochlear region is much more defined and distinguishable.

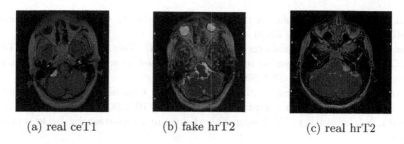

(a) real ceT1   (b) fake hrT2   (c) real hrT2

Fig. 7. Figure showing the comparison in the mapping of tumour and cochlea. Left: Real ceT1 annotated slice, Middle: Corresponding mapped slice to hrT2 domain, Right: Real hrT2 image (unpaired)

6 Conclusion

In this paper, we investigated the unsupervised domain adaptation task from ceT1 domain to hrT2 domain of brain MRI images. Two techniques have been used to leverage the unlabelled data. Firstly, a CycleGAN architecture based network is trained to create a mapping from ceT1 to hrT2 domain. This mapping is used to generate synthetic hrT2 data to train a segmentation network. Further, this segmentation network is used to predict pseudo-labels for unlabelled real hrT2 data which is used to further fine-tune the network. Finally, the highest overall dice score obtained on validation data is 0.6117 with higher recognition of tumour (≈ 0.73) than cochlea (≈ 0.49). In the future work, we will aim at improving cochlea recognition by utilising information about its position in the brain as the anatomy is expected to be consistent across all patients.

Acknowledgements. This work has been partially supported by the Spanish project PID2019-105093GB-I00 and by ICREA under the ICREA Academia programme. Additionally, this work has also been supported in part by the European Union's Horizon 2020 research and innovation programme under grant agreement No. 825903 and No. 952103.

References

1. Shapey, J., et al.: Segmentation of vestibular schwannoma from MRI, an open annotated dataset and baseline algorithm. Sci. Data **8**(1), 286 (2021). https://doi.org/10.1038/s41597-021-01064-w
2. Zhu, J.-Y., Park, T., Isola, P., Efros, A.A.: Unpaired image-to-image translation using cycle-consistent adversarial networks. CoRR, abs/1703.10593 (2017)
3. Isensee, F., et al.: nn-UNet: self-adapting framework for U-Net-based medical image segmentation. CoRR, abs/1809.10486 (2018)
4. Isensee, F., Jaeger, P.F., Full, P.M., Vollmuth, P., Maier-Hein, K.H.: nn-UNet for brain tumor segmentation. CoRR, abs/2011.00848 (2020)
5. Gretton, A., Borgwardt, K.M., Rasch, M.J., Schölkopf, B., Smola, A.J.: A kernel method for the two-sample-problem. In: Schölkopf, B., Platt, J.C., Hofmann, T. (eds.) NIPS, pp. 513–520. MIT Press (2006). ISBN: 0-262-19568-2

6. Sun, B., Feng, J., Saenko, K.: Return of frustratingly easy domain adaptation. CoRR, abs/1511.05547 (2015)
7. Damodaran, B.B., Kellenberger, B., Flamary, R., Tuia, D., Courty, N.: DeepJDOT: deep joint distribution optimal transport for unsupervised domain adaptation. CoRR, abs/1803.10081 (2018)
8. Kang, G., Jiang, L., Yang, Y., Hauptmann, A.G.: Contrastive adaptation network for unsupervised domain adaptation. CoRR, abs/1901.00976 (2019)
9. Ganin, Y., Lempitsky, V.: Unsupervised domain adaptation by backpropagation (2014)
10. Goodfellow, I., et al.: Generative Adversarial Nets. In: Ghahramani, Z., Welling, M., Cortes, C., Lawrence, N., Weinberger, K.Q. (eds.) Advances in Neural Information Processing Systems, vol. 27. Curran Associates, Inc. (2014). https:// proceedings.neurips.cc/paper/2014/file/5ca3e9b122f61f8f06494c97b1afccf3-Paper. pdf
11. Shen, J., Qu, Y., Zhang, W., Yu, Y.: Wasserstein distance guided representation learning for domain adaptation. In: McIlraith, S.A., Weinberger, K.Q. (eds.) AAAI, pp. 4058–4065. AAAI Press (2018)
12. Chen, C., Dou, Q., Chen, H., Qin, J., Heng, P.-A.: Synergistic image and feature adaptation: towards cross-modality domain adaptation for medical image segmentation. In: AAAI, pp. 865–872. AAAI Press (2019). ISBN: 978-1-57735-809-1
13. Li, Y., Wang, N., Shi, J., Liu, J., Hou, X.: Revisiting batch normalization for practical domain adaptation. In: ICLR Workshop. OpenReview.net (2017)
14. Carlucci, F.M., Porzi, L., Caputo, B., Ricci, E., Bulò, S.R.: AutoDIAL: automatic domain alignment layers. In: ICCV, pp. 5077–5085. IEEE Computer Society (2017). ISBN: 978-1-5386-1032-9
15. Saito, K., Ushiku, Y., Harada, T.: Asymmetric tri-training for unsupervised domain adaptation. In: Precup, D., Teh, Y.W. (eds) ICML, pp. 2988–2997. PMLR (2017)
16. Michieli, U., Biasetton, M., Agresti, G., Zanuttigh, P.: Adversarial learning and self-teaching techniques for domain adaptation in semantic segmentation. IEEE Trans. Intell. Veh. 5, 508–518 (2020)
17. Chang, W.L., Wang, H.P., Peng, W.H., Chiu, W.C.: All about structure: adapting structural information across domains for boosting semantic segmentation. In: CVPR, pp. 1900–1909. Computer Vision Foundation/IEEE (2019)
18. Sun, Y., Wang, X., Liu, Z., Miller, J., Efros, A., Hardt, M.: Test-time training with self-supervision for generalization under distribution shifts. In: Proceedings of the 37th International Conference on Machine Learning. Proceedings of Machine Learning Research, vol. 119, pp. 9229–9248 (2020). https://proceedings.mlr.press/ v119/sun20b.html
19. Karani, N., Chaitanya, K., Konukoglu, E.: Test-time adaptable neural networks for robust medical image segmentation. CoRR, abs/2004.04668 (2020)
20. Varsavsky, T., Orbes-Arteaga, M., Sudre, C.H., Graham, M.S., Nachev, P., Cardoso, M.J.: Test-time unsupervised domain adaptation. In: Martel, A.L., et al. (eds.) MICCAI 2020. LNCS, vol. 12261, pp. 428–436. Springer, Cham (2020). https://doi.org/10.1007/978-3-030-59710-8_42 ISBN: 978-3-030-59710-8
21. Wang, D., Shelhamer, E., Liu, S., Olshausen, B., Darrell, T.: Tent: Fully Test-Time Adaptation by Entropy Minimization. In: International Conference on Learning Representations (2021). https://openreview.net/forum?id=uXl3bZLkr3c
22. Campello, V.M., et al.: Multi-centre, multi-vendor and multi-disease cardiac segmentation: the M&Ms challenge. IEEE Trans. Med. Imaging 40(12), 3543–3554 (2021). https://doi.org/10.1109/TMI.2021.3090082

23. Dorent, R., et al.: CrossMoDA 2021 challenge: Benchmark of Cross-Modality Domain Adaptation techniques for Vestibular Schwannoma and Cochlea Segmentation (2022). arXiv: 2201.02831. https://doi.org/10.48550/arxiv.2201.02831
24. Yi, Z., Zhang, H.(Richard), Tan, P., Gong, M.: DualGAN: unsupervised dual learning for image-to-image translation. Paper presented at the meeting of the ICCV (2017)
25. Royer, A., et al.: XGAN: unsupervised image-to-image translation for many-to-many mappings. In: Singh, R., Vatsa, M., Patel, V.M., Ratha, N. (eds.) Domain Adaptation for Visual Understanding, pp. 33–49. Springer, Cham (2020). https://doi.org/10.1007/978-3-030-30671-7_3

QUBIQ

Ohio

Extending Probabilistic U-Net Using MC-Dropout to Quantify Data and Model Uncertainty

Ishaan Bhat[(✉)] and Hugo J. Kuijf

Image Sciences Institute, University Medical Center Utrecht,
Heidelberglaan 100, 3584 Utrecht, CX, The Netherlands
i.r.bhat@umcutrecht.nl

Abstract. We extend the Probabilistic U-Net using MC-Dropout to estimate model uncertainty in addition to the data uncertainty in order to improve the overall predictive uncertainty estimate. We use this model on the datasets present in the QUBIQ21 challenge and achieve a mean score of 0.719.

1   Introduction

Standard deep learning techniques only provide point estimates for their predictions, therefore fail to capture the inherent uncertainty present in the data and/or model. Recent approaches [2,5], developed specifically for segmentation tasks where multiple annotations are available, seek to remedy this by estimating data and model uncertainty using variational inference techniques.

The QUBIQ[1] challenge comprises of datasets with multiple annotations across different anatomies and image modalities. The goal of the challenge is to investigate the ability of uncertainty estimation techniques to realistically estimate the variability in manual delineations observed for different structures. Each dataset has a fixed number of tasks, each task involves segmenting a particular structure of interest within an image. For example, there are three tumor types to be segmented in the brain-tumor dataset, therefore this dataset contains three tasks.

The following datasets are present within the QUBIQ 2021 challenge:

- Brain-growth (MRI, one task, seven annotations per image)
- Brain-tumor (MRI, three tasks, three annotations per image)
- Prostate (MRI, two tasks, six annotations per image)
- Kidney (CT, one task, three annotations per image)
- Pancreas (CT, one task, two annotations per image)
- Pancreatic-lesion (CT, one task, two annotations per image)

---

[1] https://qubiq21.grand-challenge.org/.

2 Methodology

2.1 Data Pre-processing

We performed z-score normalization for the MR images (brain-growth, brain-tumor, prostate) and scaled intensities to the $[0, 1]$ range for the CT images (kidney, pancreas, pancreatic-lesions). We performed data augmentation using random flips and rotations. We also applied intensity transforms by altering contrast and brightness of images. All images were resized (via upsampling/downsampling followed by interpolation using a 3rd order B-Spline) to the nearest power of 2 to their original dimensions, therefore the brain-growth and brain-tumor images have dimensions of 256×256, while the kidney and prostate images have dimensions of 512×512. The pancreas and pancreatic-lesion datasets did not need to resized since they already had dimensions of 512×512.

2.2 Neural Network Architecture and Hyper-parameters

Our neural network architecture was based on the Probabalistic U-Net [5] that uses a low-dimensional latent space to encode different segmentation variants, making it ideal to handle datasets with multiple annotations. We deviate from the architecture in [5] by adding dropout [6] (dropout rate = 0.5) layers at the outputs of the lower-most encoder and decoder. The code is publicly available at https://github.com/kilgore92/PyTorch_ProbUNet.

Neural network hyper-parameters for all datasets are shown in Table 1. Optimization for all neural networks was performed using the ADAM [3] optimizer. We terminated training when no decrease in validation loss was observed for 100 epochs and chose the checkpoint with the lowest validation loss for inference. The neural network architecture and training scheme is shown in Fig. 1.

Table 1. Neural Network hyper-parameters

Dataset	Hyper-parameters			
	Learning Rate	Conv. filters	Batch Size	Latent vector dim.
Brain-growth	10^{-4}	[32, 64, 128, 192]	12	6
Brain-tumor	10^{-4}	[32, 64, 128, 192]	12	6
Kidney	10^{-5}	[32, 64, 128, 256, 512]	6	6
Prostate	10^{-4}	[32, 64, 128, 192]	6	6
Pancreas	10^{-5}	[32, 64, 128, 256, 512]	6	6
Pancreatic-lesion	10^{-5}	[32, 64, 128, 256, 512]	6	6

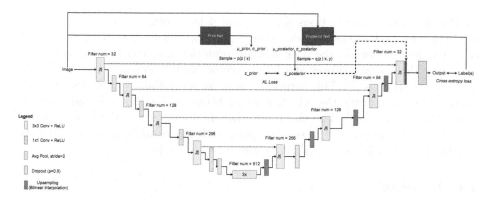

Fig. 1. Neural network architecture and training scheme. The Prior and Posterior nets have the same sequence of convolutional blocks as the encoding path of the U-Net. During inference, the Posterior net is discarded and different predictions are generated by sampling from $p(z|x)$ and combining the samples with the U-Net output.

2.3 Loss Function

The original formulation of the Probabilistic U-Net captures the uncertainty inherent in the data, by matching segmentation variants with multiple annotations available per image. We extend this method to additionally capture the model uncertainty, similar to [2]. Instead of variational dropout [4], which increases the number of model parameters, we used MC-Dropout [1] to capture the uncertainty in the model.

The key idea in variational inference is choosing an approximate posterior that is tractable. The training objective is chosen to be the minimization of the KL-divergence between the approximate posterior $(q(z, w|x, y))$ and the exact posterior $(p(z, w|x, y))$. Similar to [2], we factorize the approximate posterior as:

$$q(z, w|x, y) = q(z|x, y)q(w)$$

With this factorization we obtain the following loss function:

$$L = -\frac{1}{N} \sum_{i=1}^{N} \frac{1}{M} \sum_{j=1}^{j=M} \mathbb{E}_{q(w)q(z|x_i, y_i)} \log(p(y_{ij}|x_i, w, z))$$

$$+ \beta * \frac{1}{N} \sum_{i=1}^{N} \mathrm{KL}(q(z|x_i, y_i)||p(z|x_i)) \qquad (1)$$

$$+ \lambda * ||w||^2$$

Here N is the number of training samples (or mini-batch size) and M is the number of annotations available for a particular image. The first term (negative log-likelihood) is the average binary cross-entropy loss between the prediction(s) and the different annotations for each image. A new latent vector, conditioned on the mean over annotations y_i, is sampled from $q(z|x_i, y_i)$ to compute the prediction for each of the provided annotations, y_{ij}. The 2nd term minimizes the KL divergence between the approximate posterior and the prior (conditioned only over the image x_i) over the latent vector, with a weight term β, which is set to 10 similar to [5]. This term is computed using the Pytorch distributions package that computes the KL divergence between distributions and supports gradient computation[2]. The third term i.e. the L-2 norm of the weights arises from the KL divergence between the prior and approximate posterior over the weights i.e. $KL(q(w)\|p(w))$ [1]. We chose λ to be 5×10^{-5}.

2.4   Inference

For an image x^*, we generate the final prediction by computing the mean over predictions generated from 100 samples of the latent space ($z \sim p(z|x^*)$) and 20 samples of MC-Dropout i.e. 20 passes through the model with a different set of random weights retained during each pass.

3   Results

Table 2. Results for the QUBIQ validation data, Mean score = 0.719

Dataset	QUBIQ metric		
	Task 1	Task 2	Task 3
Brain-growth	0.896	–	–
Brain-tumor	0.940	0.694	0.614
Kidney	0.870	-	–
Prostate	0.835	0.760	–
Pancreas	0.486	–	–
Pancreatic-lesion	0.380	–	–

In Table 2, we present the results for all datasets. We computed the metric described on the QUBIQ challenge website. The qubiq metric is average of dice scores computed at thresholds $0.1, 0.2, ...0.9$ between the prediction and the mean over the different reference segmentations.

4   Conclusion

In this paper, we have presented an approach for image segmentation with multiple annotations by extending the Probabilistic U-Net framework to use MC-Dropout to capture model uncertainty in addition to data uncertainty. Our approach shows promising results on different datasets and tasks that are a part of the QUBIQ challenge.

---

[2] https://pytorch.org/docs/stable/distributions.html?highlight=kl_divergence# torch.distributions.kl.kl_divergence.

References

1. Gal, Y., Ghahramani, Z.: Dropout as a bayesian approximation: representing model uncertainty in deep learning. In: Proceedings of the 33nd International Conference on Machine Learning, ICML 2016. JMLR Workshop and Conference Proceedings, vol. 48, pp. 1050–1059. JMLR.org (2016)
2. Hu, S., Worrall, D., Knegt, S., Veeling, B., Huisman, H., Welling, M.: Supervised uncertainty quantification for segmentation with multiple annotations. In: Shen, D., Liu, T., Peters, T.M., Staib, L.H., Essert, C., Zhou, S., Yap, P.-T., Khan, A. (eds.) MICCAI 2019. LNCS, vol. 11765, pp. 137–145. Springer, Cham (2019). https://doi.org/10.1007/978-3-030-32245-8_16
3. Kingma, D.P., Ba, J.: Adam: a Method for Stochastic Optimization, January 2017. http://arxiv.org/abs/1412.6980, arXiv: 1412.6980
4. Kingma, D.P., Salimans, T., Welling, M.: Variational dropout and the local reparameterization trick. In: Proceedings of the 28th International Conference on Neural Information Processing Systems - Volume 2, NIPS 2015, pp. 2575–2583. MIT Press, Cambridge (2015)
5. Kohl, S., et al.: A Probabilistic U-Net for Segmentation of Ambiguous Images. In: Bengio, S., Wallach, H., Larochelle, H., Grauman, K., Cesa-Bianchi, N., Garnett, R. (eds.) Advances in Neural Information Processing Systems, vol. 31. Curran Associates, Inc. (2018). https://proceedings.neurips.cc/paper/2018/file/473447ac58e1cd7e96172575f48dca3b-Paper.pdf
6. Srivastava, N., Hinton, G., Krizhevsky, A., Sutskever, I., Salakhutdinov, R.: Dropout: a simple way to prevent neural networks from overfitting. J. Mach. Learn. Res. 15(56), 1929–1958 (2014)

Holistic Network for Quantifying Uncertainties in Medical Images

Jimut Bahan Pal[✉]

Ramakrishna Mission Vivekananda Educational and Research Institute,
Howrah, West Bengal 711202, India
jpal.cs@gm.rkmvu.ac.in

Abstract. Variability in delineation is an inherent property for segmenting medical imagery, when images are annotated by a variety of expert annotators. Previous methods have used adversarial training, Monte-Carlo sampling, and dropouts, which might sometimes produce a wide range of segmentation masks that differ from the styles of mask produced by a set of expert annotators. State-of-the-art method uses multiple U-Nets to capture the individual delineations, but it is computationally demanding. To mitigate this problem, a holistic network containing N-Encoder and N-Decoder is proposed, which could individually model the variability of delineation produced by the expert annotators. This will help to create segmentation masks for different tasks of the same dataset through a single network by learning the common features of multiple Encoders via a common channel and passing those features to Decoder. These create one segmentation mask. All the masks are calculated by using weighted loss at each end of the Decoders that show excellent results for some datasets.

Keywords: Holistic network · Medical image segmentation · Multiple encoder-decoders · Quantifying uncertainties · Residual networks

1 Introduction

Multiple medical domain experts label and annotate biomedical image data [24] using standard software. In medical image segmentation tasks, individual samples of manually segmented mask may have variability in delineations [13]. This variability is prominent across a wide variety of structures and pathology [5] which is influenced by imaging modality and different expert annotators. It is an inherent property of the biological problem.[1] But - as of now - it is not holistically considered in designing medical image quantification algorithms. This is because of unavailability of datasets and consensus that addresses uncertainty

---

[1] https://qubiq21.grand-challenge.org/About/.

Supported by MICCAI-QUBIQ-2021 challenge.

quantification on realistic estimates against expert annotated medical image segmentation data. This present study deals with segmenting different image structures of diagnostic relevance to quantify the variability of local delineations with the help of Deep Learning.

Unavailability of data makes an algorithm unable to model distribution of previously unseen data. So far, the researchers addressed the problem of data imbalance via extensive data augmentation. For example, using Dropouts [22] in the model, acts as an ensemble of small networks. Other methods may include L_1 and L_2 regularization [18] of kernel weights, which effectively address the problem of over-fitting, simultaneously producing better results. Using transfer learning [23] is also becoming more popular since it leverages the weights from previously trained similar task to augment the capability of network with relatively less data by fine-tuning. The general choice of weights is ImageNet [7] which is trained on natural imagery that can be used almost anywhere by applying some fine-tuning. In this experiment, we propose a model that could be trained from scratch to achieve good results without transfer learning and data augmentations. By applying transfer learning to the encoder may increase the overall capability of the network.

Sometime non-Bayesian deep learning architectures have used multiple independent networks [17] of U-Net to model radiologists and estimate segmentation uncertainties. Another type of architecture used Bayesian methods, Monte-Carlo Dropouts, that train the network with dropout [17] and generate a posterior distribution of segmentation masks at the test phase by sampling several times. This proposed work uses multiple Encoder-Decoder to provide uncertainty maps holistically across different image modalities using the sole model. This reduces the overhead for training multiple independent networks to perform similar tasks.

2   Literature Review

Supervised image segmentation in Deep Learning is carried out by an Encoder-Decoder architecture. Encoder part of the network compresses information by learning feature representation from input images of datasets during training, while the Decoder part uses this representation to get better and better at segmenting images. The most common type of architecture is U-Net [19]. Other variants of U-Net include Attention U-Net [21] which surpasses the capabilities of U-Net by adding attention modules for focusing on relevant regions of an image during training. BCDU-Net [4], an extension of U-Net uses the advantages of Bidirectional Convolutional LSTM (Long Shot Term Memory models), dense convolutions and U-Net to achieve state-of-the-art performance on few datasets. Another form of segmentation structure is Double U-Net [11] which is a combination of two U-Nets stacked on top of one-another. The first U-Net uses VGG-19 as encoder, which was previously trained on ImageNet [7] dataset to capture patterns from natural imagery, and a second U-Net was added at the bottom to capture more semantic information in Double U-Net [11]. These models have been successfully applied to segment single binary mask for unique problems.

Apart from medical images, natural images are usually segmented via semantic segmentation, where each pixel is assigned a label belonging to one class. The models are like the ones segmenting medical images, since they use a series of pooling and up-pooling layers to capture the features. An alternative form of segmentation of natural imagery is instance segmentation using Mask-RCNN [9] where each pixel of individual objects are assigned different colours. These algorithms can be used for segmenting medical images as well, except the fact that medical images require precise allocation of segmentation mask to small objects. However, these algorithms do not quantify the amount of uncertainty in segmentation mask generated by them in semantic segmentation tasks.

The next class of models deals with quantifying uncertainties by learning distribution over segmentation mask for a particular input. In case of medical images, the region of interest might not be clear from images alone, hence a group of grader produce a set of diverse segmentation mask for a single input. Probabilistic U-Net [14] is based on a generative model and conditional variational auto-encoder that can generate an unlimited number of plausible segmentation hypothesis. Other methods may use energy-based minimization by perturbing the energy function of conditional random field (CRF) [3] followed by maximum a posteriori inference (MAP). These methods provide a diverse set of segmentation masks for an input image. The proposed work captures patterns to construct segmentation masks closer to individual annotator's choice by learning the inherent distribution of masking techniques common to individual annotator, using annotator specific Encoder-Decoder that simulates the decision of expert annotators on which the model is trained on.

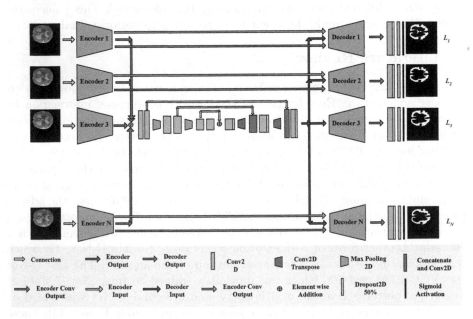

Fig. 1. The overall architecture of the proposed model with multiple Encoders and Decoders to holistically segment medical images.

3 Materials and Methods

The main purpose of designing this architecture is to model the variance of segmentation mask produced by each of the annotators. Using adversarial training, the mask generated will become too unpredictable to capture the style of masking of individual annotators for each task, hence, we propose a model to improve this by adding multiple Encoder and Decoders.

3.1 Network Architecture

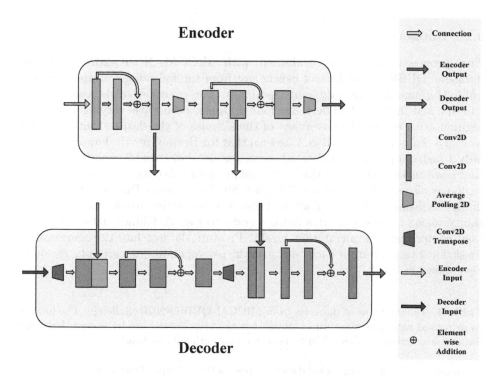

Fig. 2. The structures of Encoder (shown above) and Decoder (shown below) block of the proposed architecture.

For capturing the individual style of producing segmentation masks for annotators, a set of N Encoders and corresponding set of N Decoders is used (Fig. 1). The structure of Encoder and Decoder is shown in Fig. 2. Simple Residual blocks [10] have been used to capture the features in the Encoder by adding features from the previous convolutional layers. The features are concatenated with the Decoder to improve segmentation results, taking more information from the initial and the final layers of the Deep Learning Network. In the Decoder block,

Transpose 2-dimensional Convolution is used to match the dimension of feature space before concatenation along with up sampling.

Resulting feature volume produced by all the Encoder is added and passed to a common block, which accumulates all the important features responsible for generating the segmentation masks. This block also has a set of dropout layers [22] through which the model can regularize itself by learning an ensemble of networks. Output got from this block is passed through each of the Decoder as shown in Fig. 1. The outputs generated by the Decoder are passed through as a set of convolutional layers to generate individual segmentation masks. Loss is calculated at each of these output layers corresponding to each of the individual decoders, i.e., L_1 to L_N.

3.2   Datasets

The proposed method is evaluated with MICCAI-QUBIQ-2020 challenge datasets. QUBIQ-2020 dataset can be got from the following website (https:// qubiq21.grand-challenge.org/participation/). The overview of datasets can be summarized in Table 1. There are four datasets, each with varying tasks and segmentation masks. The overview of the samples of the dataset can be shown in Fig. 3. From the figure, it can be seen that for Brain-Growth dataset, there is only 1 task comprising 7 annotated segmentation masks, and 7 expert annotators that have annotated each of the individual mask for this dataset. The uncertainty region is also shown for all the 7 masks. Similarly, Brain-Tumor dataset has 9 mask consisting of 3 tasks. Each task has 3 segmentation mask, and the uncertainty region is shown for this dataset (refer to Fig. 3). Kidney dataset has one task comprising 3 segmentation masks. Prostate dataset has 12 segmentation mask for 2 tasks, 6 from each task and the corresponding uncertainty region is also shown in Fig. 3.

Table 1. The overview of datasets from MICCAI-QUBIQ-2020 challenge. The images were passed with the same input dimension to the proposed model except, Prostate dataset was resized to 256×256 to reduce computational overheads.

Dataset	#Training	#Validation	#Test	#Task	#Input Dimension
Brain-Growth	34	5	10	1	$256 \times 256 \times 1$
Brain-Tumor	28	4	8	3	$240 \times 240 \times 4$
Kidney	20	4	4	1	$497 \times 497 \times 1$
Prostate	48	7	13	2	$640 \times 640 \times 1$ and $960 \times 640 \times 1$

3.3   Loss Function

Loss functions can sometime access the data imbalance [2] in medical image segmentation. For segmenting binary masks, region based Tversky [20] loss function is used. All the losses (i.e., L_1 to L_N) (refer to Fig. 1) are given equal weight

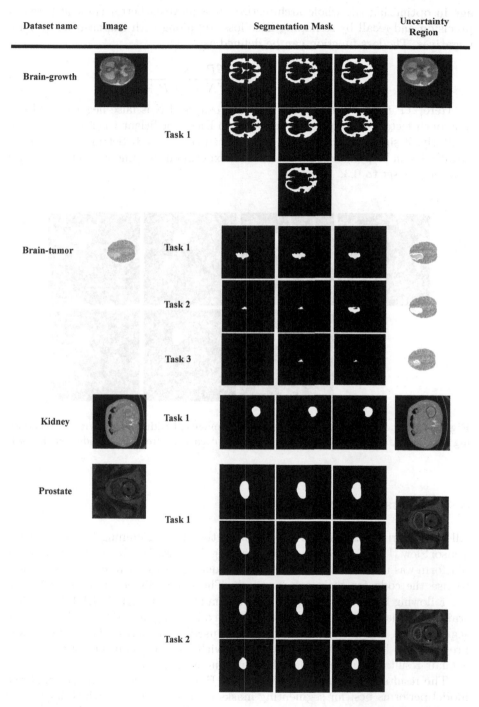

Fig. 3. Individual samples of datasets from the MICCAI-QUBIQ-2020 challenge.

age in optimizing the whole architecture. It achieves a better tradeoff between precision and recall by reshaping Dice loss [16] along with emphasizing on false negatives. The loss function can be defined as:

$$L_{Tversky} = \frac{TP + s}{TP + \alpha FN + \beta FP + s} \tag{1}$$

Here, TP is true positive, FP is false positive, FN is false negative and s is a smooth factor. The equation simplifies to Dice Coefficient when $\alpha = \beta = 0.5$, similarly, it simplifies to Jaccard Index when $\alpha = \beta = 1$. Setting $\alpha > \beta$, false negatives can be penalized more. For this experiment α value was set to 0.7 and β value was set to 0.3.

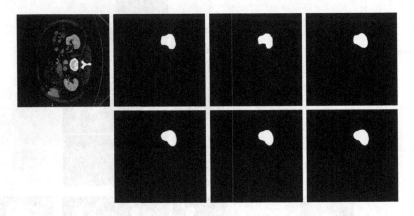

Fig. 4. The uncertainty corresponding to the images of Kidney (top) with corresponding predictions (bottom) for individual task of case 23 from the validation dataset.

4   Results and Discussions

All our experiments were carried out in Python3 programming language, using TensorFlow [1] and Keras [6] Deep Learning frameworks. Google Co-laboratory platform was used to train the models on cloud. This can help future researchers to use the code for their own research. The code will be made available on the following URL (https://github.com/Jimut123/MICCAI_QUBIQ_21). While training, Nadam [8] optimizer was used with a learning rate of 1e-05. To generate segmentation mask, Dice Coefficient was used as a metric. The dataset was preprocessed by normalizing each image with its maximum intensity value to get fair results from the model while training and testing.

The results are summarized in Table 2. From the table, we can see that the model performs best for segmenting masks for Kidney dataset which have little variability in delineations. It also performs well for Brain-Growth, which has one task and Brain-Tumor's task 1. Images corresponding to the segmentation

Table 2. The Dice Coefficient generated from validation dataset for all the available 2D image datasets from MICCAI-QUBIQ-2020 Challenge. The proposed model is compared with the previous state-of-the-art [12] method by combining several U-Nets, which shows our method performs significantly better at some tasks.

Model Name	Dataset	Task1	Task2	Task3
Proposed	**Brain-Growth**	**89.76**	–	–
Proposed	**Brain-Tumor**	**92.15**	36.68	65.69
Proposed	**Prostate**	**60.53**	38.46	–
Proposed	**Kidney**	**95.20**	–	–
U-Net Combined [15]	**Brain-Growth**	50.48	–	–
U-Net Combined [15]	**Brain-Tumor**	84.45	96.43	81.09
U-Net Combined [15]	**Prostate**	46.46	50.79	–
U-Net Combined [15]	**Kidney**	83.48	–	–

of Kidney's data sample for three tasks is shown in Fig. 4. The above row shows the individual delineations of the individual raters. Similarly, the row below has the algorithm's prediction. The images show some delineations of the individual raters simulated by the algorithm on the validation dataset. Prostate dataset has variable size images, so the model produces excellent results while training, but when the images are rescaled, the masks are out of position. The results can be further improved by fine-tuning the architecture. The results might increase significantly when more data is available. Our proposed model performs better than the previous state-of-the-art architecture in Task-1 of all the datasets.

5 Conclusions

A holistic network for quantifying uncertainties in medical images is proposed, which shows excellent results in some datasets without transfer learning and data augmentation. The main purpose of designing this architecture is to model variations in delineations in individual samples of segmentation masks produced by individual annotators via a holistic network of encoder and decoders. This model may further improve its performance by adding attention networks to focus on relevant features while training.

Acknowledgements. The author acknowledges the MICCAI-QUBIQ-2021 team to organize such a wonderful challenge by making the novel datasets available and also the reviewers for their critical discussions. Finally, the author thanks his mentors, Tamal Maharaj, Swathy Prabhu Mj, Dripta Mj and his father Dr. Jadab Kumar Pal for their suggestions.

References

1. Abadi, M., et al.: Tensorflow: a system for large-scale machine learning. In: 12th USENIX Symposium on Operating Systems Design and Implementation (OSDI 16), pp. 265–283 (2016). https://www.usenix.org/system/files/conference/osdi16/osdi16-abadi.pdf
2. Abraham, N., Khan, N.M.: A novel focal tversky loss function with improved attention u-net for lesion segmentation. In: 2019 IEEE 16th International Symposium on Biomedical Imaging (ISBI 2019), pp. 683–687 (2019). https://doi.org/10.1109/ISBI.2019.8759329
3. Alberts, E., et al.: Uncertainty quantification in brain tumor segmentation using crfs and random perturbation models. In: 13th IEEE International Symposium on Biomedical Imaging, ISBI 2016, Prague, Czech Republic, April 13–16, 2016, pp. 428–431. IEEE (2016). https://doi.org/10.1109/ISBI.2016.7493299, https://doi.org/10.1109/ISBI.2016.7493299
4. Azad, R., Asadi-Aghbolaghi, M., Fathy, M., Escalera, S.: Bi-directional convlstm u-net with densley connected convolutions. In: 2019 IEEE/CVF International Conference on Computer Vision Workshop (ICCVW), pp. 406–415 (2019)
5. Becker, A., et al.: Variability of manual segmentation of the prostate in axial t2-weighted mri: a multi-reader study. Eur. J. Radiol. **121**, 108716 (2019)
6. Chollet, F., et al.: Keras. https://github.com/fchollet/keras (2015)
7. Deng, J., Dong, W., Socher, R., Li, L.J., Li, K., Fei-Fei, L.: Imagenet: a large-scale hierarchical image database. In: 2009 IEEE Conference on Computer Vision and Pattern Recognition, pp. 248–255 (2009). https://doi.org/10.1109/CVPR.2009.5206848
8. Dozat, T.: Incorporating nesterov momentum into adam (2016)
9. He, K., Gkioxari, G., Dollár, P., Girshick, R.: Mask r-cnn. In: 2017 IEEE International Conference on Computer Vision (ICCV), pp. 2980–2988 (2017). https://doi.org/10.1109/ICCV.2017.322
10. He, K., Zhang, X., Ren, S., Sun, J.: Deep residual learning for image recognition. In: 2016 IEEE Conference on Computer Vision and Pattern Recognition (CVPR), pp. 770–778 (2016). https://doi.org/10.1109/CVPR.2016.90
11. Jha, D., Riegler, M.A., Johansen, D., Halvorsen, P., Johansen, H.D.: Doubleu-net: A deep convolutional neural network for medical image segmentation. In: 2020 IEEE 33rd International Symposium on Computer-Based Medical Systems (CBMS), pp. 558–564. IEEE Computer Society, Los Alamitos, CA, USA, July 2020. https://doi.org/10.1109/CBMS49503.2020.00111, https://doi.ieeecomputersociety.org/10.1109/CBMS49503.2020.00111
12. Ji, W., et al.: Learning calibrated medical image segmentation via multi-rater agreement modeling. In: Proceedings of the IEEE/CVF Conference on Computer Vision and Pattern Recognition (CVPR), pp. 12341–12351, June 2021
13. Joskowicz, L., Cohen, D., Caplan, N., Sosna, J.: Inter-observer variability of manual contour delineation of structures in CT. Eur. Radiol. **29**, 1391–1399 (2018)
14. Kohl, S.A.A., et al.: A probabilistic u-net for segmentation of ambiguous images. In: Proceedings of the 32nd International Conference on Neural Information Processing Systems, NIPS 2018, pp. 6965–6975. Curran Associates Inc., Red Hook (2018)
15. Ma, J.: Estimating segmentation uncertainties like radiologists (2020), qUBIQ 2020 Method Description

16. Ma, J., et al.: Loss odyssey in medical image segmentation. Medical Image Analysis **71**, 102035 (2021). https://doi.org/10.1016/j.media.2021.102035. https://www.sciencedirect.com/science/article/pii/S1361841521000815

17. Ma, J., et al.: Toward data efficient learning: a benchmark for COVID 19 CT lung and infection segmentation. Med. Phys. **48**(3), 1197–1210 (2021). https://doi.org/10.1002/mp.14676

18. Ng, A.Y.: Feature selection, <i>l</i>₁ vs. <i>l</i>₂ regularization, and rotational invariance. In: Proceedings of the Twenty-First International Conference on Machine Learning, p. 78. ICML 2004. Association for Computing Machinery, New York, NY, USA (2004). https://doi.org/10.1145/1015330.1015435, https://doi.org/10.1145/1015330.1015435

19. Ronneberger, O., Fischer, P., Brox, T.: U-Net: Convolutional Networks for Biomedical Image Segmentation. In: Navab, N., Hornegger, J., Wells, W.M., Frangi, A.F. (eds.) MICCAI 2015. LNCS, vol. 9351, pp. 234–241. Springer, Cham (2015). https://doi.org/10.1007/978-3-319-24574-4_28

20. Salehi, S.S.M., Erdogmus, D., Gholipour, A.: Tversky loss function for image segmentation using 3d fully convolutional deep networks. In: Wang, Q., Shi, Y., Suk, H.-I., Suzuki, K. (eds.) MLMI 2017. LNCS, vol. 10541, pp. 379–387. Springer, Cham (2017). https://doi.org/10.1007/978-3-319-67389-9_44

21. Schlemper, J., et al.: Attention gated networks: Learning to leverage salient regions in medical images. Med. Image Anal. **53**, 197–207 (2019). https://doi.org/10.1016/j.media.2019.01.012, https://www.sciencedirect.com/science/article/pii/S1361841518306133

22. Srivastava, N., Hinton, G., Krizhevsky, A., Sutskever, I., Salakhutdinov, R.: Dropout: a simple way to prevent neural networks from overfitting. J. Mach. Learn. Res. **15**(1), 1929–1958 (2014)

23. Tan, C., Sun, F., Kong, T., Zhang, W., Yang, C., Liu, C.: A survey on deep transfer learning. In: Kůrková, V., Manolopoulos, Y., Hammer, B., Iliadis, L., Maglogiannis, I. (eds.) ICANN 2018. LNCS, vol. 11141, pp. 270–279. Springer, Cham (2018). https://doi.org/10.1007/978-3-030-01424-7_27

24. Willemink, M.J., et al.: Preparing medical imaging data for machine learning. Radiology **295**(1), 4–15 (2020). https://doi.org/10.1148/radiol.2020192224. https://doi.org/10.1148/radiol.2020192224, pMID: 32068507

Uncertainty Quantification in Medical Image Segmentation with Multi-decoder U-Net

Yanwu Yang[1,2], Xutao Guo[1], Yiwei Pan[1], Pengcheng Shi[1], Haiyan Lv[5], and Ting Ma[1,2,3,4]($\boxtimes$)

[1] Department of Electronic and Information Engineering,
Harbin Institute of Technology at Shenzhen, Shenzhen, China
tma@hit.edu.cn
[2] Peng Cheng Lab, Shenzhen, China
[3] Advanced Innovation Center for Human Brain Protection,
Capital Medical University, Beijing, China
[4] National Clinical Research Center for Geriatric Disorders,
Xuanwu Hospital Capital Medical University, Beijing, China
[5] MindsGo Co. Ltd., Shenzhen, China

Abstract. Accurate medical image segmentation is crucial for diagnosis and analysis. However, the models without calibrated uncertainty estimates might lead to errors in downstream analysis and exhibit low levels of robustness. Estimating the uncertainty in the measurement is vital to making definite, informed conclusions. Especially, it is difficult to make accurate predictions on ambiguous areas and focus boundaries for both models and radiologists, even harder to reach a consensus with multiple annotations. In this work, the uncertainty under these areas is studied, which introduces significant information with anatomical structure and is as important as segmentation performance. We exploit the medical image segmentation uncertainty quantification by measuring segmentation performance with multiple annotations in a supervised learning manner and propose a U-Net based architecture with multiple decoders, where the image representation is encoded with the same encoder, and segmentation referring to each annotation is estimated with multiple decoders. Nevertheless, a cross loss function is proposed for bridging the gap between different branches. The proposed architecture is trained in an end-to-end manner and able to improve predictive uncertainty estimates. The model achieves comparable performance with fewer parameters to the integrated training model that ranked the runner-up in the MICCAI-QUBIQ 2020 challenge.

Keywords: Uncertainty qualification · Medical images segmentation · Multiple annotations

1 Introduction

Medical imaging segmentation plays a key role in diagnosis, monitoring, and treatment planning of the disease. In recent years, segmentation in medical imag-

A. Crimi and S. Bakas (Eds.): BrainLes 2021, LNCS 12963, pp. 570–577, 2022.
https://doi.org/10.1007/978-3-031-09002-8_50

ing achieves the state of the art with deep learning, at the same time saving physicians time and providing an accurate reproducible solution for diagnosis analysis and monitoring, even outperforming those conducted by doctors. However, despite high performance in segmentation accuracy, the modeling uncertainty is as important as accuracy, especially in medical scenarios [3]. In clinical experiments, there are biases in annotation among different doctors due to experience, understanding and so on. Although the annotation would achieve a dice score over 0.9, the uncertainty still troubles. It might be also contradictory only to improve accuracy while ignoring this uncertainty.

Uncertainty measures are a promising direction since uncertainties can provide information as to how confident the system was on performing a given task on a given patient. This information in turn can be used to leverage the decision-making process of a user, as well as to enable time-effective corrections of computer results by for instance, focusing on areas of high uncertainty[5].

Recent modules focusing on segmentation uncertainty were built based on probabilistic models, such as Bayesian neural network [7], Probabilistic U-Net [9] and so on [1,2,6,7]. These methods pinpoint the probabilistic of each pixel within the segmentation. Besides, ensemble models [10,12,14] would also obtain a considerable result to some extent, with small and simple models. However, these studies measure the uncertainty with the predictions' discrepancies in various forms, which is not intuitive and there is no exact correspondence in the image [13]. Instead, the MICCAI-QUBIQ[1] challenge proposed to use a average dice loss to measure these uncertain areas with between 3 and 7 annotations from experts, where the uncertainty is quantified with labeling and would be analyzed in a reasonable way.

In this paper, we built a U-Net based architecture with multi-decoder for medical image segmentation uncertainty quantification, exploiting all the annotations as to increase the performance of segmentation and decrease the predictive uncertainty. The contributions can be concludes as: 1) We built an end-to end architecture with multi-decoders for quantifying medical image segmentation uncertainty, where each decoder was implemented for measuring and fitting one annotation. 2) A cross loss function was carried out for optimizing, where the up-sampling information within different decoders were combined. Moreover, an auxiliary loss was carried out for improving performance. 3) Our architecture could remain high segmentation performance, at the same time measuring segmentation uncertainty. And finally we ranked second in the MICCAI-QUBIQ 2020 challenge.

2   Method

2.1   Neural Network Backbone

Our architecture is built based on U-Net, as shown in Fig. 1, where the channels of each stage are [16, 32, 48, 64, 64] respectively. Similarly, the context aggregation pathway is also implemented, which recombines multi-scale representations

---

[1] https://qubiq.grand-challenge.org/.

with shallower features to precisely localize the structures of interest. Each stage consists of two convolution groups with a residual structure. In detail, the convolution group is comprised of convolution operations with kernel size of 3, step size of 1, a relu activation function, and normalization. The upsampling is implemented by interpolation. The residual block was used for each stage, promoting the transmission of features in the network, and alleviating the gradient vanishing problem, making the network easier to train [11]. The transmitted features are combined via element-wise summation. We further replace the batch normalization with instance normalization, which takes place in the feature space, therefore it should have more profound impacts than a simple contrast normalization in the pixel space [4].

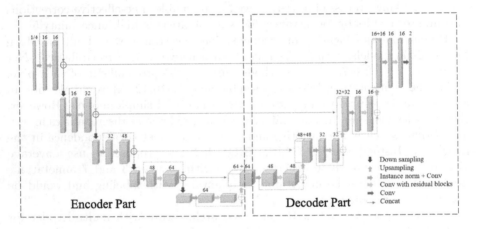

Fig. 1. The U-Net architecture implemented in our model, modified with residual blocks and instance normalization, where one decoder is shown in the figure. Our model is built upon this, with multiple decoders.

2.2   Mutli-decoder U-Net

Furthermore, multiple decoders are implemented in the architecture, where each decoder upsamples the same image representation, as shown in Fig. 2. Within the framework, multiple annotations were measured integrally at the same time, and the framework received one input and multiple labels.The framework aims to increase the predict of each branch, at the same time improve the average dice of all the metric.

A cross loss function is proposed, aiming to orient the segmentation representation with context of multiple annotations. Specially, the loss of each decoder was a combination of dice loss and cross entropy loss.

$$L_{loss}^{i} = \alpha * L_{ce}^{i,i} + L_{dc}^{i,i} + \frac{1}{n-1} \sum_{j,j \neq i}^{n} \beta_j * L_{dc}^{i,j} \tag{1}$$

$$L_{dc}^{i,j} = 1 - \frac{2}{|K|} \sum_{k \in K} \frac{\sum_{i,j}^{I} u_{i,k} * v_{j,k}}{\sum_{i}^{I} u_{i,k} + \sum_{j}^{I} v_{j,k}} \tag{2}$$

$$L_{ce}^{i,j} = - \sum_{k \in K} u_{i,k} * log(v_{j,k}) \tag{3}$$

where $u_{dc}^{i,j}$ denotes the average dice loss measured by the softmax output u_i of the ith branch, the jth denotes one hot encoding of the ground truth segmentation map v_j, $j \in n$ represents the number of the annotations, and $u_{ce}^{i,j}$ denotes the cross entropy loss in the same way. Both u and v have the same shape I by K, $k \in K$ being the classes.

In addition, an auxiliary loss that is not differentiable, is adapted for assistant training, obtained by the dice coefficient between average predictions and averaged ground truths:

$$L_{ad} = -\frac{1}{10} \sum_{\tau=0}^{1} dice(Mask(i, \tau), Mask(j, \tau)), \tag{4}$$

where τ denotes the threshold ranging from 0 to 1 by step of 0.1, and $Mask$ denotes the operation to binarize the segmentation.

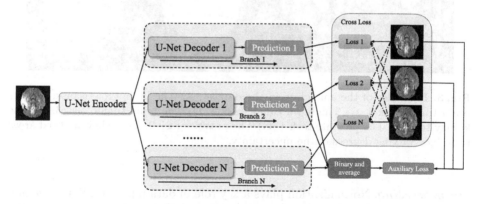

Fig. 2. The whole architecture of our multi-decoder U-Net, where each decoder is designed for predicting one annotation, and an auxiliary loss is implemented for improving training. The dotted line exhibit the training procedure, where the default dice loss is used as initialization, and the cross loss is enabled after a few epochs.

3   Experiments and Results

Dataset. The MICCAI-QUBIQ 2020 challenge provides 7 binary segmentation tasks in four different CT and MR data sets, where each task is segmented between three and seven times by different experts. In detail, the cohort includes 39 cases with 7 annotations for brain growth, 32 cases with 3 annotations for brain tumor, 24 cases with 3 annotations kidney, and 55 cases with 6 annotations for prostate. In total, there are seven binary segmentation tasks, two for prostate segmentation, one for brain growth segmentation, three for brain tumor segmentation, and one for kidney segmentation. Following the challenge, 48 cases of the prostate data, 34 cases of the brain growth data, 28 cases of the brain tumor data, and 20 cases of the kidney data are utilized as the training data. The remaining are the testing data. In addition, the data shapes within a single dataset are various, and are further padded to the same shape (Fig. 3).

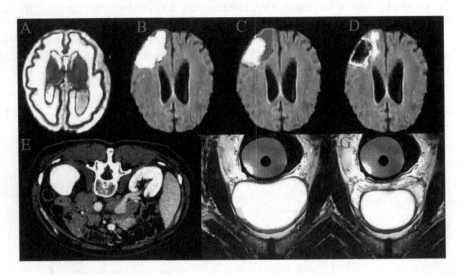

Fig. 3. Examples of the ambiguity in the dataset. A) The brain-growth task. B) The brain tumor task 1. C) The brain tumor task 2. D) The brain tumor task 3. E) The kidney task. F) The prostate task 1. G) The prostate task 2. The yellow and red areas introduce varying degrees of the uncertainty.

Preprocessing. Normalization plays a key role in data representation, specially for data acquired with various protocols. For MRI images, we conducted the z-score normalization by subtracting the mean and dividing by the standard deviation. In the CT image data, we localized the regions of interests, filtering non-sensitive parts and subsequently rescale to $[0, 1]$. Considering that the annotations came from different experts and were labeled with inconsistent rule, we relabeled the annotations by reference to the overlap of raters. For example, the tumor task includes three annotations, and the three annotations would be averaged with values of $[0.00, 0.33, 0.67, 1.00]$ and further binarized with threshold values of $[0.33, 0.67, 1.00]$ into three new labels.

Experiments. The result was conducted by the average prediction of each branch, which simulates experts to annotate the image. In this experiment, the performance is evaluated using the averaged dice score, measuring the uncertainty by binary at ten probability levels (that are 0.0, 0.1, 0.2, ..., 0.8, 0.9), as in (4).

However, the results would be seriously impacted when the convergence rate of all the branches vary, leading to non-uniform decreasing trends of losses. In terms of this, pretrained models were conducted, where all the models were trained from scratch to the same extent separately. Moreover, these models would be fine-tuned integrally. It can be estimated that although this balances the convergences of different branches, the integrated results are also impacted. In terms of this, the coefficients β_i have been modified according to the values of losses from pretrained models in the integrated training progression.

In this experiment, no external data was used and the networks were trained from scratch. We conducted the experiments using Pytorch on one Nvidia V100 GPU. The learning rate is increased to 3e−4 in 10 epochs using a linear warmup strategy. An adaptive moment estimate, Adam [8] with weight decay of 1e−5 is used as our optimizer.

Table 1. Results in comparison with different methods.

Models		U-Net	Ours	Ensemble models
Average score		0.669	0.720	**0.743**
Brain-growth		**0.483**	0.477	0.481
Brain-tumor	task01	0.821	0.852	**0.854**
	task02	0.814	0.871	**0.898**
	task03	0.825	0.832	**0.851**
Kidney		0.845	0.870	**0.872**
Prostate	task01	0.472	0.553	**0.554**
	task02	0.423	0.584	**0.689**

In terms of this novel task using multiple annotations and the average dice loss for measurement, related models are few and could hardly be implemented to achieve considerable performance. Here we designed a baseline, where several models are trained for multiple annotations. The final results were averaged with the models in the same way. Furthermore, we trained the network three times by modifying hyper-parameter of α and β_i as an ensemble to predict the respective validation and improve the generalization ability of the model. Validation set results were evaluated using the online evaluation platforms to ensure comparability with other participants (Fig. 4).

Results. The results are shown in Table 1. Our proposed multi-decoder U-Net outperforms the U-Net baseline in six tasks, with 0.852 in brain tumor task1, 0.871 in brain tumor task2, 0.832 in brain tumor task3, 0.870 in kidney, 0.553 in prostate task1, and 0584. in prostate task2. Besides, the ensemble models

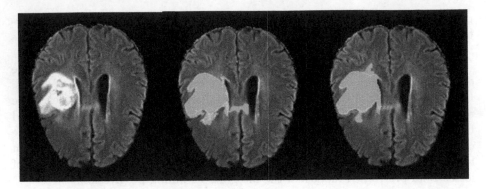

Fig. 4. Brain tumor segmentation results in comparison, which is shown as ground truth, averaged annotations and our results from left to right. The colors represent the uncertainty of the annotation and the segmentation.

performs the best. While, all the models perform badly in the brain-growth task, mainly because that the result is corresponding to the number of annotations and it is more likely that the gap between the annotations is enhanced inevitably.

4   Conclusion

In this work, we proposed a multi-decoder U-Net to calibrate the uncertainty with multiple annotations in an end-to-end manner. The novel task measuring the segmentation with multiple annotations and the averaged dice loss brings a way to further analyze and quantify the uncertainty, which has a better ability to reveal tiny and ambiguous structures and has a potential for diagnosis. Our method is simple and easy to be facilitated, where the decoder imitates the experts for labeling. The intuitive training strategy outperforms other complex models and achieves competitive results on six tasks. In order to perform a stable training, we fine-tuned the models using weights of baseline models and relabeled the labels by averaging and binarizing the annotations. The combination of the proposed model and training strategy makes contribution to the results. As future work, we would like to optimize the boundaries using multiple annotations and propose an adaptive segmentation model with uncertainty quantification.

Acknowledgements. This study is supported by grants from the National Key Research and Development Program of China (2018YFC1312000), Basic Research Foundation of Shenzhen Science and Technology Stable Support Program (GXWD20201230155427003-20200822115709001), China Postdoctoral Science Foundation funded project (2021M691686), and the National Natural Science Foundation of China (62106113).

References

1. Gal, Y., Ghahramani, Z.: Dropout as a bayesian approximation: representing model uncertainty in deep learning. In: International Conference on Machine Learning, pp. 1050–1059. PMLR (2016)
2. Gustafsson, F.K., Danelljan, M., Schon, T.B.: Evaluating scalable bayesian deep learning methods for robust computer vision. In: Proceedings of the IEEE/CVF Conference on Computer Vision and Pattern Recognition Workshops, pp. 318–319 (2020)
3. Hu, S., Worrall, D., Knegt, S., Veeling, B., Huisman, H., Welling, M.: Supervised uncertainty quantification for segmentation with multiple annotations. In: Shen, D., Liu, T., Peters, T.M., Staib, L.H., Essert, C., Zhou, S., Yap, P.-T., Khan, A. (eds.) MICCAI 2019. LNCS, vol. 11765, pp. 137–145. Springer, Cham (2019). https://doi.org/10.1007/978-3-030-32245-8_16
4. Huang, X., Belongie, S.: Arbitrary style transfer in real-time with adaptive instance normalization. In: Proceedings of the IEEE International Conference on Computer Vision, pp. 1501–1510 (2017)
5. Jungo, A., Reyes, M.: Assessing reliability and challenges of uncertainty estimations for medical image segmentation. In: Shen, D., Liu, T., Peters, T.M., Staib, L.H., Essert, C., Zhou, S., Yap, P.-T., Khan, A. (eds.) MICCAI 2019. LNCS, vol. 11765, pp. 48–56. Springer, Cham (2019). https://doi.org/10.1007/978-3-030-32245-8_6
6. Kendall, A., Gal, Y.: What uncertainties do we need in bayesian deep learning for computer vision? arXiv preprint arXiv:1703.04977 (2017)
7. Kendall, A., Badrinarayanan, V., Cipolla, R.: Bayesian segnet: model uncertainty in deep convolutional encoder-decoder architectures for scene understanding. arXiv preprint arXiv:1511.02680 (2015)
8. Kingma, D.P., Ba, J.: Adam: a method for stochastic optimization. arXiv preprint arXiv:1412.6980 (2014)
9. Kohl, S., et al.: A probabilistic u-net for segmentation of ambiguous images. In: Advances in Neural Information Processing Systems, pp. 6965–6975 (2018)
10. Lakshminarayanan, B., Pritzel, A., Blundell, C.: Simple and scalable predictive uncertainty estimation using deep ensembles. arXiv preprint arXiv:1612.01474 (2016)
11. Qiu, Y., Wang, R., Tao, D., Cheng, J.: Embedded block residual network: a recursive restoration model for single-image super-resolution. In: Proceedings of the IEEE/CVF International Conference on Computer Vision, pp. 4180–4189 (2019)
12. Ronneberger, O., Fischer, P., Brox, T.: U-Net: convolutional networks for biomedical image segmentation. In: Navab, N., Hornegger, J., Wells, W.M., Frangi, A.F. (eds.) MICCAI 2015. LNCS, vol. 9351, pp. 234–241. Springer, Cham (2015). https://doi.org/10.1007/978-3-319-24574-4_28
13. Wang, L., et al.: Medical matting: A new perspective on medical segmentation with uncertainty. arXiv preprint arXiv:2106.09887 (2021)
14. Wenzel, F., Snoek, J., Tran, D., Jenatton, R.: Hyperparameter ensembles for robustness and uncertainty quantification. arXiv preprint arXiv:2006.13570 (2020)

Meta-learning for Medical Image Segmentation Uncertainty Quantification

Sabri Can Cetindag[1(✉)], Mert Yergin[2], Deniz Alis[2,3], and Ilkay Oksuz[1,4]

[1] Department of Computer Engineering, Istanbul Technical University,
Istanbul, Turkey
cetindag21@itu.edu.tr
[2] Hevi AI, Istanbul, Turkey
[3] Radiology Department, Acibadem Mehmet Ali Aydinlar University School
of Medicine, Istanbul, Turkey
[4] School of Biomedical Engineering and Imaging Sciences, King's College London,
London, UK

Abstract. Inter-rater and intra-rater variability is a major challenge in medical image segmentation. Inconsistencies of manual segmentations between different experts can challenge development of deterministic automated medical image analysis tools. QUBIQ 2021 is a challenge to enable the successful development of automated machine learning tools, when there are inconsistencies between the labels of different annotators. In this paper, we propose to use meta-learning for quantifying uncertainty in biomedical image quantification. We first train a segmentation network for each expert separately with extensive data augmentation using the nnUnet framework. Then, a meta learner model based on a conventional U-net architecture is trained using the average of all annotators as ground truth, and output of all models that have been trained for each radiologist as input. We compared our results of meta-learning with ensemble methods for various image segmentation tasks and illustrate improved performance.

Keywords: Uncertainty quantification · Medical image segmentation · Meta-learning

1 Introduction

Medical image segmentation is fundamentally an ill-posed problem, and segmentation approaches that capable of estimating uncertainty over segmentations are consequently of great interest to the medical imaging community [5,6,9,10]. One of the best examples of the this interest is the labeling of an image by multiple experts. This poses the issue of determining which label for the image is correct. The major challenge the researchers are trying to overcome is to estimate intra- or inter-rater uncertainties of segmentations. Manual uncertainty determination is time-consuming and costly process, and therefore there is a need for automated algorithms to quantify uncertainties.

A. Crimi and S. Bakas (Eds.): BrainLes 2021, LNCS 12963, pp. 578–584, 2022.
https://doi.org/10.1007/978-3-031-09002-8_51

QUBIQ Challenge 2020 provides an extensive datasets on multiple pathology segmentation tasks [1]. The winner of the challenge proposed to train a network for each annotator and combine the results with averaging [7]. The paper proposes train a different model for each expert label and the output of each model is combined to estimate the uncertainties. In the ensembling phase, a new ensemble output is created by averaging the different model predictions generated for four experts. In our paper, we have extended the work in [7] with meta-learning. As a first step, a different model is trained for each expert label. Afterwards, predictions are obtained for that expert from the models trained for each expert label. Then, a new model is trained by combining the original image and these predictions as the modality of the original image. We call this model a *Meta-learner model*, which is based on a U-net architecture. For the predictions on the test set, firstly, predictions are obtained from the models for each expert, and then they are combined with the original image as modality and predicted in the meta-learner model. Finally, prediction of meta-learner model is used as estimation of uncertainty.

2   Methods

2.1   Network

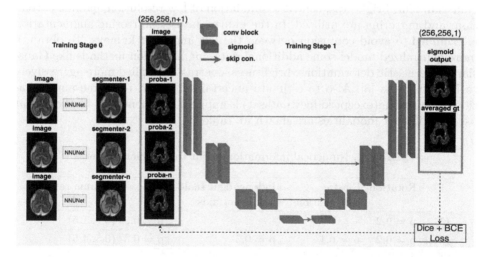

Fig. 1. Flowchart of the proposed Meta-learning scheme. We first train a separate nnUnet model [4] with extreme data augmentation for each annotator. Then, we train a meta-learner, which uses the probabilistic segmentation output of each network (n number stands for these outputs) and the input image to estimate the merged probabilistic output. The meta-learning network uses average of all annotators as ground truth. n is the segmenter number for that specific task.

The flowchart of our algorithm is shown in Fig. 1. A two step cascade deep learning method that consists of a combination of two different training stages is used. For each sub-task in the challenge, the same training pipeline is applied. In the datasets, each case contains 1 image and multiple annotations that are labeled by different experts. In training stage 0, a U-Net [8] model for each annotator is trained by using the nnUNet [4] framework. As a result, for each annotator, a U-Net model with different weights is obtained. Then, to train the model in training stage 1, a probability map of outputs of the models that are trained in training stage 0 is added to images as an additional channel (In Fig. 1, n+1 refers to the number of channels in these probability maps, whereas 1 refers to the original image). To obtain probability maps without bias 5-fold cross-validation is applied and only the output of the validation set for each fold is used in training stage 1. To generate ground truth for the model that is trained in stage 1, annotators' segmentation maps are averaged. Then the meta-learner model is trained. The output obtained at the end of stage 1 is used as the final output. As a comparison to the final output, for each task, outputs of the stage 0 models are ensembled.

2.2   Data Augmentation

Data augmentation is a technique for increasing the variety of data for training models while avoiding the need to actively collect additional data. To train the models, data augmentation methods such as rotations, scaling, Gaussian noise, Gaussian blur, brightness, contrast, simulation of low resolution, gamma correction, and mirroring are utilized. In the kidney dataset, mirroring augmentation is excluded to avoid confusion between the left and right kidneys. To obtain a more generalized model some additional data augmentation methods like Gaussian noise, elastic deformations, brightness, contrast is applied more aggressively to MRI datasets [3]. Also to estimate uncertainty better, test time augmentation by mirroring(except kidney dataset) is applied. Augmentation methods that used in different modalities are shown in Table 1.

Table 1. Numerical information about the augmentations

	Rotation	Elastic deformations	Independent scale factor per axis	Scale	Gamma range
CT	p = 0.2	-	-	p = 0.2	(0.7, 1.5)
MRI	p = 0.2	p = 0.1	p = 0.3	p = 0.3	(0.5, 1.6)

2.3   Implementation Details

Various models are trained for each dataset. The experimental settings for the model training are as follows:

- **Brain Tumor:** 2D U-Net model is implemented using nnUNet in Python. Batch size of 32 is used for 240×240 sliced pixel patches. Each model for different experts are trained for 25 epochs.

- **Brain Growth:** 2D U-Net model is implemented using nnUNet in Python. Batch size of 16 is used for 256×256 sliced pixel patches. Each model for different experts are trained for 25 epochs.
- **Prostate:** 2D U-Net model is implemented using nnUNet in Python. Batch size of 8 is used for 640×640 sliced pixel patches. Each model for different experts are trained for 25 epochs.
- **Kidney:** 2D U-Net model is implemented using nnUNet in Python. Batch size of 4 is used for 496×496 sliced pixel patches. Each model for different experts are trained for 25 epochs.
- **Pancreas:** 3D U-Net model is implemented using nnUNet in Python. Batch size of 2 is used for $28 \times 360 \times 360$ sliced pixel patches. Each model for different experts are trained for 25 epochs.
- **P. Lesion:** 3D U-Net model is implemented using nnUNet in Python. Batch size of 2 is used for $28 \times 360 \times 360$ sliced pixel patches. Each model for different experts are trained for 25 epochs.

SGD optimizer with Nesterov momentum is used for each training setup. Dice and cross-entropy is used as a loss function. Poly learning rate is used with an initial learning rate 1e−2. For each epoch 250 step size is used. Weight decay is used as 3e−5.

3   Experimental Results

3.1   Dataset

In this paper, cases of Brain Tumor, Brain Growth, Prostate, Kidney, Pancreas, Pancreatic Lesion diseases consisting of CT or MRI images with different modalities are studied. QUBIQ 2021 Challenge [2] dataset is used to train the models. Each dataset contains slices with different resolutions. Table 2 shows the details about the each individual dataset in QUBIQ 2021 Challenge.

Table 2. Numerical information about the datasets

	Training set	Validation set	Tasks	Modalities	Annotators	Slice shape
Brain Tumor	28	4	3	4	3	240×240
Brain Growth	34	5	1	1	7	256×256
Prostate	48	7	2	1	2	640×640
Kidney	20	4	1	1	3	497×497
Pancreas	40	18	1	1	2	512×512
Pancreatic Lesion	21	10	1	1	2	512×512

These datasets include different number of cases and different number of annotators. In some cases, there is a dramatic discrepancy between some experts, even in couple of cases some experts believed that there is no object to segment in the image. Three sample cases from kidney dataset is shown in Fig. 2. Each different colored line in the figure represents a different expert's label. The aim here is to estimate the uncertainty between these different experts.

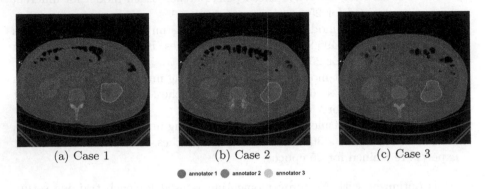

(a) Case 1   (b) Case 2   (c) Case 3

● annotator 1   ● annotator 2   ● annotator 3

Fig. 2. Example cases from kidney dataset. Disagreements between three different annotators is visible in all three cases.

3.2   Evaluation Metric

The results are obtained by calculating using the evaluation metric provided in QUBIQ 2021 Challenge between probabilistic predictions averaged ground truth labels. Briefly, probabilistic labels are obtained from ground truth labels by averaging multiple experts annotations. These values are compared using the dice metric on the probabilistic prediction for predefined thresholds (0.1, 0.2, ..., 0.9). Dice scores for all thresholds are averaged to get the final score. This evaluation metric is proposed in QUBIQ 2021 for measuring the model's uncertainty better.

3.3   Results for Different Probability Levels

Table 3. Quantitative results on kidney task on validation set

Methods/Prob. Levels	0.1	0.2	0.3	0.4	0.5	0.6	0.7	0.8	0.9	Mean
Ensemble	0.963	0.963	0.963	0.959	0.959	0.960	0.968	0.969	0.970	0.964
Meta-learner	0.968	0.974	0.975	*0.976*	0.978	0.975	0.967	0.972	0.974	0.973

As seen in Table 4, for most tasks, the meta-learner model was more successful than the ensemble of the annotators' models. As shown in Table 3 the increase was consistent between all thresholds. Figure 3 illustrates an example case from kidney Task 1, where different annotations from 3 annotators is visible. Meta-learner is capable to estimate the averaged ground truth better than the ensemble method for different probability levels.

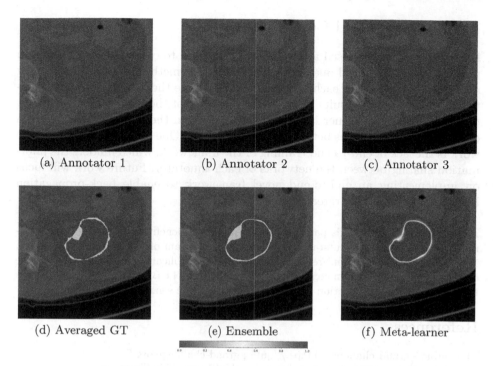

(a) Annotator 1   (b) Annotator 2   (c) Annotator 3

(d) Averaged GT   (e) Ensemble   (f) Meta-learner

Fig. 3. Results for a sample data from kidney Task 1. Top row illustrates the annotations from individual experts. Averaged ground truth (Averaged GT) is highlighting the disagreements between experts. Proposed meta-learner strategy is capable to showcase uncertainties better compared to ensemble method. Colorbar indicates the different probability levels.

3.4 Results (Meta-learner vs. Ensemble)

In Table 4, we compare the results of the proposed meta-learning technique with ensemble method. It can be observed that meta-learner framework is capable to outperform the ensemble method in most of the tasks with the exception of brain tumor task 2. As mentioned in Sect. 3.1, some tasks contain ground truth without foreground. Because of that in one task meta-learner model is not capable to outperform the ensemble model.

Table 4. Quantitative results on validation set

Methods/Dataset	B. Tumor			B. Growth	Prostate		Kidney	Pancreas	P. Lesion
Tasks	Task 1	Task 2	Task 3	Task 1	Task 1	Task 2	Task 1	Task 1	Task 1
Ensemble	0.9531	**0.8642**	0.8205	0.9293	0.9483	0.8112	0.9640	*0.6548*	*0.5418*
Proposed Meta-learner	**0.9575**	0.8185	**0.9145**	**0.9335**	**0.9579**	**0.8256**	**0.9730**	**0.7120**	**0.7261**

4 Discussion and Conclusions

In this paper, we proposed a meta-learning method to combine the information multiple annotators and quantify uncertainty. Our method is based on training an individual model for each annotator and combine the outputs using an additional network. Our results indicate that in most of the tasks in QUBIQ 2021 challenge the meta-learner is capable to outperform the ensemble technique in quantifying uncertainties between different experts. One major limitations of the work is the lack of end-to-end training of the framework, which hinders the information sharing between the networks of each annotator. Future work will focus on implementing an end-to-end novel framework to enable back-propagation between the labels generated by each annotator.

Acknowledgments. This paper has been produced benefiting from the 2232 International Fellowship for Outstanding Researchers Program of TUBITAK (Project No: 118C353). However, the entire responsibility of the publication/paper belongs to the owner of the paper. The financial support received from TUBITAK does not mean that the content of the publication is approved in a scientific sense by TUBITAK.

References

1. Qubiq - grand challenge. https://qubiq.grand-challenge.org/
2. Qubiq2021 - grand challenge. https://qubiq21.grand-challenge.org/
3. Full, P.M., Isensee, F., Jäger, P.F., Maier-Hein, K.: Studying robustness of semantic segmentation under domain shift in cardiac MRI. In: Puyol Anton, E., Pop, M., Sermesant, M., Campello, V., Lalande, A., Lekadir, K., Suinesiaputra, A., Camara, O., Young, A. (eds.) STACOM 2020. LNCS, vol. 12592, pp. 238–249. Springer, Cham (2021). https://doi.org/10.1007/978-3-030-68107-4_24
4. Isensee, F., Jaeger, P.F., Kohl, S.A., Petersen, J., Maier-Hein, K.H.: nnu-net: a self-configuring method for deep learning-based biomedical image segmentation. Nat. Methods 18(2), 203–211 (2021)
5. Jensen, M.H., Jørgensen, D.R., Jalaboi, R., Hansen, M.E., Olsen, M.A.: Improving uncertainty estimation in convolutional neural networks using inter-rater agreement. In: Shen, D., Liu, T., Peters, T.M., Staib, L.H., Essert, C., Zhou, S., Yap, P.-T., Khan, A. (eds.) MICCAI 2019. LNCS, vol. 11767, pp. 540–548. Springer, Cham (2019). https://doi.org/10.1007/978-3-030-32251-9_59
6. Kendall, A., Gal, Y.: What uncertainties do we need in bayesian deep learning for computer vision? arXiv preprint arXiv:1703.04977 (2017)
7. Ma, J.: Estimating segmentation uncertainties like radiologists. Qubiq (2015)
8. Ronneberger, O., Fischer, P., Brox, T.: U-Net: convolutional networks for biomedical image segmentation. In: Navab, N., Hornegger, J., Wells, W.M., Frangi, A.F. (eds.) MICCAI 2015. LNCS, vol. 9351, pp. 234–241. Springer, Cham (2015). https://doi.org/10.1007/978-3-319-24574-4_28
9. Wilson, R., Spann, M.: Image segmentation and uncertainty. Research Studies Press Ltd. (1988)
10. Zhang, L., et al.: Learning to segment when experts disagree. In: Martel, A.L., Abolmaesumi, P., Stoyanov, D., Mateus, D., Zuluaga, M.A., Zhou, S.K., Racoceanu, D., Joskowicz, L. (eds.) MICCAI 2020. LNCS, vol. 12261, pp. 179–190. Springer, Cham (2020). https://doi.org/10.1007/978-3-030-59710-8_18

Using Soft Labels to Model Uncertainty in Medical Image Segmentation

João Lourenço-Silva[(✉)] [iD] and Arlindo L. Oliveira [iD]

Instituto Superior Técnico/INESC-ID, Lisbon, Portugal
{joao.lourenco.silva,arlindo.oliveira}@tecnico.ulisboa.pt

Abstract. Medical image segmentation is inherently uncertain. For a given image, there may be multiple plausible segmentation hypotheses, and physicians will often disagree on lesion and organ boundaries. To be suited to real-world application, automatic segmentation systems must be able to capture this uncertainty and variability. Thus far, this has been addressed by building deep learning models that, through dropout, multiple heads, or variational inference, can produce a set - infinite, in some cases - of plausible segmentation hypotheses for any given image. However, in clinical practice, it may not be practical to browse all hypotheses. Furthermore, recent work shows that segmentation variability plateaus after a certain number of independent annotations, suggesting that a large enough group of physicians may be able to represent the whole space of possible segmentations. Inspired by this, we propose a simple method to obtain soft labels from the annotations of multiple physicians and train models that, for each image, produce a single well-calibrated output that can be thresholded at multiple confidence levels, according to each application's precision-recall requirements. We evaluate our method on the MICCAI 2021 QUBIQ challenge, showing that it performs well across multiple medical image segmentation tasks, produces well-calibrated predictions, and, on average, performs better at matching physicians' predictions than other physicians.

Keywords: Uncertainty estimation · Medical image segmentation · Soft labels

1 Introduction

Accurate segmentation of medical images is crucial in diagnosing and planning the treatment of multiple pathologies. Nevertheless, it is also very laborious and time-consuming, spurring great interest in the development of automatic segmentation mechanisms.

In the last few years, deep learning systems have achieved high performance in the segmentation of several organs and anatomical structures [30]. However, most methods do not account for the uncertainty inherent to these tasks. For a given image, there may be multiple plausible segmentations, and physicians will often disagree on the zones of interest and their contours. Thus, models should be able to capture uncertainty and express it in their predictions. Otherwise, they risk biasing physicians, which may lead to misdiagnosis and sub-optimal treatment.

To date, most work on uncertainty estimation in medical image segmentation focuses on being able to produce multiple plausible outputs for a given image [1,11,22,23,33]. However, in clinical practice, it may be impractical to browse all hypotheses. Furthermore, recent research [15] shows that, even though segmentation variability increases with the number of annotators, it plateaus after a certain data and task-dependent number of independent annotations, implying that, although multiple plausible segmentations exist for a given input, they can be encompassed by the annotations of a sufficiently large group of physicians.

In this work, we follow a trend orthogonal to that of previous work. Rather than aiming to build probabilistic models that can produce various plausible hypotheses, we propose to train deterministic models on soft labels built from the annotations of multiple physicians. We evaluated our method on datasets from the MICCAI 2021 QUBIQ challenge. The results showed that it performs well compared to alternative approaches and produces well-calibrated outputs across a range of medical image segmentation tasks and imaging modalities.

2   Related Work

Monte Carlo Dropout is a technique used by early approaches for uncertainty estimation in image segmentation, which use dropout [42] over spatial features to induce probability distributions over the models' outputs [16,17], allowing the drawing of multiple samples at test-time. However, these methods quantify uncertainty pixel-wise, leading them to produce spatially inconsistent segmentation hypotheses.

Ensembles [26,28] and *Multi-Head Neural Networks* [13,29,38] are simple methods to produce plausible and consistent output hypotheses. While they may not be able to capture diversity and learn rare variants when ensemble members and network heads are trained independently, that can be circumvented by joint training on an oracle loss [7], which only accounts for the lowest-error prediction. The main disadvantages of these approaches are their poor scaling with the number of hypotheses and the latter's requirement to be set at training time.

Variational Bayesian Inference methods, like the sPU-Net [23], HPU-Net [22] and PHiSeg [1] combine conditional variational autoencoders [19,20,36,41] with U-Net-based [37] networks to model the distribution of segmentations given an input image. Input images are encoded into multivariate normal latent spaces that the decoder samples at test-time to produce arbitrarily complex and diverse segmentation hypotheses. However, this approach requires a training-only posterior network, and the placement of the latent variables within the model entails a partial forward pass for each output hypothesis. Recent work addresses these issues with a more constrained low-rank multivariate normal distribution over the logit space, which avoids the use of a posterior network and allows efficient sampling without compromising performance [33]. Other work [11] extends the sPU-Net using variational dropout [21] to predict epistemic uncertainty, and intergrader variability as a target for supervised aleatoric uncertainty estimation.

3   Method

3.1   Motivation

For many years, due to optimization difficulties and lack of computing power, it was very difficult to train deep neural networks. Recently, however, better hardware and new architectural components, such as batch normalization [14] and residual connections [9], have enabled training increasingly deeper and wider networks [9,12,25,40,43,44], which achieve high performance in a wide range of tasks. Nevertheless, unlike their shallower and less accurate counterparts from the past, like the LeNet [27], modern neural networks are poorly calibrated, leading to a situation where the probabilities they assign to classes do not reflect their real likelihoods. Though a set of factors such as model capacity, batch normalization and lack of regularization have been put forward as possible causes for miscalibration, the use of hard labels is probably one of the causes at the heart of the problem. When training neural networks to make their predictions match a set of hard labels, which are often the only available ones, it is unreasonable to interpret them as probabilistic models and expect them to output well-calibrated confidence values.

A simple approach to address this issue would be to use soft labels conveying information about real class likelihood. These would not only allow modeling the uncertainty inherent to the data, but would also be likely to enable faster and more data-efficient training. As noted in seminal work on knowledge distillation by Hinton et al. [10], compared to hard targets, high entropy soft targets provide much more information per training case and much less variance in the gradient across samples, allowing models to be trained on much fewer data and with significantly higher learning rates. In fact, even noisy soft labels can be of great value, as showcased by recent research on semi-supervised learning [35,45].

3.2   Proposed Method

We propose to use soft labels built from multiple annotations to model uncertainty and address network calibration. Given a set of labels for an image, we average them to produce probabilistic ground-truth masks. Beyond expressing real physicians' uncertainty about zones of interest and their contours, these high entropy soft labels enable our models to enjoy the advantages pointed out by Hinton et al. [10]. Additionally, note that, for binary variables, the variance can be obtained from the mean[1]. Therefore, although it can be used as an auxiliary supervision signal, it does not need to be predicted directly by the models.

---

[1] $X = X^2 \implies \mathbf{V}(X) = \mathbf{E}(X^2) - \mathbf{E}(X)^2 = \mathbf{E}(X) - \mathbf{E}(X)^2$.

Depending on the number of annotations per image, the set S of possible ground-truth probabilities will be more or less granular. Formally, let A be the number of annotations, then $S = \{\frac{i}{A} : i \in \mathbb{N} \wedge i \leq A\}$. More annotations per image result in smoother and less noisy ground-truth, which, intuitively, should allow better segmentation performance and uncertainty modeling.

Following Hinton et al. [10], we minimize the cross-entropy between the probabilities predicted by the model, p, and the ground-truth soft targets, g. Note that the dice loss (DL) function, commonly used in segmentation tasks, is not suitable to be used with soft targets. Let C be the number of classes and N the total number of pixels. DL can be defined as

$$\mathrm{DL}(p,g) = 1 - 2\frac{\sum_{c=1}^{C}\sum_{i=1}^{N}[g_{ci}p_{ci}]}{\sum_{c=1}^{C}\sum_{i=1}^{N}[g_{ci} + p_{ci}]}. \tag{1}$$

Without loss of generalization, consider the binary classification of a single-pixel image. For $g > 0$, DL is a monotonically decreasing function of p. Hence, for $p \in [0,1]$, the minimum DL will be obtained for $p = 1$. Consequently, the model is encouraged to binarize its outputs and does not learn to predict uncertainty. This problem could be mitigated by measuring DL at multiple confidence thresholds. However, it would require defining the optimal number of thresholds and their values. Thus, we opt for the more principled cross-entropy loss. Researching overlap-based loss functions that, unlike DL, can be used to match soft targets, is a possible direction for future work.

3.3   Model Architecture

We conducted our experiments using a U-Net decoder [37] with 16-channel feature maps at the highest resolution level. As encoder, we used an EfficientNet-B0 [44], a good-performing feature extractor that makes for segmentation models whose compute scales better with input image size than the default U-Net encoder and other popular architectures [39], which can be of great value when segmenting high pixel-count medical images.

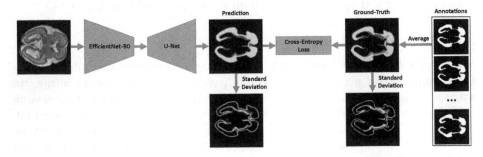

Fig. 1. Pipeline of the proposed method and segmentation model architecture. Our method allows modeling annotations without overfitting them, resulting in predictions with smooth probability and standard deviation variations.

4   Experimental Setup

4.1   Datasets and Data Augmentation

We evaluated our method on datasets from the MICCAI 2021 QUBIQ challenge[2], composed of CTs and MRIs with multiple annotations per case. Except for the four-channel brain tumor MRIs, all images are single-channel. Due to architectural constraints, the images were cropped during training to ensure their dimensions were multiples of 32. Crop sizes were set empirically to balance segmentation performance and training time. Table 1 summarizes the details of each dataset.

Table 1. Summary of the MICCAI 2021 QUBIQ challenge datasets used.

Dataset	Modality	Tasks	Annotators	Size		Cases	
				Slice	Crop	Train	Validation
Brain growth	2D MRI	1	7	256^2	256^2	34	5
Brain tumor	2D MRI	3	3	240^2	224^2	28	4
Kidney	2D CT	1	3	497^2	320^2	20	4
Prostate	2D MRI	2	6[a]	640^2	480^2	48	7
				640×960			

[a]Except for three cases, which only have 5 annotations.

Data augmentation is performed online and consists of the following sequentially applied random transformations: 1) -10% to 10% horizontal and vertical translation; 2) $-15°$ to $15°$ rotation; 3) -10% to 10% zoom; 3) horizontal flip with 50% probability; 4) vertical flip with 0% probability for the kidney dataset and 50% for the remaining. Following Fort et al. [4], we draw multiple augmentation samples per image in a growing batch regime. However, unlike them, we keep the original images in the batch, since we observed this improves performance slightly. Specifically, we augment each batch with three transformations of each image.

4.2   Evaluation Metrics

Segmentation is a spatially structured prediction task. Therefore, segmentation models' calibration must be assessed using metrics that take spatial structure into account. Hence, instead of common pixel-wise calibration metrics [2,5,34], we measured overlap and surface distance at multiple confidence thresholds. Additionally, following previous work [22,23,33], we used the generalized energy distance to measure the statistical distance between the ground-truth masks and our models' predictions at the 50% confidence threshold. Below, we briefly describe the more domain-specific metrics, which may be unknown to some readers. In addition to those, we also measured precision and recall.

---

2 Challenge information and datasets available https://qubiq21.grand-challenge.org/.

Dice Similarity Coefficient (DSC) and Intersection over Union (IoU) are measures of the overlap between two segmentations. DSC is the ratio between the area of overlap and the sum of the two areas, and is equal to $1 - DL$ (see Eq. 1). IoU is the ratio between the overlap and union areas. When both segmentation masks are empty, we set DSC and IoU to 1.

95% Hausdorff Distance (95% HD). Given two sets of points - two segmentation masks, in this context -, the Hausdorff distance is the maximum distance from a point in one set to the closest point in the other set. The 95% HD disregards the 5% most distant pairs of points, ignoring outliers, but still providing a measure of the longest distance between the two sets of points.

Generalized Energy Distance (D_{GED}) measures the statistical distance between probability distributions. As long as the function $d(\cdot, \cdot)$ is a metric, so is D_{GED}. Following previous work [22,23,33] we define $d(x,y) = 1 - IoU(x,y)$, which has been proven to be a metric [24,31]. Given the distributions of ground-truth segmentations, p, and predicted segmentations, $\hat{p}$, D_{GED}^2 is defined by

$$D_{GED}^2(p,\hat{p}) = 2\mathbb{E}_{y\sim p, \hat{y}\sim\hat{p}}[d(y,\hat{y})] - \mathbb{E}_{y,y'\sim p}[d(y,y')] - \mathbb{E}_{\hat{y},\hat{y}'\sim\hat{p}}[d(\hat{y},\hat{y}')]. \quad (2)$$

Since our models are deterministic, the formula above can be simplified to

$$D_{GED}^2(p,\hat{p}) = 2\mathbb{E}_{y\sim p}[d(y,\hat{y})] - \mathbb{E}_{y,y'\sim p}[d(y,y')], \quad (3)$$

where $\hat{y}$ is the predicted segmentation mask. The first term of Eq. 3 is the average distance between predicted and ground-truth annotations, and the second can be interpreted as a measure of ground-truth segmentation diversity.

4.3   Implementation and Training Details

We used encoders pre-trained on ImageNet [3]. Decoder hidden and output layers were initialized using Kaiming [8] and Xavier initialization [6], respectively. Models were trained for 150 epochs - 180 for the third brain tumor task -, using batches of 8 images. As optimizer, we used Adam [18], with $\beta_1 = 0.9$, $\beta_2 = 0.999$ and no weight decay. Learning rates were initialized at 10^{-2} and decreased to 10^{-4} using a cosine annealing schedule [32]. To ensure reproducibility, we trained and tested each model three times, obtaining similar results across all runs. All experiments were conducted using public PyTorch implementations [46] under an MIT license.

5   Results

To assess calibration, we started by measuring DSC, precision, recall and 95% HD between model predictions and averaged ground-truth masks at multiple confidence thresholds. Specifically, we used thresholds ranging from 10% to 90% confidence, with a step size of 10%.

The averages of these metrics across thresholds are reported in Table 2. Note that the results should be interpreted taking into account image sizes, reported in Table 1, and ground-truth area to image size ratios. For example, the prostate tasks' regions of interest are relatively large, making them easy to overlap and leading to a high DSC. However, the large size of the images - 640 × 640 and 640 × 960 - and structures leads to apparently high 95% HDs, compared to those of other tasks. On the other hand, the tiny structures in the third brain tumor segmentation task are challenging to detect and segment, hence the relatively low DSC and recall. Nevertheless, the small image size and object make low 95% HDs relatively easy to achieve.

Apart from the second brain tumor segmentation task, discussed in more detail below, our method achieves high segmentation performance in all other tasks. Furthermore, the low standard deviations indicate consistent performance across confidence thresholds and, therefore, good model calibration. This can be visualized in Fig. 2, where despite performing better at confidence values near 50%, our model does well across a range of thresholds, allowing the latter to be selected according to each application's precision and recall requirements.

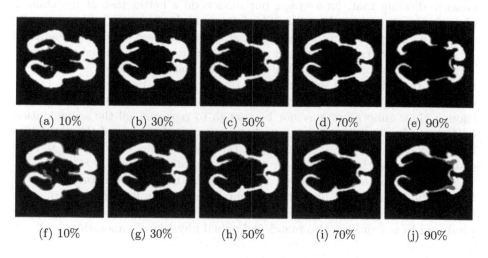

| (a) 10% | (b) 30% | (c) 50% | (d) 70% | (e) 90% |
| (f) 10% | (g) 30% | (h) 50% | (i) 70% | (j) 90% |

Fig. 2. Annotation average (top row) and model prediction (bottom row) thresholded at multiple confidence thresholds. In the bottom row, the zones in red and green correspond to false positives and false negatives, respectively. (Color figure online)

To further assess calibration and uncertainty modeling, we followed previous work [22,23,33] and measured the generalized energy distance (D_{GED}) between the multiple ground-truth annotations and the models' predictions at the 50% confidence threshold. Additionally, we measured the expected value of the DSC between predictions at 50% confidence and each physician's annotations - which is not equivalent to measuring the DSC between model predictions and average ground-truth masks at the same threshold. Results are reported in Table 3.

Table 2. Dice score, precision, recall, 95% Hausdorff distance and ground-truth area to image size ratio, averaged across confidence thresholds ranging from 10% to 90%, with a step size of 10%. Results presented as mean ± standard deviation.

Task	Dice score [%]	Precision [%]	Recall [%]	95% HD [pixels]	$\frac{\text{Ground-Truth Area}}{\text{Image Size}}$ [%]
Brain growth	93.19 ± 1.83	93.33 ± 2.55	93.16 ± 1.84	3.53 ± 0.73	8.33 ± 1.57
Brain tumor 1	92.90 ± 1.09	93.79 ± 1.01	89.04 ± 2.30	6.84 ± 2.37	3.50 ± 0.31
Brain tumor 2	65.06 ± 20.27	67.18 ± 21.75	63.74 ± 19.57	15.15 ± 13.18	1.33 ± 1.47
Brain tumor 3	85.73 ± 4.88	97.67 ± 1.78	78.34 ± 6.67	2.27 ± 2.15	0.29 ± 0.04
Kidney	96.04 ± 1.43	96.57 ± 1.64	95.65 ± 2.53	7.67 ± 3.65	1.90 ± 0.12
Prostate 1	95.64 ± 0.04	94.13 ± 1.05	97.43 ± 0.78	16.18 ± 7.58	8.87 ± 0.68
Prostate 2	93.56 ± 4.58	91.78 ± 4.09	95.70 ± 5.32	12.48 ± 5.46	5.49 ± 0.58

Except for the second brain tumor segmentation task, the remaining tasks' D_{GED}^2 is very low, meaning the models' predictions closely match the distributions of ground-truth annotations. In fact, in most cases, the expected value of the IoU distance between model predictions and ground-truth annotations is lower than that of the IoU distance between annotations by different physicians, indicating that, on average, our models do a better task at matching a physician's annotations than other physicians do, which is remarkable, especially considering the small dimension of the datasets, composed of 20 to 48 samples.

The overall worse performances are registered for the second and third brain tumor segmentation tasks. For the latter, the lower performance is largely justified by the difficulty of segmenting its tiny structures. However, in the former case, the difficulty lies in the high variability between ground-truth masks. Even though three annotators may not be enough to represent all the segmentation hypotheses in this task, we suspect the annotations from one of the physicians to be incorrect, as their average IoU distance to the others is 94.15%, and the distance between the other two physicians' annotations is only 19.82%.

Finally, note that the expected value of the DSC between predictions at 50% confidence and each physician's annotations is generally high, meaning that beyond matching the averaged predictions of multiple physicians, the masks produced by our models also match individual physicians' annotations well.

Table 3. From the 2nd to the 5th column: squared generalized energy distance; expected IoU distance between predictions and ground-truth masks; ground-truth diversity; expected DSC between predictions at 50% confidence and each physician's annotations. Results presented as mean ± standard deviation.

Task	D_{GED}^2	$\mathbb{E}_{y \sim p}[1 - \text{IoU}(y, \hat{y})]$	$\mathbb{E}_{y,y' \sim p}[1 - \text{IoU}(y, y')]$	$\mathbb{E}_{y \sim p}[\text{DSC}(y, \hat{y})]$
Brain Growth	0.1323 ± 0.0077	0.1876 ± 0.0087	0.2429 ± 0.0124	89.63 ± 01.60
Brain Tumor 1	0.1455 ± 0.0622	0.1393 ± 0.0492	0.1330 ± 0.0497	92.39 ± 03.78
Brain Tumor 2	0.6731 ± 0.5631	0.6843 ± 0.3167	0.6955 ± 0.0835	34.27 ± 43.45
Brain Tumor 3	0.2515 ± 0.1928	0.2272 ± 0.1523	0.2030 ± 0.1306	86.25 ± 10.22
Kidney	0.0613 ± 0.0077	0.0814 ± 0.0105	0.1015 ± 0.0150	95.73 ± 01.59
Prostate 1	0.0950 ± 0.0692	0.1096 ± 0.0569	0.1242 ± 0.0478	94.07 ± 03.80
Prostate 2	0.0988 ± 0.0907	0.1431 ± 0.0679	0.1874 ± 0.0828	90.99 ± 15.25

6   Discussion

We proposed a new way of approaching uncertainty modeling in image segmentation. Instead of building models that learn independently from the annotations of multiple physicians and can produce multiple segmentation hypotheses for a given image, we train deliberately deterministic models on the joint predictions of physician ensembles, using the averages of their predictions as soft labels.

We evaluated our method on datasets from the MICCAI 2021 QUBIQ challenge, showing that it results in well-calibrated models that, on average, match physicians' predictions better than other physicians. The results show that our system exhibits a good performance on this task, competitive with other approaches.

A limitation of our method is that annotation averaging leads to loss of information about the spatial correlation between pixels, which could be valuable to train better and more accurate models. Additionally, by relying on annotation averaging to model uncertainty, our method's applicability is limited to datasets with more than one label per image, and the quality of its results is particularly dependent on the granularity of the ground-truth probabilistic targets.

In future work, we plan to test this technique on larger datasets and more challenging tasks with multiple classes, possibly including problems outside the scope of medical image segmentation. Additionally, we intend to investigate if the soft labels used in our method allow the more data-efficient training generic soft labels do [10]. Finally, given soft labels' role in recent teacher-student semi-supervised learning methods [35, 45], we plan to assess if networks trained on soft labels, like ours, can be better teachers than those trained on hard labels.

Acknowledgments. This work was supported by national funds through Fundação para a Ciência e Tecnologia (FCT), under the project with reference UIDB/50021/2020 and the project PRELUNA, with the reference PTDC/CCI-INF/4703/2021.

References

1. Baumgartner, C.F., et al.: PHiSeg: capturing uncertainty in medical image segmentation. In: Shen, D., Liu, T., Peters, T.M., Staib, L.H., Essert, C., Zhou, S., Yap, P.-T., Khan, A. (eds.) MICCAI 2019. LNCS, vol. 11765, pp. 119–127. Springer, Cham (2019). https://doi.org/10.1007/978-3-030-32245-8_14
2. Brier, G.W., et al.: Verification of forecasts expressed in terms of probability. Mon. Weather Rev. **78**(1), 1–3 (1950)
3. Deng, J., Dong, W., Socher, R., Li, L.J., Li, K., Fei-Fei, L.: ImageNet: a large-scale hierarchical image database. In: Proceedings of the IEEE Conference on Computer Vision and Pattern Recognition. pp. 248–255. IEEE (2009)
4. Fort, S., Brock, A., Pascanu, R., De, S., Smith, S.L.: Drawing multiple augmentation samples per image during training efficiently decreases test error. arXiv preprint 2105.13343 (2021)
5. Friedman, J., Hastie, T., Tibshirani, R., et al.: The elements of statistical learning, vol. 1. Springer Series in Statistics New York (2001)

6. Glorot, X., Bengio, Y.: Understanding the difficulty of training deep feedforward neural networks. In: Proceedings of the Thirteenth International Conference on Artificial Intelligence and Statistics, pp. 249–256. JMLR Workshop and Conference Proceedings (2010)

7. Guzman-Rivera, A., Batra, D., Kohli, P.: Multiple choice learning: learning to produce multiple structured outputs. In: Advances in Neural Information Processing Systems, vol. 1, p. 3 (2012)

8. He, K., Zhang, X., Ren, S., Sun, J.: Delving deep into rectifiers: surpassing human-level performance on imagenet classification. In: Proceedings of the IEEE International Conference on Computer Vision, pp. 1026–1034. IEEE (2015)

9. He, K., Zhang, X., Ren, S., Sun, J.: Deep residual learning for image recognition. In: Proceedings of the IEEE Conference on Computer Vision and Pattern Recognition, pp. 770–778 (2016)

10. Hinton, G., Vinyals, O., Dean, J.: Distilling the knowledge in a neural network. arXiv preprint 1503.02531 (2015)

11. Hu, S., Worrall, D., Knegt, S., Veeling, B., Huisman, H., Welling, M.: Supervised uncertainty quantification for segmentation with multiple annotations. In: Shen, D., et al. (eds.) MICCAI 2019. LNCS, vol. 11765, pp. 137–145. Springer, Cham (2019). https://doi.org/10.1007/978-3-030-32245-8_16

12. Huang, G., Liu, Z., Van Der Maaten, L., Weinberger, K.Q.: Densely connected convolutional networks. In: Proceedings of the IEEE Conference on Computer Vision and Pattern Recognition, pp. 4700–4708 (2017)

13. Ilg, E., Çiçek, Ö., Galesso, S., Klein, A., Makansi, O., Hutter, F., Brox, T.: Uncertainty estimates for optical flow with multi-hypotheses networks. arXiv preprint 1802.07095 p. 81 (2018)

14. Ioffe, S., Szegedy, C.: Batch normalization: accelerating deep network training by reducing internal covariate shift. In: International Conference on Machine Learning, pp. 448–456 (2015)

15. Joskowicz, L., Cohen, D., Caplan, N., Sosna, J.: Inter-observer variability of manual contour delineation of structures in ct. Eur. Radiol. **29**(3), 1391–1399 (2019)

16. Kendall, A., Badrinarayanan, V., Cipolla, R.: Bayesian SegNet: Model uncertainty in deep convolutional encoder-decoder architectures for scene understanding. arXiv preprint 1511.02680 (2015)

17. Kendall, A., Gal, Y.: What uncertainties do we need in Bayesian deep learning for computer vision? arXiv preprint 1703.04977 (2017)

18. Kingma, D.P., Ba, J.: Adam: A method for stochastic optimization. arXiv preprint 1412.6980 (2014)

19. Kingma, D.P., Mohamed, S., Rezende, D.J., Welling, M.: Semi-supervised learning with deep generative models. In: Advances in Neural Information Processing Systems, pp. 3581–3589 (2014)

20. Kingma, D.P., Welling, M.: Auto-encoding variational Bayes. arXiv preprint **1312**, 6114 (2013)

21. Kingma, D.P., Salimans, T., Welling, M.: Variational dropout and the local reparameterization trick. Adv. Neural. Inf. Process. Syst. **28**, 2575–2583 (2015)

22. Kohl, S.A., et al.: A hierarchical probabilistic U-Net for modeling multi-scale ambiguities. arXiv preprint 1905.13077 (2019)

23. Kohl, S.A., et al.: A probabilistic U-Net for segmentation of ambiguous images. arXiv preprint 1806.05034 (2018)

24. Kosub, S.: A note on the triangle inequality for the Jaccard distance. Pattern Recogn. Lett. **120**, 36–38 (2019)

25. Krizhevsky, A., Sutskever, I., Hinton, G.E.: ImageNet classification with deep convolutional neural networks. Adv. Neural. Inf. Process. Syst. **25**, 1097–1105 (2012)
26. Lakshminarayanan, B., Pritzel, A., Blundell, C.: Simple and scalable predictive uncertainty estimation using deep ensembles. arXiv preprint 1612.01474 (2016)
27. LeCun, Y., Bottou, L., Bengio, Y., Haffner, P.: Gradient-based learning applied to document recognition. Proc. IEEE **86**(11), 2278–2324 (1998)
28. Lee, S., Prakash, S.P.S., Cogswell, M., Ranjan, V., Crandall, D., Batra, D.: Stochastic multiple choice learning for training diverse deep ensembles. In: Advances in Neural Information Processing Systems, pp. 2119–2127 (2016)
29. Lee, S., Purushwalkam, S., Cogswell, M., Crandall, D., Batra, D.: Why M heads are better than one: training a diverse ensemble of deep networks. arXiv preprint 1511.06314 (2015)
30. Lei, T., Wang, R., Wan, Y., Zhang, B., Meng, H., Nandi, A.K.: Medical image segmentation using deep learning: a survey. arXiv preprint 2009.13120 (2020)
31. Lipkus, A.H.: A proof of the triangle inequality for the Tanimoto distance. J. Math. Chem. **26**(1), 263–265 (1999)
32. Loshchilov, I., Hutter, F.: Sgdr: Stochastic gradient descent with warm restarts. arXiv preprint 1608.03983 (2016)
33. Monteiro, M., Folgoc, L.L., de Castro, D.C., Pawlowski, N., Marques, B., Kamnitsas, K., van der Wilk, M., Glocker, B.: Stochastic segmentation networks: modelling spatially correlated aleatoric uncertainty. arXiv preprint 2006.06015 (2020)
34. Naeini, M.P., Cooper, G., Hauskrecht, M.: Obtaining well calibrated probabilities using Bayesian binning. In: Twenty-Ninth AAAI Conference on Artificial Intelligence (2015)
35. Pham, H., Dai, Z., Xie, Q., Luong, M.T., Le, Q.V.: Meta pseudo labels (2021)
36. Rezende, D.J., Mohamed, S., Wierstra, D.: Stochastic backpropagation and approximate inference in deep generative models. In: International Conference on Machine Learning, pp. 1278–1286. PMLR (2014)
37. Ronneberger, O., Fischer, P., Brox, T.: U-Net: convolutional networks for biomedical image segmentation. In: Navab, N., Hornegger, J., Wells, W.M., Frangi, A.F. (eds.) MICCAI 2015. LNCS, vol. 9351, pp. 234–241. Springer, Cham (2015). https://doi.org/10.1007/978-3-319-24574-4_28
38. Rupprecht, C., Laina, I., DiPietro, R., Baust, M., Tombari, F., Navab, N., Hager, G.D.: Learning in an uncertain world: representing ambiguity through multiple hypotheses. In: Proceedings of the IEEE International Conference on Computer Vision, pp. 3591–3600 (2017)
39. Silva, J.L., Menezes, M.N., Rodrigues, T., Silva, B., Pinto, F.J., Oliveira, A.L.: Encoder-decoder architectures for clinically relevant coronary artery segmentation. arXiv preprint 2106.11447 (2021)
40. Simonyan, K., Zisserman, A.: Very deep convolutional networks for large-scale image recognition. arXiv preprint 1409.1556 (2014)
41. Sohn, K., Lee, H., Yan, X.: Learning structured output representation using deep conditional generative models. Adv. Neural. Inf. Process. Syst. **28**, 3483–3491 (2015)
42. Srivastava, N., Hinton, G., Krizhevsky, A., Sutskever, I., Salakhutdinov, R.: Dropout: a simple way to prevent neural networks from overfitting. J. Mach. Learn. Res. **15**(1), 1929–1958 (2014)
43. Szegedy, C., et al.: Going deeper with convolutions. In: Proceedings of the IEEE Conference on Computer Vision and Pattern Recognition, pp. 1–9 (2015)
44. Tan, M., Le, Q.: EfficientNet: rethinking model scaling for convolutional neural networks. In: International Conference on Machine Learning, pp. 6105–6114 (2019)

596   J. Lourenço-Silva and A. L. Oliveira

45. Xie, Q., Luong, M.T., Hovy, E., Le, Q.V.: Self-training with noisy student improves ImageNet classification. In: Proceedings of the IEEE/CVF Conference on Computer Vision and Pattern Recognition, pp. 10687–10698 (2020)
46. Yakubovskiy, P.: Segmentation models pytorch (2020). https://github.com/qubvel/segmentation_models.pytorch

Author Index

Printed in the United States
by Baker & Taylor Publisher Services